Exercise Prescription

Kamala Shankar, MD

Clinical Faculty, Division of Physical Medicine
  and Rehabilitation
Department of Functional Restoration
Stanford University Medical Center
Stanford, California
Physical Medicine and Rehabilitation Service
VA Palo Alto Health Care System
Palo Alto, California
Assistant Clinical Professor
Department of Physical Medicine and Rehabilitation
University of California, Davis, School of Medicine
Davis, California

904

'04

HANLEY & BELFUS, INC./Philadelphia

Publisher: HANLEY & BELFUS, INC.
              Medical Publishers
              210 South 13th Street
              Philadelphia, PA 19107
              215-546-7293; 800-962-1892
              FAX 215-790-9330
              Web site: http://www.hanleyandbelfus.com

Library of Congress Cataloging-in-Publication Data

Exercise prescription / edited by Kamala Shankar.
      p.   cm.
    Includes bibliographical references and index.
    ISBN 1-56053-258-0 (alk. paper)
    1. Exercise therapy.   I. Shankar, Kamala, 1955–
    [DNLM: 1. Exercise Therapy.   2. Exercise.   WB 541 E9543
    1998]
    RM725.E936   1998
    615.8′2—dc21
    DNLM/DLC
    for Library of Congress   98-3976
                                                     CIP

EXERCISE PRESCRIPTION   ISBN 1-56053-258-0

Last number is the print number: 9 8 7 6 5 4 3 2 1

CONTENTS

94869

III. NEUROLOGIC ASPECTS

IV. MUSCULOSKELETAL ASPECTS

V. SPECIAL GROUPS

CONTRIBUTORS

Karen L. Andrews, M.D.
Assistant Professor, Department of Physical Medicine and Rehabilitation, Mayo Foundation; Mayo Clinic, Rochester, Minnesota

Sharon Broadbent, M.D.
Department of Physical Medicine and Rehabilitation, UCLA Multicampus Physical Medicine and Rehabilitation Residency, Los Angeles, California

Stephen Burns, M.D.
Department of Rehabilitation Medicine, University of Washington School of Medicine; Spinal Cord Injury Service, Veterans Affairs Puget Sound Health Care System, Seattle, Washington

Rene Cailliet, M.D.
Chairman and Professor Emeritus, Department of Physical Medicine and Rehabilitation, University of Southern California School of Medicine; Clinical Professor, Department of Physical Medicine and Rehabilitation, University of California, Los Angeles, UCLA School of Medicine, Los Angeles; UCLA Santa Monica Hospital, Santa Monica, California

Denise I. Campagnolo, M.D., M.S.
Assistant Professor, Department of Physical Medicine and Rehabilitation, UMDNJ-New Jersey Medical School; University Hospital, Newark, New Jersey

Hans L. Carlson, M.D.
Assistant Professor, Department of Orthopedics and Rehabilitation, Oregon Health Sciences University, Portland, Oregon

Nels L. Carlson, M.D.
Clinical Neurophysiology Fellow, Department of Neurology, Harvard Medical School; Associate Neurologist, Brigham and Women's Hospital, Boston, Massachusetts

Charles B. Corbin, Ph.D.
Professor, Department of Exercise Science and Physical Education, Arizona State University, Tempe, Arizona

Robert DiGiacomo, P.T.
Regional Amputee Rehabilitation Center, Moss Rehabilitation Hospital, Philadelphia, Pennsylvania

Alberto Esquenazi, M.D.
Associate Professor, Department of Physical Medicine and Rehabilitation, Temple University School of Medicine; Director, Regional Amputee Rehabilitation Center, Moss Rehabilitation Hospital, Philadelphia, Pennsylvania

Walter R. Frontera, M.D., Ph.D.
Associate Professor and Chairman, Department of Physical Medicine and Rehabilitation, Harvard Medical School; Chief, Department of Physical Medicine and Rehabilitation, Spaulding Rehabilitation Hospital; Massachusetts General Hospital, Boston, Massachusetts

David R. Gater, M.D., Ph.D.
Assistant Professor, Department of Physical Medicine and Rehabilitation, University of Kentucky College of Medicine; Chandler Medical Center; Lexington Veterans Affairs Medical Center; Cardinal Hill Rehabilitation Hospital, Lexington, Kentucky

Stuart J. Glassman, M.D.
Clinical Assistant Professor, Department of Rehabilitation Medicine, University of Medicine and Dentistry of New Jersey, Robert Wood Johnson Medical School, New Brunswick, New Jersey; Medical Director, HealthSouth Rehabilitation Hospital, Concord, New Hampshire

Lance Goetz, M.D.
Spinal Cord Injury Service, Dallas Veterans Affairs Medical Center, Dallas, Texas

Barry Goldstein, M.D., Ph.D.
Associate Professor, Department of Rehabilitation Medicine, University of Washington School of Medicine; Department of Rehabilitation Medicine, Harborview Medical Center, Seattle, Washington

John A. Horton III, M.D.
Department of Physical Medicine and Rehabilitation, UMDNJ-New Jersey Medical School, Newark, New Jersey

Tissa Kappagoda, MBBS, Ph.D.
Professor, Department of Cardiovascular Medicine, University of California, Davis, School of Medicine, Davis; Department of Cardiovascular Medicine, University of California, Davis, Medical Center, Sacramento, California

David D. Kilmer, M.D.
Associate Professor, Department of Physical Medicine and Rehabilitation, University of California, Davis, School of Medicine, Davis; Department of Physical Medicine and Rehabilitation, University of California, Davis, Medical Center, Sacramento, California

Tanja L. Kujac, M.D.
Department of Physical Medicine and Rehabilitation, Stanford University School of Medicine, Stanford, California

Rajeswari Kumar, M.D.
Clinical Professor, Department of Medicine, University of California, Los Angeles, UCLA School of Medicine, Los Angeles; Staff Physician, Veterans Affairs Medical Center, West Los Angeles, California

Geoffrey E. Moore, M.D.
Assistant Professor, Department of Internal Medicine, University of Pittsburgh School of Medicine; University of Pittsburgh Medical Center, Pittsburgh, Pennsylvania

Jonathan N. Myers, Ph.D.
Clinical Assistant Professor, Division of Cardiovascular Medicine, Stanford University School of Medicine, Stanford; Department of Cardiology, Palo Alto Veterans Affairs Health Care System, Palo Alto, California

Nirmala N. Nayak, M.D.
Assistant Professor, Department of Physical Medicine and Rehabilitation, University of California, Davis, School of Medicine, Davis; Department of Physical Medicine and Rehabilitation, University of California, Davis, Medical Center, Sacramento; Chief, Department of Physical Medicine and Rehabilitation, Veterans Affairs Northern California Health Care System, Davis, California

John J. Nicholas, M.D.
Professor and Chairman, Department of Physical Medicine and Rehabilitation, Rush Medical College; Attending Physician, Rush-Presbyterian-St. Luke's Medical Center; Attending Physician, Grant Hospital, Chicago, Illinois

Robert P. Pangrazi, Ph.D.
Professor, Department of Exercise Science and Physical Education, Arizona State University, Tempe, Arizona

Kenneth David Randall, M.P.T., A.T.C.
Physical Therapist, Livermore, California

Arjun Shankar
Pleasanton, California

Kamala Shankar, M.D.
Clinical Faculty, Division of Physical Medicine and Rehabilitation, Department of
Functional Restoration, Stanford University School of Medicine, Stanford; Assistant
Clinical Professor, Department of Physical Medicine and Rehabilitation, University of
California, Davis, School of Medicine, Davis; Department of Physical Medicine and
Rehabilitation, Palo Alto Veterans Affairs Health Care System, Palo Alto, California

Kazuko L. Shem, M.D.
Department of Physical Medicine and Rehabilitation, Palo Alto Veterans Affairs
Health Care System, Palo Alto, California

Marc Owen Sherman, M.D.
Assistant Professor, Department of Physical Medicine and Rehabilitation, University
of Cincinnati College of Medicine; Medical Director, Spine and Sports Care, Drake
Center, Inc., Cincinnati, Ohio

Steven Stiens, M.D.
Department of Rehabilitation Medicine, University of Washington School of Medi-
cine; Spinal Cord Injury Service, Veterans Affairs Puget Sound Health Care System,
Seattle, Washington

Viviane Ugalde, M.D.
Assistant Professor, Department of Physical Medicine and Rehabilitation, University
of California, Davis, School of Medicine, Davis; Department of Physical Medicine
and Rehabilitation, University of California, Davis, Medical Center, Sacramento,
California

Vincent J. Yacyshyn, M.D.
Department of Cardiovascular Diseases, Mayo Foundation; Mayo Clinic, Rochester,
Minnesota

Jennifer Young, M.S., P.T.
Spinal Cord Injury Service, Veterans Affairs Puget Sound Health Care System,
Seattle, Washington

FOREWORD

Like a medieval baron going to war, a book editor must recruit a phalanx of ideal knights/authors, investing them with appropriate titles and practical tools. Dr. Shankar began this enterprise with obvious enthusiasm and uncanny skill. This excellent start is reflected by her choices of authoritative authors who are in complete control of their assigned fields. The sections that I have had the privilege of reading in manuscript are excellent. As an editor/author of many works on therapeutic exercise, I freely admit that this book will be the leader in its chosen province—the clinical art of prescribing and supervising exercise.

My use of the word *art* above is no accident, for it is an art in the sense that Hippocrates articulated 2,600 years ago in his immortal lines that began: *Life is short, the art long* . . . . Indeed, the healing art is very long and it dominates all that we do clinically.

Like all the arts, there is a continuous evolution of the healing art. And there are many crossroads to negotiate. But, beware! Hippocrates then continued: . . . *opportunity is fleeting, experience treacherous and judgment difficult.* Is this statement a conundrum? Or is it a profound forecast of the current storm of scientific searches (in which I have been swept up) for ideal, scientifically based therapy?

We cannot avoid concluding the Hippocrates was never satisfied with the status quo, even in an era when statistics and double-blind research were not dreamt of. Today, they are not dreams: they are essentials. Before we can discover and set off on the high road of valid research of various types of therapeutic exercise, we must first establish clear definitions of recommended practices. That is what this book offers us at the crossroads: the prescription of exercises, their supervision, and their hoped-for outcomes. Only then can we choose the high road to the validity of therapeutic outcomes and the scientific proof of success or failure. This book is a fine guide for our first steps.

John V. Basmajian, O.C., O.Ont., M.D.,
FRCP (Can), FRCPS (Glasgow)
Professor Emeritus in Medicine and Anatomy
McMaster University
Hamilton, Ontario, Canada

PREFACE

This book on exercise prescription focuses on the use of exercise as a therapeutic modality for health promotion and maintenance of functional independence. Exercise is defined as "activity that is performed or practiced in order to develop or improve a specific power or skill, or bodily exertion for the sake of developing and maintaining physical fitness." Prescription is "the written direction for preparation, compounding, and administration of a drug or other therapy."

Exercise, like medications, should be prescribed by a physician or an appropriately trained health care professional and should be monitored, titrated, and maintained to achieve a stable dose. As with drugs and other management interventions, while prescribing exercise as a therapeutic agent all other available interventions should be considered. When necessary, exercise can be used to complement these other interventions.

Throughout this book, attempts have been made to elaborate on the various components of exercise prescription. When a person follows an exercise program, consideration of that person's health status, presence of illness or impairments, previous exercise level, and precautions are important. It is advisable to discuss these factors with the person's physician. Once an exercise program is started, motivation, persistence, and compliance are very important for long-term benefits. Health professionals should also take into account the environment in which exercises are performed, because hazards in the environment may affect exercise performance or place the person at risk for injury.

Before exercise prescription is made, effects of exercise on organ systems should be well understood. In the first section of this book, topics such as the effects of exercise, foundations of exercise classification, historical aspects, and exercise testing are described. In the second section medical conditions such as cardiac and pulmonary illness and multiple chronic medical illness and exercise considerations are described. Section three focuses on neurologic impairments and exercise considerations. Section four focuses on musculoskeletal disorders and repetitive motion disorders with exercise consideration. In the last section, exercise consideration for special groups, such as postmenopausal women, youth, and elderly, is addressed.

I appreciate the time and efforts taken by the authors in preparation of the chapters. I would like to thank all the authors who have contributed to this book. My special thanks to my beloved family for supporting me through this project.

Kamala Shankar, M.D.

This book is dedicated in memory of my father, Mr. R. Sivaswamy.

KAZUKO L. SHEM, MD

KAMALA SHANKAR, MD

1

History of Therapeutic Exercise

"If a well appointed gymnasium is at hand, the physician should be as well able to prescribe the exact use of its different apparatus as he is to write for doses from the adjoining drug store . . . If no gymnasium is at hand, the doctor should still be as well able to advise about . . . the various forms of exercise without apparatus as about the use of other domestic remedies."[89]
—Dr. Alfred Worchester, 1883

Therapeutic exercise has been defined as "the prescription of bodily movement to improve function, relieve symptoms, or maintain a state of well-being."[58] It is an integral part of the practice of physical medicine and rehabilitation. Since early recorded history, humans have recognized and explored the relationship among exercise, health, and rehabilitation.

The history of exercise in medicine begins before the time of Christ and continues to the present day. Although the exact origin of therapeutic exercise is difficult to establish, the earliest known writing on therapeutic exercise is the *Cong Fou* of ancient China.[3,20,65] Promoted by a Chinese surgeon, Hua T'o, the Cong Fou consisted of a series of ritualistic motions based on the movement of animals and was prescribed by Buddhist monks for the relief of pain and other symptoms.[53] The Cong Fou was practiced in schools throughout China and reached the height of its popularity during the Chou dynasty (1151 BC).[3]

The Chinese believed that inactivity caused disease.[3] In 400 BC, a Chinese medical text, the *Huang Di Nei Jing,* discussed the importance of functional restoration.[95] Remedies for the loss of mobility and sensation included acupuncture, massage, therapeutic exercises, and heat packs. The Confucian value of filial piety led to an interest in geriatric rehabilitation. Therapeutic exercise became a regular part of medical care and treatment of hemiplegia, arteriosclerosis, diabetes, rheumatoid arthritis, dizziness, and other conditions.[95] Chinese medicine, in addition to therapeutic exercise, acupuncture, and massage, also originated moxibustion and breathing-relaxation-meditation techniques called Qiqong.[53] Tai Chi Chuan, increasing in popularity in the United States today, was also developed in China in the 13th century.

Although most historians of therapeutic exercise recognize Chinese Cong Fu as the earliest therapeutic exercise, in India the importance of exercise for good health was emphasized in writings dating back to 3000 BC.[35] The practitioners at that time established exercise guidelines in the ancient medical texts, the *Susurate Charaka, et al* and *Astang Hridays Samhi,* as follows:

1. Do not exercise after meals.

2. Exercise should be performed daily.

3. Exercises should be appropriate to the individual's age, physical condition, and capacity.

4. Do not exercise to the point of fatigue, as evidenced by the amount of perspiration or mouth dryness.[35]

Similar to early Chinese medicine, diseases, which were thought to be caused by inactivity, were treated with exercise.

Ancient India's best-known influence on modern therapeutic exercise is yoga.[3] A system of physical, mental, and spiritual exercise, yoga has been practiced since ancient times. Yoga exercises promote control of mental and bodily functions. Its practice can arrest many of the ailments or degenerative symptoms of old age. Yoga exercises strengthen the weak parts of the body without the use of aerobically taxing activities. Ailments such as asthma, arthritis, constipation, and obesity are believed to be relieved by yoga. The yoga system of exercises is not intended to combat disease but to condition the body and mind.[93] Some now believe that Chinese Cong Fou may have been adapted from yoga.[65]

In ancient Greece, Herodicus, considered by some as the father of therapeutic exercise, was the first to write on the subject of "remedial exercises."[3,20,84] Herodicus was a wrestling and boxing instructor who recognized that exercise made his weaker athletes stronger.[11] Exercises for medical purposes were often called "therapeutic gymnastics" or "gymnastic medicine."[11] The Greeks, including Aristotle, Socrates, and Plato, emphasized the importance of physical well being, fitness, and a healthy active life.[3,20,65] The best known of the Greek physicians was Hippocrates, and he used the word *analepsis* to mean "medical rehabilitation."[20] His saying, "Exercise strengthens and inactivity wastes" is an underlying principle in rehabilitation today.[71] Hippocrates and many of his followers used exercise to strengthen weak muscles, hasten recovery, and increase mental fortitude.[9,63,65,71]

As the Greek civilization declined, the Roman civilization rose, adapting portions of Greek medicine.[3] Not only did the Roman physicians recognize the value of moderate exercise, but they also used strenuous exercise to treat many acute diseases. Galen, a prominent name in Roman medicine, classified exercises according to the body parts involved, vigorousness, duration, frequency, and the use of apparatus.[9,33] In describing exercise in his book, *On Hygiene,* he wrote: "Those movements which do not alter the respiration are not called exercise."[37] To Galen, the goals of exercise included promoting muscle tone and regular bowel movements.

Other Romans recommended exercises for treating conditions such as epilepsy, gout, headaches, vertigo, dyspepsia, paralysis, and arthritis.[9,11,30] Another Roman, Pliny, recognized that the mind is "stimulated by movements of the body."[30] Celsus and Asclepiades also advocated the use of postoperative exercises and avoidance of "disuse" in nonacutely ill patients. First "graded" exercise was also described by the Romans.[9] In 500 BC, one of the followers of Galen, Aurileanus, published his concepts on aquatic therapy, suspension, and kinesiotherapy with pulleys and weights in his book, *On Chronic Diseases*.[3,20]

After the fall of the Roman empire and during the Arabian control of the southern Europe, progress in medicine and rehabilitation stalled due to Arabian laws against dissection. During the Middle Ages, exercise was abandoned because the Christians of that period disapproved of the Roman-type athletic spectacles and renounced materialism, including preservation of the body. Medicine was practiced minimally during this period, since the Christians believed that "man was placed on earth to suffer."[3] The advent of the Renaissance brought a renewed interest in medicine and rehabilitation. The ideals of physical education and works of Hippocrates and Galen were reintroduced in the 15th century.[3,9,20]

In the 16th century, the first important book on therapeutic exercise from the Renaissance period, *De Arte Gymnastica,* was written by Hieronymus Mercurialis.[3] He created a set of principles, including the following:

1. Each exercise should preserve the existing healthy state.

2. Exercises should be suited to each part of the body.

3. All healthy people should exercise regularly.

4. Sick people should not be given exercises that might exacerbate existing conditions.

5. Special exercises should be prescribed for convalescent patients on an individual basis.

6. Persons who lead a sedentary life urgently need exercise.

In the 18th century, the most significant contribution to advancement of therapeutic exercise was made by Joseph-Clement Tissot. In 1780, 33-year-old Tissot wrote the book *Gymnastique Medicinale et Chirurgicale.*[63] An army surgeon, Tissot broke from traditions of that time and recommended mobilization of postsurgical patients. He was a vigorous opponent of prolonged bed rest. According to Licht, Tissot recognized that the most important objectives of rehabilitation were to improve "the ability to make a living" and "the opportunity to enjoy living."[63] He founded occupational therapy by advising the disabled to exercise through "craft" work and wrote: "Most craft activities place the muscle of the upper extremities in almost continual contraction. According to their use, some activate certain muscles more than others."[9] He adapted sports as a recreational therapy and wrote on the use of fencing as a "means of strengthening the extremities, increasing the range of the joints as well as the circulation of the viscera."[9]

He further made recommendations on management of respiratory diseases, decubitus ulcers, hemiplegics, and arthritis that were advanced for his time and almost contemporary.[9] John Hunter, a renowned surgeon around the same time, also advocated frequent mild exercise for healing joints.[71]

Rapid advancement of therapeutic exercise in the 19th century may be credited to Sweden's Pehr Henri Ling (1776–1839).[43,48] After experiencing an improvement in his right shoulder joint pain after fencing, he concluded that exercise might cure illness.[48] His main objective was to demonstrate that movements could heal diseases and correct bodily deficits. He defined "medical gymnastics" as "gymnastics through which a man either through his own power and in a suitable position, or by the help of others and effective exercises can try to lessen or overcome illnesses that have invaded his body owing to abnormal circumstances."[48] He was observant and precise in describing therapeutic movements and categorized exercises into three groups: (1) totally passive, (2) half passive, and (3) active-passive.[43] Furthermore, he described the movements of the arms to be along the "perpendicular, anteroposterior, and transverse" diameters of the body. The concepts of "eccentric and concentric movement" and of physiologic phenomenon of fatigue were also introduced by Ling. His greatest contribution may have been his method of dosage, counting, and detailed directions for exercises.[43,48] In 1813, he founded the Royal Gymnastic Central Institute in Stockholm.[59] Mary McMillan noted in 1932 that "It is Peter Henry Ling and the Swedish systematized order that we owe much today . . . in the field of . . . therapeutic exercises."[43] The teachings of Ling were further disseminated by his pupils. In fact, it was one of Ling's pupils, George Taylor, who in 1868 wrote a textbook on therapeutic exercise, *An Exposition of the Swedish Movement Cure.*[59]

However, Ling's system of exercise required expensive and intense individualized attention by a therapist. Gustav Zander of Sweden instead used levers, wheels, and weights, and designed 71 different types of apparatus for active, assistive, and resistive exercises.[9] By using weights of known sizes and levers with graduated rulers, "dosage" of exercises became more exact. Zander's apparatuses were used in the "Zander Institutes" not only throughout Europe and in the United States but as far away as Egypt and Argentina. In the early 1800s, British engineer William Cubitt designed a "stepping wheel," a forerunner to the modern treadmill, upon which prisoners would walk as a punishment.[34] By the mid 1800s, measurement of respiratory and metabolic responses to treadmill exercise laid the groundwork for future studies in evaluating exercise performance in patients with coronary artery disease.

In 1865, a book on medicine and exercise, *Gimnastica, Hygienica, Medica y Ortopedica,* was written in Spain by Torro Busquey. According to Licht, the word "rehabilitation" was possibly used for the first time in its modern context.[9] Busquey wrote about exercises that he referred to as "orthopedic gymnastics," and he established that ". . . such movements as may directly rehabilitate the muscle groups which are weak, and at the same time calling attention to the fact that the failure to use such special exercises is the cause of alterations in alignment and even of deformities."[9]

From the time of Hippocrates to the 18th century, most physicians were pessimistic about treating hemiplegic patients.[64] One of the first reports on stroke rehabilitation was made by Thomas Hun in 1851.[63] One aphasic patient was retrained by his wife, who had him repeatedly speak, read, and spell words. H. S. Frenkel indirectly contributed to the development of modern rehabilitation for hemiplegic patients when he recognized that coordination could be improved with practice. Frenkel, in 1887, observed a patient with tabes dorsalis performing the finger-to-nose test poorly and told the patient that he did not "pass" the test.[63] At his next visit one month later, the patient showed a significant improvement. The patient had "practiced" so that he could pass the text. Based on this experience, Frenkel rented a house and asked his patients to practice with equipment to improve their coordination. In 1889, Frenkel presented his revolutionary exercise program for ataxic patients in a conference in Germany. This program involved "repeated exercises" to let the central nervous system differentiate stimuli of minute intensity.[36,43] Incidentally, the word *exercise* was derived from the Latin word for practice, *exercitum*.[63]

Frenkel, however, was only interested in treating tabetic patients. After Frenkel presented his findings, Fulgence Raymond and Rubens Hirschberg expanded on Frenkel's exercise and established rehabilitation for hemiplegic patients.[63] Raymond was a successor to Charcot, the best known neurologist in France at the time. He sent Hirschberg to Switzerland to observe Frenkel's work and introduced the concept of Frenkel's exercise program by using the name "functional rehabilitation."[63] In 1896, Raymond established in France possibly the first hospital gymnasium ever. He named and defined "rehabilitation" as "programmed gymnastics which attempts to reestablish normal relationships between a conscious perception and the will."[63]

The history of therapeutic exercises from ancient Greece to the 1800s has been well researched and documented by Dr. Licht in his multiple publications, especially in a chapter in the text *Therapeutic Exercise*.[9] Dr. Licht had access to a collection of historical publications on therapeutic exercises and even translated Tissot's *Gymnastique Medicinale et Chirurgicale*.[1] His wife, Elizabeth Licht, in supporting her husband's work, published many historical books on therapeutic exercises.[1] Practitioners in the field of physical medicine and rehabilitation owe a debt of gratitude to Dr. Licht for his contribution. Many of the historical notes in this chapter are attributable to Dr. Licht.

In the late 1800s, "graded activity" was developed in a German tuberculosis sanatorium. Graded activity has two essential characteristics: (1) tasks are classified by degree of difficulty and (2) patients begin working at a level appropriate for their current abilities and move to other levels as function changes.[23] The graded activity was initially conceptualized to build general endurance in patients with chronic conditions, but it was further used to treat burns, fractures, peripheral nerve injuries, heart disease, and industrial injuries. The principle was further expanded to include graded manual work and crafts in occupational therapy. Visually impaired patients were first given larger objects that could be placed in their hands, and gradually smaller objects were used to train the hands for finer work.[23] In 1914 Sir William Osler further described the use of "graded exercise" as follows: "The distance walked each day is marked off and is gradually lengthened. In this way the heart is systematically exercised and strengthened."[33] In addition to using graded exercise for patients with tuberculosis, he noted that exercise in moderation is "helpful" for treating constipation.

In the United States, the need for physical activity was recognized in the late 1700s by such prominent Americans as Benjamin Franklin, Thomas Jefferson, and Noah Webster. Franklin was quoted as saying, "...a little exercise a quarter of an hour before meals, as to swing a weight, or swing your arms about with a small weight in each hand: to leap, or the like, for that stirs the muscles of the breast."[33] Jefferson encouraged people to devote more than 2 hours per day to exercise. The Americans were influenced by the European recognition of the need for physical activity for health. In the 1800s, Catherine Beecher, Dudley Sargent, and Edward Hitchcock established guidelines for prescribing therapeutic exercise.[3]

At the beginning of the 20th century, the attention of medical profession was directed to outbreaks of poliomyelitis.[43,70] The first epidemic of polio in the United States occurred in 1894, and it stimulated the development of physical therapy.[20] Sir Colin McKenzie advocated rest and splints during early phase of paralysis and started voluntary muscle exercises as soon as the acute stage of infection was over. The process of recovery was called "reeducation" for the first time by McKenzie.[41] Sister Kenny, an Australian nurse, then attempted "restoration of muscle function" by simultaneously reeducating both afferent and efferent pathways.[62] For example, she advocated the use of warm moist heat in combination with early muscle training.[58,70] Sister Kenny traveled throughout Europe and the United States to demonstrate and teach her techniques, but she met with resistance from her predominantly male colleagues.[51] Later on, hydrotherapy was recommended for exercising paralyzed patients. Wilhelmine Wright also developed many exercise techniques for training quadriplegic polio patients to ambulate using crutches.[9] The manual muscle test, which was developed in the early 1900s to evaluate polio patients, had a significant influence on the development of therapeutic exercises.[43]

In 1903, Brissaud advocated having hemiplegic patients exercise as soon as possible and walk while moving their hands "purposefully" twice a day.[64] In the same year, Hirschberg distinguished three phases of therapy for hemiplegia as absolute rest in the first phase, passive motion to "avoid ankylosis" in the second phase, and "muscle reeducation" and "action motion" to move part of body and oppose it with resistance in the third phase.[9]

From the 1920s to 1930s, Coulter and Clayton developed detailed exercise programs for hemiplegic patients.[5,91] Their exercise programs were arbitrary in their approaches, but portions of their programs adhered to the principles of normal motor development and emphasized exercising proximal parts of the limbs. Coordination was not emphasized in the early part of the exercise program but was superimposed after selected movement returned. In *Physiotherapy in General Practice,* published in 1924, Clayton outlined this program as follows:

1. Practice active movements in single joints.

2. Hold one joint stable while moving another.

3. Attempt to control the entire limb.

4. Use the sound arm to assist the affected arm in two-handed stick exercise.

5. Use pulley exercises and weight to overcome spasticity.

6. Use ball exercises for the fingers.

7. Train the use of individual fingers.

8. Teach rhythmic movements using music.

9. Teach normal use of limbs through practicing self-care.[91]

In the 1950s, Deaver advocated a reeducation program similar to that used for polio patients for stroke patients with flaccid arm.[24]

By World War II, the muscle training exercises developed for polio patients proved inadequate for trauma patients, especially those with brain injuries. Attention was shifted to using "pathological reflexes" to work for the benefit of patients. In the middle of this century, various methods of physical therapy with different approaches and philosophies of therapeutic exercise were studied. The theoretical basis for facilitation techniques widely used in therapeutic exercise can be traced to Sherrington's discovery of the concept of facilitation.[85] In the 1940s, Herman Kabat introduced a new principle that "proprioceptive stimulation resulting from increased tension facilitates the voluntary motor mechanism."[47] He called his method *central facilitation* and applied the program in the treatment of patients with paralysis at Kabat-Kaiser Institute. He employed "maximal resistance, stretch, mass movement patterns, reflexes, and reversal of antagonists" and took exercises out of the cardinal plane by introducing spiral and diagonal composite movements.[43]

In the 1950s, Margaret Rood, having treated children with cerebral palsy, introduced a therapeutic approach of retracing steps of normal developmental sequences.[82,83] She used gentle mechanical or superficial thermal stimulation to obtain localized facilitating effects. The application of these "brushing" and "icing" stimuli to discrete areas of the skin, she thought, would modify the tone and promote contractions of underlying muscles.

Temple Fay, a neurosurgeon who also worked extensively with children with cerebral palsy in the 1950s, thought that the control of basic reflexes was essential before more advanced coordination could be learned.[58] He then claimed that by incorporating pathologic reflexes, the "spontaneous reflex pattern movement" of the limbs would eventually become the basis of true coordinated patterns of walking. He suggested that the twice daily induction of these pathologic reflexes would improve spastic muscle function and decrease the level of spasticity.[32]

The Bobaths, from the 1950s to the 1970s, developed a "neurodevelopmental approach" initially for patients with cerebral palsy and then later applied it to stroke patients.[12–16] They used involuntary responses such as postural reflexes and equilibrium reactions of the head and body to modify muscle tone and elicit desired movements.[58] Brunnstrom further combined central facilitation, peripheral proprioceptive stimulation, and peripheral cutaneous stimulation to take a stroke patient from the initial stage of synergistic reactions to the next stage of voluntary motion dominated by synergies.[19] Another approach to facilitation was the proprioceptive neuromuscular facilitation (PNF) of Knott and Voss.[52] PNF attempts to facilitate the contraction of muscle groups in a synergistic pattern of diagonal-spiral movements by placing the muscles to be facilitated under the maximal stretch and ending with the muscles at the maximally shortened end of their range. The goal of PNF is to improve range of motion, flexibility, and neuromuscular function.[3]

In the early 1900s, therapeutic exercise was the domain of the orthopedic surgeons and neurologists. After World War I, "restorative exercise" and physical measures were used increasingly in the military hospitals.[9,57] In 1921, the term "rehabilitation" was used possibly for the first time in the United States by E. Maxine Call, author of a paper entitled "Problems in the Rehabilitation of Victims of War."[20] The paper provided a detailed account of management of amputees after World War I. In 1938, the term "physiatrist" was proposed by Frank Krusen to identify physicians specializing in physical medicine.[75]

Not until World War II did therapeutic exercise become an important part of physical medicine. A European surgeon, Earnest Nicoll, established a set of remedial exercise principles to be applied after traumatic injury.[73] His principles stated that therapeutic exercise be:

1. Both focal and general.

2. Administered with due regard to dosage.

3. Rhythmic with regard to contraction and relaxation.

4. Progressive in range, power, and time.

5. Variable in form in "gymnastic" (current equivalent of physical therapy), occupational, and recreational therapies.

England's success with "corrective therapy" in treating casualties of World War II came to the attention of the American military. In 1943, nonphysicians in the military were enrolled in Army schools for "physical reconditioning" to be trained in exercises for the treatment of medical, surgical, and convalescent patients. Those trained in "corrective physical rehabilitation" were called "corrective therapists" in the United States and "medical gymnasts" in England.[18]

In the United States, Howard Rusk, who is considered to be the father of modern rehabilitation medicine, conducted a controlled experiment in which he showed that early ambulation after surgery, aggressive therapy, and recreational activities for injured soldiers were superior to inactive convalescence.[55] Rusk and Henry Kessler made a significant contribution in the field of rehabilitation. They introduced the principle of integrating medical, psychological, and social issues to restore a patient's independence.[46] In 1941, "physical medicine" was defined by the American Council of Physical Medicine as "the employment of physical and other effective properties of light, heat, cold, water, electricity, massage, manipulation, exercise and mechanical devices in physical and occupational therapy in the diagnosis and treatment of disease."[6] In 1947, Frank Krusen and his colleagues established the American Board of Physical Medicine, and physical medicine and rehabilitation was recognized as a specialized field in medicine.[75]

The field of exercises for strengthening and endurance also began during and after World War I, when isometric exercise was introduced.[3] Use of resistance was not a new concept in therapeutic exercise, but Thomas DeLorme developed a system that is still being practiced.[28] While assigned to a military hospital, DeLorme noticed that the quadriceps can be restored to full strength postoperatively by increasing the resistance applied to exercise muscles.[9] He noted that there are different methods of exercise depending on which part of muscles (such as power, endurance, speed, or coordination) one is interested in developing. His exercise principle states that high-resistance and low-repetition exercise builds muscle *power* and that low-resistance, high-repetition exercise builds *endurance*.

In 1951, DeLorme published a book on his exercise method, progressive resistance exercise, which was rapidly adopted into the field of exercise.[29,47] His method required determination of 10 RM (highest weight that can be lifted through the full range of motion ten times only), and in an exercise session, the subject lifts a series of fraction of the 10 RM for 10 repetitions. DeLateur's work in 1968, however, suggested that both strength and endurance would be built as long as the subject continues repetitions to "the point of fatigue."[25] Another method called the "Oxford technique," also known as regressive resistive exercise, was developed as a modification of DeLorme's method.[96] It recommended reducing the weight lifted after setting the 10 RM and diminished resistance as muscles fatigued so that the subjects could lift for more repetitions. This method was proven ineffective by Hellenbrandt's overload principle in 1958.[39]

The concept of isometric exercise began to be used in therapeutic exercise after the work of Hettinger and Muller in 1953.[3] Hellenbrandt and Houtz further showed that the work capacity of a muscle is enhanced by increasing the rate of training, even if the weight is kept constant.[40] The effectiveness of isotonic versus isometric exercise was further examined by DeLateur in 1972.[26] The "double-shift transfer-of-training" design showed that the best training for a given type of exercise is that type of exercise itself, but some delayed transfer may occur.[26] The Knight technique of daily adjustable progressive resistance exercise was then developed to objectively quantify the resistance to be used in an isotonic strengthening program. More recently, circuit training was introduced in 1970s and has enjoyed increased popularity.[35]

Biofeedback has been applied in rehabilitation medicine since sensory feedback was proven to be effective in motor learning. Marinacci and Horande first described the use of electromyography (EMG) in a biofeedback training method called "audio-neuromuscular reeducation" in 1960.[45] In the 1960s, more studies were conducted to explore the use of EMG to control a limited number of motor units.[8] Since then it has been used to provide auditory and visual cues as a dynamic method of training motor units.[45,86] In stroke patients with foot drop, biofeedback training with EMG was shown not only to increase strength but also to improve range of motion.[10] Reverse application of EMG feedback to relax spastic muscles in hemiplegic patients was also advocated.[45]

Some therapeutic exercises using reflexes and facilitation, as advocated by Sister Kenny and Kabat earlier, may result in incoordination. In the 1930s, Coulter noted that "muscle reeducation" is a form of exercise for muscles in which "neuromuscular coordination" has become impaired.[5] In the 1950s, Phelps, while developing exercise programs for cerebral palsy patients, realized that practicing a desired movement pattern improved the performance of that pattern, but he was not aware of the concept of "engrams."[58] Later, Kottke specifically emphasized the need for repetitions to develop "engrams" (i.e., development of a pattern of performance) for coordination.[56] The exercise program for coordination as advocated by Kottke included:

1. "Perceptual feedback" to correct performance errors.

2. "Precision" at every level of training.

3. "Perpetual practice" of more than millions of repetitions.

4. Practicing performance at a level just below the "peak of performance."

5. "Progression" of performance as ability increases.

After World War II, in addition to physical and occupational therapists, other subspecializations were becoming recognized as important participants of the rehabilitation team. Around this time, cardiac and pulmonary rehabilitation were founded, and treatment techniques were becoming more specialized. In the 1970s and 1980s, studies were conducted to prove the effectiveness of exercises in treating chronic diseases such as coronary artery disease, chronic obstructive pulmonary disease, cystic fibrosis, rheumatoid and degenerative arthritis, osteoporosis, end-stage renal disease, cancer, chronic pain, obesity, Parkinson's disease, and muscular dystrophy.[29,54,66,78,81,88,94]

Some innovative uses of therapeutic exercise in treating chronic diseases were developed in Europe and introduced to the United States later. Frenkel's exercise, first presented in 1889 in Dresden, was brought to the United States in 1897 by an American physician, Bettman.[63] John Coulter, one of the pioneers of modern rehabilitation in the United States, also may have been influenced by Frenkel's exercise while he was at French military hospitals.[63] In 1939, Danish physician Holger Bisgaard first presented the use of massage and exercise in the treatment of lower extremity static edema. In 1956, the "Bisgaard treatment" was brought to the United States by Stillwell, a Canadian physician.[87]

In the field of hand rehabilitation, Wertz recognized the importance of the hand position of function as early as the 1500s.[20] In the 17th century, Friedrich Hoffman made a contribution to the field of "kinetic" occupational therapy.[3] In 1780, Tissot recommended the use of arts, crafts, and occupations for disability of the musculoskeleton following disease or injury. Dunton, who has been called the father of occupational therapy, provided ideas for graded exercises. Throughout and after World War II, the concept of the team approach was developed specifically for hand rehabilitation, and there was rapid spread of the field from military centers to civilian practice.[20]

James Parkinson in 1817 first described parkinsonism as a disease that he called "shaking palsy."[18] A century later, in the early 1900s, came the world pandemic of influenza, which was followed by the epidemic of encephalitis, mostly in young people.[18,78] These patients had symptoms similar to those of the older parkinsonian patients. First, stretching exercise was recommended. Then it was noted that patients seemed to do better in a group setting with background music. Gotthard Booth recommended ball games, dancing, and swimming according to each patient's preference.[18]

Multiple sclerosis was first described in 1870 by a French neurologist, Jean Martin Charcot. It was considered to be a rare disease and not clearly defined until the 1940s.[18,21] Once patients with multiple sclerosis were recognized as possible candidates for rehabilitation, muscle reeducation exercise was recommended. Because cerebellar dysfunction is common in multiple sclerosis, Frenkel's exercise, which was developed for tabetic ataxia, was applied to patients with cerebellar ataxia.[62]

After myocardial infarction was first described in 1912, patients were confined to bed rest for 2 months.[76] By the late 1940s, the use of "chair therapy" was advocated as one of the first departures from the practice of strict bed rest.[40] In the middle of the century, the efficacy and safety of an early graded activity and early ambulation were reported. In 1952, Newman et al. described in detail a 6-week exercise program for patients with myocardial infarction.[72] Even after coronary bypass surgery, exercise for 36–48 months has been shown to improve functional capacity in those patients.[74,76,90] Borg's rating of perceived exertion was developed in 1970 to be used by the patient to rate the intensity of exercise.[17]

As early as the Roman era, Galen noted that "deep breathing" is a specific exercise for the "thorax and lungs."[37] Diaphragmatic breathing was described by Cooper in 1839 and Duchenne in 1867, and pursed-lip breathing was described by Hofbauer.[7] In more modern times, the use of breathing and postural exercises as treatments for emphysema appeared in 1925.[77] By 1935, physical therapy as an adjunct to other treatments for asthma, emphysema, and chronic pulmonary disorders was suggested in Europe.[69] In the 1960s, there was greater than 100% increase in the number of cases of lung diseases and a significant increase in patients with disability related to lung diseases.[44] Abdominal breathing and reconditioning exercise programs were recommended to increase endurance and to relieve some physical disabilities.[7,44,69]

The application of physical therapeutic measures to treat rheumatoid arthritis has been recommended since the 1940s.[6,31,79,80] The goals of exercise in rheumatoid arthritis are to maintain or increase the range of motion and the strength of weakened muscles. To protect and stabilize arthritic joints, adequate muscular control and strength were considered to be important, and progressive resistive exercise was again promoted.[31,80] "Corrective exercises" were described in detail by Hill in 1955, and specific precautions for patients with arthritis engaging in exercise were described by Rae and Bender.[42,79,80] Exercise for osteoarthritic patients was encouraged as early as the 1950s.[89]

By the early 1900s, difficulty in diagnosing and treating back pain was recognized.[68,92] In 1931, Mennell wrote in his book *Backache* that exercises that exacerbate symptoms should be omitted and exercises to "re-educate the postural reflexes" should be included.[68] In the 1950s, Paul C. Williams thought that lower lumbar intervertebral disc degeneration may be the cause of back pain, and he described a series of postural exercises to strengthen the back flexor muscles to reduce the lumbosacral angle and to restore proper posture.[92] His exercise program is called the "Williams flexion exercise," as opposed to the McKenzie back exercise program, which is commonly known as a "hyperextension" exercise. However, the original book written by McKenzie described both extension and flexion exercises to treat extension and flexion dysfunction.[67]

In the 1950s a conservative treatment to treat muscle "spasms" started with heat. Iontophoresis was recommended to control pain before starting to exercise. Then exercise was to be performed as long as pain did not accompany the movements.[59] However, in 1955 Krusen showed that active neck exercise in addition to modalities and massage was therapeutic in patients with neck and shoulder pain with acute "fibrositis."[59] More recently, postisometric relaxation has been used to treat myofascial pain.[61] For shoulder pain, Ernest A. Codman noted that the arm is moved painlessly under the influence of gravity. From this concept, the pendulum or stooping exercises that bear the name of Codman were developed.[22]

The word *scoliosis* was used by Hippocrates to describe the condition of the spine that is "twisting" or "bending."[30] In the 1800s, Jacques-Mathieu Delpech, an orthopedic surgeon in France, resurrected interest in scoliosis.[63] In 1821, Delpech established a school for girls with scoliosis, which can be considered to be the first inpatient rehabilitation center. At the center, patients participated in aquatic therapy and other therapeutic programs, reportedly up to 14 hours a day. In the early 1900s, scoliosis was considered to be the result of "faulty growth" and gravitational force on the vertebral column.[30,38] Thus, many detailed exercises to counteract the gravitational force have been described for the treatment of scoliosis.[30,38,59] In the 1920s, Rudolph Klapp described an exercise program of creeping and crawling for children with scoliosis.[3] Unfortunately, scoliosis is one musculoskeletal disorder upon which exercise has been proven to have no effect. However, exercises are still being advocated for postural correction and faulty body mechanics.[50]

In the field of osteoporosis, the first major contribution was made in 1892 by Julius Wolff, who stated that bones adjust to the habitual loads placed on them by altering their amount and distribution of bone mass. By the 1960s osteoporosis had been shown to be caused by bed rest, inactivity, and disuse secondary to disabling conditions such as stroke, amputation, and spinal cord injury.[2] By the end of the 1970s, multiple studies proved that exercise can prevent osteoporosis in postmenopausal women and in the geriatric population.[2,4]

In today's managed care environment, there has been an increasing need to prove the efficacy and cost-effectiveness of any medical treatment. Many treatments in rehabilitation, including modalities and therapeutic exercises, have been advocated by clinical experiences, anecdotes, and retrospective or case-control studies. Effectiveness of therapeutic exercise must be proven by randomized controlled studies. Physiatrists and other rehabilitation professionals are encouraged to continue research efforts to prove the efficacy of therapeutic exercises. Furthermore, general rehabilitation patients have shorter hospital stays, and patients with musculoskeletal and chronic pain are rarely hospitalized today. With decreasing financial resources, physiatrists must be able not only to prescribe exercise programs but also to instruct patients in exercises that can be performed at home.

REFERENCES

1. 1969 Gold Key Award (Elizabeth Licht). Arch Phys Med Rehabil 50:668–669, 1969.
2. Abramson AS, Delagi EF: Influence of weight-bearing and muscle contraction on disuse osteoporosis. Arch Phys Med Rehabil March:147–151, 1961.
3. Adams RC, McCubbin JA: Games, Sports, and Exercises for the Physically Disabled, 4th ed. Philadelphia, Lea & Febiger, 1991.
4. Aloia JF, Cohn SH, Ostuni JA, et al: Prevention of involutional bone loss by exercise. Ann Intern Med 89:356–358, 1978.
5. American Medical Association: Handbook of Physical Therapy. Chicago, American Medical Association, 1932.
6. Bach F: Physical medicine and the rheumatism. Br J Phys Med 10:66–69, 1947.
7. Barach AL: Breathing exercises in pulmonary emphysema and allied chronic respiratory disease. Arch Phys Med Rehabil 36:379–390, 1955.
8. Basmajian JV: Control and training of individual motor units. Science 141:440–441, 1963.
9. Basmajian JV: Therapeutic Exercise, 4th ed. Baltimore, Williams & Wilkins, 1984.
10. Basmajian JV, Kukulka CG, Narayan MG, Takabe K: Biofeedback treatment of footdrop after stroke compared with standard rehabilitation technique: Effects of voluntary control and strength. Arch Phys Med Rehabil 56:231–236, 1975.
11. Berryman JW: The tradition of the "six things non-natural:" Exercise and medicine from Hippocrates through ante-bellum America. Exerc Sports Sci Rev 17:515–559, 1989.
12. Bobath B: A study of abnormal postural reflex activity in patients with lesions of the central nervous system. Part I. Physiotherapy 40:259–267, 1954.
13. Bobath B: A study of abnormal postural reflex activity in patients with lesions of the central nervous system. Part II. Physiotherapy 40:295–300, 1954.
14. Bobath B: A study of abnormal postural reflex activity in patients with lesions of the central nervous system. Part III. Physiotherapy 40:326–334, 1954.
15. Bobath B: A study of abnormal postural reflex activity in patients with lesions of the central nervous system. Part IV. Physiotherapy 40:368–373, 1954.
16. Bobath K, Bobath B: The facilitation of normal postural reactions and movements in the treatment of cerebral palsy. Physiotherapy 50:246–262, 1964.
17. Borg G: Perceived exertion as an indicator of somatic stress. Scand J Rehabil Med 2:92–98, 1970.
18. Brenner JH: Therapeutic Exercises for the Treatment of the Neurologically Disabled. Springfield, IL, Charles C Thomas, 1957.
19. Brunnstrom S: Movement Therapy in Hemiplegia. New York, Harper & Row, 1970.
20. Bush DC, William DA: Hand rehabilitation—retrospective. Clin Plast Surg 13:293–300, 1986.
21. Cailliet R: Therapeutic exercises for multiple sclerosis. J Phys Ment Rehabil 3(30):9–10, 1949.
22. Codman EA: The Shoulder. Boston, Thomas Todd, 1934.
23. Creighton C: Graded activity: Legacy of the sanatorium. Am J Occup Ther 47:745–748, 1993.
24. Deaver GG: The rehabilitation of the hemiplegic patient. J Phys Ment Rehabil 4(6):9–12, 1951.
25. DeLateur BJ, Lehman JF, Fordyce WE: A test of the DeLorme axiom. Arch Phys Med Rehabil 49:245–248, 1968.
26. DeLateur B, Lehman J, Stonebridge J, Warren CG: Isotonic versus isometric exercise: A double-shift transfer-of-training study. Arch Phys Med Rehabil 53:212–216, 1972.
27. DeLorme TL: Restoration of muscle power with heavy resistance exercise. J Bone Joint Surg 27:645, 1945.
28. DeLorme TL: Progressive Resistance Exercise: Technique and Medical Application. New York, Appleton-Century-Crofts, 1951.
29. Doshay LJ, Boshes LD: Parkinson's disease in general practice. Med Clin North Am 45:1595–1603, 1961.
30. Drew LC: Individual Gymnastics. Philadelphia, Lea & Febiger, 1926.
31. Duthie JJR: The fundamental treatment of rheumatoid arthritis. Practitioner 166:22–31, 1951.
32. Fay T: The use of pathological and unlocking reflexes in the rehabilitation of spastics. Am J Phys Med 33:347–352, 1954.

33. Fletcher GF: The history of exercise in the practice of medicine. J Med Assoc Ga 72:35–40, 1983.
34. Ganorkar SW, Mandal HV: Medicine and physical exercise in ancient India. J Sports Med Phys Fitness 13:134–136, 1973.
35. Gettman LR, Ayres JJ, Pollock ML, et al: Physiologic effects on adult men of circuit strength training and jogging. Arch Phys Med Rehabil 60:115–120, 1979.
36. Granger FB: Physical Therapeutic Technic. Philadelphia, WB Saunders, 1929.
37. Green RM: A Translation of Galen's Hygiene. Springfield, IL, Charles C Thomas, 1951.
38. Hawley G: The Kinesiology of Corrective Exercise. Philadelphia, Lea & Febiger, 1937.
39. Hellenbrandt FA, Houtz SJ: Methods of muscle training: The influence of pacing. Phys Ther Rev 38:319–322, 1958.
40. Hellerstein HK, Golston E: Rehabilitation of patients with heart disease. Postgrad Med 30:265–278, 1954.
41. Hembrow CH: Sir Colin McKenzie and his contribution to the treatment of poliomyelitis. Med J Aust 1:194–198, 1973.
42. Hill D: Basic treatment in rheumatoid arthritis. Med Clin North Am 39:393–403, 1955.
43. Hirt S: Exploratory and analytical survey of therapeutic exercise. Historical bases for therapeutic exercise. Am J Phys Med 46:32–38, 1967.
44. Hoffman FP: Rehabilitation of chronic obstructive lung diseases. Rehabil Lit 29:34–39, 1968.
45. Johnson HE, Garton WH: Muscle re-education in hemiplegia by use of electromyographic device. Arch Phys Med Rehabil 54:320–322, 1973.
46. Joke E: The Scope of Exercises in Rehabilitation. Springfield, IL, Charles C Thomas, 1964.
47. Kabat H: Studies of neuromuscular dysfunction: XV. The role of central facilitation in restoration of motor function in paralysis. Arch Phys Med September:521–533, 1952.
48. Karling K: Per Henrik Ling and Swedish medical gymnastics. Physiotherapy 40:335–338, 1954.
49. Katch FI, Drumm SS: Effects of different modes of strength training on body composition and anthropometry. Clin Sports Med 5:413–459, 1986.
50. Kendall HO, Kendall FP, Boynton DA: Posture and Pain. Baltimore, Williams & Wilkins, 1952.
51. Kenny E: And They Shall Walk. New York, Dodd, Mead & Co., 1944.
52. Knott M, Voss DE: Proprioceptive Neuromuscular Facilitation. New York, Harper & Row, 1956.
53. Koh TC: Chinese medicine and martial arts. Am J Chin Med 9:181–186, 1981.
54. Kottke FJ: From reflex to skill: The training of coordination. Arch Phys Med Rehabil 61:551–561, 1980.
55. Kottke TE, Caspersen CJ, Hill CS: Exercise in the management and rehabilitation of selected chronic diseases. Prevent Med 13:47–65, 1984.
56. Kotteke FJ, Halpern D, Easton JK, et al: The training of coordination. Arch Phys Med Rehabil 59:567–572, 1978.
57. Kottke FJ, Knapp ME: The development of physiatry before 1950. Arch Phys Med Rehabil 69(spec no):4–14, 1988.
58. Kottke FJ, Lehman JF: Krusen's Handbook of Physical Medicine and Rehabilitation. Philadelphia, WB Saunders, 1990.
59. Kraus H: Principles and Practice of Therapeutic Exercises. Springfield, IL, Charles C Thomas, 1949.
60. Krusen EM: Pain in the neck and shoulder, common causes and response to therapy. JAMA 159:1282–1285, 1955.
61. Lewit K, Simons DG: Myofascial pain. Relief by post-isometric relaxation. Arch Phys Med Rehabil 65:452–456, 1984.
62. Licht S: Therapeutic Exercise. Baltimore, Waverly Press, 1958.
63. Licht S: Rehabilitation medicine: Definition and origin. Arch Phys Med Rehabil 51:619–624, 1970.
64. Licht S: Stroke: A history of its rehabilitation. Walter J. Zeiter Lecture. Arch Phys Med Rehabil 54:10–18, 1973.
65. MacAuley D: A history of physical activity, health and medicine. J R Soc Med 87:32–35, 1994.
66. McGavack TH: Treatment of uncomplicated obesity. Med Clin North Am 45:1515–1522, 1961.
67. McKenzie RA: The lumbar spine: Mechanical diagnosis and therapy. New Zealand, Spinal Publications Limited, 1981.

68. Mennell J: Backache. Philadelphia, P. Blakiston's Son & Co., 1931.
69. Miller WF: Physical therapeutic measures in the treatment of chronic bronchopulmonary disorders. Am J Med 24:929–939, 1958.
70. Mulder DW: Clinical observations on acute poliomyelitis. Ann N Y Acad Sci 753:1–10, 1995.
71. Moss CN: Rehabilitation and occupational medicine. J Occup Med 16:81–85, 1974.
72. Newman LB, Andrews MF, Koblish MO, Baker LA: Physical medicine and rehabilitation in acute myocardial infarction. Arch Intern Med 89:552–561, 1952.
73. Nicoll EA: Principles of exercise therapy. BMJ June:747–750, 1943.
74. Oldridge NB, Nagle FJ, Balke B, et al: Aortocoronary bypass surgery: Effects of surgery and 32 months of physical conditioning on treadmill performance. Arch Phys Med Rehabil 59:268–275, 1978.
75. Optiz JL, Folz TJ, Gelfman R, Peters J: The history of physical medicine and rehabilitation as recorded in the diary of Dr. Frank Krusen: Part 1. Gathering momentum (the years before 1942). Arch Phys Med Rehabil 78:442–445, 1997.
76. Pashkow FJ: Issues on contemporary cardiac rehabilitation: A historical perspective. J Am Coll Cardiol 21:822–834, 1993.
77. Petty T: Physical therapy: Introduction. Am Rev Respir Dis 110:129–131, 1974.
78. Rabiner AM, Hand MH: Activity as a therapeutic measures in Parkinsonian syndromes. N Y State J Med 43:1033–1034, 1943.
79. Rae JW, Bender LF: Treatment of patients with rheumatoid arthritis by physical means. JAMA 160:611–613, 1956.
80. Rae JW, Bender LF: Physical therapy in rheumatoid arthritis. J Chron Dis 5:706–711, 1957.
81. Robertson R: A therapeutic program for muscular dystrophy. Am Corr Ther J 31:70–74, 1977.
82. Rood M: Neurophysiological reactions as a basis for physical therapy. Phys Ther Rev 34:444–449, 1954.
83. Rood MS: Neurophysiological mechanisms utilized in the treatment of neuromuscular dysfunction. Am J Occup Ther 10:220–225, 1956.
84. Rosen NB: The role of sports in rehabilitation of the handicapped. 1A. Historical. Md State Med J 22:30–32, 1973.
85. Sherrington CS: Flexion-reflex of the limb, crossed extension-reflex, and reflex stepping and standing. J Physiol (Lond) 40:28–121, 1910.
86. Simard TG, Basmajian JV: Methods in training the conscious control of motor units. Arch Phys Med Rehabil 48:2–19, 1967.
87. Stillwell DM: Bisgaard treatment for static edema and its sequelae in the lower extremity. Arch Phys Med Rehabil 37:693–698, 1956.
88. Traut EF: Degenerative arthritis: Its causes, recognition and management. Med Clin North Am 40:63–78, 1956.
89. Vertinsky P: "Of no use without health:" Late nineteenth century medical prescriptions for female exercise through the left span. Women Health 14:89–115, 1988.
90. Weiner DA, McCabe CH, Roth RL, et al: Serial exercise testing after coronary artery bypass surgery. Am Heart J 101:149–154, 1981.
91. Wescott EJ: Traditional exercise regimens for the hemiplegic patient. Am J Phys Med 46:1012–1023, 1967.
92. Williams PC: Examination and conservative treatment for disk lesions of the lower spine. Clin Orthop 5:28–40, 1955.
93. Yogeswar T: Simple Yoga and Therapy. Madras, India, 1986.
94. Young P: A pilot scheme in rehabilitation for the cancer patient. Physiotherapy 57:125–126, 1971.
95. Zhou DH: The contribution of traditional Chinese medicine to rehabilitation medicine. Chin Med J 94:593–596, 1981.
96. Zinofieff AN: Heavy resistance exercises: The "Oxford technique." Br J Phys Med 14:129–132, 1951.

KAMALA SHANKAR, MD
NIRMALA N. NAYAK, MD

2

Effects of Exercise on Organ Systems

The effects of exercise on the human body have been studied for centuries. This chapter describes adaptations and effects of exercise on selected organ systems. Although the effects on the organ systems have been described individually, the effects are often interrelated. For instance, skeletal muscles, the cardiovascular system, and the respiratory system work together to provide homeostatic gas exchange between external environment and working muscle fibers. Pathologies in any one of these organ systems can cause lowering of exercise tolerance. Both acute effects and chronic adaptations occur in response to exercise. Understanding the effects of exercise on various organ systems is prudent before exercise prescription is considered.

MUSCULOSKELETAL SYSTEM

Animal and human muscles contain two different types of muscle fibers. Type I muscle fiber, known also as slow oxidative slow-twitch, are the fatigue-resistant red fibers. Type II fibers, or fast-twitch fibers, have two different characteristics. Type IIa, which are bigger and faster than type I, are also fatigue-resistant and are referred to as fast oxidative glycolytic, or FOG, fibers. Type IIb are the classical white fibers, which lack aerobic enzymes and therefore fatigue rapidly (Table I).

Each muscle contains type I and II fibers in various proportions. The basic distribution of fiber types is probably an inherited characteristic.[3,62] Muscle fibers form part of motor units, and within any one motor unit the fibers are of the same type.[3]

Although distribution varies among individuals, the average ratio of fast- to slow-twitch fibers is 50:50.[62] Individuals trained in endurance activities usually have a higher proportion of slow-twitch fibers, and those trained for high-intensity, high-speed activities such as sprinting mainly have high-twitch fibers.[52] The oxidative capacity of both fibers can be greatly increased by endurance training, but the glycolytic capacity and contractile properties are not modified.[21]

Fibers are recruited selectively during exercise. Slow-twitch fibers are supplied by small neurons with a low threshold of activation and are preferentially used during ex-

TABLE 1. Muscle Fiber Types and Their Characteristics

	Type I	Type IIa	Type IIb
Fiber size	Small	Intermediate	Large
Color	Red	Red	White
Oxidative enzymes	High	High	Low
Rate of fatigue	Low	Intermediate	High
Lipid content	High	Intermediate	Low
Glycogen content	Low	Intermediate	High
Contraction speed	Slow	Fast	Fast

ercise of low intensity. Fast-twitch fibers are innervated by larger neurons with a higher threshold of stimulation. These are activated during high-intensity exercises. Both fiber types are active during heavy exercise.

The biochemical processes occurring during aerobic and anaerobic exercises are depicted in Figure 1. Glycogen, glucose, and free fatty acids are the major source of energy. Aerobic oxidation yields ten times as much adenosine triphosphate (ATP) and energy than the anaerobic process, which produces pyruvate and lactate. The duration and intensity of exercise determines which of these pathways will be used. Equal amounts of energy are derived aerobically from fats and carbohydrates at rest. During low levels of exercise, free fatty acids form the main fuel source, but the proportion of energy derived from carbohydrates increases steeply with increasing effort levels. Only carbohydrates are used during maximal work. A well-trained individual, at any given submaximal level of energy expenditure, uses more fat and less carbohydrates than the untrained person.[1,19]

The transition from aerobic to anaerobic metabolism is a gradual process. Anaerobic metabolism of glucose and glycogen is the main source of energy early in exercise when high-energy phosphates (ATP and creatine phosphate) are depleted and the blood flow has not reached levels high enough to sustain aerobic metabolism. Anaerobic metabolism can be used only to a limited extent. Maximum exercise of less than a minute is mainly supported by anaerobic mechanisms. This proportion decreases rapidly with increasing duration of the effort, e.g., 20% at 5 minutes, to less than 10%

Anaerobic

1. ATP $\leftrightarrow$ ADP + phosphate + free energy
2. Creatine phosphate + ADP $\leftrightarrow$ creatine + ATP
3. Glycogen or glucose + P + ADP $\rightarrow$ lactate + ATP

Aerobic

1. Glycogen or glucose + P + ADP + O_2 $\rightarrow$ CO_2 + H_2O + ATP
2. Free fatty acids + P + ADP + O_2 $\rightarrow$ CO_2 + H_2O + ATP

FIGURE 1. Energy for muscular contraction.

at 10 minutes, and 1% at 1 hour.[62] The exact mechanisms limiting anaerobic mechanisms are poorly defined. However, there is a strong correlation between lactate accumulation and toxicity.

There is considerable controversy concerning the ability of the muscle fiber to change fiber type. The conventional view that an individual inherits a specific pattern of fast- and slow-twitch fibers that remains constant throughout life may be challenged by studies done in animals.[14,48,50] These studies have shown that all biochemical and physiologic parameters can be changed by electrical stimulation and that twitch speed may be related to the frequency and pattern of electrical stimulation.[14,51] There also appears to be widespread consensus that the metabolic capacity of fibers can be changed, as evidenced by the increase in oxidative capacity of the muscle fibers with training.

Muscle function can be described in terms of strength and endurance. Strength can be defined in several ways depending on the specific method of measurement. In absolute terms, muscle strength is related to the diameter of the muscle fiber. Muscle fiber hypertrophy has been consistently shown to occur with strength training.[52] This occurs in all fiber types but somewhat more in fast-twitch fibers,[40,61] and it appears to result from an increase in myofibrils in a given muscle fiber.[14] Muscle fibers with large diameters (type II) have more myofibrils and more actin-myosin bridges to produce force. The strength of the whole muscle is related to the cross-sectional area of the muscle when measured perpendicular to the length of the muscle fibers.[13] The cross-sectional measurement changes with contraction and relaxation.

Endurance can be measured as the ability to work over time. Local muscle endurance should be distinguished from general body endurance. Activities such as running, jogging, and swimming involve general body endurance. In contrast, local muscle endurance refers to the ability of an isolated muscle group to continue a prescribed task.[22]

A hyperbolic mathematical relationship exists between strength and endurance. The hyperbolic relationship may be related to the relative contributions from anaerobic and aerobic metabolism.[13]

Significant strength gains are possible in all populations, including children, women, and the elderly when exposed to an adequate strength-training program. Strength gains occur from enhanced neuromuscular activation over the initial 8 weeks and from increased fiber density and hypertrophy during subsequent weeks.[34] Even in the aged population, resistance and endurance training appear to attenuate age-related alterations in skeletal muscle properties if the stimulus is of sufficient intensity and duration.[60]

Fatigue, the inability to continue to maintain a given activity, can be general or local. To avoid fatigue, adequate tissue ATP levels must be maintained to supply the energy that is required. High-intensity exercises involve an energy demand that may exceed the individual's maximal aerobic power and thus require a high level of anaerobic metabolism. As fatigue develops, levels of ATP, phosphocreatine, and high-energy phosphates decrease, and levels of lactate, adenosine diphosphate, inorganic phosphates, and hydrogen ions increase. All of these changes are possible fatigue agents. During endurance exercises, numerous factors have been linked to opment of fatigue, including depletion of muscle and liver glycogen, decreases in blood glucose, dehydration, and increases in body temperature.

Osteoporosis is a loss of bone mass per unit volume with retention of a normal ratio of mineral to matrix. The major factor in osteogenesis is weightbearing activity. Intensity of load, area of application of load, and the relative newness of the activity are important factors. Studies of immobility have noted that bone loss occurs primarily from weightbearing bones, including the vertebrae, femur, calcaneous, and metacarpals.

The relationship between bone mass and activity is well established. Complete immobilization results in rapid onset of accelerated bone resorption as evidenced by an increase in urine calcium and hydroxyproline levels and increased osteoclastic activity. At the same time, osteoblastic activity and bone formation are reduced. Similar events occur in weightlessness. Bone mass recovers when activity resumes, but whether bone loss is completely reversible is unknown.

Exercise also affects joints. Immobilization leads to changes in collagen, ligaments, and muscles next to the joint, causing reduced motion. Internal changes in the joint with atrophy of synovium and deterioration of subchondral bone also can occur. Early mobilization and maintenance of range of motion through active and passive exercise at least twice a day decreases the changes of contracture formation.

Acute and chronic musculoskeletal injuries such as sprains and degenerative joint changes are negative effects of exercise. The incidence of injuries can be reduced by limiting the frequency and duration of exercise during the initial stages and gradually increasing them until fitness is achieved.[36]

CARDIOVASCULAR SYSTEM

Exercise training in all age groups results in numerous physiologic benefits, including cardiac adaptation, hemodynamic alterations, and improvements in metabolic efficiency. Many of the physiologic changes that occur in older adults can be limited by increasing physical activity. Primary and secondary causes of cardiovascular disease are similarly reduced with regular exercise.[22]

The extent of improvement is determined in part by the type of exercise; frequency, intensity, and duration of the exercise session; and the initial level of fitness.

The effect of exercise on the cardiac parameters can be summarized as follows: with graded exercise, the heart rate (HR) for both sedentary and conditioned individuals increases in a linear fashion. HR increases first by augmentation of sympathetic neural input to the sinoatrial node. Following aerobic conditioning, resting heart rate is reduced by 10–15 beats per minute, which is primarily attributed to enhanced parasympathetic tone. Decreased sympathetic discharge and a decreased rate of firing of the sinoatrial node also may contribute to the reduction in heart rate.[47] Maximal HR is unchanged or only slightly reduced after aerobic conditioning.

Stroke volume is defined as the average volume of blood ejected per heartbeat. In the resting state, stroke volume is higher in supine than in the upright posture as a result of greater venous return. Stroke volume generally is increased as a result of augmented diastolic filling (preload) via the Starling mechanism and is reduced by increased arterial blood pressure and other factors that raise impedance to aortic blood flow (after load). With graded exercise, stroke volume increases in a linear fashion and is attributed to increased myocardial contractibility and sympathetic neural stimulation resulting in an increase in ejection fraction.

Cardiac output is the product of HR and stroke volume. This parameter also rises linearly with graded exercise; it is achieved by a combination of sympathetic ionotropic and chronotropic influences on contractile force of the ventricle and the rate of ejection, respectively. Coronary blood flow during exercise increases in proportion to the cardiac output but remains the same on a percentage basis.[47]

The Starling mechanism of the venous return tends to increase left ventricular end diastolic pressure and hence increases the initial length of the ventricular fibers. In 1918 Starling stated that "if a man starts to run, his muscular movements pump more blood into the heart, as a result the heart is overfilled. Its volume both in systole and diastole enlarge progressively until by the lengthening of the muscle fibers so much more active surfaces are brought into play within the fibers that the energy of contraction becomes sufficient to drive on into the aorta during each systole, the largely increased volume of blood entering the heart from the veins during diastole."[30]

Blood pressure (BP) is the product of cardiac output and peripheral resistance. Acute increases in BP occur with both resistance and endurance exercises. The BP response to resistance training can be much greater than with endurance training, which suggests caution in prescribing resistance exercise to patients with significant hypertension or those at risk for cerebral bleeding. Another effect of exercise on BP is post-exercise hypertension, which can occur with both endurance and resistance exercise. It begins shortly after exercise and lasts up to 3 hours.[24]

Long-term effects of exercise in general support the concept that BP is related inversely to the level of physical activity. Irrespective of age, there is a decline in BP with endurance training, with the greatest decline occurring among the elderly and hypertensive persons.[24] The usual drop is 6–10 mm Hg in systolic and 4–6 mm Hg in diastolic BP. The BP response begins within the first few weeks and continues to show improvement over the year as long as the exercise is continued. The benefits of exercise cease once exercise is discontinued. The intensity of exercise in most studies for lowering BP is aimed between 50 and 70% of maximal aerobic power ($VO_{2\,max}$) three times a week for 30–40 minutes.

$VO_{2\,max}$ is the oxygen uptake of an individual under maximal aerobic exercise conditions and is the product of peak output and maximum oxygen extraction from the tissues. The most fundamental systemic characteristic of the trained state includes (1) an increase in $VO_{2\,max}$ and (2) a resting and submaximal exercise bradycardia. As a general rule at least 50% of training-induced increase in $VO_{2\,max}$ can be attributed to an increase in maximal stroke volume (SV_{max}). Augmented SV_{max} secondary to a chronic exercise paradigm is almost always associated with an increase in left ventricular diastolic dimensions. This increase in the trained state may be achieved by a variety of mechanisms: (1) an increase in the intrinsic compliance of the myocardium, (2) an increase in end diastolic filling pressure, and (3) an increase in left ventricular chamber dimensions resulting from myocyte growth.[41]

A relative bradycardia during rest and submaximal exercise is a classic hallmark of the trained state. This reduction of resting and submaximum HR in the trained state is generally thought to be caused by factors extrinsic and intrinsic to the heart. With respect to the extrinsic factors, increased parasympathetic and decreased sympathetic drive are possible contributing mechanisms. In many but not all studies, chronic exercise has been shown to elicit increases in the contractile performance of the ventricular myocardium in both humans and animals.[41] Alterations in cellular energy metabolism, calcium regulation, contractile element composition, and signal transduction pathways have been implicated as factors that may contribute to training-induced changes in intrinsic cardiac contractile function.

The positive effects of training on performance of the heart have been well documented in a number of cardiopathologic states. In certain hypertensive states and with advanced age, a number of cellular systems that appear to show diminished function respond positively to programs of chronic exercise.

Medications used in cardiac disorders influence exercise capacity. Many studies have been conducted on the effects of beta-blockers. The earliest β-blockers blocked both β_1 and β_2 receptors. The more recent agents are relatively selective, producing greater effect on β_1 and β_2 receptors. This results in fewer side effects such as bronchospasm and peripheral vasodilatation. β-blockers generally produce lower HR and BP at rest and during exercise, thus reducing myocardial oxygen demand. This usually allows a higher achieved workload. β_1 selective blockers appear to have advantages over nonselective blockers for patients with high systolic BP during exercise and those with impaired myocardial oxygen delivery.[24,30]

On the other hand, using β-blockers in physically active patients with uncomplicated hypertension may have disadvantages, including reducing exercise capacity[41] and possibly having negative effects on exercise training.

Calcium channel blockers produce decreased BP during rest and exercise. This class of drugs is as an alternative to β-blockers for supressing an excessive rise in BP during exercise. Nitrates may improve exercise capacity by increasing the anginal threshold.

PULMONARY SYSTEM

There is no direct information regarding the amplitude and pattern of activation of inspiratory and expiratory muscles at different levels of exercise. Henke et al. inferred the action of abdominal muscles during graded exercise from changes in gastric pressure. Their data indicate activation of these muscles at low levels of exercise with progressive increase at higher levels. Over low and moderate exercise ventilation increases primarily due to increases in tidal volume. End-expiratory volume (EEV) appears to slowly, progressively decrease, reaching about 1 L below resting level with heavy exercise. Increases in EEV are common in healthy older subjects.[63]

Spirometric changes with progressive exercise are as follows: oxygen consumption, minute ventilation, and tidal volume progressively increase; inspiratory capacity changes slightly; inspiratory duration and expiratory duration decrease slightly; and end-expiratory lung volume decreases.

As with other skeletal muscles, the ability of respiratory muscles to sustain high levels of ventilation is limited. The highest level of ventilation can be sustained only for several seconds, with the endurance time increasing as ventilation decreases.

The increased metabolism associated with exercise results in delivery of more carbon dioxide (CO_2) to the lungs and requires more oxygen uptake (VO_2) from the lungs compared with the resting state. To maintain constancy of Pa_{CO_2} (partial pressure of carbon dioxide in arterial blood) when the CO_2 production has increased, alveolar ventilation increases in proportion to increase in CO_2 output.

To meet the demand for increased alveolar ventilation, ventilatory muscles must generate total ventilation (VE) greater than alveolar ventilation by the amount needed to ventilate the anatomic dead space (upper airways and bronchi) and alveolar dead space (unperfused alveoli). The ventilatory muscles move the rib cage and the diaphragm to achieve cyclical inflation and deflation of the lungs, thereby producing air flow. If the lungs had unlimited ability to support air flow, the only limitation would be the ventilatory muscles and chest wall. Intrinsic lung disease of the chest wall can cause further limitation. The increased ventilatory demands of exercise are met in most healthy individuals by increasing tidal volume at low levels of exercise, followed by increased breathing frequency near maximal exercise, with tidal volume increasing to about 60% of vital capacity. Similarly VE_{max} approaches 60% maximal ventilatory volume. In elite athletes VE_{max} may approach maximal ventilatory volume, suggesting a ventilatory limitation.[63]

In normal individuals, maximum exercise is limited by hemodynamic factors, particularly the levels to which the cardiac output can be elevated efficiently, and by the ability of muscles to generate sufficient metabolic energy. In normal subjects, low levels of exercise result in an increase in (1) cardiac output, primarily due to an increase in heart rate, (2) a widening of the arterial mixed venous oxygen difference, and (3) an increase in oxygen consumption and production of CO_2. The minute ventilation increases sufficiently to maintain the alveolar ventilation at a level great enough to remove all the CO_2 produced; therefore the Pa_{CO_2} remains within normal limits. Initially, with exercise the pulmonary blood flow increases; pulmonary perfusion becomes evenly distributed; there is improvement in the ventilation perfusion relationship; and the oxygen gradient is decreased. As the exercise level is increased, the blood flow to the exercising muscles ultimately becomes inadequate to provide sufficient oxygen to maintain pure aerobic metabolism. At that point, anaerobic glycolytic metabolism occurs. Lactic acid enters the venous circulation and the blood pH falls. When the acid produced is buffered by bicarbonate, an additional amount of CO_2 is produced.

At higher levels of exercise, the pH falls sufficiently to drive VE out of proportion to CO_2 production, causing a fall in Pa_{CO_2}. However, Pa_{CO_2} remains within normal limits. Thus, cardiac output and the resultant increase in muscle blood flow are the primary factors limiting exercise in normal subjects.[6] In patients with pulmonary disease due to ventilatory limitations or pulmonary gas exchange compromise, the classic relationships among VO_2, HR, and VE are not followed. Because the limitation to exercise in pulmonary patients is not of hemodynamic origin, the use of HR or oxygen consumption to guide maximum exercise is not safe. Also, such patients rarely achieve anaerobic threshold because they are forced by dyspnea to discontinue exercise well before the anerobic threshold is reached. Even in the older adults, the response to alveolar ventilation to exercise is adequate for CO_2 elimination (even during maximal exercise), and arterial homeostasis is generally maintained.[28]

Studies have shown that the respiratory system becomes an exercise-limiting factor during an endurance test in normal sedentary subjects[7] and normal endurance-trained subjects.[8] Exercise can be deleterious in individuals prone to exercise-induced bronchospasm and exercise-induced anaphylaxis.[32] The mechanisms of these syndromes are unclear, but it is helpful to avoid an excessively cold, dry environment and use a prolonged warm-up period and bronchodilators prior to exercise.

GASTROINTESTINAL SYSTEM

Exercise is characterized by a shift in blood flow away from the gastrointestinal (GI) tract toward the active muscle and the lungs. Changes in the nervous activity, circulating hormones, peptides, and metabolic end products lead to changes in GI motility, blood flow, absorption, and secretion. The gut is not an athletic organ in that it adapts to increased exercise-induced physiologic stress.[9] However, adequate training leads to a less dramatic decrease of GI blood flow at submaximal exercise intensities and is important in the prevention of GI symptoms.[49]

One complication that occasionally occurs following prolonged exercise is GI bleeding, probably mediated by visceral ischemia.[44] Diarrhea, incontinence, and rectal bleeding sometimes occur in runners.[45] In exhausting endurance events, 30–50% of participants may develop one or more GI symptoms, such as stomachache, vomiting, reflux, and heartburn. There is no evidence that ingestion of nonhypertonic drinks during exercise induces GI stress or diarrhea. Dehydration because of insufficient fluid replacement has been shown to increase the frequency of GI symptoms. Physical activity appears to occasionally protect against colorectal cancer and colorectal adenomas.[54]

The rate of exercise on the GI motor function and, in particular, on transit time is a matter of debate.[29] In a study on the effects of exercise on mouth-to-cecum transit in trained athletes, Kayaleh et al. observed that (1) mouth-to-cecum transit time is not affected by short-term intense exercise in trained athletes; (2) bouncing of the abdominal contents in the case of running probably does not change the transit time; and (3) the impact of moderate to intense short-term exercise on the mouth-to-cecum transit is not influenced by the subject's fitness state. In another study in soccer players, no overall difference in large bowel transit was observed; however, only regional differences such as right colon transit were slower, but left colon and rectal transit were accelerated.[55] Similarly, the effects of exercise on esophageal motility and gastroesophageal reflux were similar in trained and untrained subjects performing similar percentages of $VO_{2\ max}$, even though the absolute levels of exercise achieved in each group were different.[58] Other studies also have shown that there is no consistent effect on large bowel function with exercise under a constant diet.[5,11] Conversely, physical inactivity caused significant prolongation of colonic transit time,[37] calling for increasing activity and exercise among physically inactive individuals.

NERVOUS SYSTEM

The literature related to the nervous system can be categorized in two ways. First, there are anecdotal reports related to the effects of exercise on analgesia, mood, and general improved quality of life.[59] Second, there are attempts to explain these effects based on physiologic changes. Exercise research is fraught with methodologic and practical problems. In interpreting results, it is difficult to distinguish between the effects of exercise per se and those of other components that might themselves be beneficial.

Research has been aimed at finding powerful pain-relieving substances that are free of the hazards of existing opiate analgesics, such as depressed respiration and potential for addiction. The discovery of neuropeptides was initially reported in 1975 by Hughes, Smith, Kosterlitz, et al.[26] Neuropeptides have since been shown to have the same properties as opiates, such as inhibition of isolated smooth muscle contraction and blockage of its action by opiate antagonists.

At least three families of endogenous opioid peptides are now generally distinguished: encephalins, endorphins, and dynorphins. The link between exercise and endorphins has been well publicized by the media and in superficial reports in the literature. It has been observed that pain perception can decrease during periods of stress or great emotional excitement as well as under the influence of opioid drugs. Experimental pain sensitivity has been studied in long-distance runners,[27] in whom pain thresholds increased following a run. The plasma levels of beta-endorphins, adrenocorticotropic hormone, prolactin, and growth hormone also increased.

The biologic significance of rises in plasma levels of endogenous opioids with exercise is unclear. In addition, exercise is accompanied by numerous other physiologic and biochemical changes that are linked with catecholamine activity. In normal subjects, plasma norepinephrine rises only modestly during exercise below the anaerobic threshold,[18] suggesting that the neural response to low-level exercise is related largely to vagal withdrawal. Above this aerobic threshold, the plasma norepinephrine level rises rapidly to levels at peak oxygen consumption of 3000–5000 pg/ml. It is possible that the endogenous opioids inhibit the release of catecholamine induced by any form of severe stress. Exercise may be only one of a number of stressors that may interact with the opioid systems.

Work by Morgan[43] on the influence of cognition on exercise metabolism adds to the complexity of exercise research. His methods, although indirect through hypnosis, show a relationship between perception of the intensity of the exercise and the physiologic changes in HR, ventilatory volume, and CO_2 production. Hypnotic suggestions of light and heavy exercise in resting subjects yielded physiologic changes proportionate to the perceived exertion. Many individuals employ various methods of cognitive strategies during athletic events.[42] Some, for example, employ a "disassociation" cognitive strategy in an effort to reduce the discomfort associated with exercise stress, and others focus closely on the sensory input during stress. These strategies are known to be associated with different physiologic responses and levels of performance.

The physiologic and psychological effects of exercise may be closely linked. Morgan and Goldstein described four main hypotheses for the psychological effects of exercise: (1) the endorphin hypothesis, which results in improved mood from release of endorphins; (2) the monoamine hypothesis, which suggests that monoamine levels are related to norepinephrine levels, which increases during exercise; (3) the thermogenic hypothesis, in which a temporary increase in body temperature during exercise produces a pyrogenic effect that contributes to decreased muscle tension, elevated mood, reduced anxiety, and improved sleep patterns; and (4) the distraction hypothesis, which explains that exercise provides distraction from symptoms.

Although clear-cut studies on the mechanism of the psychological benefits of exercise are not available, clinical observation has shown that regular physical activity benefits patients with anxiety and depression.[36]

Exercise for treatment of vestibular disorders was introduced in the 1940s. Attempts have been made to manage dizziness and vertigo from vestibular dysfunction through exercise. The treatment approach for patients with complete loss of vestibular function involves the use of exercise that promotes the substitution of the visual and somatosensory cues that can be used to maintain balance. Patients with some remaining vestibular function can benefit from vestibular adaptation exercises, which enhance the remaining function.[23]

Patients with complete bilateral vestibular loss may not be able to return to activities such as driving because they have gaze instability. Those with some preservation of vestibular function have a better prognosis.

IMMUNE SYSTEM

The immune system, which does not fall into the category of an organ system, nevertheless plays an important role in health and fitness. In the ever-expanding knowledge of psychoneuroimmunology, almost any stress seems capable of altering immune function.

Much of the research interest in exercise-associated changes centers around the alteration of numbers and changes in lymphocytes and the implications for interactions with viral infections, especially infection with the human immunodeficiency virus.

There is an increase in white blood cell (WBC) count proportionate to the effort exerted during brisk exercise.[15] The exercise-related increase in WBCs is thought to be largely mediated by the mechanical effects of an increased cardiac output and the physiologic effects of a surge in blood and adrenaline concentration.[15] During exercise, WBCs enter the blood from the reserve pools in the lung, liver, and especially the spleen.

The rise of WBCs consists of granulocytes (mainly polymorphonuclear neutrophils [PMNs]), monocytes, and lymphocytes.[56] Among the lymphocytes, the number of natural killer (NK) cells increases the most.

Whether the function or activity of NK cells also increases is unclear. In a randomized, controlled study of 15 weeks of moderate exercise training among 36 women ages 25–45, training seemed to increase NK activity at the 6-week point, but, by the end of 15 weeks, the NK activity in both the exercise and no exercise groups was enhanced to the same extent. The authors speculated that the increase in the latter group may have been a "seasonal" effect.[46]

It has long been known that exercise triggers a rise in blood level in PMNs,[39] especially in exercises that have an eccentric component, such as downhill running. If the exercise goes beyond about 30 minutes, there tends to be a second rise in PMNs over the next 2–4 hours, while the exerciser is at rest. This delayed rise in PMNs is probably mediated in part by cortisol, which influences release of PMNs from the bone marrow and restricts egress of PMNs from the bloodstream. Diverse cytokines released from the damaged muscles also may contribute to leukocytosis after exercise.

After brief, gentle exercise, the PMN count soon returns to baseline; however, after prolonged, strenuous exercise, this return to normal may be delayed 24 hours or longer.[15] As with the lymphocytes, it is unclear whether there is enhanced function of PMNs with exercise. Research is sparse and contradictory. One study suggests that increased resistance to infection occurs by priming the killing capacity of the PMNs after vigorous activity, but after prolonged periods of intensive training it may have the opposite effect.[57]

Little research has been done on exercise-related changes in serum immunoglobulins. One study suggests that moderate exercise training may slightly increase serum immunoglobulin levels; another suggests that exhausting endurance exercise may slightly decrease such levels.[15] Salivary immunoglobulins, which have been studied more than serum immunoglobulins, also show mixed results, e.g., a decline in immonoglobulin A (IgA) levels during swimming but not during running. Salivary IgA levels may be low in the elite cross-country skiers at rest and seem to fall further after a race. In contrast, IgA levels, while normal at rest in cyclists, decline during 2 hours of strenuous indoor cycling.

Other immune factors[10] show a complex cascade of reactions caused by strenuous exercise, which can damage enough tissue to evoke the "acute phase response." This response can conceivably modulate immune defense by activating complement and spurring release of tumor necrosis factor, interferons, interleukins, and other cytokines. Much more research is needed, however, before we can understand the implication of exercise-induced immunologic changes.

ENDOCRINE SYSTEM

This section addresses fuel homeostasis, including lipids, glucose, metabolism, and obesity.

Many studies have shown that, after cardiac rehabilitation, significant improvements occur in exercise capacity, percent body fat, high-density lipoprotein (HDL) cholesterol, triglycerides, and quality of life parameters.[23,33,38] In another study, physically disabled men with coronary artery disease participated in a home exercise training program and showed significantly improved left ventricular ejection fraction and a significant increase in HDL cholesterol.[17] Similarly, in postmenopausal women, exercise alone without estrogen therapy had a significant effect: total cholesterol, triglycerides, and low-density lipoprotein cholesterol were reduced, and HDL cholesterol was increased.[35]

Endurance exercise training can favorably modify the abdominal fat distribution profile that is typical in older men and women and can reduce abdominal obesity.[31]

Physically active men and women may be less likely than their sedentary peers to become overweight. The American College of Sports Medicine recommends that people should engage in regular physical activity that promotes a daily energy expenditure of at least 300 calories per day and to choose from a variety of activities, particularly those that are enjoyable and that can be continued for life. Insulin resistance is frequently associated with abdominal obesity and probably plays an important role in the pathophysiology of triglyceridemia, low levels of plasma HDL cholesterol, hypertension, and reduced fibrinolytic activity. Exercise training may counteract the aberrant metabolic profile associated with abdominal obesity, both directly and as a consequence of body fat loss. Changes in the activity of insulin-sensitive glucose transporters and of the skeletal muscle lipoprotein lipase are some of the possible explanations for the increased insulin sensitivity and improved blood lipid profile. The effect of exercise alone on body fat mass is variable and is less efficient than diminishing caloric intake. Exercise helps to accelerate fat loss and maintain lean body mass. There is a reduction in waist:hip ratio with increased exercise. Exercise programs of low to moderate intensity, long duration, and high frequency seem to be most beneficial, with the most popular forms of exercise being walking or jogging, cycling, and swimming.

The relationship between obesity and non–insulin-dependent diabetes mellitus (type 2) is well established, and most type 2 diabetics are classified as obese. Although the pathogenesis of type 2 diabetes mellitus is not fully understood, it is known that multiple organ systems are involved, including abnormalities of insulin secretion, peripheral insulin resistance, and hepatic insulin resistance.[64] A single exercise session improves and partially normalizes both insulin responsiveness and sensitivity for glucose utilization. A single bout of physical activity often results in decreased plasma glucose levels, which persist after exercise. Improved hemoglobin A_{1C} and glucose tolerance tests following physical training programs are also noted. Physical training increases insulin action in skeletal muscle in healthy men. In a study by Dela et al. in type 2 diabetes, in response to training, muscle lactate production and glucose storage and glycogen synthetase messenger RNA increased. Improvements in the whole body glucose clearance rate involve enhancement of an insulin-mediated increase in muscle blood flow and the ability to extract glucose.[12] Exercise may also benefit women with gestational diabetes mellitus by acting as an adjunct to preventing excessive weight gain and preventing or decreasing the severity of hypertension or hyperlipidemia during pregnancy.[25]

There are numerous benefits of exercise for patients with type 1 or insulin-dependent diabetes mellitus, including increases in insulin sensitivity and reductions of blood glucose levels. The type 1 diabetic is especially prone to exercise-induced hypoglycemia. In nondiabetics, the enhancement of skeletal muscle glucose intake, which increases 20- to 30-fold, is compensated for by enhanced hepatic glucose production. This is mediated primarily by a fall in circulating insulin levels consequent to an exercise-induced catecholamine discharge, which inhibits B cell secretion. Such regulation is impossible in the insulin-treated diabetic, whose subcutaneous depot not only continues to release insulin during exercise but also shows an accelerated absorption rate when the injection site is in close proximity to the muscles being exercised. When this occurs, increased levels of circulating insulin compromise the hepatic output of glucose. To prevent hypoglycemia, insulin-treated diabetics must be advised to avoid injection into areas adjacent to muscles most involved in the particular exercise or to reduce the insulin dose appropriately. To prevent insulin-induced hypoglycemia in patients treated with insulin infusion pumps, a reduction or omission of the premeal bolus may be required. To prevent hypoglycemia, the insulin dose may need to be reduced 30–50% before exercise. Avoiding regular insulin at bedtime and reducing the evening dose may help prevent nocturnal hypoglycemia.[16]

Precautions need to be taken by diabetics during exercise. With proliferative retinopathy, exercise may result in retinal or vitreous hemorrhage.[25] Strenuous exercise or exercise associated with Valsalva-like maneuvers are particularly dangerous and should be avoided by patients with proliferative retinopathy. Exercise involving jarring or rapid head motion may precipitate hemorrhage or retinal detachment. Other complications can include soft tissue or joint injuries in persons with peripheral neuropathy.[4] If autonomic neuropathy is present, the capacity for high-intensity exercise may be impaired due to decreased maximum HR and aerobic capacity. Impaired response to dehydration and problems with postural hypotension also may occur.

To summarize, with proper precautions, exercise is beneficial in persons with both types of diabetes. A regular exercise program can produce positive changes in the lipid profile, reduce blood pressure, reduce weight, and improve other cardiovascular risk factors.

CONCLUSION

Several studies in recent years have shown benefits of exercise in various organ systems, particularly in the areas of cardiac wellness, improved serum lipids and glucose tolerance, better control of hypertension, and prevention of osteoporosis. Almost all of the organ systems appear to benefit from effectively used exercise programs.

ACKNOWLEDGMENTS   We gratefully acknowledge the assistance of Ronald McLeod and Virginia Carrillo.

REFERENCES

1. Astrand PO, Rodahl K: Textbook of Work Physiology, 2nd ed. New York, McGraw Hill, 1977.
2. Barnard RJ: Effects of life style modification on serum lipids. Arch Intern Med 151:1389–1394, 1991.
3. Basmajian JV: Therapeutic Exercise. Baltimore, Williams & Wilkins, 1990.
4. Bell DS: Exercise for patients with diabetes. Benefits, risks, precautions. Postgrad Medicine. 92:183–184, 187–190, 195–198, 1992.
5. Bingham SA, Cummings SM: Effects of exercise and physical fitness on large intestinal function. Gastroenterology 97:1389–1399, 1989.
6. Bordon RA, Moser KM: Manual of clinical problems in pulmonary medicine. Boston, Little, Brown & Co., 1985.
7. Boutellier V, Buchel R, Kundert A, Spengler C: The respiratory system as an exercise limiting factor in normal trained subjects. Eur J Appl Physiol 65:347–353, 1992.
8. Boutellier V, Piwko P: The respiratory system as an exercise limiting factor in normal sedentary subjects. Eur J Appl Physiol 64:145–152, 1992.

9. Brouns F, Beckers E: Is the gut an athletic organ? Digestion, absorption and exercise. Sports Med 15:242–257, 1993.
10. Cannon JG, Kluger MJ: Endogenous pyrogen activity in human plasma after exercise. Science 220:617–619, 1983.
11. Coenen C, Wegener M, Wedmann B, et al: Does physical exercise influence bowel transit time in healthy young men? A J Gastroenterol 87:292–295, 1992.
12. Dela F, Larson JJ, Mikines KJ, et al: Insulin stimulated muscle glucose clearance in patients with NIDDM. Effects of one legged physical training. Diabetes 44:1010–1020, 1995.
13. Joynt RL: Therapeutic exercise. In DeLisa JA (ed): Rehabilitation Medicine: Principles and Practice. Philadelphia, JB Lippincott, 1988, pp 346–387.
14. Edrstrom L, Grimby L: Effect of exercise on the motor unit. Muscle Nerve 9:104–126, 1986.
15. Eichner RA, Calabrese LH: Immunology and exercise. Med Clin North Am 78:377–388, 1994.
16. Fahey PJ, Stallkamp ET, Kwatra S: The athlete with type I diabetes: Managing insulin, diet and exercise. Am Fam Phys 53:1611–1624, 1996.
17. Fletcher BJ, Dumbar SB, Felner JM, et al: Exercise testing and training in physically disabled men with clinical evidence of coronary artery disease. Am J Cardiol 73:170–174, 1994.
18. Francis GS, Goldsmith SR, Ziesche SM, Cohn JN: Response of plasma norepinephrine and epinephrine to dynamic exercise in patients with congestive heart failure. Am J Cardiol 49:1152–1159, 1982.
19. Gollnick PD, Saltin B: Significance of skeletal muscle oxidative enzyme enhancement with endurance training. Clin Physiol 2:1–12, 1982.
20. Gollnick PD, Hermansen L: Biochemical adaptations to exercise: Anaerobic metabolism. In Wilmore JH (ed): Exercise and Sports Reviews. Vol 1. New York, Academic Press, 1973.
21. Gollnick PD, Sembrowich WL: Adaptations in Human Skeletal Muscle as a Result of Training. Exercise in Cardiovascular Health and Disease. New York, Yorke Medical Books, 1977.
22. Halar E: Cardiac rehabilitation. Part II. Phys Med Rehabil Clin North Am 6:225–241, 1995.
23. Herdman JS: Vestibular Rehabilitation. Philadelphia, FA Davis, 1994.
24. Hirth VA, Schwartz RS: The effects of endurance and resistance training on blood pressure. Phys Med Rehabil Clin North Am 5:317–336, 1994.
25. Horton ES: Exercise in the treatment of NIDDM. Applications for GDM? Diabetes 40 (suppl 2): 175–178, 1991.
26. Hughes J, Smith TW, Kosterlitz HW, et al: Identification of two related pentapeptides from the brain with potent opiate agonist activity. Nature 258:577–579, 1975.
27. Janal MN, Colt EWD, Clark WC, Glusman M: Pain sensitivity, mood and plasma endocrine levels in man following long distance running: Effects of naloxone. Pain 19:13–25, 1984.
28. Johnson BD, Badr MS, Dempsey JA: Impact of aging pulmonary system on the response to exercise. Clin Chest Med 15:229–246, 1994.
29. Kayaleh RA, Meshkinpour M, Avinashi A, Tamadon A: Effect of exercise on mouth to cecum transit in trained athletes: A case against the role of runner's abdominal bouncing. J Sports Med Phys Fitness 36:271–274, 1996.
30. Keele CA, Neil E: Samson Wright's Applied Physiology, 12th ed. New York, Oxford University Press, 1971, pp 104–106.
31. Kohrt WM, Obert KA, Holloszy JO: Exercise training improves fat distribution patterns in 60 to 70 year old men and women. J Gerontol 47:M99–105, 1992.
32. Kyle JM: Exercise induced pulmonary syndrome. Med Clin North Am 78:413–421, 1994.
33. Lavie CJ, Milani RV: Effects of cardiac rehabilitation and exercise training programs in patients > or = 75 years of age. Am J Cardiol 78:675–677, 1996.
34. Lillegard WA, Terrio JD: Appropriate strength training. Med Clin North Am 78:457–477, 1994.
35. Lindheim SL, Notelovitz M, Feldman FB, et al: The independent effects of exercise and estrogen on lipids and lipoprotein in post menopausal women. Obstet Gynecol 83:167–172, 1994.
36. Goldberg L, Elliot D: Exercise for Prevention and Treatment of Illness. Philadelphia, FA Davis, 1994.
37. Liu F, Kondo T, Toda Y: Brief physical inactivity prolongs colonic transit time in elderly active men. Int J Sports Med 14:465–467, 1993.

38. Maines TV, Lavie CJ, Melani RV, et al: Effects of cardiac rehabilitation and exercise programs on exercise capacity, coronary risk factors, behavior, and quality of life in patients with coronary artery disease. South Med J 90:43–49, 1997.
39. McCarthy DA, Dale MM: The leukocytosis of exercise. Sports Med 6:333–363, 1988.
40. MacDougall JD, Elder GCB, Sake DG, et al: Effects of strength training and immobilization of human muscle fibers. Eur J Appl Physiol 43:25–34, 1980.
41. Moore LR, Korzich HD: Cellular adaptation of myocardium to chronic exercise. Progr Cardiovasc Dis 37:371–396, 1995.
42. Morgan WP, Pollock ML: Psychologic characterization of the elite distance runner. Ann NY Acad Sci 301:382–403, 1977.
43. Morgan WP, Goldston SE: Exercise and Mental Health. New York, Hemisphere, 1987.
44. Moses FM: Gastrointestinal bleeding and the athlete. Am J Gastroenterol 89:1157–1159, 1994.
45. Moses FM: The effect of exercise on gastrointestinal tract. Sports Med 9:159–172, 1990.
46. Nieman DC, Nehlsen-Cannarella SL, Maykoff PA, et al: The effects of moderate exercise training on natural killer cells and acute respiratory tract infections. Int J Sports Med 11:467, 1990.
47. Pate R, Blair SN, Durstine JL, et al: Guideline for Exercise Testing and Prescription, 4th ed. Philadelphia, Lea & Febiger, 1991.
48. Pette D, Vrbova G: Invited review: Neural control of phenotype expression in mammalian muscle fibers. Muscle Nerve 8:676–686, 1985.
49. Robertson G, Meshkinpour H, Vanderberg K, et al: Effects of exercise on total and segmental colon transit. J Clin Gastroenterol 16:300–303, 1993.
50. Rubinstein N, Mabuchi K, Pepe F, et al: Use of specific antimyosins to demonstrate the transformation of individual fibers in chronically stimulated rabbit fast muscles. J Cell Biol 79:252–261, 1978.
51. Salmon S, Hendrikson J: The adaptive response of skeletal muscles to increased use. Muscle Nerve 4:94–105, 1981.
52. Saltin B, Gollnick PD: Skeletal muscle adaptability: Significance for metabolism and performance. In Peachey LD, Adrian RH, Geiger SR (eds): Handbook of Physiology. Section 10: Skeletal Muscle. Bethesda, MD, American Physiological Society, 1983, pp 555–631.
53. Saltin B, Hendrikson J, Nygaard E, et al: Fiber types and metabolic potentials of skeletal muscles in sedentary man and endurance runners. Ann N Y Acad Sci 301–303, 1977.
54. Sandler RS, Pritchard ML, Bangdiwala S: Physical activity and the risk of colorectal adenomas. Epidemiology 6:602–606, 1995.
55. Sesboue B, Arhan P, Devroede G, et al: Colonic transition in soccer players. J Clin Gastroenterol 20:211–214, 1995.
56. Shinkai S, Shore S, Shek PN, Shepard RJ: Acute exercise and immune system. Int J Sports Med 13:452, 1992.
57. Smith JA, Telford RD, Mason IB, Weidermann MJ: Exercise, training and neutrophil microbicidal activity. Int J Sports Med 11:179–187, 1990.
58. Soffer EE, Wilson J, Duethman G, et al: Effect of graded exercise on esophageal mobility and gastroesophageal reflux in nontrained subjects. Dig Dis Sci 39:193–198, 1994.
59. Steptoe A, Cox S: Acute effects of aerobic exercise on mood. Health Psychol 7:329–340, 1988.
60. Thompson LV: Effects of age and training on skeletal muscle physiology and performance. Phys Ther 74:71–81, 1994.
61. Thorstensson A: Muscle strength, fiber types and enzyme activities in man. Acta Physiol Scand (Suppl) 443:1–45, 1976.
62. Blomquist CG: Clinical exercise physiology. In Wenger KN, Hellerstein KH (eds): Rehabilitation of the Coronary Patient, 2nd ed. New York, John Wiley & Sons, 1984, pp 179–196.
63. Whipp BJ, Wasserman K: Exercise: Pulmonary Physiology and Pathophysiology. New York, Marcel Dekker, 1991.
64. Zierath JR, Wallberg, Henrikson H: Exercise training in obese diabetic patients. Special considerations. Sports Med 14:171–189, 1992.

MARC OWEN SHERMAN, MD

3

Foundations of Therapeutic Exercise Classification and Prescription

The benefits of exercise are continuously touted by both the scientific community and the lay press.[86] Yet, exercise presents both benefits and risks. This balance can be easily maneuvered toward the benefit side of the equation with an optimal exercise prescription, which can be reached by conducting a thorough and accurate evaluation of the patient's aerobic, medical, and biomechanical condition. This chapter does not attempt to teach the important cornerstones of diagnosis and assessment. Rather, it describes the various types of exercises that are prescribed. Fundamental basic science principles underlying each type of exercise are essential in understanding the various categories of exercises and how to prescribe them. Simple concepts such as stretching are reviewed as well as the more advanced strengthening program techniques and self-mobilization. Clinical examples are given to illustrate the principles of the types of prescribed exercises.

STRETCHING

Flexibility and motion are critical determinants of the performance of activity. Stretching is one of the most important categories of exercises that can be prescribed to maintain and restore normal balance in each of these parameters. Muscle, fascia, tendon, and ligament all may exhibit a degree of increased tightness that leads to nonoptimal functioning at a given joint secondary to restricting available range of motion.[50] Muscle spasm and scarring can further limit available motion and therefore curtail overall functioning of the musculoskeletal system, hereafter referred to as the "kinetic chain." Simply stated, the correct application of a stretching program improves biomechanical performance. The basic science behind stretching exercise involves an understanding of the properties of tendon, muscle, and connective tissue.[64,65] Each of these have different properties of extensibility. Extensibility describes a resistance to stretch. A given musculotendinous unit, for example, may have varying extensibility between a given muscle and its tendon, and this determines the location of failure should overstretch occur. Resistance to stretch tends to be greater in the tendon than in a muscular zone of similar cross-sectional area. Therefore, when tensile stress is applied to overload, the musculotendinous junction becomes a potential site of failure. This underscores the potential for injury during stretch.[74]

Force, rate, and duration of stretch should be specified in the exercise prescription. All of these factors play a role in determining both effectiveness of the stretch and tendency toward overload and potential injury.[24] An effective stretch achieves a longer tissue length. The stretch-contractile response should be avoided because it could result in reactive shortening of the tissue being stretched, particularly as is applied to muscular stretch. Excessive speed of shortening elicits the contractile response. Therefore, the concept of holding a gentle prolonged stretch should be communicated to the patient clearly.[98] A muscle, for example, is put on length just to the point of the feeling of non-painful tightness and is held at that point. The passively held stretch should be maintained 15–120 seconds.[90] This author has found efficacy in holding stretches for 30–60 seconds in patients without central nervous system injury. Heating prior to stretching has been shown to be effective in promoting muscular lengthening.[66] Studies of length-failure relationships show that a heated muscle fails at a greater length than it would in a nonheated state.[94] Therefore, an optimal stretching program could include the application of superficial heat 10–20 minutes prior to a 30-second gentle prolonged stretch. Some deeper muscle groups, such as the piriformis, may be more affected by deep heating modalities than superficial ones. In general, superficial heating can be taught to patients; self-application could decrease the time and, hence, the cost of physical therapy sessions.

Scar tissue is a type of connective tissue that tends toward shortening if left in the immobile position. Therefore, attention directed toward stretching of scar tissue helps collagen turnover as well as length improvement. This occurs largely through stimulation of collagen breakdown and by staying ahead of the formation of cross-linking by the collagen,[64] which, in the relatively immobile patient, promotes shortening. Overall then, stretching has many benefits, including improving flexibility, relaxing muscles, preventing adhesive scar formation, and decreasing muscle soreness.

Specific examples of stretching techniques highlight general stretching exercises. The actual performance and position of the stretch is important to its success. Muscles should be relaxed during stretching. Thus, the stretching of lumbar extensors, for example, is better done in the prone position than in the standing position. Just as respiratory illnesses produce predictive patterning of presentation, described as "pink puffers" and "blue bloaters," so does the kinetic chain examination show typical patterns of inflexibility. Several authors have explored these patterns in the spine, hip, and pelvis region.[12,38,68] Areas prone to tightness include the hip adductors, hamstring muscles, the tensor fascia lata and iliotibial band (Figs. 1–3), and the hip flexors (rectus femoris and iliopsoas). The latissimus dorsi muscle is important to evaluate for tightness (Fig. 4) due to its long attachments as it arises from lumbar, sacral, and the lower six thoracic vertebrae as well as the iliac crest to insert on the lateral lip of the bicipital grove. Tightness of this muscle has a dramatic effect on spine posture and function. The cervical spine is also a frequent source of muscular tightness on clinical presentation. Long muscles that

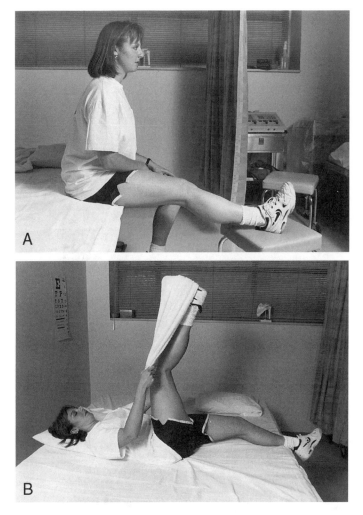

FIGURE 1. *A,* Proximal fiber hamstring stretching. *B,* Distal fiber hamstring stretching.

often benefit from stretching in this area include the levator scapulae, upper trapezius fibers, sternocleidomastoid, and the scalene group (Figs. 5 and 6).

A word of caution should be made regarding the risks of overstretching a given muscle group. Every muscle has its normal desired length for function. Exceeding this length, however, may predispose to injury and increase the energy necessary for a given activity. Muscular activity around a lax joint may be increased just to maintain stability at that joint. An instability should not be created by overstretching. Physician follow-up and observation of the overall exercise program is important in this regard. Routine assessment should prevent exceeding the normal range. For example, consider the hamstring group; in testing hamstring length, a finding of 90° is considered the maximum

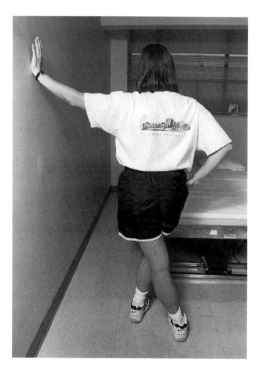

FIGURE 2. Position for initiating iliotibial band stretch on the left side of the body. The patient would lean into the wall from this position to accentuate the stretch.

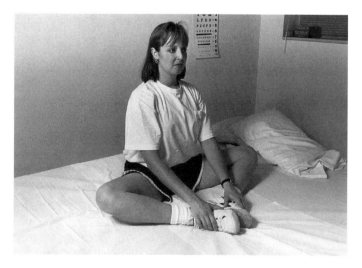

FIGURE 3. Adductor stretch.

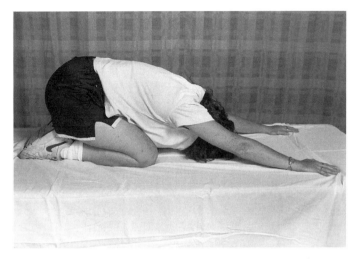

FIGURE 4. A combination self-stretch, including lengthening of the latissimus dorsi muscle.

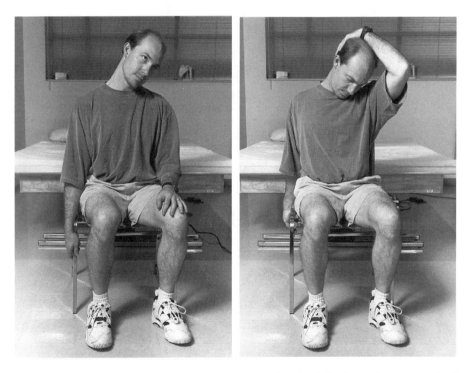

FIGURE 5. Upper trapezius stretch. Notice hand positioning.

FIGURE 6. Stretch for the levator scapulae. Hand position maximizes stretch, both for anchoring on the chair as well as head traction oriented parallel to the muscle fibers to be stretched.

normal range. A greater range is simply too loose. Therefore, at some point in a stretching program, a patient may require encouragement to deemphasize certain stretching routines to avoid overstretch. The overall goal with stretching is not stretching isolated groups to their limit but, rather, to balance flexibility in the kinetic chain in relation to other joints and muscle groups.

One method of achieving muscular lengthening related closely to stretching is referred to as "postisometric relaxation."[79] In this model, there is an assumption that a hypertonic muscle, often seen in combination with spinal segmental motion restrictions, is kept hypertonic by the combined actions of constant alpha motor firing and gamma efferent impulses. This leads to spindle shortening and extrafusal muscle contraction. An isometric contraction has a relaxing effect on some of the spindle fibers, because certain sensory structures are elongated as the overall muscle length does not change. The central mechanism responsible for this is referred to as synaptic fatigue or resetting the gamma gain.[79] In this technique, the patient performs a 3–5 second isometric contraction. The contraction is then released, giving a postisometric relaxation phase lasting at least 1 second. During this phase, the muscle fiber elongates without causing sensory-ending stimulation, thus eliminating the stimulus for maintaining the shortened muscle length.

Let us look at one example involving the use of this principle in improving length of the gluteus maximus. The gluteus maximus, a powerful spine and hip extensor, originates from the sacrum, sacroiliac ligaments, ilium, and the sacrotuberous ligaments. It then inserts on the fascia lata and gluteal tuberosity. Therefore, tightness of this single joint muscle can have effects on the spine, hip, and pelvis simultaneously. To produce postisometric relaxation, the patient is placed in a supine position, and the hip and knee are flexed together with the patient in neutral spine. As the physician or therapist moves the leg into a knee-to-chest position, at some point the feather edge of tightness or resistance to movement is felt. At this point, the flexed leg is held by the physician at the anterior portion of the knee and the patient keeps his leg totally relaxed. The patient is then asked to attempt to extend his hip against the physician's hand, effecting an isometric contraction of the gluteus maximus. At the same time, the physician is providing a balancing counterforce, enabling isometric contraction only. This is held for 5 seconds, and the patient is then asked to relax, with the physician continuing to hold the patient's limb at the anterior knee. After 1 second of relaxation, the patient is moved into a further degree of hip flexion (with the knee still bent) until resistance is felt. This sequence is generally repeated three to five times, ending with the relaxation phase and the physician passively bringing the leg back to its extended position at completion of the exercise. This type of exercise is best used for chronically shortened muscle as opposed to the muscle involved in acute spasm.

RANGE OF MOTION EXERCISE

Range of motion exercise is complementary to stretching techniques[89] and allows the addition of active movement of a given joint through available range when performed nonpassively. There are instances, however, when more passive range of motion with assistance is required. In fact, if motion is acutely painful at the knee (e.g., as seen in active rheumatoid arthritis), complete assistance may be needed. In this case, the physician or therapist provides the energy necessary to move the joint through its available range.

The purpose of prescribing passive range of motion is to avoid increasing loss of range or to maintain current range and to do so in a relatively pain-free manner.[103] Passive range of motion allows complete patient relaxation and is particularly useful when treating the acutely inflamed joint. Active-assistive range of motion allows the patient to actively move a joint through pain-free range with some assistance at the end-range of the joint. It is possible to teach a patient to perform this himself. For example, using a wand held in both hands, the affected shoulder is actively moved into abduction, and the contralateral arm is then allowed to move the wand into further abduction at the ipsilateral injured shoulder to achieve the target range. The prescription of active range of motion allows the patient to perform the activity himself. The joint is put through the full range under the patient's own power. Recommendations include putting all major joints of the body through available range at least twice daily as part of a routine exercise program.

However, there are some activity-specific joint restrictions that impact range of motion exercise, such as occur in baseball pitchers.[71] Knowing the characteristics of a given activity enables the physician to provide and direct the highest function-achieving range of motion prescription. This becomes particularly important as our population ages and maintains a relatively high level of physical activity. Range of motion exercises should be limited or eliminated in cases of unstable fractures, osteoporosis, and deep venous thrombosis. In addition, with regard to spine exercise for range of motion, isolated measurements of range of the lumbar spine do not correlate with a given patient's functional abilities.[52,57] This is largely secondary to the importance of the biomechanical function of the pelvis and its corelationship with the spine in motion, such as in forward bending and other motions.

PROPRIOCEPTION

Proprioception refers to joint position sense, but its function is not limited strictly to the joint. With intact proprioception, the kinetic chain performs in an organized, smooth, and coordinated fashion, with all of the musculoskeletal components communicating to achieve functional activity and balanced posture. It also improves reaction time. The location of all of the components of the nervous system involved with proprioception are not completely understood, but proprioceptive endings have been identified in ligaments, joint capsular structures, and the vestibular system.[8,33,61,73] Pacinian corpuscles and Golgi tendon organs are thought to be able to transmit proprioceptive information and have been located in the outer anular layer of vertebral discs.[10,11,48,77] When the proprioceptive function is impaired, predisposition to further injury occurs.[34,100]

Presumably, injury to this important sensory system leads to a relative incoordination of muscle groups in the related functional area; therefore, the extremity cannot react in a coordinated fashion when confronted by a stress or demand. Exercise for the proprioceptive system involves encouraging control of an extremity based on applied postural and positional challenges of gradually increasing difficulty. Common areas treated by this form of exercise include the knee, ankle, shoulder, and spine. Spine care, for example, may begin in the supported supine position, using pelvic positioning to increase positional awareness, and finally leading to the well-known Swiss ball exercises, a more dynamic challenge to truncal awareness. Knee proprioception also can be trained using an inflated plastic ball, and ankle disc training is frequently used as a method to focus on ankle proprioception. In the latter instance, the patient is progressed from using the ankle disc in sitting to standing, controlling the motion of the disc in various directions. Proprioceptive exercises for the shoulder are receiving increasing amounts of attention, because the shoulder depends a great deal on dynamic, as opposed to static, stability (Fig. 7). The same principles apply with regard to progressive challenge to shoulder stability and positioning, initially using static pressure and progressing to control of shoulder motion when confronted by an unstable surface (Fig. 8).

STRENGTHENING EXERCISE

Strengthening receives a great deal of attention as a form of exercise. Factors involving strength training are numerous and complex and span cellular and macroscopic levels. This section approaches strengthening from both the cellular and muscular levels. Aspects of the scientific basis of strength training are reviewed, and strength training programs and approaches are described.

Strengthening exerts its effects on skeletal muscle, upon which we rely to move the static aspects of the kinetic chain, which is largely a system of bony levers. The muscle

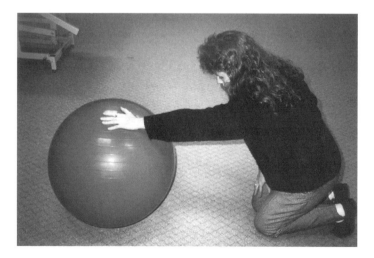

FIGURE 7. Early shoulder proprioceptive retraining. The patient controls the direction of the ball from her shoulder.

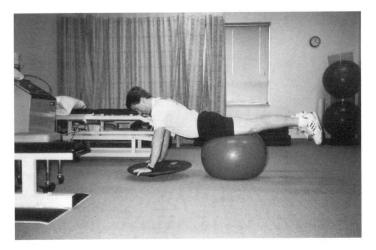

FIGURE 8. Advanced proprioceptive exercise. Challenges are presented to the shoulder and trunk as the patient controls joint motion while moving the wobble board in different controlled directions. The difficulty of the exercise can be modified by moving the ball distally or proximally.

can be trained in contraction, relaxation, and stretch, showing itself to be quite adaptable. Remember as well that structure is closely related to function, and skeletal muscle exists in a variety of shapes that help us to understand their function.[35] For instance, muscle can have one, two, or three heads. Individual fibers within a given muscle may be oriented in different patterns, described as parallel, convergent, or pinnate. The muscles that are organized in parallel are often long, and the term "parallel" defines the muscle in relation to its line of action. An example is the tensor fascia lata muscle. Convergent muscle types take origin from a wide surface area only to attach to a more focused site. Consider the pectoralis major with its multifaceted origin but common insertion on the lateral lip of the bicipital grove of the humerus. "Pinnate" refers to muscle orientation in which the fibers of the same muscle lie at varying angles to the overall line of pull of the muscle. Therefore, as the muscle contracts, a changing rotation in relation to the line of pull occurs. These factors all have impact for how strengthening may be carried out for a given muscle.

Muscular contraction during strengthening exercise involves cellular events: muscles are composed of fibers that in turn are composed of myofibrils that are themselves made up of sarcomeres, the basic contractile unit.[53] The functional contractile proteins, actin and myosin, are arranged as seen in Figure 9. Actin attaches to the outer margin of the unit, and myosin is associated with a midline structure called the "M" line. There is overlap between actin and myosin, and the variance of the percentage of this overlap is directly related to the force generation produced in a given muscle.[83,95] Macroscopically, this can be thought of as the muscle length-tension concept. The actin and myosin are associated with cross-bridges, and this association increases or decreases depending on the degree of overlap attained during a muscle shortening or lengthening contraction.[5,25,46] The events surrounding muscular contraction have been well de-

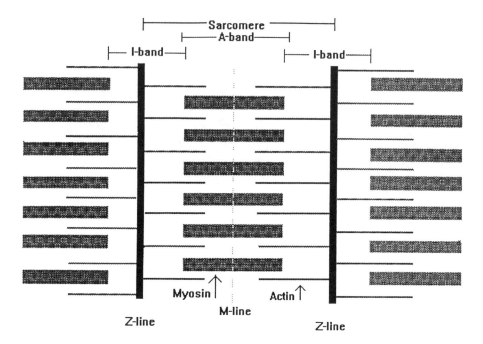

FIGURE 9. Schematic representation of the sarcomere in striated muscle.

fined.[2,62,67] A T-tubular system, the sarcoplasmic reticulum, is positioned longitudinally in association with the myofibril. Neural initiation enables release of calcium, which promotes an interaction with the troponin-C complex, inducing a change in shape of this molecule. This conformational change exposes the actin binding sites, and as myosin binds, overlap increases and the contractile unit shortens. Finally, when considering the musculotendinous unit as a whole, one must remember that viscoelastic properties allow potential energy storage that can add to the contractile force total. This has implications for the types of muscular contractions prescribed in strength training, particularly as it applies to plyometric strengthening.[9]

When strength training occurs, muscle is adapting and changing. An understanding of the determinants of strength are prerequisite to prescribing the form of training. Cross-sectional area of a muscle is the first determinant of strength. This area is directly related to the ability to generate contractile force.[31] Increases in muscle fiber size imply increases in muscle force.[87] Recalling that muscle contractile force depends on actin and myosin quantity and crossover bridging, the discussion of cross-sectional area merely is a reflection of cellular events. Through training stimulus, contractile proteins are upregulated, leading to increases in muscle size.[43,102] This muscle response to strength training is called *hypertrophy*. The idea of hyperplasia (increase in muscle fiber number as opposed to increase in size) as a source of increased cross-sectional area as well as fiber splitting both have some scientific support, but the overwhelming evidence points to hypertrophy as the major response to strength training as it applies to increases in cross-sectional area.[39,42,81,99]

Muscular activation is an additional determinant of strength. Force is proportional to the number of motor units firing and the rate of that firing. Neural factors are clearly related to force production, and a training effect may occur as one habituates to a specific exercise series.[28,75]

Muscle length also determines strength. As movement occurs, joint angle and muscle length change. This interdependent relationship between joint and muscle causes variance between muscle groups and shapes as to their optimal length relationship. However, there is a muscle-specific optimal length for a given sarcomere, which allows for maximum actin-myosin cross-bridging. Therefore, one can conclude that force generation is dependent on position and length. It follows that overall muscle length can be changed by adding or subtracting sarcomeres, and this has relevance as seen in immobilized muscles, as sarcomere dropout occurs. Training position should take muscle length into account because muscle will adopt the appropriate number of sarcomeres to provide maximal contraction at the trained length. The optimal muscle length for force production is usually at or just above a muscle's resting length.

Muscle fiber type also plays a role in strength determination. These varying muscle fiber types are differentiated by their contractile and metabolic properties. Type I fibers are described as slow twitch, smaller, and responsible for low-intensity work.[7] An example is the tonic postural musculature. Type II fibers are fast twitch, characterized by rapid calcium release, and can generate more force, even when lifting the same isometric weight.[37] These fibers are found in phasic muscles used in short burst activity such as sprinting, and they generate larger amounts of tension than the type I fibers in less time. Type II fibers are divided into subtypes A, B, and C. Type IIB are classically described above. Type IIA fibers have intermediate properties between types I and II. Type IIC is used to describe undifferentiated muscle fibers. Therefore, specific types of training exercises will predispose use of one type of muscle fiber versus another. Interconvertability of muscle fiber types is controversial, but evidence does exist to support the concept.[1,44,54] Study of athletes reveals characteristic fiber type predominance based on an athlete's given sport.[92] For example, marathon runners tend to have type I fiber predominance in their gastrocnemius-soleus complex.

Speed of shortening and training is the last factor to be considered. Strength is defined as force over velocity; training effects are velocity-specific.[18,55,80] Faster contraction gives less time for cross-bridging to occur, and therefore decreased force generation is seen at faster velocities in concentric contractions. In general, the greatest force generation occurs at the slowest speeds of movement. The exception is consideration of eccentric lengthening contractions, in which greater force is produced at faster velocities.[5,46]

TYPES OF MUSCULAR CONTRACTIONS

The clinician has the option of prescribing different types of muscle contractions as part of the exercise program. This specification is important in achieving goals and avoiding injury. In thinking about the various categories of muscular contractions, one must consider what happens to the muscle length as work is being done against external resistance (Table 1).

For example, a concentric muscular contraction occurs when the force generated by a given muscle overcomes the applied external resistance. When performing elbow flexion with a handheld weight, the brachioradialis muscle shortens as the elbow flexes. This exercise begins in the anatomically neutral position, and the muscle is said to have contracted concentrically as the shortening occurs.

An eccentric contraction is seen when the external resistance exceeds the muscular contractile force. The muscle lengthens as tension is generated. Consider the performance of a prone hamstring curl: as the weight is brought closer to the trunk, the hamstrings shorten concentrically, but as the weight is slowly returned to its starting position, the hamstring musculature lengthens. Eccentric contractions also occur frequently with shock absorption, such as landing from a jump. Eccentric contractions produce greater force than their isometric and concentric counterparts and therefore are commonly used in strengthening programs. Because of increased overload potential, the development of delayed-onset muscle soreness is more likely with this form of training.

It is possible for work to be done as tension is developed without change in muscle length; this is called an isometric contraction. Resistance is not overcome, and a given body segment is not moved, such as occurs when a person pulls an object that does not move. Clinically, isometric contractions are useful in the acutely inflamed joint, as seen in rheumatoid arthritis. Repetitive resistive joint motion may worsen joint inflammation.[27,96,97] Such flare-ups can be avoided by the use of brief maximal isometric exercise.[69] Although implications for functional muscle use remain unclear, the improvement in static strength is probably helpful in maintaining tone and preparing the patient for more functional strengthening and activity when the disease process allows.

Isokinetic muscle contraction implies tension development at the same velocity throughout a given range. Notoriety regarding this type of contraction derives from exercise testing equipment that measures torque values as a joint applies force against a lever arm controlled to move at a single angular velocity (Fig. 10). This generates graphical data that are statistically interesting but of questionable functional value, given that isokinetic muscular contraction almost never occurs outside specific artificial testing conditions.[56]

TABLE 1. Classification of Muscle Contractions

Type of Contraction	Effect on Muscle Length
Isometric	Tension without muscle length change
Isodynamic	Tension with similar resistance throughout range
Isokinetic	Tension with same velocity throughout range
Concentric	Tension with muscle shortening
Eccentric	Tension with muscle lengthening
Plyometric	Tension with lengthening prior to shortening

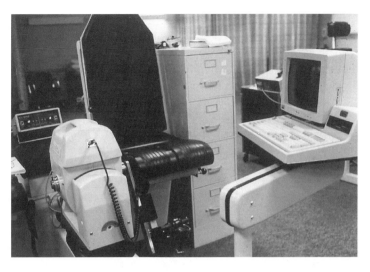

FIGURE 10. Typical isokinetic testing equipment.

Isodynamic exercise occurs when tension is generated in a given muscle through-out a given range of motion. Eccentric and concentric strengthening could be considered forms of isodynamic exercise. In reality, tension does not likely remain identical throughout all angles in a given joint motion. Isotonic exercise is a related term that literally refers to identical tension exercise. Since this is not likely to occur, the term "isodynamic" is probably more accurate.

Another specific muscle action is a plyometric contraction. Recall that a muscle and its tendon contain a certain amount of viscoelastic energy-storing properties. By applying a prestretch to the muscle, energy can be stored in these elastic elements and then released. Specifically, an eccentric lengthening preload allows more energy to be released during the immediately following concentric contraction, leading to greater force generation by a given muscle. Muscle recruitment also may be enhanced. One popular type of plyometric exercise is known as jump training. On landing from a jump, eccentric lengthening of the Achilles mechanism occurs; during completion of the jump, the calf group shortens in the concentric phase. Because this type of exercise may predispose to injury, adequate strength, achieved through less stressful exercise, and adequate muscle length must be present before this type of strengthening is prescribed. In addition, apophyseal injury may occur, particularly in children and adolescents.

OPEN AND CLOSED KINETIC CHAIN STRENGTHENING

Advances have been made in the understanding of the human body as working in a "kinetic chain" model. From a purely biomechanical standpoint, this means that bones, joints, muscles, and ligaments work together in functional movement and that motion at one link of the chain affects other links.[70] During gait, knee, ankle, and hip motion are intimately related. The obvious corollary is that dysfunction at one area of the chain places potentially greater stress, motion requirements, or strength production at another link in the chain. Therefore, the terms "closed" and "open" kinetic chain strengthening are frequently used, and an understanding of these terms is key in the description of these types of exercises.

"Kinetic chain" was originally an engineering term described in 1875 by Realoux as two metallic rods linked together by a pin joint in which movement at one rod obligated movement at the other.[43a] Steindler refined the definition, describing two types of contractions based on their differing limb loading characteristics.[92a] In the closed kinetic chain (CKC) model, the foot or hand meets a considerable, usually fixed resistance, giving recruitment and joint motion patterns distinctly different than the condition in which little or no resistance is met. These patterns generally occur in a predictable pattern. Examples include a pull-up or rising from a squat. In the open kinetic chain (OKC) system, the peripheral joint of an extremity can move freely. Examples include hand waving or foot movement during the swing phase of the gait cycle.

The development of the understanding of the closed kinetic chain exercise takes origin in the injury and reconstruction of the anterior cruciate ligament (ACL). This literature begins with clinical observation and can be traced sequentially through detailed experimental conditions.[16,26,84] It is shown that CKC exercise at the knee in the form of squats and leg presses results in decreased patellofemoral joint reaction forces and decreased stress on the ACL and ACL graft relative to OKC isolated knee extension exercise.[70] Essentially in closed kinetic chain exercise, the coactivation of the hamstring and quadriceps together produces the beneficial effects (Fig. 11).[91] Inclusion of the gastrocnemius-soleus complex may also give benefit. Randomized studies now support their clinical efficacy.[104] Table 2 compares open and closed kinetic exercise.

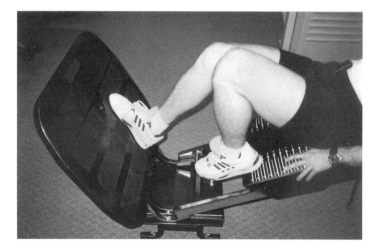

FIGURE 11. Closed kinetic chain exercise: single leg on leg press machine.

TABLE 2. Comparison of Open Kinetic Chain and Closed Kinetic Chain Exercises

	Open Kinetic Chain Exercises			Closed Kinetic Chain Exercises		
	Characteristics	Advantages	Disadvantages	Characteristics	Advantages	Disadvantages
	Single muscle group	Isolated recruitment	Limited function	Multiple muscle groups	Functional recruitment	Difficult to isolate
	Single axis and plane	Simple movement	Less proprioception and joint stability with increased joint shear forces	Multiple axes and planes	Functional movement patterns	Compressive forces at articular surface
	Emphasize concentric contraction	Minimal joint compression		Balance of concentric and eccentric contractions	Functional contractions	
	Nonweightbearing			Weightbearing exercise	Increase proprioception and joint stability	

In considering closed kinetic chain exercise for the shoulder, several facts are important. The shoulder relies on dynamic stability for optimal function. Position and motion of the scapula is important in shoulder rehabilitation. CKC exercises should be used in shoulder rehabilitation because the shoulder transfers forces from the trunk and coactivation of shoulder muscle groups enhances dynamic stability.[58] In addition, the use of CKC exercise promotes scapular stability and places less tensile stress on ligaments and tendons. There is also enhanced proprioception during the exercise. CKC exercise at the shoulder includes placing the hand against a wall and contracting against resistance in different directions. Progressive degrees of difficulty can be introduced (Fig. 12) as the surface changes from a wall, to a small gymball between the hand and a wall, to the use of a wobble board to challenge stability at both the shoulder and the trunk. The aquatic environment serves as an intermediary situation between pure open and closed kinetic chain exercise, as is discussed in the section on aquatic exercise.

PROGRAMS FOR STRENGTH TRAINING

This section describes general principles of strength training programs and uses several illustrative examples. Gains experienced during strength training have multiple origins. The term "training effect" refers to gains made of neural origin in which patterns and efficiency of motor recruitment improve to allow functional strength gains.

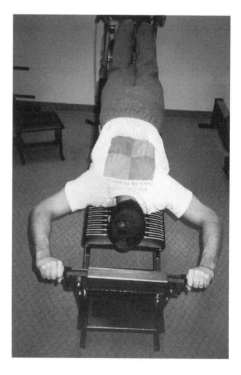

FIGURE 12. Closed kinetic chain exercise for the shoulder on an inclined sliding track system.

At the cellular level, myofibrillar cross-sectional area and size increase. The number of actual myofibrils also may increase. In general, training programs tend to be based on the overload principle, which holds that the exercise program needs to exceed the demands of daily activity in general and cause fatigue of muscle tissue in specific. Greater overload may give greater gains, although the risk of injury is evident. One should also remember the SAID principle: "specific adaptation to imposed demand." The SAID principle implies that a given muscle adapts to its exercise, in this case strengthening, but that the adaptation is exercise-specific to a certain degree and not directly applicable to demands not related to the exercise mode and pattern. There is no one single best method of strength training.

The DeLorme method of strengthening is a heavy resistance technique that uses sets of repetitions moving heavy weight through a full range of motion.[20–22] The amount of weight used is based on the concept of the ten-repetition maximum: the maximum weight that can be lifted through full range of motion ten times. The classic DeLorme method calls for four days of training followed by a rest day. More recently, every-other-day recommendations have been promoted. Competitive bodybuilders may work out six days a week. The number of sets in a given workout session typically is three, with 50%, 75% and finally 100% of the ten-repetition maximum weight used for a total of three sets of ten repetitions of gradually increasing demand. The first two sets are often referred to as "warm-up sets."

The Oxford method is related to the DeLorme method, but the order is reversed so that maximum resistance is worked against first, with gradual decreases to 50% of the ten-repetition maximum weight used on the third set. Earl Elkins in 1946 showed no difference between the two programs in 12 subjects. Both tend to cause muscular work by the overload principle on a regular basis, and this is probably the most important fact. The daily adjustable progressive resistive exercise technique (DAPRE) allows adjusting working weights to keep the trainee working at his capacity even within a single workout. This program includes four exercise sessions, and the number of repetitions in the third set determines the working weight in the fourth set, according to standard guidelines. If ten repetitions were the maximum number in the third set, the weight is increased by 5–10 pounds for the fourth set. If only two repetitions were accomplished in the third set, the fourth set is decreased by 5–10 pounds.[60]

Other techniques involve combining types of strengthening exercises such as isometric and isodynamic contractions. Moreover, weighted vests for running and balls for throwing give an overload condition during performance of the desired activity; however, the benefit of this type of functional overload has not been demonstrated conclusively (Fig. 13).

Circuit training involves the use of 6–15 stations. Each station enables a different group of muscles to be strengthened than the previous station; no group is directly challenged on consecutive stations.

Periodization strength training is a potentially important form of exercise programming. It is a global training plan that has variability in the form of training at regularly spaced periods of time. Benefits include peaking at a certain time, perhaps associated with a specific sporting event, as well as gains in muscle strength, endurance,

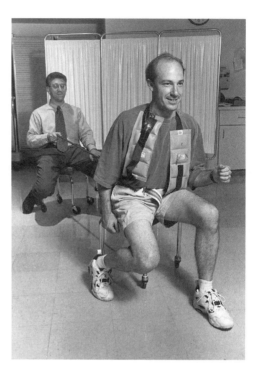

FIGURE 13. Functional overload. The patient works against added resistance while performing a functional activity.

and power. The changes in exercise intensity, frequency, and mode may avoid boredom and, if planned properly, could prevent injury and also prevent the recreational athlete from becoming stale. Periodization training has been directly compared to DeLorme-type strength training programs in several studies, and results over a period of months show statistically significant benefit.[93] The overload principle, as previously discussed, is fundamental to periodization strength training. Muscle hypertrophy is promoted by regular use of resistance, set to at least 60% of the one repetition maximum. However, central to the periodization schedule is planned relative rest to allow a phase where strength improvements can occur. Heavy workouts are followed by immediate fatigue and therefore weakness. The use of relative rest allows positive strength gains in the form of muscular adaptations to occur.

The variety in the periodization program can include light, moderate, and heavy workout days during a given week, or heavy versus light weeks over a given month. Although the periodization programs are individually designed, heavy training periods often are followed by short periods of detraining. The variability in the program occurs with focus on number of repetitions per given set, the weight in a given set, and the number of sets themselves. The exact regions of the body that are exercised and the order of the performed exercises are also modulated. Rest periods between sets in a given workout as well as between training sessions also are varied. In general, three to six sets are used in a given muscle group workout, and the body regions worked on vary by day. The specifics of the program vary based on the goals of training, but often training occurs 4–6 days per week.

Day 1 may include exercise sets for the calves and thighs, while day 2 focuses on spine extensors and abdominal muscles, with day 5 for rest. Seven-day cycles also are used. This is done against a backdrop of seasonal planning, often to match athletic seasons.

Thus, various phases, identified as preparation, first transition, competition, and second transition, each are composed of differing levels of strengthening intensity, in which the volume, speed, and resistance in a given workout are modulated to give an overall cycle, termed a macrocycle, or year of training. The preparation (hypertrophy) phase uses a high-repetition, low-intensity workout, and the first transition phase (strength) moves into higher resistance training with lower volume. The competition phase shows peak intensity with minimal volume of strengthening exercise. Finally, the second transition or off-season (recovery) is a period of relative rest, in which some differing form of lower intensity exercise is performed. Tables 3–6 show sample periodization training schedules. For further study regarding periodization, the reader is referred to Fleck and Kraemer.[30]

AQUATIC EXERCISE

The use of water as an exercise medium is not a new idea. However, with a growing understanding of the exercise response in both aerobic and kinetic chain terms, the use of aquatic exercise is growing rapidly. As our aging population works to maintain activity

TABLE 3. Sample Weekly Training Schedule

	Intensity	Volume	Muscle Group
Monday	High	Low	Legs, calves, thighs
Tuesday	—	—	—
Wednesday	Medium	Medium	Arms, shoulder, abdominals
Thursday	—	—	—
Friday	Low	High	Back, chest
Saturday	—	—	—
Sunday	—	—	—

TABLE 4. Sample Daily Workout Log

Exercise Type	3 Sets of. . .	Results
Bench press	10 reps at 150 lbs.	3 x 10, 10, 10
Hamstring curl	10 reps at 40 lbs.	3 x 10, 9, 7
Biceps curl	8 reps at 40 lbs.	3 x 8, 6, 4
Triceps extension	8 reps at 30 lbs.	3 x 8, 8, 8
Lateral pull-downs	8 reps at 110 lbs.	3 x 8, 8, 7

Results could be used to raise or lower weights at the next training session.

TABLE 5. Characteristics to Consider When Planning Multiple Weeks in a Given Phase of Training

Volume/Intensity
Number of sessions per week
Number and type of exercises
Number of sets and repetitions
Length of rest period between sets
Total number of weeks in a phase

TABLE 6. Typical General Schedule for 1 Year of Periodization for a Competitive Team Sport Played in January and February

Month	Training Goal	Volume/Intensity
January	Competitive season	Low/Moderate
February	Hypertrophy	High/Low
March	Strength	Moderate/Moderate
April	Hypertrophy	High/Low
May	Hypertrophy	High/Low
June	Strength	Moderate/Moderate
July	Power	Low/Moderate
August	Recovery	Low/Low
September	Hypertrophy	High/Moderate
October	Strength	Moderate/High
November	Power	Low/High
December	Competitive season	Low/Moderate

---

and fitness, the use of a therapeutic pool will continue to grow by sheer numbers. This section serves several purposes. To promote a complete understanding, we discuss the principles of water as well as how being in water affects the body's systems and the response to exercise in water. Before discussing specific exercise programs, contraindications to the use of pool therapy are reviewed. Readers should develop an understanding of the breadth of patient populations that can benefit from aquatic exercise.

PRINCIPLES OF WATER

The idea of buoyancy is critical to understanding aquatic exercise. Buoyancy is defined as an upward force acting opposite to the force of gravity, related to the volume of water displaced by the human body.[23] Recalling that density equals mass over volume, as we inhale air, our density decreases, and we tend to float more. Exhalation is accompanied by a relative sinking in the water. We are able to float because, in most instances, human density is less than one, and the density of water is one.

Arms tend to be less dense than legs, which presents the opportunity to use various devices to help float a patient. Buoyancy can be used in a progressive water-based strengthening program. Consider hip abduction. In a side-lying position, if the uppermost leg starts from a lower position in the water and is moved toward the surface, this abduction motion is "buoyancy assisted." If, however, the patient is again in side-lying and the inferior leg is abducted to a greater depth of water, the exercise is "buoyancy resisted." In general, buoyancy can help unload joints by decreasing the joint reactive force. Less muscular activation is needed to support a given limb, whether upper or lower, and therefore movement is made easier. This has significant implications for several classes of patients, including patients with osteoarthritis of the hip or patients with a post-humeral fracture. Any patient with a sensitivity to weightbearing may benefit from the principle of buoyancy, with the possible exception of patients with joint instability.

When immersed, hydrostatic pressure affects the human body.[29] Essentially, water has a certain property of incompressibility and therefore has the ability to exert a force on the surface area of an immersed body. This pressure tends to increase with increasing depth and can be calculated. This has clinical relevance: the calculated pressure reaches a value similar to that of typical diastolic pressures in the human body, helping with resolution of edema in a body part. However, it also leads to a tendency toward diuresis as well as requiring greater effort from muscles of respiration, such as the intercostals, as water resists chest expansion.

Viscosity refers to the friction between molecules as a body moves through it. Because water is more viscous than air, its resistance to movement of the body is greater than that of land-based exercises.[78] A greater velocity in the water gives a greater resistance, and this principle affects varying degrees of gradation of an aquatic therapy prescription.

EFFECTS OF WATER ON SYSTEMS OF THE BODY

The circulatory system is affected when a body is in water largely because hydrostatic pressure exceeds venous pressure and tends to increase venous return to the heart. This represents a fluid shift from the extremities more centrally. The end-diastolic volume increases, and mean stroke volume has been shown to increase up to 35% with neck level immersion.[4] Effects on cardiac filling and stroke volume have implications for cardiac conditioning.[88] Benefits have been shown in patients with infarct and myopathy.[76] From a pulmonary standpoint, water increases the work of breathing. With regard to the musculoskeletal system, immersion decreases the need for peripheral vasoconstriction and can improve muscular blood flow and metabolic waste removal. Renal blood flow improves with immersion and therefore affects the levels of antidiuretic hormone, renin, and aldosterone.[29] The significance for the medicated cardiac patient is obvious. Also, water can serve as a useful method of heat transfer to the immersed body. The temperature of the water can be adjusted in many therapeutic pools and can serve as a heat sink or a heat source, essentially delivering a heating or cold modality to the body, helping to achieve desired therapeutic effects.

CONTRAINDICATIONS

Caution should be urged in certain patient populations. Not everyone is an appropriate candidate for aquatic rehabilitation or exercise. For example, placing patients with cardiac failure in water would increase the stress on the central circulatory system. Patients who are using catheters or who have infectious conditions such as open wounds, urinary tract infections, draining herpetic lesions, and known incontinence are not appropriate candidates for aquatic rehabilitation. Other conditions that also raise concern and should be closely scrutinized as to the appropriateness of aquatic exercise include epilepsy, multiple sclerosis, severe deconditioning, and unstable blood pressure.[82]

GENERAL CLINICAL USES OF AQUATIC REHABILITATION

Common problems that occur in outpatients with musculoskeletal conditions include pain, increased muscle tone and spasm, decreased joint range of motion, and muscular inflexibility. Decreased strength and stability also occur. Patients with abnormal movement patterns such as poor posture, body mechanics, and gait deviations can be aided. Pain relief is effected by unweighting of the joints and relaxation. As muscle spasm decreases, range of motion and flexibility improves. The aquatic environment is ideal for improving trunk stability and extremity strength, particularly for persons needing the assistance of buoyancy to achieve correct physiologic muscular coordination and appropriate prefunctional spine extremity postures. This can be thought of as facilitating normal movement patterns by enabling improvements in coordination, alignment, and body mechanics. Improvements also can occur in circulation, endurance, and even motivation.

Aquatic rehabilitation for spine-based pain has received a great deal of attention. For many of the aforementioned reasons, water offers an excellent environment for promoting therapeutic exercise in patients with back pain. These programs can be used in conjunction with well-known land-based lumbar stabilization programs.[17] Treatment plans are individualized based on a complete structural and anatomic diagnosis, but several general comments can be made. Flexibility, strength, and aerobic conditioning all can be achieved in water. The importance of muscular dynamic stabilization has been studied in detail.[63] By optimizing spine stabilizer musculature, potential for injury to a given motion segment is reduced, and injured motion segments can heal and undergo less stress, perhaps decreasing the rate of progress of the degenerative cascade described by Kirkaldy-Willis.[59] This cascade describes a predictable sequence of spine segment injury changes caused by static structure overload. The static structures referred to include the intervertebral disc, its two related vertebral bodies, and the posterior segmental elements such as the zygapophyseal joints. The overall goal of the aquatic program is to achieve motion segment stabilization dynamically, therefore improving lumbar motion control and decreasing potentially harmful shearing forces across the motion segment. In addition, when working on the entire trunk, the entire spinal axis, including transition zones between the cervical, thoracic, and lumbar zones, can likewise improve.

The techniques used in spine stabilization have been well described.[17] Essentially, we want to build a program of progressive difficulty. This is often done through a core group of six exercises, including tasks such as walking forward and backward and wall-sitting. While these exercises may seem easy, the maintenance of a neutral spine and variance in length of the exercise as well as the resistance that is used offer the ability to change the grade of difficulty. Walking forward challenges the abdominals, and walking backward conditions the spinal extensors. Wall-sitting trains the quadriceps, hamstrings, and abdominals. These three exercises serve as basic examples, and others parallel varying positions used in land-based stabilization programs.

Other ideas for trunk stabilization include having the patient float supine while the therapist applies resistance to trunk spinning motion. The patient could also float prone while wearing a snorkel and actively move the upper and lower extremities in set sequences while maintaining neutral spine and trunk posture. The Bad Ragaz ring method, originally described in the 1930s, has found use in rehabilitation for neurologic disorders but also may have applicability to the spine patient.[14] The therapist is in the water with the patient. Via hand placements and positioning relative to the patient, the therapist serves as a point of stability, guiding the patient through specific motion sequences that serve to increase range of motion and strength. While classically used to facilitate extremity movement patterns, similar techniques can be used to foster trunk strengthening and coordination, such as by moving the patient's trunk through the water and asking the patient to tighten and coordinate trunk muscle in order to maintain posture and respond to therapist-produced directional changes.

The benefits of using a water environment for rehabilitation of shoulder disorders is worthy of greater appreciation. Goals for shoulder rehabilitation include elimination of pain, full range of motion at the glenohumeral joint, complete tissue healing, strength balance, and good flexibility. Performing range of motion exercises for the shoulder in the water requires less muscular effort and energy and will decrease glenohumeral joint reaction forces during exercise, helping the patient reach his or her goals. Normal movement patterns become easier to restore, and rehabilitation simply proceeds more quickly. Thus, dynamic joint stability and coactivation can be promoted with reduced stress and increased proprioceptive emphasis. Simple range can be prescribed, and pool wall-resisted contraction can be promoted. Pectoralis stretching can occur, and activity-specific motions can be re-created throughout the program, leading to functional and finally land-based activities.

Aqua running can be prescribed to improve and maintain aerobic fitness depending on the needs of the individual. This may be useful in athletes with musculoskeletal injury or in those simply desiring to decrease the impact of a workout. Essentially the running or jogging motion is re-created in deep water. Flotation belts can be used, and the mouth is kept above water. Arm and leg motions are similar to running and jogging, with the exception that hip flexion angles may reach up to 80°, exceeding usual running values. The neutral spine is maintained, therefore reinforcing the importance of spine stabilization. Quantities of individual effort and exercise intensity can be graded using the Borg scale (see Fig. 4 in chapter 4) or the more recent Brennan scale developed by Brennan and Wilder specifically for aqua running.[15] The Brennan scale numbers from one to five, with level 1 being equivalent to a light jog and level 5 to a 100-meter sprint. Heart rates can be monitored in the water, and achievement of 55–90% maximum heart rate is recommended for exercise training. The overall workout program can be segmented into different levels of exertion in a given workout. This means that one can swim with maximum intensity during one part of the workout and have intermittent rest periods, in effect creating a periodization scheme within a given workout.[101]

A word should be mentioned regarding closed versus open kinetic chain exercise as it relates to the aquatic environment. Both can be prescribed in water, and a medium also can be seen. If the foot is on the bottom of the pool, a closed system exists although the lower limb may weigh less than on land because of buoyancy. Therefore, coactivation and reduced joint reaction forces occur and normal recruitment can be established in an isolated way before increasing the level of difficulty. On the other hand, and arm can be lifted out of the water and worked in an OKC fashion, with the trunk benefiting from water support. With an immersed limb not on the pool floor, however, an in-between state occurs where some terminal resistance is present; this can vary but is not fixed. Thus, the closed chain can be approximated using paddles or other devices that would, in effect, increase resistance to motion, and an intermediate state can be used.

AEROBIC EXERCISE

"Every US adult should accumulate 30 minutes or more of moderate-intensity physical activity, on most, and preferably all, days of the week."[85] This type of advice is frequently seen in journal articles and texts, but how should aerobic activity be prescribed? This section defines aerobic terminology, the affected bodily systems, and discusses the assessment, planning, and execution of the aerobic exercise prescription.

In prescribing aerobic activity, the health care practitioner must have some knowledge base in exercise physiology (Table 7). The maximal oxygen uptake ($VO_{2\,max}$) is an important term in defining aerobic capacity in a given individual. Essentially, as work activity increases, the demand at the cellular level for energy production also increases. This is dependent on oxygen uptake. At the $VO_{2\,max}$, oxygen uptake cannot keep pace with demand, and a component of anaerobic metabolism ensues.[72] Improvement in aerobic capacity and conditioning is synonymous with improvement in $VO_{2\,max}$. Heart rate and $VO_{2\,max}$ are related in a linear fashion, therefore allowing measurement of heart rate during exercise to serve as a reflection of a given individual's $VO_{2\,max}$, or aerobic fitness. From a more general standpoint, one must understand that the two major systems used in aerobic activity include the central circulatory/pulmonary system and also the specific muscular aerobic capacity system. Positive adaptations to aerobic exercise are many and include mild increase in left ventricular capacity and heart wall size; increased plasma volume, allowing improvement in thermoregulatory dynamics and exercise oxygen delivery; decreased resting and exercise heart rates, improved stroke volume, cardiac output, and muscular oxygen extraction; decreases in both systolic and diastolic pressures; and improved pulmonary function.[49,51]

To evaluate the aerobic level of fitness of a patient, a simple step test can be used. The person steps up and down off a stair or block for 3 minutes. This is often done to the beat of a metronome, at about 96 beats a minute, with a total single cycle consisting of four metronome beats (left up, right up, left down, right down). At the end of 3 minutes, the pulse is recorded. Table 8 shows separate conditions for varying levels of fitness. For the less fit individual, perhaps a sedentary person, the step test workload represents a greater stress on the cardiovascular system relative to the trained individual. In addition, a recovery heart rate taken after 1 minute of exercise can be recorded. The unfit individual often will not return to baseline pulse as quickly as the fit individual. The baseline data are helpful in a general classification of aerobic levels of fitness and also serve as an easy gauge that can be checked at monthly intervals as a monitor of aerobic fitness progress.

The actual prescription of aerobic exercise necessitates specification of frequency, intensity, duration, and mode. Remember that aerobic exercise is trying to take advantage of the flexibility of the body's aerobic system to adapt to an imposed demand. A minimum frequency is necessary to create that stimulus for change. The frequency minimum for the average individual is approximately three times per week. However, there is variability. An unfit individual may make gains at a lesser frequency of exercise while a highly trained individual may require more frequent training sessions to achieve gains. The body generally requires 6 weeks of aerobic training at the minimum frequency to achieve significant gains, and studies in this area should therefore progress for at least 6 weeks.

Duration defines the length of a given training session. The specific optimal length of time per training session varies among people and even in the same person depending on his or her level of fitness. In general, benefit can be achieved with 20–30 minutes per day. In unfit individuals, preserving the total amount of time but breaking it into smaller blocks of time is still helpful, particularly when one first initiates training. Eventually, however, longer training sessions may be necessary to continue to

---

TABLE 7. Key Facts about Aerobic Conditioning

Aerobic capacity is classified based on age
Maximum VO$_2$ can improve with aerobic training
Percent of maximum heart rate and percent maximum VO$_2$ are directly related
After aerobic training, a significant reduction in exercise heart rate occurs

---

TABLE 8. Heart Rates Associated with Step Test Exercise in Three Levels of Fitness

	Superior Fitness	Average Fitness	Poor Fitness
Initial Heart Rate	60	70	80
3-Minute Heart Rate	120	145	170
Recovery Heart Rate (one minute after exercise)	65	80	95

achieve gains in aerobic fitness. Duration often depends on the next factor of training—intensity.

Intensity may be the single most important determinant to the stress and therefore the effect of aerobic exercise. Intensity is defined in several concrete parameters, including heart rate or percentage of maximum age-related heart rate, percent $VO_{2\,max}$, calories expended per unit time, or even in terms of factors of the metabolic resting rate, called METs, or metabolic equivalents. This last manner of measuring exercise intensity has particular impact on the postmyocardial infarction patient, as the various stages of cardiac rehabilitation are targeted and restricted at certain METs, both for goal setting as well as protection.[32] A common method of setting the exercise intensity for a patient is the maximum heart rate method. Although there are many methods for calculating a target heart rate, the maximum rate is generally described as 220 − age.[3] The target heart range for aerobic exercise is 70–90% of this calculated maximum heart rate. Therefore, in a 40-year-old with a maximum rate of 180 beats per minute, the target range for training would be 126–162 beats per minute. These values can be used for both men and women. The other important method of intensity monitoring is the use of the Borg RPE (rate of perceived exertion) scale (see Fig. 4 in chapter 4).[13] This scale gives a visual and verbal description of effort. A rating of 13–14 is equivalent to the heart rate threshold value, and the RPE scale also correlates with $VO_{2\,max}$. This type of monitoring becomes particularly important in the diabetic population, where monitoring of heart rate may be less reliable given potential autonomic dysfunction.

The mode portion of the exercise prescription tells exactly how the exercise will be performed. Swimming, jogging, an exercise bike, and rowing machines are a small sampling of available modes. Certain patients, however, may be more suited to one mode over another. For instance, a patient with spinal stenosis may need to avoid exercise in a prolonged extended position, and therefore a bicycle would be preferable to jogging or using a ski machine. A patient with knee osteoarthritis is generally more suited to aquatic aerobics, because the relative unweighting of the knee allows more exercise to occur with less pain and cartilaginous loading. A patient with bilateral lower extremity amputations may be better served by incorporating upper extremity exercise.[19]

The use of upper extremity exercise and swimming are topics unto themselves with regard to aerobic conditioning. In general, the maximum heart rate is lowered by a value of 13 beats per minute when calculating the target heart range.[72] Arm work is essentially not as efficient as leg work and, therefore, in comparing arm and leg exercise, at a given workload a greater VO_2 is achieved. Given the linear relationship between heart rate and VO_2, a lesser heart rate is therefore needed in arm exercise to achieve the same $VO_{2\,max}$ with leg exercise.[5]

Venous pooling in the legs after aerobic exercise is worthy of note. Specifically, a cooling down period after aerobic exercise is important. Therefore, after a cross-country race, runners must keep moving at a less strenuous pace, such as simple walking, to avoid blood pooling in the lower extremities. Sudden stopping or lying down after a race could cause a drop in blood pressure that could lead to decreased circulation to the brain and heart and to potential loss of consciousness, arrhythmia, and other less severe but related symptoms.

Aerobic conditioning also can be used for weight loss in overweight patients.[36] This is often accomplished by lengthening the duration of the exercise and lessening the intensity. The body's systems have a sequence of energy source utilization, and to mobilize free-fatty acids as an energy source, duration should be at least 30 minutes, with benefit for fat mobilization with longer duration.[47] Also, as aerobic conditioning causes the bodily systems to adapt, lipid metabolism increases as improved blood flow and fatty enzyme systems increase and become more efficient.

SELF-MOBILIZATION EXERCISE

One of the major goals of the physiatrist is to help patients achieve independence in home management. Some patients may have recurrent difficulties with somatic dysfunctions, which include regional tenderness, restricted and asymmetric motion, and associated tissue texture changes on physical examination, often associated with patient-reported discomfort. In the setting of known recurrent somatic dysfunctions, self-mobilization exercises can be taught, but the patient must be warned of several caveats. If exercises are not performed accurately, pain may increase. Therefore, the patient should stop exercising if any persisting increase in pain occurs. If a herniated disc is present, leading to unrecognized radicular symptoms, some self-mobilization could lead to clinical worsening.

The cervical spine is fraught with sensitivity to motion restrictions. Whether it is the occasional kink in the neck or a more chronic limitation in motion, self-mobilization can be helpful. Knowledge in segmental evaluation of the spine is paramount in diagnostically specific exercise prescription. [12,45,68] In self-mobilization of the atlantooccipital joint, the head is turned to rotational limits to "lock out" C1-2 motion. The patient brings the head into maximal available flexion and then in concert with the breathing cycle gives a firm motion into flexion at the end of exhalation (Fig. 14). For improving retroflexion motion, the opposite occurs. The remainder of the cervical spine can be mobilized for improved flexion and extension by having the patient place his hands around the back of the neck with the ulnar edge of the hands positioned at the segment to be mobilized (at the lower vertebra). The limit of cervical extension is reached and the hands gently perform oscillation forward. This promotes obligatory cervical extension (Fig. 15). To promote flexion, the hands are placed on the upper vertebrae of the restricted segment, and the oscillatory motions are performed after the cervical spine segment is flexed to its limit (Fig. 16).

For treating limitations in cervical rotation, a small towel is often useful. The towel is placed around the back of the neck at the lower vertebrae of the restricted segment. If the limitation is in left rotation, the patient crosses his arms in front of his face, left arm over right, and holds each end of the towel, with the left hand holding the right side of the towel. The distraction motion occurs along the planes of the cervical facet joints, with an upward motion occurring in concert with a left rotation. The upper arm tends to control the rotation, and the lower arm and towel side stabilize the overall motion (Fig. 17). The position of the towel can be modified to treat different levels of the cervical spine.

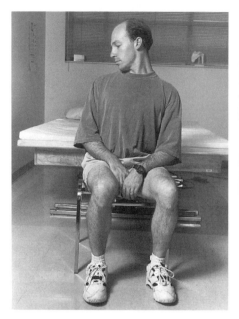

FIGURE 14. Atlantooccipital self-mobilization.

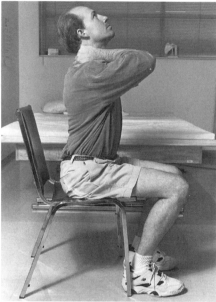

FIGURE 15. Self-mobilization for cervical extension.

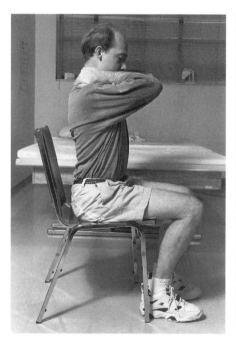

FIGURE 16. Self-mobilization for cervical flexion.

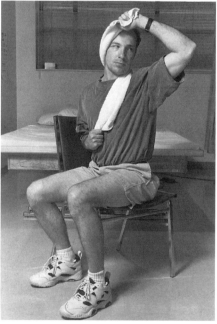

FIGURE 17. Towel-assisted cervical rotation mobilization.

The cervicothoracic junction is a difficult area to treat if restricted. Self-mobilization treatment requires action by the patient that involves the cervical and thoracic spine, both segmentally and by using muscles that cross the junction. With the arms in 90° of abduction and elbows extended, the hands are alternately rotated into pronation and supination, each hand opposite the other (Fig. 18A). This is combined with cervical rotation motion as the patient turns her head in combination with moving her arms alternatively into pronation and supination. The cervical spine rotates in the direction of hand pronation (Fig. 18B). This gives a repetitive mobilization of segments and musculature across the cervicothoracic junction. Upper thoracic rotation can be accomplished when the patient places one hand on her ipsilateral shoulder with the elbow bent and the other arm holding the bent elbow. The fingers of the active arm can be placed along the upper thoracic paraspinal area close to the midline, and this operator arm pulls the elbow laterally and slightly inferior (Fig. 19).

The thoracic spine also can be put through a general elongation exercise, with bending at the waist and hands outstretched to touch a nearby wall. The performance of an anterior pelvic tilt in this position enables a sense of elongation. A typical cat stretch and hyperextension help with those motions (Fig. 20). In addition, the use of foam rollers or golf balls can be used to help with thoracic extension and can be segmentally specific (Figs. 21 and 22).

The lumbar spine is a frequent area of dysfunction and complaints of tightness and stiffness. The usual self-treatment is based on flexion/extension and rotation. Two aspects of the spine should be mentioned. Patients with segmental hypermobility should be approached with caution, particularly with the rotational exercises. Patients will need to learn how to stabilize their hypermobile segments while mobilizing hypomobile segments if they are to be successful. Self-mobilization techniques are in general, however, quite helpful. If the patient is restricted in extension, for example, at L4-5, a belt can be placed around the L4 vertebra. The patient would then move into his extension limit as he pulls up on the belt and forward (Fig. 23). The movement is directed anteriorly and superiorly toward the face. A similar technique without a belt uses the patient's own fist as a fulcrum, again moving into extension as the fist is moved cranio-anteriorly. This can be considered as an active form of lumbar support.

Lumbar spine rotation exercises include the well-known lumbar rolls.[11,13,101] The patient lies on her side, generally with the lower leg straight and the upper leg bent at varying degrees of hip and knee flexion. The knee often comes off the table, and the upper ankle is positioned just behind the lower knee for stabilization. The patient's head is rotated to the opposite side of the side-lying, and the upper arm grasps the table for support. The lower arm places pressure on the upper knee, causing a torque at the spine and producing the desired rotation (Figs. 24 and 25). In most cases, the side of dysfunction of the lumbar segment is positioned closer to the table; if a lumbar segment is rotated to the right, manifesting as a right-sided posteriorly prominent transverse process, the patient would be lying on her right side.

Sacroiliac joint restrictions are relatively common and cause a variety of functional difficulties, including gait disturbances and pain on transitioning from various spine postures, such as moving from the seated to the standing position. Three exercises may be helpful in treating a wide variety of dysfunctions. One includes kneeling on both

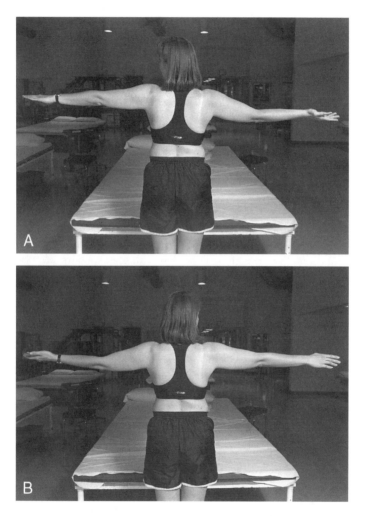

FIGURE 18. *A,* Positioning for cervicothoracic mobilization. *B,* As the head is rotated, the palms alternate between pronation and supination, matching a single cervical rotation to a single direction change for the wrist and palm. The neck is always turned to the pronated side.

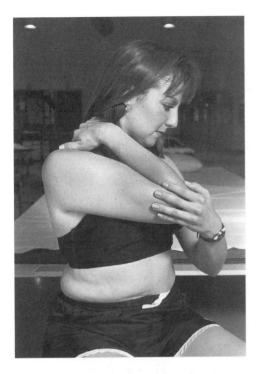

FIGURE 19. Upper thoracic rotation is assisted as the right hand, positioned along the upper thoracic right transverse processes, is pulled anteriolaterally and downward.

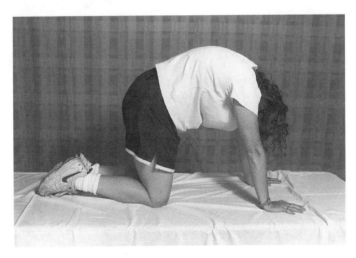

FIGURE 20.   General thoracic flexion exercise.

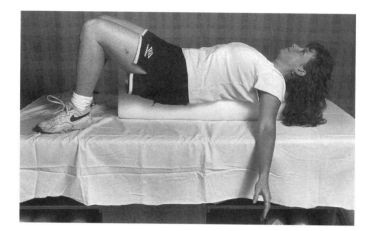

FIGURE 21.   General thoracic extension exercise.

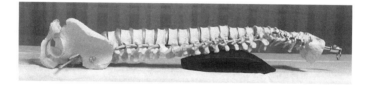

FIGURE 22.   A mobilization device can be positioned at a specific segment prior to mobilization motion.

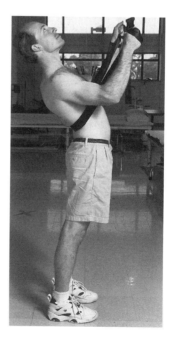

FIGURE 23.   Belt-assisted lumbar extension mobilization.

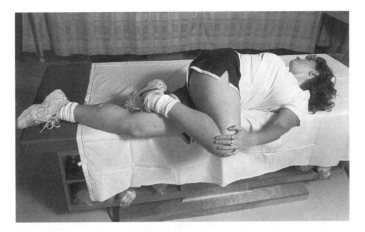

FIGURE 24. Lumbar roll technique.

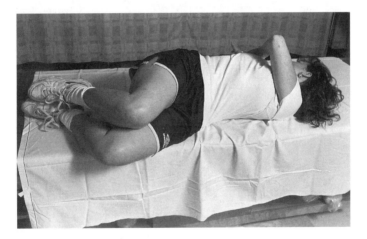

FIGURE 25. Alternative form of lumbar roll, requiring less baseline rotation motion than in Figure 24.

arms and legs close to the edge of a table and allowing the knee on the unaffected side to be dropped over the edge of the table while the foot of the unsupported limb is hooked over the ankle of the supported limb. The patient can bring the unsupported knee downward toward the floor in a progressive fashion of small but definite downward movements. This has the effect of mobilizing the area on the supported side (Fig. 26). A piriformis stretch (Fig. 27) encourages the upper poles of the sacrum to extend, particularly on the ipsilateral side. The patient also can perform an opposite maneuver to encourage the sacrum to move in the opposite direction. The patient is prone with one leg off the table touching the floor. From this position, the patient can extend the spine, creating a force that promotes relative flexion of the upper sacral pole ipsilaterally (Fig. 28).

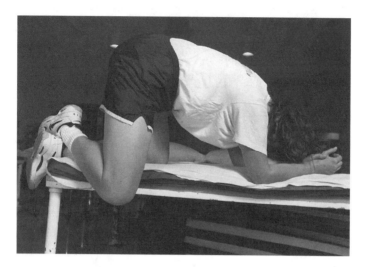

FIGURE 26. The left sacroiliac joint is mobilized as the right knee is brought toward the floor. The pelvis remains stable during the exercise.

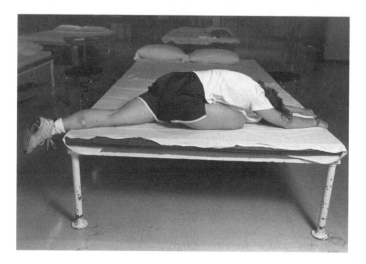

FIGURE 27. Mobilization of the upper poles of the sacrum posteriorly, encouraging the sacral base toward sacral extension, or counternutation.

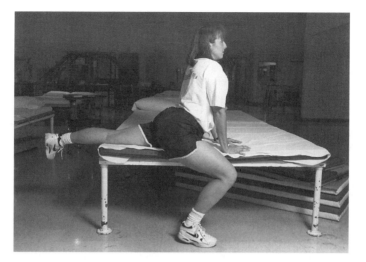

FIGURE 28. Promoting nutation, or sacral flexion.

CONCLUSION

This chapter has described the major categories of exercise to provide fundamental understanding of the principles effecting therapeutic programming. Patients' highest functional level is most commonly obtained with the optimal combination of exercise techniques. This chapter is designed to educate, increase awareness, and provoke thought regarding the creative construction and progression of exercise as we guide our patients to desired activities, goals, and athletic endeavors in a safe fashion.

REFERENCES

1. Abernethy PJ, Thayer R, Taylor AW: Acute and chronic responses of skeletal muscle to endurance and sprint exercise. Sports Med 10:365–389, 1990.
2. Adelstein RS, Eisenberg E: Regulation and kinetics of the actin-myosin-ATP interaction. Annu Rev Biochem 49:921–956, 1980.
3. American College of Sports Medicine: Guidelines for Exercise Testing and Prescription, 4th ed. Philadelphia, Lea & Febiger, 1991.
4. Arborelius M, Balldin UI, Lilja B, et al: Hemodynamic changes in man during immersion with the head above water. Aerospace Med 43:593–599, 1972.
5. Astrand PO, Rodahl K: Textbook of Work Physiology. New York, McGraw Hill, 1986.
6. [reference deleted]
7. Baldwin KM, Winder WW, Terjung RL, et al: Glycolytic enzyme in different types of skeletal muscle: Adaptation to exercise. Am J Physiol 225:962–966, 1973.
8. Barrack RL, Skinner HB, Buckley SL: Proprioception in the anterior cruciate deficient knee. Am J Sports Med 17:1–6, 1989.
9. Bobbert MF: Drop jumping as a training method in jumping ability. Sports Med 9:7–22, 1990.
10. Bogduk N, Twomey LT: Clinical anatomy of the lumbar spine, 2nd ed. New York, Churchill Livingstone, 1991.

11. Bogduk N, Windsor H, Inglis A: The innervation of the cervical intervertebral discs. Spine 13:2–8, 1988.
12. Bookhout MR: Examination and treatment of muscle imbalances. In Bourdillon JF, Day EA, Bookhout MR (eds): Spinal Manipulation, 5th ed. London, Butterworth, 1992, pp 313–334.
13. Borg G: Perceived exertion as an indicator of somatic distress. Scand J Rehabil Med 2-3:92–98, 1970.
14. Boyle AM: The Bad Ragaz ring method. Physiotherapy 67:265–268, 1981.
15. Brennan DK, Wider RP: Aqua Running: An Instructor's Manual. Houston, Houston International Running Center, 1990.
16. Bynum EB, Barrack RL: Open versus closed kinetic chain exercises after anterior cruciate ligament reconstruction: A prospective randomized study. Am J Sports Med 23:401–406, 1995.
17. Cole AJ, Eagleston RE, Moschetti M: Swimming. In White AH, Schofferman JA (eds): Spine Care. St. Louis, Mosby, 1995, pp 727–745.
18. Councilman JE: The importance of speed in exercise. Athletic J 72–75, 1976.
19. Davidoff GN, Lampman RM, Westbury L, et al: Exercise testing and training of persons with dysvascular amputation: Safety and efficacy of arm ergometry. Arch Phys Med Rehabil 73:334–338, 1992.
20. DeLorme TL, Watkins AL: Techniques of progressive resistance exercise. Arch Phys Med Rehabil 29:263–273, 1948.
21. DeLorme TL, West FE, Shriber WJ: Influence of progressive-resistance exercises on knee function following femoral fractures. J Bone Joint Surg 32A:910–924, 1950.
22. DeLorme TL: Restoration of muscle power by heavy resistance exercises. J Bone Joint Surg 27:645–667, 1945.
23. Department of Health and Human Services: Aqua Dynamics: Water Exercises Are the New Way to Stay in Shape. Washington, DC, Department of Health and Human Services, 1986.
24. Devries HA: Evaluation of static stretching procedures for improvement of flexibility. Res Q 33:222–229, 1962.
25. Dillingham MF: Strength training. Phys Med Rehabil State Art Rev 1:555–568, 1987.
26. Draganich LF, Jaeger RJ, Krajl AR: Coactivation of the hamstrings and quadriceps during extension of the knee. J Bone Joint Surg, 71A:1075–1081, 1989.
27. Ehrlich CE: Rest and splinting. In Total Management of the Arthritis Patient. Philadelphia, JB Lippincott, 1973.
28. Enoka RM: Muscle strength and its development: New perspectives. Sports Med 6:146–168, 1988.
29. Epstein M: Cardiovascular and renal effects of headout water immersion in man. Circ Res 39:619–628, 1976.
30. Fleck SJ, Kraemer WJ: Periodization Breakthrough! The Ultimate Training System. New York, Advanced Research Press, 1996.
31. Fleck SJ, Kraemer WJ: Resistance training: Physiological responses and adaptations. Phys Sportsmed 16:108–124, 1988.
32. Flores AM, Zohman LR: Rehabilitation of the cardiac patient. In Delisa J, Gans B (eds): Rehabilitation Medicine: Principles and Practice. Philadelphia, JB Lippincott, 1993.
33. Frederickson JM, Schwarz D, Kornhuber HH: Convergence and interaction of vestibular and deep somatic afferents upon neurons in the vestibular nuclei of the cat. Acta Otolaryngol 61:168–188, 1966.
34. Freeman MR, Dean ME, Hanman IF: The etiology and prevention of functional instability of the foot. J Bone Joint Surg 47B:678–682, 1965.
35. Gans C: Fiber architecture and muscle function. Exerc Sport Sci Rev, 19:160–207, 1982.
36. Garrow JS: Effects of exercise on obesity. Acta Med Scand S711:67–74, 1986.
37. Gauthier GF, Lowey S: Distribution of myosin isozymes among skeletal muscle fiber types. J Cell Biol 81:10–25, 1981.
38. Geraci MC: Rehabilitation of pelvis, hip, and thigh injuries in sports. Phys Med Rehabil Clin North Am 5:157–173, 1994.
39. Gollnick PD, Parsons D, Riedy M, Moore RL: Fiber number and size in overloaded chicken anterior latissimus dorsi muscle. J Appl Physiol 54:1292–1297, 1983.
40. Gollnick PD, Timson BF, Riedy M, Moore RL: Muscular enlargement and number of fibers in skeletal muscle of rats. J Appl Physiol 50:936–943, 1981.

41. Gonyea WJ, Sale DG, Gonyea FB, Mikesky A: Exercise induced increases in skeletal muscle fiber number. Eur J Appl Physiol 55:137–141, 1986.
42. Gonyea WJ: Role of exercise in inducing increases in skeletal muscle fiber number. J Appl Physiol 48:421–426, 1980.
43. Goodman MN: Amino acid and protein metabolism. In Horton ES, Terjung RL (eds): Exercise, Nutrition, and Energy Metabolism, New York, Macmillan, 1988, pp 89–99.
43a. Gowitzke BA, Millner S: Scientific Basis of Human Movement. Baltimore, Williams & Wilkins, 1988.
44. Green HJ, Klug GA, Reichmann H, et al: Exercise-induced fiber type transitions with regard to myosin, parvalbumin, and sarcoplasmic reticulum in muscle of the rat. Pflugers Arch 400:432–438, 1984.
45. Greenman PE: Principles of Manual Medicine. Baltimore, Williams and Wilkins, 1989.
46. Guyton AC: Textbook of Medical Physiology, 8th ed., Philadelphia, WB Saunders, 1991.
47. Haskell WL: The influence of exercise training on plasma lipids and lipoproteins in health and disease. Acta Med Scand S711:25–38, 1986.
48. Hickey D, Hukins D: Relation between the structure of the annulus fibrosus and the function and failure of the intervertebral disk. Spine 5:100–116, 1980.
49. Hickson RC, Hagberg JM, Ehsani AA, Holloszy JO: Time course of adaptive responses of aerobic power and heart rate to training. Med Sci Sports Exerc 13:17–20, 1981.
50. Holland GJ: The physiology of flexibility: A review of the literature. Kinesiol Rev 49–62, 1968.
51. Holloszy JO: Metabolic consequences of endurance training. In Horton ES, Terjung RL (eds): Exercise, Nutrition, and Energy Metabolism. New York, Macmillan, 1988.
52. Horn TJ: Presented at the 17th annual meeting of the International Society for Study of the Lumbar Spine, Heidelberg, Germany, 1990.
53. Huxley AF: Muscular contraction. J Physiol 243:1–43, 1974.
54. Jansson E, Sjodin B, Tesch P: Changes in muscle fibre type distribution in man after physical training. Acta Physiol Scand 104:235–237, 1978.
55. Kanehisa H, Miyashita M: Specificity of velocity in strength training. Eur J Appl Physiol 52:104–106, 1983.
56. Kannus P: Isokinetic evaluation of muscular performance: Implications of muscle testing and rehabilitation. Int J Sports Med 15(suppl 1): S11–S18, 1994.
57. Keeley J, Mayer TG, Cox R, et al: Quantification of lumbar function. Part 5. Reliability of range of motion measures in the sagital plane and an in vivo torso rotation measurement technique. Spine 11:31–42, 1986.
58. Kibler WB, Livingston BK, Bruce R: Current concepts in shoulder rehabilitation. Arch Phys Med Rehabil 3:249–300, 1995.
59. Kirkaldy-Willis WH: Managing Low Back Pain. New York, Churchill Livingstone, 1983.
60. Knight KL: Knee rehabilitation by the daily adjustable progressive resistive exercise technique. Am J Sports Med 7:336–337, 1979.
61. Komendantov GL: Proprioceptive reflexes of the eye and head in rabbits. Fiziol Zh 31:62, 1945.
62. Komi PV (ed): Strength and Power in Sport. London, Blackwell Scientific Publications, 1992.
63. Kong WZ, Goel VK, Gilbertson LG, Weinstein JN: Effects of muscle dysfunction on lumbar spine mechanics. Spine 21:2197–2207, 1996.
64. Kottke FJ, Pauley DL, Ptak RA, et al: The rationale for prolonged stretching for correction of shortening of connective tissue. Arch Phys Med Rehabil 47:345–352, 1966.
65. LeBan MM: Collagen tissue: Implications of its response to stress in vitro. Arch Phys Med Rehabil 47:345–352, 1962.
66. Lehmann JP, DeLateur BJ: Diathermy and superficial heat and cold therapy. In Kottke FJ, Stillwell GK, Lehmann JF (eds): Krusen's Handbook of Physical Medicine and Rehabilitation, 3rd ed. Philadelphia, WB Saunders, 1982, pp 275–350.
67. Lehmkuhl LD, Smith LK: Brunnstrom's Clinical Kinesiology, 4th ed. Philadelphia, FA Davis, 1985.
68. Lewit K: Examination of locomotor function and its disturbance. In Lewit K: Manipulative Therapy in Rehabilitation of the Locomotor System, 2nd ed. Oxford, Butterworth-Heinemann, 1991, pp 78–132.
69. Liberson WT, Asa MM: Further studies of brief isometric exercise. Arch Phys Med Rehabil 40:330–336, 1959.

70. Lutz GE, Palmitier RP, An K, Chao EY: Biomechanical analysis of kinetic chain exercises. Arch Phys Med Rehabil 72:804, 1991.
71. Magnusson P, Gleim G, Kolbe P, et al: Shoulder weakness in professional baseball pitchers. Med Sci Sports Exerc 24:s37, 1992.
72. McArdle WD, Katch FI, Katch VL: Essentials of Exercise Physiology. Philadelphia, Lea & Febiger, 1994.
73. McCouch GP, Deering ID, Ling TH: Location of receptors for tonic neck reflexes. J Neurophysiol 15:191–196, 1951.
74. McCully KK, Faulkner JA: Injury to Skeletal muscle fibers of mice following lengthening contractions. J Appl Physiol 59:119–126, 1985.
75. McDonagh MN, Davies CM: Adaptive response of mammalian skeletal muscle to exercise with high loads. Eur J Appl Physiol 52:139–155, 1984.
76. McMurray RG, Fieselman CC, Avery KE, Sheps DS: Exercise hemodynamics in water and on land in patients with coronary artery disease. Cardiopulm Rehabil 8:69–75, 1988.
77. Mendel T, Wink CS, Zimney M: Neural elements in human cervical intervertebral discs. Spine 17:132–135, 1992.
78. Miller F: Fluids. In College Physics, 4th ed. New York, Harcourt, Brace, Jovanovich, 1977.
79. Mitchell FL: The elements of muscle energy technique. In The Muscle Energy Manual, Vol 1. East Lansing, MI, MET Press, 1995, pp 3–24.
80. Moffroid MT, Whipple RH: Specificity of speed and exercise. J Am Phys Ther Assoc 50:1699–1704, 1970.
81. Moritani T, deVries HA: Neural factors versus hypertrophy in the time course of muscle strength gain. Am J Phys Med 58:115–130, 1979.
82. Moschetti M, Cole AJ: Aquatics: Risk management strategies for the therapy pool. Musculoskel Rehabil 4:265–272, 1994.
83. Noble MM, Pollack GH: Molecular mechanisms of contraction. Circ Res 40:333–342, 1977.
84. Noyes PR, Mathews DS, Moar PA, Grood ES: The Symptomatic anterior cruciate deficient knee. Part 2: The results of the rehabilitation activity modification, and counseling on functional disability. J Bone Joint Surg 65A:163–174, 1983.
85. Pate RR, Pratt M, Blair SN, et al: Physical activity and public health. JAMA 273:402–407, 1995.
86. Physical Activity and Cardiovascular Health, NIH Consensus Statement 13:3, pp. 1–33, 1995.
87. Rasch PJ, Morehouse LE: Effect of static and dynamic exercise on muscular strength and hypertrophy. J Appl Physiol. 11:29–32, 1957.
88. Risch WD, Koubenec HJ, Beckmann U, et al: The effect of graded immersion on heart volume, central venous pressure, pulmonary blood distribution, and heart rate in man. Pflugers Arch 374:115–118, 1978.
89. Sapega AA, Quendenfeld TC, Moyer RA, et al: Biophysical factors in range-of-motion exercise. Physician Sportsmed 19:57–60, 1991.
90. Schultz P: Flexibility: Day of static stretch. Physician Sportsmed 7:109–117, 1979.
91. Solomnow M, Baratta R, D'Ambrosia R: The role of the hamstrings in the rehabilitation of the anterior cruciate deficient knee in athletes. Sports Med 7:42–48, 1989.
92. Staron RS, Malicky ES, Leonardi MJ, et al: Muscle hypertrophy and fast fiber type conversions in heavy-resistance trained women. Eur J Appl Physiol 59:1716–1720, 1990.
92a. Steindler A: Kinesiology of the Human Body under Normal and Pathological Conditions. Springfield, IL, Charles C. Thomas, 1973.
93. Stone MH, O'Bryant H, Garhammer JG: A hypothetical model for strength training. J Sports Med Phys Fitness 21:342–351, 1981.
94. Strickler T, Malone T, Garrett WE: The effects of passive warming on muscle injury. Am J Sports Med 18:141–145, 1990.
95. Sug H, Pollack GH: Crossbridge Mechanism in Muscle Contraction. Baltimore, University Park Press, 1979.
96. Swaim LT: The orthopedic and physical therapeutic treatment of chronic arthritis. JAMA 103:1589–1592, 1934.
97. Swezey R: Essentials of physical management and rehabilitation in arthritis. Arthritis Rheum

3:349–368, 1974.

98. Taylor DC, Dalton JD, Seaber AV, et al: Viscoelastic properties of muscle-tendon units: The biomechanical effects of stretching. Am J Sports Med 18:300–309, 1990.

99. Timson BF, Bowlin BK, Dudenhoefer GA: Fiber number, area, and composition of mouse soleus muscle following enlargement. J Appl Physiol 58:619–624, 1985.

100. Tropp H, Askling C, Gillquist J: Prevention of ankle sprains. Am J Sports Med 13:259–262, 1985.

101. Wilder RP, Brennan DK: Fundamentals and techniques of aqua running for athletic rehabilitation. J Back Musculoskel Rehabil 4:287–296, 1994.

102. Wong TS, Booth FW: Protein metabolism in rat tibialis anterior muscle after stimulated eccentric exercise. J Appl Physiol 69:1718–1724, 1990.

103. Wright V, Johns RJ: Physical factors concerned with the stiffness of normal and diseased joints. Bull Johns Hopkins Hosp 106:215, 1960.

104. Yack HJ, Collins CE: Comparison of closed and open kinetic chain exercise in the anterior-cruciate deficient knee. Am J Sports Med 21:49–54, 1993.

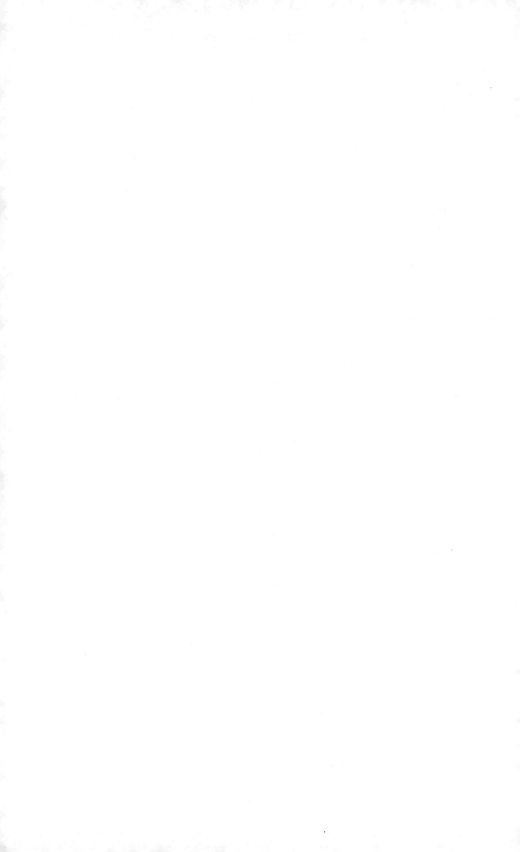

JONATHAN N. MYERS, PhD

4

Exercise Testing

Exercise testing is a noninvasive procedure that provides diagnostic, prognostic, and functional information for a wide spectrum of patients with cardiovascular, pulmonary, and even neurologic disorders. Few procedures yield as high a volume of clinically useful information as the exercise test. The exercise test is widely used in the evaluation of therapy, the assessment of interventions, and as a first-choice diagnostic modalilty, a role in which it functions as a gatekeeper to more expensive and invasive procedures. In the latter role, the test has become even more important in the current era of health care cost containment. In cardiac rehabilitation, the exercise test is the cornerstone on which the exercise prescription is based and is the primary method by which the efficacy of training is assessed. This chapter provides an overview of basic applications, methodology, and principles of exercise testing.

EXERCISE TESTING PERSONNEL

In 1990, a joint statement by the American College of Chest Physicians, the American College of Cardiology, and the American Heart Association regarding physician competence in exercise testing was issued.[41] This position statement was the first of its type and outlined the necessary cognitive skills needed to perform exercise testing, including knowledge of indications and contraindications to testing, basic exercise physiology, principles of interpretation, and emergency procedures. The committee suggested that at least 50 procedures were required during training to achieve these skills. The American College of Sports Medicine (ACSM) has developed certification programs for competency in exercise testing and training.[1] ACSM certification has been strongly recommended for technicians, nurses, or physiologists who oversee exercise testing and training. Because surveys have shown that complications during exercise testing are extremely rare, particularly in recent years,[50] the question has been raised as to whether physician supervision is required for all exercise testing. Most authorities continue to advocate physician presence when testing individuals who have cardiovascular or pulmonary disease or who are at high risk for its development. The ACSM also has outlined general guidelines for conditions for which physician supervision is recommended.[1]

EXERCISE TEST SELECTION

The purpose of the test, the health and fitness of the subject, the exercise modality, and the exercise protocol are fundamental considerations of testing. In many exercise laboratories, these issues are determined by the availability of equipment and custom, but each can have a profound effect on the response of the exercise test.

EXERCISE TESTING MODE

An ideal exercise mode increases total body and myocardial oxygen demand in progressive, equal, and modest increments and brings the subject to a maximal level within a reasonable time (an optimal test duration has been suggested to be 8–12 minutes).[7,11,30] This requires a dynamic exercise device that uses major muscle groups, permitting large increases in cardiac output, oxygen delivery, and gas exchange. Many modalities have been used for diagnostic testing, but the most common are the treadmill and the cycle ergometer. In the last decade, pharmacologic stress also has become a commonly used mode for echocardiographic and nuclear imaging.

Since the 1950s, numerous studies have compared exercise responses to the treadmill and cycle ergometer.[7,15,19,30,53] Relative to the treadmill, the cycle ergometer is generally less expensive, occupies less space, and is more quiet. Upper body motion is minimized, increasing the stability of blood pressure and electrocardiographic recordings. The workload administered by simple, mechanically braked bicycle ergometers is not always accurate and depends on pedaling speed, causing variations in the work performed. More expensive electronically braked ergometers maintain the workload at a specified level over a wide range of pedaling speeds and are therefore superior for quantifying work. Work rates are generally expressed differently for the cycle ergometer and the treadmill, but any work rate on either mode can be converted to metabolic equivalents (METs—a common clinical expression of exercise capacity representing a multiple of the resting metabolic rate) using standardized equations.[1]

The treadmill is used most often for exercise testing in North American.[47] It is usually more expensive than the cycle ergometer, is relatively immobile, and makes more noise. An advantage of the treadmill is that most subjects are more accustomed to walking than cycling. Researchers comparing treadmill and bicycle ergometer exercise tests have reported maximal oxygen uptake to be 10–20% higher (range 6–25%) and maximal heart rate to be 5–20% higher on the treadmill.[7,15,19,30,53] The frequency of ST segment changes has been reported to be similar or slightly higher,[53] and angina is elicited more frequently during treadmill testing than with the cycle ergometer.[15,30] Exercise-induced myocardial ischemia by thallium scintigraphy was recently reported to be greater after treadmill testing than cycle ergometry.[15] Although most of the differences are minor, if assessing the true functional limits of the patient and optimizing the diagnostic information from the test are important objectives, the treadmill may be preferable.

Dynamic arm exercise testing is necessary for patients in whom neurologic or orthopedic impairments of the lower extremities preclude walking on a treadmill or pedaling a cycle ergometer. Because the upper extremities have a smaller muscle mass than the lower extremities, the peak workload achieved is considerably lower for arm exercise.[3,4,9,42,45] However, for any given matched work rate, heart rate and systolic blood pressure tend to be higher for arm exercise, again owing to the smaller muscle mass and consequently a comparatively higher peripheral resistance in the working muscle. Studies on the sensitivity of arm ergometry have been mixed, but sensitivity generally has been reported to be comparatively low.[3,4,9,42,45] Balady and coworkers reported a sensitivity of 40% for arm ergometry versus 80% for leg exercise, but the peak rate-pressure product did not differ.[3] For concordantly positive tests, oxygen uptake at the onset of ischemia was lower for arm testing than for leg testing (12 vs 17 ml/kg/min, respectively). Arm testing appears to be a reasonable, but not an equivalent, alternative to leg exercise testing for patients who cannot perform treadmill or cycle ergometry.

Pharmacologic stress is an intriguing and relatively new area with important applications for echo and nuclear techniques, but only limited data are available directly comparing pharmacologic stress testing to standard exercise testing. Dipyridamole, adenosine, dobutamine, and, recently, arbutamine are the major pharmacologic agents that have been used for this purpose, and dipyridamole (Persantine) has been used the most. Comparisons between dipyridamole and standard exercise testing have demonstrated dipyridamole to have similar[44] or slightly better[5] diagnostic accuracy than standard exercise testing. Pharmacologic stress techniques are advantageous for patients who are unable to exercise on a treadmill or cycle ergometer to an adequate level. Patients who may be appropriate candidates for this approach include those with peripheral vascular disease or neurologic or musculoskeletal disorders. The disadvantages of dipyridamole stress testing include minor side effects, in 40–50% of patients,[38] and lack of cardiovascular response, in about 10% of patients.[54]

EXERCISE PROTOCOLS

Because the exercise test can be performed for various indications, such as the evaluation of chest pain (diagnostic), functional assessment, risk stratification, or some combination of these, the protocol should be chosen to fit the individual being tested and the purpose of the test. That so many exercise protocols are in use has led to some confusion regarding how to compare tests between patients. In 1980, Stuart and Ellestad surveyed 1375 exercise laboratories in North America and reported that, of those performing treadmill testing, 65.5% used the Bruce protocol for routine clinical testing.[47] Since then, an appreciation for more gradual, individualized approaches has occurred. Arguments in favor of more gradual approaches come from several directions. Large and unequal work increments have been shown to result in less accurate estimates of exercise capacity, particularly for patients with cardiac disease. Recent investigations have demonstrated that work rate increments that are too large or rapid result in a tendency to overestimate exercise capacity, less reliability for studying the effects of therapy, and lowered sensitivity for detecting coronary disease.[11,17,30,32,36,40,48,49,51] Individualizing the protocol by considering the subject and purpose of the test, rather than employing the same protocol for every subject, appears to offer several advantages for cardiopulmonary assessment.

Protocols suitable for clinical testing should include a low-intensity warm-up phase followed by progressive, continuous exercise in which the demand is elevated to a patient's maximal level within a total duration of 8–12 minutes.[7,11,30] For patients with cardiovascular disease, modifications of the Balke-Ware protocol are recommended because of its constant treadmill speed between 2 and 3.3 miles per hour (mph), equal increments in grade (2.5% or 5%), and equal (one or two) increases in METs. In the absence of gas exchange techniques, it is important to report exercise capacity in METs rather than treadmill time, so that exercise capacity can be compared uniformly between protocols. METs can be estimated from any protocol using standardized equations that have been put into tabular form[1] (Fig. 1). In general, 1 MET represents an increment on the treadmill of roughly 1 mph or 2.5% grade. On a cycle ergometer, 1 MET represents an increment of roughly 20 W (120 kg/min) for a 70-kg person. The assumptions necessary for predicting MET levels from treadmill or cycle ergometer work rates (including not holding the handrails, that oxygen uptake is constant [steady state], that the subject is healthy, and that all individuals are similar in their walking efficiency) raise uncertainties as to the accuracy of estimating the work performed for an individual patient. For example, the steady state requirement is rarely met for the majority of patients on most exercise protocols; most clinical testing is performed in patients with varying degrees of cardiovascular or pulmonary disease; and individuals vary widely in their walking efficiency.[27] It has therefore been recommended that a patient be ascribed a MET level only for stages in which all or most of a given stage duration has been completed.

FUNCTIONAL CLASS	CLINICAL STATUS	O₂ COST ml/kg/min	METS	BICYCLE ERGOMETER (1 WATT = 6.1 Kpm/min; FOR 70 KG BODY WEIGHT Kpm/min)	BRUCE 3 MIN STAGES MPH / %GR	BALKE-WARE % GRADE AT 3.3 MPH 1 MIN STAGES	USAFSAM MPH / %GR	"SLOW" USAFSAM MPH / %GR	McHENRY MPH / %GR	STANFORD %GR AT 3 MPH / %GR AT 2 MPH	ACIP MPH / %GR	CHF MPH / %GR	METS
NORMAL AND I (HEALTHY, DEPENDENT ON AGE ACTIVITY)		56.0	16		5.5 / 20	26							16
		52.5	15		5.0 / 18	25	3.3 / 25				3.4 / 24.0		15
		49.0	14	1500	4.2 / 16	24 / 23			3.3 / 21				14
		45.5	13			22 / 21	3.3 / 20				3.1 / 24.0		13
	SEDENTARY HEALTHY	42.0	12	1350		20 / 19 / 18			3.3 / 18	22.5	3.0 / 21.0		12
		38.5	11	1200	3.4 / 14	17 / 16	3.3 / 15	2 / 25		20.0	3.0 / 17.5	3.4 / 14.0	11
		35.0	10	1050		15 / 14			3.3 / 15	17.5	3.0 / 14.0	3.0 / 15.0	10
		31.5	9	900		13 / 12	3.3 / 10	2 / 20	3.3 / 12	15.0	3.0 / 10.5	3.0 / 12.5	9
	LIMITED	28.0	8	750		11 / 10				12.5		3.0 / 10.0	8
II		24.5	7		2.5 / 12	9 / 8	3.3 / 5	2 / 15	3.3 / 9	10.0 / 17.5		3.0 / 10.0	7
		21.0	6	600	1.7 / 10	7 / 6		2 / 10	3.3 / 6	7.5 / 14.0	3.0 / 7.0	3.0 / 7.5	6
	SYMPTOMATIC	17.5	5	450		5 / 4		2 / 5		5.0 / 10.5	3.0 / 3.0	2.0 / 10.5	5
III		14.0	4	300	1.7 / 5	3	3.3 / 0	2 / 0		2.5 / 7.0	2.5 / 2.0	2.0 / 7.0	4
		10.5	3	150	1.7 / 0	2 / 1	2.0 / 0		2.0 / 3	0 / 3.5	2.0 / 0.0	2.0 / 3.5	3
		7.0	2									1.5 / 0.0	2
IV		3.5	1									1.0 / 0.0	

USAFSAM = United States Air Force School of Aerospace Medicine
ACIP = Asymptomatic Cardiac Ischemia Pilot
CHF = Congestive Heart Failure (Modified Naughton)
Kpm/min = Kilopond meters/minute
%GR = percent grade
MPH = miles per hour

FIGURE 1. The oxygen cost per stage of some commonly used protocols. (Adapted from Froelicher VF, Myers J, Follansbe W, et al: Exercise and the Heart. St. Louis, CV Mosby, 1993.)

An approach to exercise testing that has gained interest in recent years is the ramp protocol, in which work increases constantly and continuously. In 1981, Whipp et al. first described cardiopulmonary responses to a ramp test on a cycle ergometer,[52] and many of the gas exchange manufacturers now include ramp software. Recently, treadmills have been adapted to conduct ramp tests.[29,30] The recent call for "optimizing" exercise testing[7,11,30,32,51] would appear to be facilitated by the ramp approach, because large work increments are avoided and increases in work are individualized, permitting test duration to be targeted. Because there are no stages, the errors associated with predicting exercise capacity as mentioned above are lessened.[29]

Submaximal exercise testing is most appropriate clinically for predischarge, post-myocardial infarction evaluations, and for patients with orthopedic or neurologic disorders whose cardiovascular status is uncertain. For the former, submaximal testing has been shown to be important in risk stratification.[12,43] Submaximal testing can be useful for making appropriate activity recommendations, for recognition of the need for modification of the medical regimen or the need for further interventions. Submaximal testing is also appropriate for patients with a high probability of serious arrhythmias. A submaximal, predischarge test appears to be as predictive for future events as a symptom-limited test among patients less than 1 month following myocardial infarction. Testing endpoints for submaximal testing have traditionally been arbitrary but should always be based on clinical judgment. A heart rate limit of 140 beats per minute and a MET level of 7 are often used for patients younger than 40, and limits of 130 beats per minute and a MET level of 5 are often used for patients older than 40. For patients taking beta-blockers, a Borg perceived exertion level in the range of 7 to 8 (1–10 scale) or 15 to 16 (6 to 20 scale) is a conservative endpoint. These limits are somewhat arbitrary and should be superseded by clinical judgment. Maximal testing is probably more appropriate more than 1 month following myocardial infarction, but submaximal testing has been used effectively and safely for risk stratification among patients less than 1 month after an infarction.

PATIENT PREPARATION

Exercise testing should be an extension of the history and physical examination, and an important role of the physician supervising the test involves patient assessment prior to beginning. Indications (Table 1) and contraindications for testing (Table 2) should be carefully considered. If doubt exists as to the purpose or safety of the test, it should not be performed. The referring physician should be contacted if the reason for the test is not clear. Specific questioning should determine which medications are being taken, and potential electrolyte abnormalities should be considered. For routine testing, withdrawal of cardiac medicines is usually not recommended; the potential dangers of withdrawing medical therapy generally do not outweigh gains in test performance.[1,11] If withdrawal of medications is considered necessary for diagnostic testing in a particular patient, this process should be carefully supervised by a physician or nurse.

The patient should come to the laboratory appropriately dressed for exercise and be instructed not to eat, drink caffeinated beverages, or smoke for at least 3 hours prior

---

TABLE 1. Indications for Exercise Testing

Evaluating chest pain
Screening for ischemic heart disease in at-risk asymptomatic males
Evaluating dysrhythmias
Determining functional capacity
Generating an exercise prescription
Establishing the severity/prognosis of ischemic heart disease to stratify those who need additional
    intervention with angioplasty or coronary artery bypass graft
Evaluating antianginal or antihypertensive therapy
Evaluating antiarrhythmic therapy
Evaluating the patient after myocardial infarction for risk stratification

---

TABLE 2. Absolute and Relative Contraindications to Exercise Testing

Absolute Contraindications	Relative Contraindications*
Acute myocardial infarction (within 3-5 days)	Left main coronary stenosis or its equivalent
Unstable angina	Moderate stenotic valvular heart disease
Uncontrolled cardiac arrhythmias causing symptoms or hemodynamic compromise	Electrolyte abnormalities
	Significant arterial or pulmonary hypertension
Active endocarditis	Tachyarrhythmias or bradyarrhythmias
Symptomatic severe aortic stenosis	Hypertrophic cardiomyopathy
Uncontrolled symptomatic heart failure	Mental impairment leading to inability
Acute pulmonary embolus or pulmonary infarction	to cooperate
Acute noncardiac disorder that may affect exercise performance or be aggravated by exercise (infection, renal failure, thyrotoxicosis)	High-degree atrioventricular block
Acute myocarditis or pericarditis	
Physical disability that would preclude safe and adequate test performance	
Thrombosis of lower extremity	

*Relative contraindications can be superseded if benefits outweigh risks of exercise.

to the test. The adverse hemodynamic and symptomatic effects of food, caffeine, and tobacco in close proximity to the exercise test among patients with heart disease are well known.[31] Those supervising the test should carefully explain the potential discomforts and risks to the patient. The explanation should include a demonstration of how to perform the test and how to terminate the test if the patient wishes to do so. Universal agreement on the necessity of signed informed consent is lacking. While this may depend on the setting, there is sufficient case law to recommend informed consent prior to exercise testing.[18]

These issues are less important when testing apparently healthy individuals or athletes. In such individuals, diagnostic testing is of minimal value; the test is more commonly performed to assess fitness and efficacy of training. As such, the focus is commonly placed on gas exchange and lactate responses, running economy, endurance evaluations, and research. On rare occasions, initial screening of athletes raises questions regarding subclinical heart disease, and the exercise test is indicated as part of further examination. When routine testing of young, healthy individuals is performed, it is generally not necessary to have a physician present.[1] As with patients, the protocol and sequence of the test should be carefully explained. Contraindications to testing are the same for athletes as for the general population.

HEART RATE AND ELECTROCARDIOGRAPHY

Heart rate increases linearly with oxygen uptake during exercise. Of the two major components of cardiac output, heart rate and stroke volume, heart rate is responsible for most of the increase in cardiac output during exercise, particularly at higher levels. Thus, maximal heart rate achieved is a major determinant of exercise capacity.[16,27] The inability to appropriately increase heart rate during exercise ("chronotropic incompetence") has been associated with the presence of heart disease and a worse prognosis.[16] Although maximal heart rate has been difficult to explain physiologically,[14] it is affected by age, gender, health, type of exercise, body position, blood volume, and environment. Of these factors, age is the most important. There is an inverse relationship between maximal heart rate and age, with correlation coefficients in the order of -0.40. However, the scatter around the regression line is quite large, with standard deviations ranging from 10–15 beats per minute (Fig. 2). Thus, age-predicted maximal heart rate is a limited measurement for clinical purposes and should not be used as an endpoint for exercise testing.[11,16]

Diagnostically, the electrocardiographic response is the cornerstone of the clinical exercise test. Thus, reliable test interpretation and patient safety mandate a quality exercise electrocardiogram (ECG). Critical to obtaining a high-quality ECG tracing is proper skin preparation and precise electrode placement. The goal of skin preparation is to decrease the resistance at the skin-electrode interface and thus improve the signal-to-noise ratio. After removing hair from the general areas of placement, each site should be vigorously rubbed with an alcohol pad to remove skin oil. The skin should be abraded using abrasive pads, gels, or other products designed to further reduce resistance by removing the superficial layers of skin. Finally, each electrode should be carefully placed in the proper location to ensure good skin contact with both the conducting gel and adhesive surfaces of the electrode.

The Mason-Likar limb lead placement[24] (Fig. 3) is the standard configuration clinically since it provides a 12-lead ECG with less artifact and less restriction to movement than the standard limb placement. However, the Mason-Likar placement can result in differences in electrocardiographic amplitude and axis when compared to the standard limb placement.[13,21,39] Because these shifts may be misinterpreted as diagnostic changes, it is often recommended that a resting supine ECG be recorded using the standard limb lead placement. It is also important to note that position changes may alter the interpretation of the ECG. For this reason, diagnostic ST segment changes

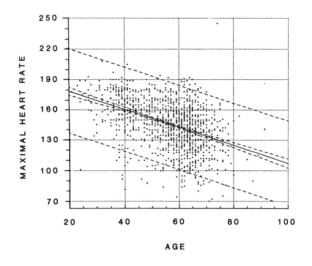

FIGURE 2. Relationship between maximal heart rate and age among 1,388 patients referred for exercise testing for clinical reasons. Inner lines represent the standard error; outer lines represent 95% confidence limits. (From Morris CK, Myers J, Froelicher VF, et al: J Am Coll Cardiol 22:175–182, 1993, with permission.)

should always be made relative to the resting exercise baseline position (i.e., upright rather than supine for treadmill and cycle ergometry).

The variety of medications taken by patients referred for exercise testing can have profound effects on the response to exercise. The medications can affect heart rate, blood pressure, myocardial contractility, cardiac rhythm, electrocardiographic responses, and exercise capacity. The group of medications having the most dramatic effects are the beta blockers, which attenuate heart rate, blood pressure, and cardiac output at rest and during exercise. Nitrates tend to increase heart rate, lower blood pressure, and reduce ischemic responses to exercise, whereas other vasodilators may have widely varying effects on the exercise ECG. Most antiarrhythmic agents have minimal effects on hemodynamic responses to exercise; quinidine may cause false negative ECG responses, and procainamide can cause false positive responses. Digoxin increases myocardial contractility but is known to cause ST segment depression independent of myocardial ischemia. It is useful to note the potential effects of the medicines being taken by a given patient prior to beginning the test. The effects of these medicines on heart rate are an additional reason that the age-predicted maximal heart rate should not be used as a test endpoint.

BLOOD PRESSURE

Assessment of systolic and diastolic blood pressure at rest and during the exercise test is important for patient safety and can provide important diagnostic and prognostic information. Properly trained personnel can obtain accurate and reliable blood pressures using noninvasive auscultory techniques, and guidelines have been developed for this

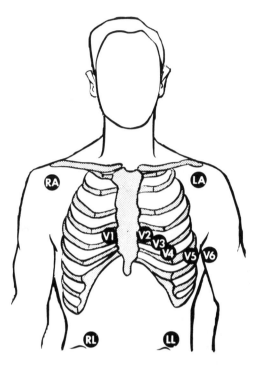

Figure 3.   The Mason-Likar simulated 12-lead electrode placement for exercise testing. (From Froelicher VF, Myers J, Follansbe W, et al: Exercise and the Heart. St. Louis, CV Mosby, 1993, with permission.)

purpose.[2,20] Blood pressure should be measured at rest prior to the test in both the supine and standing positions. When measured prior to an exercise test, resting blood pressure may be elevated compared to normal resting conditions due to pretest anxiety. Uncontrolled hypertension is a relative contraindication to exercise testing.[1,11] However, if blood pressure is elevated due to anxiety, a slight drop in blood pressure during the initial stage of an exercise test, when the workloads are light, is common and of no concern. A drop in systolic blood pressure below baseline during exercise has been associated with a poor prognosis.[10] Systolic and diastolic blood pressure should be assessed during the last minute of each exercise stage and more frequently if hypo- or hypertensive responses are observed. Normally, systolic blood pressure increases parallel with an increase in work rate. It is not uncommon in healthy individuals to exceed 200 mm Hg. In general, a value above 260 mm Hg is an indication to terminate the exercise test.[1,11] Diastolic pressure normally stays the same or increases slightly during exercise. The fifth Korotkoff sound, however, can frequently be heard all the way to zero in a young, healthy individual. A diastolic blood pressure exceeding 115 mm Hg is an indication to terminate the exercise test.[1,11] A drop in systolic blood pressure with increasing workloads should be remeasured immediately and, particularly when accompanied by symptoms, should result in termination of the test.

EXPIRED GAS ANALYSIS

The measurement of gas exchange and ventilatory variables provides an added dimension to the exercise test and yields additional information regarding the patient's cardiopulmonary function. Gas exchange techniques have been shown to provide a more precise and reproducible measure of exercise tolerance when compared to estimating work from treadmill speed and grade.[27] The use of these techniques, however, requires added attention to detail and a working knowledge of the equipment and basic physiology. This is particularly important given the recent advances in automation for the collection and calculation of expired gases.

Maximal oxygen uptake is the most common and generally the most useful measurement derived from gas exchange data during an exercise test. Maximal oxygen uptake defines the upper limits of the cardiopulmonary system and is dependent on the capacity to increase heart rate, augment stroke volume, and increase the extraction of oxygen by the active muscles. The inaccuracies associated with predicting MET levels from treadmill and cycle ergometer workloads alluded to earlier can only be resolved by the use of gas exchange techniques. Gas exchange techniques can provide a great deal of additional information regarding the capacity of the heart and lungs to deliver oxygen to the working muscle during exercise. The clinical importance of an objective and accurate measurement of exercise capacity is underscored by studies on prognosis in patients with heart disease. In a 1991 review, exercise capacity was identified more frequently than any other variable, including clinical history, markers of ischemia, and other exercise test variables, as a significant determinant of survival.[26] In patients with congestive heart failure, peak oxygen consumption has been identified as one of the best predictors of survival and is now widely used to help optimize the timing of heart transplantation.[22]

Heart and lung diseases frequently manifest themselves through gas exchange abnormalities during exercise, and the information obtained is increasingly employed in clinical trials. In addition to oxygen uptake, the influence of an intervention on ventilatory efficiency, the ventilatory threshold, and oxygen kinetics can provide useful information concerning the intervention. Modern metabolic systems tabulate and display these measurements online.

ASSESSING MAXIMAL EFFORT

Although many efforts have been made to objectify maximal effort, such as age-predicted maximal heart rate, a plateau in oxygen uptake, exceeding the ventilatory threshold, or a respiratory exchange ratio greater than unity, all have considerable measurement error and intersubject variability.[33–35,46] These problems are true irrespective of the population being tested. The 95% confidence limits for maximal heart rate based on age, for example, range considerably (see Fig. 2); therefore, this endpoint is maximal for some and submaximal for others.[16] The classic index of one's cardiopulmonary limits, a plateau in oxygen uptake, is not observed in many patients, is poorly reproducible, and has been confused by the many different criteria applied.[33–35] Though subjective, the Borg perceived exertion scale is helpful for assessing exercise effort[6] (Fig. 4). Good judgment on the part of the physician remains the most effective criteria for terminating exercise.

Table 3 lists clinical indications for stopping an exercise test.[1,11] Most problems can be avoided by having an experienced physician, nurse, or exercise physiologist standing next to the patient, measuring blood pressure, and assessing the patient's appearance during the test. The exercise technician should operate the recorder and treadmill, take appropriate tracings, enter data on a form, and alert the physician to any abnormalities that may appear on the monitor. If the patient's appearance is worrisome, systolic blood pressure plateaus or drops, marked electrocardiographic changes occur, chest pain becomes worse than the patient's usual pain, or if a patient wants to stop the test for any reason, the test should be stopped, even at apparent submaximal levels.

A great deal of effort has been directed toward the assessment of chest pain during exercise testing.[28] Our preference has been to use a 1 to 4 scaling system (Fig. 5) in which the test is terminated at a rating of 3, indicating the patient has reached a moderately severe level of chest discomfort or a point at which the patient would stop and rest or take a sublingual nitroglycerin pill during normal daily activities. This scale is particularly useful when using gas exchange techniques because chest pain can be expressed nonverbally with simple hand signals. In most instances, a symptom-limited maximal test is preferred, but it is usually advisable to stop if 0.2 mV of ST segment elevation occurs or if 0.2 mV flat or downsloping ST depression occurs.[11]

6	No exertion at all
7	Extremely light
8	
9	Very light
10	
11	Light
12	
13	Somewhat hard
14	
15	Hard
16	
17	Very hard
18	
19	Extremely hard
20	Maximal exertion

FIGURE 4. The Borg 6-20 perceived exertion scale. (From Borg GAV: Psychophysical bases of perceived exertion. Med Sci Sports Exerc 14:377–381, 1982, with permission.)

TABLE 3. Absolute and Relative Indications for Termination of an Exercise Test

Absolute Indications	Relative Indications
Acute myocardial infarction or suspicion of a myocardial infarction	Pronounced ECG changes from baseline (> 2 mm of horizontal or downsloping ST-segment depression, or > 2 mm of ST-segment elevation, except in AVR)
Onset of moderate to severe angina	Any chest pain that is increasing
Drop in systolic blood pressure with increasing workload accompanied by signs or symptoms or drop below standing resting pressure	Physical or verbal manifestations of severe fatigue or shortness of breath
Serious arrhythmias (e.g., second- or third-degree AV block, sustained ventricular tachycardia or increasing premature ventricular contractions, atrial fibrillation with fast ventricular response)	Wheezing
	Leg cramps or intermittent claudication (grade 3 on 4-point scale)
Signs of poor perfusion, including pallor, cyanosis, or cold and clammy skin	Hypertensive response (systolic blood pressure > 260 mmHg; diastolic blood pressure > 115 mmHg)
Unusual or severe shortness of breath	Less serious arrhythmias such as supraventricular tachycardia
Central nervous system symptoms, including ataxia, vertigo, visual or gait problems, or confusion	Exercise-induced bundle branch block that cannot be distinguished from ventricular tachycardia
Technical inability to monitor the ECG	
Patient's request	

The occurrence of "serious" arrhythmias during exercise, although rare, are indications to terminate the exercise test. Arrhythmias may be overt, such as ventricular tachycardia, or more subtle, such as unifocal premature ventricular contractions (PVCs) increasing in frequency, or a period of supraventricular tachycardia. Arrhythmias for which there should be no debate about stopping the test include second- or third-degree heart block and ventricular tachycardia of any duration. When in doubt as to the nature or origin of the arrhythmia, the test should be stopped. Isolated PVCs, even when they occur frequently, are not as ominous as previously thought. Recent studies have demonstrated that the occurrence of PVCs during an exercise test have minimal prognostic impact.[55] PVCs should be interpreted in context, such that the decision to terminate the test is made based on the patient's history and whether the patient remains hemodynamically stable or the arrhythmias are accompanied by symptoms.

Dyspnea may be the prominent symptom in some patients with coronary artery disease (CAD), but it is more often associated with reduced left ventricular function and chronic obstructive pulmonary disease (COPD). In the former, it is usually accompanied by poor exercise capacity and can occur with impaired systolic blood pressure responses to exercise. Dyspnea is also appropriately quantified using a 1 to 4 point scale.[1]

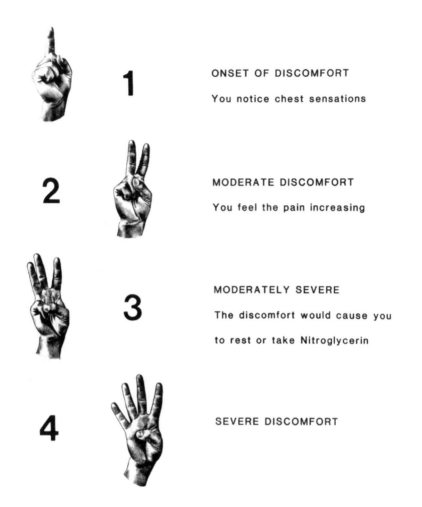

FIGURE 5. Rating scale for exertional chest discomfort. A rating of three is the appropriate endpoint. (From Myers NJ: Perception of chest pain during exercise testing in patients with coronary artery disease. Med Sci Sports Exerc 26:1082–1086, 1994, with permission.)

INTERPRETATION OF EXERCISE TEST RESPONSES

The most common reason that individuals undergo exercise testing is to diagnose CAD. Most of these patients are referred for testing for the evaluation of chest pain. In this role, the test serves the important purpose of screening those who should or should not undergo additional procedures. How accurately the exercise test distinguishes individuals with disease from those without disease depends on the population being tested, the definition of disease, and the criteria used for an abnormal test.

TABLE 4. Terms Used to Express the Diagnostic Value of a Test

Sensitivity = $\dfrac{TP}{TP + FN} \times 100$

Specificity = $\dfrac{TP}{TN + FP} \times 100$

Positive Predictive Value = $\dfrac{TN}{FP + TN} \times 100$

Negative Predictive Value = $\dfrac{TP}{FP + TN} \times 100$

TP = True positives, or those with abnormal test results and with disease
FN = False negatives, or those with normal test results and with disease
FP = False positives, or those with abnormal test results and no disease
TN = True negatives, or those with normal test results and no disease

The most common terms used to describe test accuracy are *sensitivity* and *specificity*. Sensitivity is the percentage of times a test correctly identifies those with CAD. Specificity is the percentage of times a test correctly identifies those without cardiovascular disease. Sensitivity and specificity are inversely related and are affected by both the population being tested and the choice of discriminant value for abnormal. For example, if the population of individuals has a greater severity of disease (such as triple vessel or left main coronary disease), the test will have a higher sensitivity. Alternatively, the test will have a higher specificity when performed in a group of younger, healthier subjects.

Another important term that helps define the diagnostic value of a test is the *predictive value*. The predictive value of an abnormal test (positive predictive value) is the percentage of persons with an abnormal test result who have disease. Conversely, the predictive value of a normal test (negative predictive value) is the percentage of persons with a normal test result who do not have disease. The predictive value of a test cannot be determined directly from the sensitivity and specificity but are strongly associated with the prevalence of disease in the population being tested. Table 4 presents the calculations used to determine sensitivity, specificity, and predictive value.

Ever since ECG changes were first associated with myocardial ischemia in the 1920s, the diagnostic ECG criteria and leads that exhibit abnormalities during exercise have been the source of significant debate. Numerous ECG criteria, including complex mathematical constructs, combined scores, and ST areas during exercise and recovery have been proposed to optimally diagnose the presence of CAD. Few of these studies, however, have followed accepted rules for evaluating a diagnostic test.[37] Most published guidelines continue to suggest the application of a traditional criterion, 1.0 mm or greater ST segment depression that is horizontal or downsloping. ST segment changes greater than 1.0 mm that are downsloping generally are indicative of more severe CAD. ST segment elevation occuring over leads *without* Q waves is indicative of severe transmural ischemia. ST segment elevation over leads *with* Q waves is more common and is related to the presence of dyskinetic areas. Probably more than 90% of ST changes will occur in the lateral precordial leads.[11] Although it has historically been thought that the diagnostic performance of the test was incomplete without all 12 leads, recent studies suggest that ST segment changes isolated to the inferior leads are frequently false positive responses.[25]

Diagnostically, the distinction between typical and atypical angina is important. Typical angina tends to be consistent in its presentation and location, is brought on by a physical or emotional stress, and is relieved by rest or nitroglycerin. Atypical angina refers to pain that has an unusual location, prolonged duration, or inconsistent precipitating factors that are unresponsive to nitroglycerin. Exercise-induced chest discomfort that has the characteristics of stable, typical angina provides better confirmation of the presence of CAD than any other test response. A patient exhibiting the combination of typical angina and an abnormal ST response has a 98% probability of having significant CAD. An indication to stop the exercise test is moderately severe angina or pain that would normally cause the patient to stop daily activities or take nitroglycerin.[1,11,28] (see Fig. 5).

FALSE POSITIVE AND FALSE NEGATIVE RESPONSES

The factors that can be associated with a false positive or false negative response should be considered prior to the test. A false positive response is defined as an abnormal exercise test response in an individual without significant heart disease, and it causes the specificity to be decreased. A false negative response occurs when the test is normal in an individual with disease, and it causes the sensitivity of the test to be reduced. Table 5 lists factors that have been associated with false positive and false negative responses. In some individuals, an alternative procedure, such as an exercise or pharmacologic echocardiogram, or a radionuclide test, may be appropriate.

TABLE 5. Causes of False Negative and False Positive Tests

False Positive	False Negative
Resting repolarization abnormalities	Failure to reach ischemic threshold, secondary to medications
Cardiac hypertrophy	Monitoring an insufficient number of leads to detect ECG changes
Accelerated conduction defects	
Digitalis	Angiographically significant disease compensated by collateral circulation
Nonischemic cardiomyopathy	
Hypokalemia	Musculoskeletal limitations preceding cardiac abnormalities
Vasoregulatory abnormalities	
Mitral valve prolapse	
Pericardial disease	
Coronary spasm in absence of CAD	
Anemia	
Female gender	

PROGNOSIS

One of the most important clinical applications of the exercise test is the identification of low-risk patients in whom catheterization (and revascularization) can be safely deferred. Numerous studies have shown that the exercise test has value for estimating prognosis in patients with or suspected of having cardiovascular disease.[8] There are several reasons why accurately establishing prognosis is important. An estimate of prognosis provides answers to patients' questions regarding the probable outcome of their illness, which may be useful to the patient in planning return to work/disability, recreational activities, and finances. A second reason to estimate prognosis is to identify patients for whom interventions might improve outcome. Combining clinical and exercise test information into scores has been shown to improve the estimation of risk among men and women undergoing exercise testing.[8]

CONCLUSION

Although important strides have been made in related procedures, the exercise test remains an invaluable tool in the assessment of patients with diseases of the heart, lungs, and other neurologic, orthopedic, and organ system disorders. Few tools clinically yield as great a volume of diagnostic, prognostic, and functional information. Access to limited health care resources often hinges on the test's results.[23] The exercise test is the cornerstone of the exercise prescription and is often the basis by which therapeutic decisions are made for patients with cardiovascular disease. Just as the exercise prescription and therapy are individualized, so too should the exercise test. Optimizing the information yield from the test requires attention to proper methodology and an understanding of issues related to basic physiology of exercise, safety, interpretation of electrocardiographic and hemodynamic responses, and, finally, a familiarity with the related professional guidelines.

Appendix A:
Case Studies

DEGENERATIVE JOINT DISEASE

Degenerative joint disease (DJD) is a localized osteoarthritic condition caused by cartilage destruction. DJD is characterized by pain, stiffness, weakness, swelling, and restricted mobility of the joints. Exercise testing in DJD can be influenced by the severity of pain, and performance may be limited by associated conditions such as inflammatory processes in the heart, lung, and the peripheral arterial or nervous systems. Abnormal gait often necessitates the use of a cycle ergometer rather than a treadmill. In patients whose pain is so severe that exercise cannot be tolerated, an alternative procedure (nuclear or echocardiographic stress) is indicated. The exercise test should be preceded by light range of motion exercises and/or stretching.

The following patient was referred for exercise testing for functional assessment and the evaluation of disability. He is a 61-year-old man with a history of moderate DJD in both knees, hypertension, and bypass surgery 6 years ago. His cardiovascular status has been stable, but he recently reported an increase in the frequency and severity of knee pain that interferes with his ability to work as a real estate agent and perform his daily activities. Given his joint pain, he was tested on a cycle ergometer using a ramp protocol (10 W/min). He is taking losartan for hypertension and aspirin.

Rest   The ECG showed a heart rate of 76 with normal sinus rhythm and inferior Q waves. His blood pressure was 128/86.

Exercise   The test was terminated after 5 minutes and 36 seconds due to knee pain. No chest pain or shortness of breath was reported. Maximal heart rate was 142, and no significant ECG changes or arrhythmias were observed during exercise or recovery. Maximum blood pressure was 176/82. He achieved a peak workload of 56 W, and the maximum MET level achieved was 4.2 (50% of predicted for age).

Interpretation   The patient demonstrated a normal cardiovascular response to exercise, but the limitation due to DJD was as expected. It was suggested that he begin an exercise program to improve muscle strength, flexibility, and endurance.

STROKE

Strokes occur as a result of vascular insufficiency in the brain. There are three general categories of stroke: (1) thrombosis or embolism, (2) progressive atherosclerosis, and (3) hemorrhage. In all three cases cell death results in impairment of the central nervous system. Most strokes occur in the elderly, with the incidence increasing in the sixth, seventh, and eight decades. Following a stroke, the degree of neurologic impairment is related to both the size and location of the ischemic area. The individual may present with motor and sensory impairment, visual deficits, impaired ability to communicate, confusion, and impaired learning and performance of voluntary movements.

Because most strokes involve atherosclerosis, exercise testing often involves evaluation of coexisting CAD. The mode of exercise testing should consider the severity and location of neurologic impairment. Treadmill testing would be appropriate only for individuals who have minimal motor impairment and ambulate independently without a walker or cane. A cycle ergometer is more appropriate for patients who have difficulty with balance, gait, or both. It is usually advisable to secure the affected lower limb to the pedal with toe clips or straps. Lack of motor function can hinder exercise performance considerably. Thus, with the use of either exercise mode, the protocol should be individualized and incremented more gradually than usual.

The following is a test report from a 69-year-old woman referred for exercise testing as a follow-up evaluation for functional capacity and evaluation of coronary disease. She recently reported transient, sharp pains in the chest and back. She has minor right-sided weakness. She was tested on a cycle ergometer (8 W/min ramp) with both feet secured to the toe clips. She was taking only aspirin.

Rest   The ECG showed a heart rate of 67, with normal sinus rhythm and a right bundle branch block. Her blood pressure was 134/80.

Exercise   The test was terminated after 9 minutes and 10 seconds due to leg fatigue. The maximal heart rate was 118, and 0.5 mm of upsloping ST depression was observed laterally, normalizing in recovery. The maximum blood pressure was 165/80. A peak workload of 75 W was achieved, corresponding to a maximum MET level of 5.1 (80% of predicted for age).

Interpretation   Given the patient's condition, she exhibited a reasonably good exercise tolerance. The ST segment changes were not significant, and she did not demonstrate symptoms that might indicate ischemia, suggesting that significant coronary disease is unlikely. The patient was reassured that it would be safe to return to normal daily activities.

PULMONARY DISEASE

Chronic pulmonary disease imposes a multitude of impairments, including, in addition to ventilatory and gas exchange problems, those involving the cardiovascular and muscular systems. Ventilatory impairments contributing to exercise intolerance may include increased airway resistance, reduced lung compliance, ventilatory inefficiency, and ventilatory muscle weakness and fatigue. Gas exchange abnormalities often include both ventilation and perfusion inequality and breakdown of the alveolar-capillary membrane. These abnormalities usually lead to secondary cardiovascular and skeletal muscle deconditioning due to a reduction in physical activity. Often, a patient has combined pulmonary and cardiovascular disease. During exercise testing patients may be limited by a true ventilatory limitation (in which maximal ventilation during exercise approaches the maximal voluntary ventilation at rest) or cardiovascular factors such as reduced left ventricular function, reduced pulmonary blood flow, hypoxemia, and deconditioning. Dyspnea is the hallmark symptom.

The following patient was referred to a pulmonary department for worsening symptoms of dyspnea. He is a retired 70-year-old man with a history of COPD that has been stable for about 4 years. He has no history of heart disease and, although not a current smoker, he has a 50-pack-year history of cigarette smoking. Resting pulmonary function tests were performed, and exercise testing was performed using ventilatory gas exchange techniques on a treadmill. Since he reported experiencing worsening symptoms at home during activities approximating 4 METs, the ramp rate on the treadmill was set such that a 4-MET workload was achieved in about 10 minutes. He is taking albuterol and hydrochlorothiazide.

Rest   The ECG shows a heart rate of 80, low voltage, and right atrial enlargement. His blood pressure was 130/74.

Pulmonary functions were as follows:

FVC,l	3.10 (66% of normal)
FEV_1 l	1.97 (54% of normal)
MVV, l/min	43.8 (31% of normal)
FEV_1/FVC, %	63.5 (81% of normal)

Exercise   The test was terminated after 9 minutes and 23 seconds due to dyspnea. No chest pain was reported. Maximal heart rate was 131, and no significant ECG changes were observed during exercise or recovery. The maximum blood pressure achieved was 160/80. The peak workload achieved was 2.5 mph/5% grade; the maximum estimated METs was 4.6 (60% of age predicted).

Ventilation and Gas Exchange

Peak VO_2: 13.3 ml/kg/min (3.8 METs, 54% of predicted for age)

Peak VE: 42.1 l/min

RER: 1.21

VCO_2: 1.126 l/min

VE/VO_2: 45.1

VE/MVV: 0.96

Interpretation   His pulmonary function data suggest moderate obstructive lung disease, but the values represent no change from his previous test approximately one year ago. Gas exchange techniques provide a precise and reproducible measure of exercise capacity, so it is important to note that his peak VO_2 is also similar to his previous test. The values for VE/VO_2 and the ratio of maximal exercise ventilation to maximal voluntary ventilation (VE/MVV) are typical of a patient with pulmonary disease. The VE/MVV suggests a true ventilatory limitation (96%), and the high VE/VO_2 confirms the ventilatory inefficiency commonly seen in pulmonary disease (normal value is 30–40). Given that there has been no apparent worsening of his pulmonary function or exercise capacity, no further testing was recommended. He was continued on albuterol and was placed on low-dose prednisone. He enjoys working in his garden, and was encouraged to remain active in this and other physical activities, and to return to the clinic if symptoms worsen.

SPINAL CORD INJURY

Spinal cord injury (SCI) is defined by damage to the neural elements within the spinal canal. Depending on the level (cervical, thoracic, or sacral) and extent of the injury, there is partial or total loss of motor and sensory function in the trunk and extremities. Muscular paralysis and sympathetic nervous system impairment reduce the patient's capacity to voluntarily perform exercise of the large muscle groups and also impair the ability of the nervous system to stimulate cardiovascular function to support higher rates of aerobic work. Common abnormal responses to exercise include venous pooling, orthostatic and exercise hypotension, limited positive chronotropic and inotropic states, autonomic dysreflexia, and exercise intolerance.

For paraplegic patients, in whom paralysis is limited to the lower body, lower extremity exercise such as walking and leg cycling are precluded. Exercise testing with upper arm ergometry has been shown to be reasonably sensitive for the detection of coronary disease. Maximal exercise ECG changes are best interpreted immediately after exercise due to noise associated with upper body motion. Despite its limitations, exercise testing remains the first-choice modality for evaluating chest pain in patients with SCI. However, the smaller muscle mass used restricts peak values achieved for work rate, cardiac output, and oxygen uptake. In patients with quadriplegia, in whom injuries to the spinal cord are more extensive, upper body exercise responses will be even more limited, and exercise may not be tolerated at all due to paralysis and because of orthostatic and exercise hypotension. Exercise testing in some patients has been performed with the assistance of electrical stimulation or leg exercise combined with arm exercise. In many individuals, however, pharmacologic stress using echocardiographic or nuclear techniques is indicated.

The following 50-year-old man was referred for exercise testing for the evaluation of chest pain. He had a lower thoracic SCI and thus had relatively good upper body strength, and he was physically active. He had no history of cardiovascular disease but had been a smoker for 20 years. He was tested on an arm ergometer using a ramp rate of 8 W/min. He was taking no medications.

Rest   The ECG showed a heart rate of 65 and was normal. His blood pressure was 116/68.

Exercise   The test was terminated after 8 minutes and 16 seconds due to arm fatigue, and the patient reported moderate chest tightness beginning at about 6 minutes. Maximal heart rate was 130, maximal blood pressure was 152/86, and there was 1.5 mm horizontal ST depression in the lateral leads. The ST changes did not resolve until about 6 minutes into recovery. A peak workload of 70 W was achieved, which represents an estimated MET level of 6.1.

Interpretation   The patient exhibited relatively good exercise tolerance for paraplegia. The symptoms he exhibited combined with ischemic ST segment changes during exercise and recovery strongly suggest the presence of significant CAD. He was referred for nuclear testing, which demonstrated reversible ischemia, and coronary angiogram showed three-vessel coronary disease.

CORONARY ARTERY DISEASE

Chest pain is the most common condition for which individuals are referred for exercise testing clinically. The test is performed to help establish the presence or absence of CAD.

The following patient is a 68-year-old male inpatient referred for evaluation after a myocardial infarction was ruled out. He experiences atypical angina, is taking nitrates, and is a heavy smoker. He has a family history of CAD but has had no events himself.

Rest   The resting ECG is normal and shows only minor ST segment elevation in the inferior limb leads. His resting blood pressure is 134/86.

Exercise   Maximal heart rate was 136, and maximal blood pressure was 160/84. He achieved 4 METs on the treadmill, which represents 50% of his expected exercise capacity for age. Typical angina occurred during both exercise and recovery. The ECG showed about 3 mm of horizontal ST segment depression in leads V2–V6 (Fig. 6). These ST segments became downsloping in recovery, which persisted beyond 5 minutes after exercise.

Interpretation   The profound ST segment depression and symptoms observed are

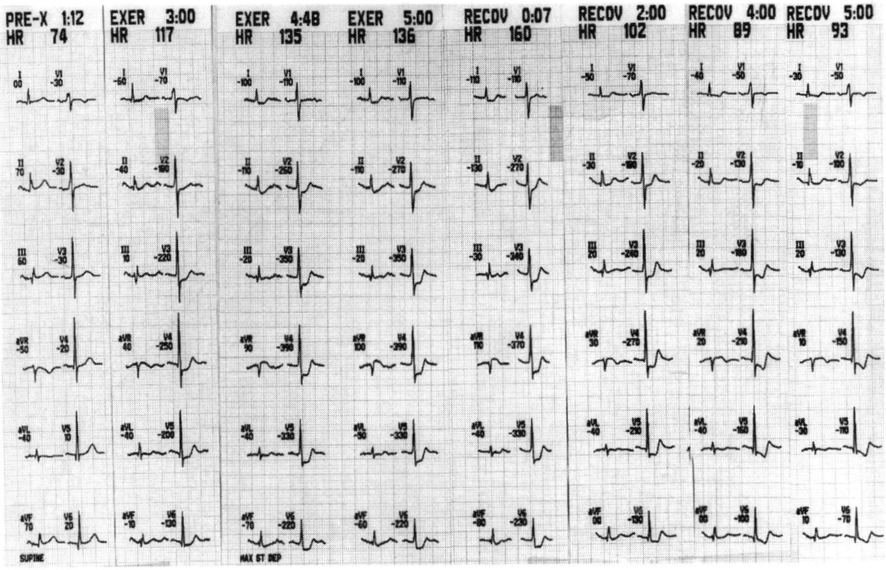

FIGURE 6.   Electrocardiogram showing about 3 mm of horizontal ST segment depression in leads V2–V6.

consistent with multivessel coronary disease. He was urged to undergo cardiac catheterization and was found to have triple-vessel disease with good left ventricular function. He has since done well with surgery and has increased his exercise capacity.

REFERENCES

 1. American College of Sports Medicine: Guidelines for Exercise Testing and Exercise Prescription, 5th ed. Baltimore, Williams & Wilkins, 1995.
 2. Bailey RH, Bauer JH: A review of common errors in the indirect measurement of blood pressure. Arch Intern Med 153:2741–2748, 1993.
 3. Balady GJ, Weiner DA, McCabe CH, Ryan TJ: Value of arm exercise testing in detecting coronary artery disease. Am J Cardiol 55:37–39, 1985.
 4. Bevegard S, Freyschoss U, Strandell T: Circulatory adaptation to arm and leg exercise in supine and sitting position. J Appl Physiol 21:37–46, 1966.
 5. Bolognese L, Sarasso G, Aralda D, et al: High dose dipyridamole echocardiography early after uncomplicated acute myocardial infarction: Correlation with exercise testing and coronary angiography. J Am Coll Cardiol 14:357–363, 1989.
 6. Borg GAV: Psychophysical bases of perceived exertion. Med Sci Sports Exerc 14:377–381, 1982.
 7. Buchfuhrer MJ, Hansen JE, Robinson TE, et al: Optimizing the exercise protocol for cardiopulmonary assessment. J Appl Physiol 55:1558–1564, 1983.
 8. Chang JA, Froelicher VF: Clinical and exercise test markers of prognosis in patients with stable coronary artery disease. Curr Probl Cardiol 19:533–538, 1994.
 9. DeBusk R, Valdez R, Houston N, Haskell W: Cardiovascular responses to dynamic and stable effort soon after myocardial infarction. Circulation 58:368–375, 1978.
10. Dubach P, Froelicher VF, Klein J, et al: Exercise induced hypotension in a male population: Criteria, causes, and prognosis. Circulation 78:1380–1387, 1988.
11. Fletcher GF, Froelicher VF, Hartley LH, et al. Exercise standards: A statement for health professionals from the American Heart Association. Circulation 91:580–615, 1995.
12. Froelicher VF, Purdue S, Pewen W, Risch M: Application of meta-analysis using an electronic spreadsheet to exercise testing in patients after myocardial infarction. Am J Med 83:1045–1054, 1987.
13. Gamble P, McManus H, Jensen D, Froelicher VF: A comparison of the standard 12-lead electrocardiogram to exercise electrode placement. Chest 85:616–622, 1984.
14. Graettinger W, Smith D, Neutel J, et al: Relationship of left ventricular structure to maximal heart rate during exercise. Chest 107:341–345, 1995.
15. Hambrecht R, Schuler GC, Muth T, et al: Greater diagnostic sensitivity of treadmill versus cycle exercise testing of asymptomatic men with coronary artery disease. Am J Cardiol 70:141–146, 1992.
16. Hammond K, Froelicher VF: Normal and abnormal heart rate responses to exercise. Prog Cardiovasc Dis 27:271–296, 1985.
17. Haskell W, Savin N, Oldrige R: Factors influencing oxygen uptake during exercise testing soon after myocardial infarction. Am J Cardiol 50:299–304, 1982.
18. Herbert DL, Herbert WG: Legal Aspects of Preventive Rehabilitative, and Recreational Exercise Programs. Canton, OH, PRC Publishers, 1993.
19 Hermansen L, Saltin B: Oxygen uptake during maximal treadmill and bicycle exercise. J Appl Physiol 26:31–37, 1969.
20. Iyriboz Y, Hearon CM: Blood pressure measurement at rest and during exercise: Controversies, guidelines, and procedures. J Cardiopulm Rehabil 12:277–287, 1992.
21. Kleiner JP, Nelson WP, Boland MJ: The 12 lead electrocardiogram in exercise testing. Arch Intern Med 138:1572–1573, 1978.
22. Mancini DM, Eisen H, Kussmaul W, et al. Value of peak exercise oxygen consumption for optimal timing of cardiac transplantation in ambulatory patients with heart failure. Circulation 83:778–786, 1991.
23. Marcus R, Lowe R, Froelicher VF, Do D: The exercise test as gatekeeper: Limiting access or appropriately directing resources? Chest 107:1442–1446, 1995.

24. Mason RE, Likar I: A new system of multiple-lead exercise electrocardiography. Am Heart J 71: 196–205, 1966.
25. Miranda CP, Liu J, Kadar A, et al: Usefulness of exercise-induced ST-segment depression in the inferior leads during exercise testing as a marker for coronary artery disease. Am J Cardiol 69:303–307, 1992.
26. Morris CK, Ueshima K, Kawaguchi T, et al: The prognostic value of exercise capacity: A review of the literature. Am Heart J 122:1423–1431, 1991.
27. Myers J: Essentials of Cardiopulmonary Exercise Testing. Champaign, IL, Human Kinetics, 1996.
28. Myers NJ: Perception of chest pain during exercise testing in patients with coronary artery disease. Med Sci Sports Exerc 26:1082–1086, 1994.
29. Myers J, Buchanan N, Smith D, et al: Individualized ramp treadmill: Observations on a new protocol. Chest 101:2305–2415, 1992.
30. Myers J, Buchanan N, Walsh D, et al: Comparison of the ramp versus standard exercise protocols. J Am Coll Cardiol 17:1334–1342, 1991.
31. Myers J, Froelicher VF: Optimizing the exercise test for pharmacologic studies in patients with angina pectoris. In Ardissino D, Savonitto S, Opie LH (eds): Drug Evaluation in Angina Pectoris. Pavia, Italy, Kluwer Academic, 1994, pp 41–52.
32. Myers J, Froelicher VF: Optimizing the exercise test for pharmacological investigations. Circulation 82:1839–1846, 1990.
33. Myers J, Walsh D, Buchanan N, et al: Can maximal cardiopulmonary capacity be recognized by a plateau in oxygen uptake? Chest 96:1312–1316, 1989.
34. Myers J, Walsh D, Sullivan M, et al: Effect of sampling on variability and plateau in oxygen uptake. J Appl Physiol 68:404–410, 1990.
35. Noakes T: Implications of exercise testing for prediction of athletic performance: A contemporary perspective. Med Sci Sports Exerc 20:319–330, 1988.
36. Panza J, Quyyumi AA, Diodati JG, et al: Prediction of the frequency and duration of ambulatory myocardial ischemia in patients with stable coronary disease by determination of the ischemia threshold from exercise testing: Importance of the exercise protocol. J Am Coll Cardiol 17:657–663, 1991.
37. Philbrick JT, Horowitz RJ, Feinstein AR: Methodological problems of exercise testing for coronary artery disease: Groups, analysis and bias. Am J Cardiol 64:1117–1122, 1989.
38. Ranhosky A, Kempthorne-Rawson J: The safety of intravenous dipyridamole thallium myocardial perfusion imaging. Circulation 81:1205–1209, 1990.
39. Rautaharju PM, Prineas RJ, Crow RS, et al: The effect of modified limb positions on electrocardiographic wave amplitudes. J Electrocardiol 13:109–114, 1980.
40. Redwood DR, Rosing DR, Goldstein RE, et al: Importance of the design of an exercise protocol in the evaluation of patients with angina pectoris. Circulation 43:618–628, 1971.
41. Schlant R, Friesinger GC, Leonard JJ: Clinical competence in exercise testing: A statement for physicians from the ACP/ACC/AHA Task Force on clinical privileges in cardiology. Circulation 82:1884–1888, 1990.
42. Schwade J, Blomqvist G, Shapiro W: A comparison of the response to arm and leg work in patients with ischemic heart disease. Am Heart J 94:203–208, 1977.
43. Senaratne MPJ, Hsu L, Rossall RE, Kappagoda T: Exercise testing after myocardial infarction: Relative values of the low-level pre-discharge and the post-discharge exercise test. J Am Coll Cardiol 12:141–146, 1988.
44. Severi S, Picano E, Michelassi C, et al: Diagnostic and prognostic value of dipyridamole echocardiography in patients with suspected coronary artery disease: Comparison with exercise electrocardiography. Circulation 89:1160–1173, 1994.
45. Shaw DJ, Crawford MS, Karliner JS, et al: Arm-crank ergometry: A new method for the evaluation of coronary heart disease. Am J Cardiol 33:801–805, 1974.
46. Stachenfeld NS, Eskenazi M, Gleim GW, et al: Predictive accuracy of criteria used to assess maximal oxygen consumption. Am Heart J 123:922, 1992.
47. Stuart RJ, Ellestad MH: National survey of exercise stress testing facilities. Chest 77:94–97, 1980.

48. Sullivan M, McKirnan MD: Errors in predicting functional capacity for postmyocardial infarction patients using a modified Bruce protocol. Am Heart J 107:486–491, 1984.

49. Tamesis B, Stelken A, Byers S, et al: Comparison of the asymptomatic cardiac ischemia pilot versus Bruce and Cornell exercise protocols. Am J Cardiol 72:715–720, 1993.

50. Thompson P: The safety of exercise testing and participation. In American College of Sports Medicine: Resource Manual for Guidelines for Exercise Testing and Prescription, 2nd ed. Philadelphia, Lea & Febiger, 1993, pp 359–363.

51. Webster MWI, Sharpe DN: Exercise testing in angina pectoris: The importance of protocol design in clinical trials. Am Heart J 117:505–508, 1989.

52. Whipp BJ, Davis JA, Torres F, Wasserman K: A test to determine parameters of aerobic function during exercise. J Appl Physiol 50:217–221, 1981.

53. Wicks JR, Sutton JR, Oldridge NB, Jones NL: Comparison of the electrocardiographic changes induced by maximum exercise testing with treadmill and cycle ergometer. Circulation 57:1066–1069, 1978.

54. Wilson RF, Laughlin DE, Ackell PH, et al: Transluminal, subselective measurement of coronary artery blood flow velocity and vasodilator reserve in man. Circulation 72:82–92, 1985.

55. Yang JC, Wesley RC, Froelicher VF: Ventricular tachycardia during routine treadmill testing: Risk and prognosis. Arch Intern Med 151:349–353, 1991.

NELS L. CARLSON, MD

HANS L. CARLSON, MD

WALTER FRONTERA, MD, PhD

5

Cardiac Dysfunction

CARDIAC REHABILITATION AND EXERCISE PROTOCOLS

Coronary artery disease is the leading cause of morbidity and mortality in the United States.[37] Myocardial infarction (MI) is the most significant ischemic syndrome of the heart. Postmyocardial infarction exercise programs can improve quality of life, exercise tolerance, risk factors, and return to work status.[26] For these reasons cardiac rehabilitation programs are recommended for patients with coronary artery disease and MI, but they also can benefit patients with other cardiac problems. This chapter presents a set of general guidelines regarding exercise prescription in cardiac rehabilitation. The reader is encouraged to review the many sources that detail the fundamentals of exercise testing, prescription, monitoring, and follow-up involved in cardiac rehabilitation programs.[1,2,22,46,47]

EPIDEMIOLOGY, PATHOLOGY, AND PATHOPHYSIOLOGY OF CORONARY ARTERY DISEASE

Risk factors for coronary artery disease can be thought of as modifiable and nonmodifiable. The risk factors that cannot be altered are male gender, age, a positive family history of coronary artery disease in a close relative before the age of 55, or a positive past history of previous coronary artery disease, peripheral vascular disease, or cerebrovascular disease. The modifiable risk factors that offer the opportunity for intervention include hypertension, cigarette smoking, low high-density lipoprotein cholesterol, hypertriglyceridemia, hypercholesterolemia, high lipoprotein A, obesity, diabetes, and inactivity.[37]

The major mechanism of MI is coronary atherosclerosis. Atherosclerotic plaques most commonly affect the coronary arteries, popliteal arteries, internal carotid arteries, and abdominal and thoracic aorta.[48] An initial endothelial injury may lead to the development of the atherosclerosis. This injury may be caused by trauma, hyperlipidemia, hypertension, tobacco use, or vessel injury related to diabetes.[48] The atheromatous plaques form as a response to the endothelial injury and are made of superficial connective tissue, smooth muscle cells, and leukocytes with a necrotic center.[48]

Myocardial ischemia, a result of myocardial oxygen supply not meeting myocardial oxygen demand, can be caused by decreased coronary blood flow related to atherosclerosis or vasospasm. Increased myocardial oxygen demand can be caused by hypertrophy, tachycardia, periods of high stress, or digestion after meals.[30] Decreased oxygen transport can result from respiratory disease, anemia, carbon monoxide poisoning, or other factors.[48] Ischemic heart disease can present as angina, MI, or sudden cardiac death. MIs can be transmural or subendocardial.

HISTORY OF CARDIAC REHABILITATION

Job-related exercise was noted to decrease the incidence of coronary disease in public transportation and postal workers in England in the 1950s. It was also found that people with more sedentary jobs could have lower risk of coronary heart disease if their physical activity away from work was more intense.[3] Similar results were discovered with longshoreman in San Francisco. Workers in high activity levels had less risk of coronary heart disease than sedentary workers independent of other risk factors or previous MI.[3] These observations, among others, provided a basis for exercise as a primary prevention for coronary artery disease.

Lifestyle risk factors for developing coronary artery disease have been identified, and there is evidence that behavioral changes can affect the progression of atherosclerosis. Exercise after MI developed with early mobilization programs during the acute hospitalization. These programs were shown to give both psychological and physical benefits without increasing the risk of cardiac complications.[26] Risk stratification is needed to identify the level of activity appropriate for these patients.[2]

Secondary prevention of coronary artery disease and other cardiac problems in the form of a structured, comprehensive cardiac rehabilitation program can have many benefits. It is estimated that up to two-thirds of patients who may benefit from cardiac rehabilitation do not take part in a program, possibly due to lack of access, referral, interest, or funding.[59] With the increased aging population, more patients with coronary artery disease and cardiac dysfunction will be candidates for cardiac rehabilitation programs. More primary care physicians are playing a role and may be needed with cardiac rehabilitation programs. There is opportunity for risk factor modification and exercise guideline intervention in many patients in the outpatient setting.[38]

COMPONENTS OF CARDIAC REHABILITATION

Cardiac rehabilitation incorporates several key program components into different phases of a patient's event and rehabilitation progression. The components of cardiac rehabilitation are exercise training, risk factor modification, and education and counseling regarding the patient's return to normal activities.[7] The phases of rehabilitation are generally described after MI or coronary artery bypass graft (CABG) procedures. Phase 1 is the inpatient phase. Phase 2 incorporates the progression of exercise training, return to full activity, and diet and lifestyle changes. Phase 3, the maintenance phase, includes continuation of the exercise program, risk factor modifications, and other adjustments for leisure and work activities.[37]

There are several benefits of exercise in patients with cardiac problems. An exercise training program shows trends for improved survival following MI.[7] Exercise training can improve peak functional capacity as well as submaximal capacity.[7] This allows a patient to perform a similar workload at a lower myocardial oxygen demand or rate-pressure product, which can translate to decreased ischemia at submaximal activities.[7] Return to work may be facilitated as the patient's perception of his or her activity level can be favorable with an exercise program. Exercise can favorably affect other coronary risk factors in conjunction with alterations in diet and a weight reduction program, including in patients with abnormal lipid profiles, hypertension, or diabetes.

Risk factor modification is an essential part of the cardiac rehabilitation program. Altering the cholesterol, triglyceride, and lipoprotein levels in conjunction with the rest of a cardiac rehabilitation program may decrease recurrent events and lead to improvement of atherosclerosis.[7,37] Management of lipid levels is optimized with a program of diet, nutritional counseling, exercise, weight reduction, and medications. Specific nutritional programs have been developed, and rehabilitation programs can benefit from the input and recommendations of a dietitian.[7] Smoking cessation is another priority of the rehabilitation program. This may be a requirement prior to entry to a program or facilitated during the program. Smoking cessation can be enhanced by interventions including education, medical treatments, and counseling.

Patients and their families need to make many adaptations following cardiac dysfunction. Depression and anxiety are not uncommon following MI.[7] There also may be problems of sexual dysfunction or anxiety, stress, vocational concerns, alcohol or drug abuse, or family or marital problems. These issues can adversely affect compliance and success with rehabilitation, return to work, morbidity, and mortality.[1] The rehabilitation program should offer resources to assess, counsel, and refer to more specialized interventions when necessary.[1]

Phase 1 of cardiac rehabilitation begins at admission and continues until discharge. The goals of this phase of rehabilitation are to provide the patient with education regarding his or her illness, the benefit of medication, exercise, and risk factor modification and to assess cardiovascular function and optimize the treatment plan. Early mobilization and self-care skills and daily physical activity guidelines and work restrictions are required prior to discharge.[1] The duration of this stage is variable.

Phase 2 is typically thought of as the structured outpatient phase. Although some protocols divide this into an immediate and an intermediate phase,[1] but for this overview, they are considered a single phase. The goals of the structured outpatient phase is to begin and monitor exercise training, lifestyle changes, and return to normal activity. Initially after discharge the exercise program is supervised with electrocardiogram (ECG) monitoring as well as intense risk factor modification and education programs. As the rehabilitation progresses, exercise monitoring may be needed if the patient is symptomatic. Patients are taught to follow their heart rate, perceived exertion, or level of metabolic equivalents (METs) for the safe level of activity with exercise or work. Further risk factor reduction and psychological support is given.

Phase 3, or the maintenance phase of cardiac rehabilitation, is the final and ongoing part of the program. During this stage it is up to the patient to follow his or her exercise program, diet, and activity modifications and restrictions, if necessary. Follow-up is required on occasion to alter components of the program. Compliance is dependent on the patient's previous medical history, occupation, use of leisure time, and cigarette smoking.[7] Program-dependent factors include convenience of follow-up and the ability to meet the specific concerns and provide adequate follow-up to the patient.[7]

INDICATIONS FOR CARDIAC REHABILITATION

Patients who can benefit from cardiac rehabilitation include those with MI that was followed by CABG, cardiac transplantation, valvular surgery, or percutaneous transluminal coronary angioplasty, or those with heart failure or coronary artery disease. Patients with several modifiable cardiac risk factors or decreased exercise tolerance to meet activities of daily living can benefit from a structured cardiac rehabilitation program.[7]

Cardiac rehabilitation is most commonly used following MI. Early mobilization has the benefits of decreased anxiety and depression and helping to prevent deconditioning.[26,37] Exercise training can allow the patient to increase his or her exercise tolerance. This is secondary to a decreased rate-pressure product.[26] Other potential benefits of exercise training include improved myocardial oxygen uptake by improved myocardial arteriovenous oxygen difference, improved collateral circulation, and decreased atherosclerotic plaques when combined with dieting.[26] An exercise program can help to decrease modifiable risk factors and improve return to work status.[37]

For patients with angina, cardiac rehabilitation helps to increase their work capacity. These patients also can benefit from lifestyle changes and risk factor modifications.[37] Patients with variant angina may benefit from a structured cardiac rehabilitation program following medical management.[26]

There are many benefits of cardiac rehabilitation following coronary artery bypass surgery. Early mobilization can begin 24 hours after grafting and will prevent the deleterious effects of bed rest and decrease the risk of deep venous thrombosis.[26] These patients generally have been without recent MIs prior to surgery and make good candidates for rehabilitation.

For many of the same reasons, patients who have undergone percutaneous transluminal angioplasty may undergo an exercise training and risk factor modification program. Restenoses can occur with angioplasty, and the rehabilitation program will improve the patient's work capacity and decrease the factors associated with atherosclerosis.[26]

Although patients with poor ejection fractions have not been felt to do well with exercise, a carefully graded exercise program may be beneficial.[26] Improved oxygen extraction efficiency, increased work capacity, and decreased submaximal heart rates can give patients improved exercise tolerance.[37] Patients also may do well after surgical repair of valvular heart disease; they may be quite deconditioned as a result of their poor function prior to repair. Patients taking anticoagulants may not be able to participate in vigorous exercise.[26]

Cardiac transplantation patients have unique challenges following surgery. The resting heart rate will be higher and the heart rate with exercise will be lower than normals.[37] At maximal effort the patients will have a lower work capacity, which can be improved with exercise training.[37]

While the above groups of patients may do well with exercise and lifestyle changes, some groups of patients should not begin an exercise program, including patients with unstable angina, severe aortic outflow obstruction, acute myocarditis or pericarditis, uncontrolled complex arrhythmias, active congestive heart failure, recent thrombophlebitis or pulmonary embolism, untreated third-degree heart block, unresponsive severe hypertension, uncontrolled diabetes, and acute infections.[26]

HISTORY AND PHYSICAL EXAMINATION

A careful history and physical examination is necessary to help determine the need for rehabilitation, to assess the risk for complications during an exercise program, and to guide the type and intensity of the exercise prescription.

Key components to the history include the patient's family history of cardiac abnormalities, the patient's history of cardiac risk factors, symptoms of cardiac dysfunction, activity level, previous medical problems, and work-up and current medications. An assessment of the family history should include coronary artery disease before age 55, hypercholesterolemia, sudden death, arrhythmias, and congenital abnormalities such as Marfan's disease or hypertrophic cardiomyopathies. An evaluation of the patient's current or previous smoking history as well as lifestyle and alcohol or other substance abuse should be taken. Questions directed to screening for possible cardiac conditions include a history of chest pain, hypertension, shortness of breath, paroxysmal nocturnal dyspnea, fatigue, heart palpitations, dizziness, lightheadedness or syncopal episodes, and the associated activity level. Also necessary is a careful history of current and previous medications.[37]

The history unrelated to cardiovascular abnormalities also will be helpful in guiding the exercise program. Patients with orthopedic, neurologic, or other disabilities may need modifications to the type and duration of exercise.[8]

The physical examination is an essential part of patient assessment prior to beginning an exercise program. The key components of the cardiac examination include the hemodynamic status and evaluation for orthostasis. Cardiac auscultation provides information on rhythm, valvular, or septal irregularities. Assessment of the neck veins for jugular venous distention, the extremities for edema, and the lung fields for rales can indicate congestive heart failure. Beyond the cardiac examination, the physical examination can provide information relevant to potential complications with exercise. Congenital syndromes with characteristic signs such as Down syndrome and Marfan's syndrome can have cardiac abnormalities. Signs of thyroid disease, lipid abnormalities, or vascular disorders can be detected on physical examination.[37]

RISK STRATIFICATION

Risk stratification to classify patients according to the likelihood of having an adverse cardiac event is important prior to beginning an exercise program. Stratification may be based on an initial health factor screening process. Initial risk stratification is useful for early triage of patients into appropriate diagnostic or therapeutic pathways.

Major coronary risk factors are as follows:

- Age—men older than 45 and women older than 55

- Family history of myocardial infarction or sudden death before age 55 in father or other male first-degree male relative; or before age 65 in mother or other first-degree female relative

- Current cigarette smoking

- Hypertension—blood pressure ≥ 140/90 or on antihypertensive medication

- Hypercholesterolemia—total serum cholesterol > 200 mg/dL or high-density lipoprotein < 35 mg/dL

- Diabetes mellitus

TABLE 1. Risk Stratification Guidelines

Low Risk:	Uncomplicated clinical hospital course
	No evidence of myocardial ischemia
	Functional capacity ≥ 7 METs
	Normal left ventricular function (EF > 50%)
	Absence of significant ventricular ectopy
Moderate Risk:	ST segment depression ≥ 2 mm flat or downsloping
	Reversible thallium defects
	Moderate to good left ventricular function (EF 35–49%)
	Changing pattern of or new development of angina pectoris
High Risk:	Prior myocardial infarction or infarct involving ≥ 35% of left ventricle
	EF < 35% at rest
	Fall in exercise systolic blood pressure or failure of systolic blood pressure to rise more than 10 mm Hg on exercise tolerance test
	Persistent or recurrent ischemic pain 24 hours or more after hospital admission
	Functional capacity < 5 METs with hypotensive blood pressure response or ≥ 1 mm ST segment depression
	Congestive heart failure syndrome in hospital
	ST segment depression ≥ 2 mm at peak heart rate ≤ 135 bpm
	High-grade ventricular ectopy

EF = ejection fraction
bpm = beats per minute
Adapted from American Association of Cardiovascular and Pulmonary Rehabilitation: Guidelines for Cardiac Rehabilitation Programs. Champaign, IL, Human Kinetics, 1995.

- Sedentary lifestyle and physical inactivity.[2] Signs or symptoms of cardiopulmonary disease include (1) pain, discomfort, or anginal equivalent in the chest, neck, jaw, or arm; (2) shortness of breath at rest or with mild exertion; (3) dizziness or syncope; (4) orthopnea or paroxysmal nocturnal dyspnea; (5) ankle edema; (6) palpitations or tachycardia; (7) intermittent claudication; (8) known heart failure; or (9) unusual fatigue or shortness of breath with usual activities.[2]

When patients have known cardiac disease, risk stratification is important in assessing the level of risk for a future cardiac event during cardiac rehabilitation. Risk stratification will help to determine the duration, frequency, intensity, and type of the exercise involved in the rehabilitation program and the supervision and monitoring that will be required. Risk stratification is based on a variety of factors, including extent of myocardial damage, left ventricular function, presence or absence of residual myocardial ischemia, and ventricular arrhythmias. Guidelines for assessing risk include ECG findings, exercise testing, echocardiography, and ambulatory ECG monitoring.[14,15] An example of a set of guidelines for risk stratification for cardiac patients from the American Association of Cardiovascular and Pulmonary Rehabilitation is shown in Table 1.

Risk stratification is not only important for appropriately prescribing exercise, but it is also important in determining further work-up. Patients at higher risk also may require additional diagnostic and therapeutic interventions.

EXERCISE PRESCRIPTION

The components of exercise prescription are outlined in the American College of Sports Medicine's *Guidelines for Exercise Testing and Prescription.*[2] The exercise should be any activity that is aerobic, is rhythmic, uses large muscle groups, and can be maintained over time. The intensity of the exercise will depend on the phase of rehabilitation and can be prescribed by heart rate, rating of perceived exertion, or METs. The duration will vary from 3–5 minutes in the inpatient phase, to 20–30 minutes as an outpatient, and may progress to more than an hour. The frequency as an inpatient may be one to three sessions per day. In the outpatient and maintenance phases, frequency may be scaled back to a minimum of three times per week with a rest day and a longer-duration exercise program. The rate of progression will depend on the patient's exercise tolerance and goals. It may be increased by duration initially and by intensity later.[2]

Resistance training once was felt to be unsafe in cardiac rehabilitation in light of the risk of ischemia and ventricular arrhythmias with increased blood pressure of dynamic and isometric muscle contractions.[1] There may be specific cardiac benefits to resistance training, including decreased rate-pressure product and myocardial oxygen consumption as a result of a decreased heart rate with maximal resistance training.[1] Resistance training may help control risk factors such as hypertension, glucose tolerance, insulin sensitivity, and lipid and lipoprotein levels.[1] Guidelines for a resistance training program should be similar to those of the aerobic exercise program in that they should be individualized, monitored for hemodynamic status and ECG abnormalities, and the perceived exertion and rate-pressure product should not be higher than the aerobic exercise.[1,2] Contraindications for resistance training include congestive heart failure, uncontrolled arrhythmias, severe valvular disease, uncontrolled hypertension, or an aerobic capacity of less than five METs.[1]

In general, the exercise prescription consists of mode of exercise, frequency, duration, and intensity. The exercise program needs to be continuously reevaluated to progress these components of the rehabilitation program.

MODE

The mode of exercise is the activity or activities in which the patient will be participating. The exercise mode should be specific for the type of physiologic gains that are to be achieved. Because specificity of training is important, exercises that overload the oxygen transport system, require the use of large muscle groups, and are continuous in nature are well suited for cardiovascular conditioning.[22] The greatest gains in maximal oxygen uptake are derived from these types of activities.[2] Examples include walking, jogging, running, swimming, bicycling, and aerobics. The American College of Sports Medicine divides cardiorespiratory endurance activities into three categories (Table 2). It may be helpful to start with group 1 activities when prescribing an exercise program for a novice.

Important considerations in selecting the mode of exercise include facilities and equipment, safety, and compliance. Activities such as walking or jogging require little equipment except a comfortable pair of athletic shoes. On the other hand, bicycling and swimming are more demanding in terms of equipment, facilities, and safety. For example, before beginning a swimming program, care should be taken to ensure that the patient is an adequate swimmer. Before beginning a road cycling program, the patient should be well versed in traffic safety, bicycle hand signals, and protective equipment such as helmets, reflectors, and lights. Compliance is also an often overlooked but important issue. The best planned exercise program is of little use if the patient does not regularly participate in it. If the exercise program involves activities that interest the patient, compliance will likely be improved. Cross-training also may be a useful technique not only to increase compliance by altering the daily activities but to minimize musculoskeletal overload.[4] Resistance training may be beneficial in exercise prescription in cardiac rehabilitation, but one must understand the physiologic effects of these activities. Increased maximal oxygen uptake, the primary objective in order to increase cardiorespiratory endurance, is not achieved with weight training.[2] Left ventricular volume overload is achieved through continuous, aerobic-type activities such as walking or running. These activities decrease peripheral resistance, increase cardiac output, and improve ventricular function. Left ventricular pressure overload occurs with heavy resistance or isometric activities. Increased pressor responses, Valsalva maneuvers, and arrhythmias also may occur with heavy resistance activities.[22]

The need for proper instruction in resistance training technique is well illustrated in a recent study of breathing techniques on blood pressure responses in healthy individuals. During resistance training with Valsalva maneuvers, an average blood pressure response of 311/284 mm Hg was observed during maximal lifting. This was reduced to 198/175 mm Hg with exhalation during the lifting phase.[39] Circuit resistance train-

TABLE 2. Grouping of Cardiorespiratory Endurance Activities

Group 1	Group 2	Group 3
Interindividual variation in energy expenditure is relatively low. Desirable for more precise control of exercise intensity. Examples of these activities are walking and cycling, especially treadmill and cycle ergometry.	The rate of energy expenditure is highly related to skill. Examples include swimming and cross-country skiing.	Activities where both skill and intensity of exercise are highly variable. Examples of these activities are racquet sports and basketball.

Adapted from American College of Sports Medicine: ACSM's Guidelines for Exercise Testing and Prescription. Baltimore, Williams & Wilkins, 1995.

ing is an important component in an exercise program[2] and should be considered as an addition to any exercise regime. In secondary prevention of coronary artery disease, low-resistance activities have beneficial effects for high-risk cardiac patients.[20,25,52)

FREQUENCY

The frequency of the exercise program for asymptomatic healthy adults is generally recommended to be three to five sessions per week.[2,4,58] Recent guidelines suggest that, for primary prevention, the person should exercise on most or all days of the week for at least 30 minutes at moderate intensity.[54] Training regimens of less than 2 days per week do not show meaningful increases in cardiopulmonary function measured as maximal oxygen uptake.[6] Maximal oxygen uptake is considered to be the best measurement of cardiorespiratory fitness.[54] Improvements in maximal oxygen intake begin to level off with training more than three times per week and are negligible with more than five sessions per week.[6] Increasing frequency also increases the risk of musculoskeletal injury.[43]

Despite the minimal gains in cardiorespiratory improvement noted with exercise more than 3 days per week, more frequent sessions may be desirable if weight reduction is also a goal of the exercise prescription. Exercising fewer than 3 days per week leads to little or no loss of body weight or body fat.[5,44] In asymptomatic patients with low baseline fitness levels, exercise frequency may be two or more short sessions every day. Another option is to alternate into the exercise program less vigorous exercise sessions, such as slow walking and stretching every other session.[47] Patients in the initial phase of cardiac rehabilitation also may require more frequent, shorter-duration exercise sessions. During early rehabilitation after a cardiac event, the frequency of mobilization in the first 1–3 days may be three to four sessions of short duration each day. This can gradually be reduced to about two sessions of longer duration each day.[2]

DURATION

The duration of the exercise session (Table 3) depends on the frequency and intensity of the program and whether the goal is primary or secondary prevention of cardiac disease. General guidelines for healthy adults are 20–60 minutes of continuous aerobic activity per session.[6] In patients with coronary artery disease, warm-up and cool-down periods of at least 10 minutes with an intervening exercise duration of 20–40 minutes is recommended.[4] The warm-up and cool-down periods are very important and should not be neglected. Undesirable effects of sudden, abrupt onset of vigorous exercise that decrease with an adequate warm-up period include ischemic ST depression,[10] ventricular ectopy,[11] and decreased left ventricular ejection fraction.[23] The cool-down period is important to maintain venous return, remove lactic acid, facilitate heat dissipation, and reduce the potential for hypotension.[58]

Early in the course of the exercise program, it may be beneficial to increase the duration of the activity and decrease the intensity in order to condition the musculoskeletal system and to avoid injuries.[22] The total workload should remain the same.

INTENSITY

Intensity may be the single most important factor in exercise prescription for primary and secondary prevention of cardiovascular disease. Exercise intensity can be described in many ways, the most common being percentage of heart rate, perceived exertion, and amount of energy expenditure. When prescribing the intensity of exercise, it should be remembered that total work performed is a function of both intensity and duration; therefore, a lower-intensity, longer-duration activity will provide a similar amount of total energy expenditure as a higher-intensity, shorter-duration activity. Because higher-intensity exercise has been associated with increased cardiovascular risk, increased likelihood of orthopedic injuries, and lower compliance, exercise of low to moderate intensity and longer-duration activities are usually prescribed.[6] For improving cardiorespiratory fitness, the exercise intensity should exceed 60% of the maximal heart rate or 50% of the maximal oxygen uptake. Recommended intensity levels there-

TABLE 3.   Cardiac Rehabilitation: Duration of Components in the Exercise Program

Component	Phase	Duration (min)
Warm-up	1	15–20
	2, 3	10–15
Muscular conditioning	2, 3	10–20
Aerobic exercise	1	5–20
	2	10–60
	2, 3	30–60
Cool-down	1, 3	5–15

From Pollock ML, Schmidt DH: Heart Disease and Rehabilitation. Champaign, IL, Human Kinetics, 1995, with permission.

fore are 60–90% of maximal heart rate or 50–85% of maximal oxygen uptake.[6] Intensities below these levels may be beneficial to increase cardiorespiratory endurance in individuals with low initial fitness levels.[47]

Heart Rate

Heart rate is the common standard for exercise intensity prescription in cardiac disease prevention and rehabilitation.[2,6,47] Target heart rates are usually set at 60–90% of the maximal heart rate for healthy, asymptomatic adults[2] and 55–90% of the maximal heart rate for patients with coronary artery disease.[4] One of the advantages of heart rate monitoring for exercise intensity is that it is an easily obtainable, objective measurement. The heart rate is also a useful guide to exercise intensity due to the relatively linear relationship between heart rate and maximal oxygen consumption.[2] In determining the intensity of exercise as a function of heart rate, the maximal heart rate needs to be established. One method is to estimate the maximal heart rate using the age-adjusted equation of 220 minus the patient's age: $HR_{max} = 220 - age$.[58] The variability of predicted maximal heart rate using this method is high, and it therefore may significantly under- or overestimate the maximal heart rate. This method is not recommended in cardiac patients.[27] The maximal heart rate is usually determined by an exercise test,[2,6,7,35] which is best used when the exercise test is stopped because the patient is fatigued. If the test is stopped at a submaximal level due to cardiac signs or symptoms, a heart rate of five to ten beats per minute (bpm) less than that at which onset of signs or symptoms occurs is recommended. The target heart rate may then be set as the exercise test-determined maximal heart rate multiplied by the desired training percentage.[27] This target heart rate can be about 70–85% of the maximal heart rate in cardiac patients.[33] A more accurate estimation of maximal oxygen uptake is the heart rate reserve method, also known as the Karvonen formula.[45] In the Karvonen formula, the target heart rate is equal to the product of the maximal heart rate as determined by an exercise test, minus the resting heart rate, multiplied by the training percent (in this case 60–80%), and then added to the resting heart rate: $THR = [(HR_{max} - HR_{rest}) \times (0.60 \text{ to } 0.80)] + HR_{rest}$.[32]

Perceived Exertion

The second method of prescribing exercise intensity uses ratings of perceived exertion (RPE). There are limitations to heart rate prescription. Heart rate response may be altered by emotional response or by medication.[16] Measured maximum heart rates also may show a large degree of variation.[34] If an RPE is to be used, however, it should be used in addition to target heart rate and not as a substitution for target heart rate.[2] Prescribing exercise intensity in a patient with a heart transplant may be based on perceived exertion because the heart is denervated.[9] A commonly used system is the Borg RPE scale.[12,40] The usual exercise intensity associated with physiologic adaptation on the Borg RPE scale is 12–16. In inpatient cardiac rehabilitation, the Borg RPE should be less than 13.[2]

The target RPE may be determined from a maximal exercise test as the RPE that corresponds to the desired percentage of maximum heart rate or oxygen consumption. For example, if the desired training intensity is at 70% of the maximal heart rate and the patient's perceived exertion at this heart rate during a maximal treadmill test is 14, the target RPE is 14. A method of determining target RPE from submaximal treadmill tests has been described and validated on cardiac rehabilitation patients.[18,19]

Energy Expenditure

The third method of prescribing exercise intensity uses energy expenditure. Maximal oxygen uptake can be determined during a graded exercise test by analyzing expired oxygen and carbon dioxide. Maximal oxygen uptake is measured as ml O_2/kg lean body weight/min. In this method the target heart rate is set as the heart rate that corresponds to 60–70% of the maximal oxygen uptake.[58] METs may also be used to set a target heart rate. One MET is equal to 3.5 ml O_2/kg/min.[57] METs can be estimated from the workload achieved on a graded exercise test.[42] Energy costs of many activities have been studied, and tables exist that detail these costs.[2] For a baseline of about 60% of functional capacity, the target MET level is equal to 0.60 multiplied by the maximal MET level divided by 100, and that product is then multiplied by the maximal MET level: target METs = (0.60 × max METs/100) × max MET. Exercise intensity based on absolute values of energy expenditure, such as in MET tables, is not recommended for preventive and rehabilitation programs because the original data cannot be extrapolated to 20- to 60-minute regimens of exercise training.[6] If target MET values are to be used to direct intensity of training, additional heart rate monitoring is suggested because MET tables may not accurately reflect an individual patient's energy expenditures.[58]

SUMMARY

The exercise prescription for primary prevention of cardiac disease (Table 4) should be participation in an aerobic, continuous activity using large muscle groups for three to five sessions per week, 20–60 minutes per session, at 60–90% of maximum heart rate. In cardiac populations, exercise should be aerobic, continuous activities using large muscle groups three to five times per week, 20–40 minutes per session, with an additional 10–20 minutes of warm-up and 10 minutes of cool-down, at about 55–90% of maximal heart rate as determined by a maximal graded exercise test.

PROGRESSION OF THE EXERCISE PROGRAM

HEALTHY ADULTS

Progression of the exercise program is an important part of the exercise prescription. In healthy adults, the rate of progression is influenced by the patient's functional capacity, medical status, age, and goals.[2] The three stages of progression in the endurance portion of the exercise prescription are the initial stage, the improvement stage, and the maintenance stage.[2] In cardiac patients, the initial training workload will be lower, and the rate of progression will be slower than in healthy adults.[47]

The initial stage in healthy adults usually lasts 4–6 weeks and should be focused on developing low levels of muscular endurance with modes of activity that avoid muscle soreness, discomfort, and injury. The intensity of the exercise should be approximately

TABLE 4. General Guidelines for Exercise Prescription

	Primary Prevention	Secondary Prevention
Activity:	Continuous, aerobic, involving large muscle groups (e.g., walking, biking, jogging, swimming, running, weight training)	Activities for Primary Prevention also apply here
Duration:	20–60 minutes per session	20–40 minutes per session with a 10-minute warm-up period and a 10-minute cool-down period
Frequency:	Most/all days of week	3–5 sessions per week
Intensity:		
1. Heart Rate:	Max HR may be determined by 220 − age = max HR 60–90% of max HR, (usually ~ 70–85% max HR) - or - Karvonen formula: HR = (max HR − rest HR) × (0.60 to 0.90) + rest HR - or - HR at 60–80% of maximal oxygen uptake	General inpatient criteria if no maximal exercise test Post myocardial infarction: HR < 120 bpm or rest HR + 20 bpm Post-coronary artery bypass graft: HR rest + 30 bpm HR based on maximal exercise test limited by cardiac signs/symptoms: HR 10 bpm below anginal or ischemic threshold HR based on maximal exercise test limited by fatigue: ~70–85% of max HR
2. Perceived Exertion:	RPE of 12–16 on on Borg scale	Intensity should not be based on RPE alone but used in conjunction with HR monitoring Inpatients: RPE < 13 on Borg scale Outpatients: RPE that corresponds to ~ 70–85% of max HR determined by maximal exercise test

HR = heart rate
bpm = beats per minute
RPE = rating of perceived exertion

40–60% of maximal oxygen uptake or heart rate reserve, as calculated by the Karvonen formula. Frequency of sessions should be three times per week on nonconsecutive days with an initial duration of 12–15 minutes that gradually increases to 20 minutes.[2]

The improvement stage of the program usually lasts 4–5 months. Intensity should be approximately 65–85% of maximal oxygen uptake or heart rate reserve. Duration of sessions should be gradually increased over 2- to 3-week periods until each session is 20–30 minutes of continuous aerobic exercise. Exercise frequency should gradually

---

TABLE 5. Guidelines for Exercise Prescriptions for Cardiac Patients

Phase	Frequency	Intensity	Duration	Activity
1	2–3 times/day	MI: RHR + 20 CABG: RHR + 20	MI: 5–20 min CABG: 10–30 min	Range of motion, bike, treadmill, one flight stairs
2	1–2 times/day	MI: RHR + 20, RPE 13 CABG: RHR + 20, RPE 13 (6–8 weeks after surgery or event, intensity is based on 70% maximum heart rate reserve, using a symptom-limited exercise treadmill test to determine maximum heart rate)	MI: 20–60 min CABG: 30–60 min	Range of motion, bike, treadmill, weight training, arm ergometry
3	3–5 times/week	70–85% maximum heart rate reserve	30–60 min	Walk, bike, swim, weight training, calisthenics, endurance sports

MI = myocardial infarction
CABG = coronary artery bypass graft
RHR = resting heart rate
RPE = rating of perceived exertion
Adapted from Pollock ML, Schmidt DH: Heart Disease and Rehabilitation. Champaign, IL, Human Kinetics, 1995.

---

be increased from three to four sessions per week at the beginning of the improvement stage to four to five sessions per week at the end of the improvement stage.[2]

The maintenance stage begins about 6 months into the exercise program. Activities are designed for cardiorespiratory endurance, such as walking, jogging, biking, and rowing. Additional activities, such as resistance training, may be added or expanded upon based on the individual's goals. The escalation in conditioning stimulus may be continued or tapered off, depending on the participant's interest. The goal of this stage is to maintain the participant's level of conditioning, which can be done by developing an exercise program that has a similar energy cost to the last level of the improvement stage. Incorporating activities that the patient enjoys into the exercise program helps to keep the participant interested in the program.[2] Therefore, the prescription for this stage includes continuous aerobic activities using large muscle groups at intensities of about 70–85% of heart rate reserve, duration of 30–45 minutes, and frequency of at least three and up to four to five times per week.

CARDIAC PATIENTS

In cardiac patients, progression is again dependent on the patient's age, baseline fitness level, and state of health. As with healthy patients, progression can be divided into three stages: initial or starter stage, improvement or progression stage, and maintenance stage.

The initial stage introduces patients to a low-level exercise program and helps patients to adapt physiologically to that program while avoiding injury and excessive muscle soreness. This stage begins at low intensities and includes stretching, light calisthenics, and low-level aerobic exercise. Progression is done by first increasing the frequency and duration of the activity and then increasing the intensity.[47]

The progression stage should be slow, with an increase in duration and intensity of activity. The increase should occur in one or both factors approximately every 1–4 weeks. The ability of the patient to adapt to the program will dictate the rate of progression.[47] The patient initially should be placed at a level that is appropriate for his or her current functional capacity and then advanced if stable at that level for at least 1–2 weeks.[45] Progression for the cardiac patient is longer than for the healthy adult and may take 6–18 months.[47]

The maintenance stage for the cardiac patient is comparable to that for the healthy patient, except that the frequency and duration of training are greater—about 5 days per week for 30–60 minutes—to make up for the relatively decreased intensity.[47]

Rates of progression will vary depending on the condition being treated. In patients who have had an MI, the training program should not progress until 6–8 weeks after the event, and the patient should progress at a more conservative rate than a patient who has had a CABG. After this time, the intensity of the activity may increase and the exercise program may progress,[47] because scar tissue has adequately formed on the heart about 6–8 weeks after an MI.[60] In patients having undergone CABG, progression may occur more rapidly, but lifting should be limited to less than 20–25 pounds, with no more than 10 pounds being lifted overhead, in the first 6–8 weeks. This allows time for the sternum to heal properly. Patients who have had perioperative infarcts during CABG surgery should be progressed like MI patients, with conservative progression in the first 6–8 weeks.[47]

Patients who are able to achieve a functional capacity of > 5 METs (maximal oxygen uptake of 17.5 ml O_2/kg/min) prior to discharge will be able to safely participate in most activities at home and be able to respond to a faster rate of progression of the exercise program. Patients with lower functional capacities will progress more slowly; they will require shorter bouts of lower-intensity activities with intermittent rest periods.[2]

CLASSIFICATION OF CARDIAC REHABILITATION PROGRAMS

Cardiac rehabilitation has been divided into three clinical phases: phase 1 (inpatient), phase 2 (2–3 months of supervised, monitored outpatient exercise), and phase 3 (variable-length community-level supervision with intermittent or no ECG monitoring).[2,47] Additionally, some classification systems divide phase 3 into two phases, with phase IV being an outpatient exercise program with no ECG monitoring and limited supervision.[2] Table 5 summarizes the components of a cardiac rehabilitation exercise prescription for phases 1–3.

PHASE 1

Phase 1 of the cardiac rehabilitation program is implemented during the inpatient period. It typically consists of low-level exercise and patient education. A major goal of phase 1 is to reduce deconditioning brought on by prolonged bed rest.[1] Due to the decreased length of hospital stays, phase 1 has been condensed, and education and counseling regarding exercise, diet, and risk factor modification and assessment of functional tolerance to activities of daily living is becoming increasingly important.[2] Phase 1 is primarily for patients who have had an MI or have undergone a CABG. It may also include patients with stable angina or coronary artery disease risk factors or patients who have had angioplasty, heart valve surgery, or cardiac transplant.[22] The objectives of phase 1 include assisting the patient to become ambulatory, preparing the patient and family for a healthy lifestyle, reducing psychological and emotional disorders, facilitating adjustment to the environment, identifying and modifying risk factors, and creating a positive attitude to motivate the patient to make a long-term commitment.[22]

In phase 1, education and counseling are initiated immediately;[1] in the case of CABG or other planned surgery, education may begin preoperatively.[22] Exercise should begin as soon as the patient is stable, usually 1–2 days after CABG and 1–4 days after an uncomplicated MI.[22,47] Most phase 1 activities can be accomplished in the patient's room or adjacent corridors or stairwells with little more than 1- to 2-pound weights.[22]

Inpatient exercise (Table 6) must begin with the help of a physician.[22] Physical activity early in the course of cardiac rehabilitation has been shown to reduce the risk of thrombi, decrease the incidence of orthostatic hypotension, and maintain muscle tone

TABLE 6. Exercise Prescription Guidelines for Inpatient Cardiac Rehabilitation

Intensity	Duration	Frequency	Progression
RPE < 13 (6–20 scale) Post myocardial infarction: HR rest < 120 bpm or HR rest + 20 bpm (arbitrary targets) Post-Surgery: HR rest + 30 bpm (arbitrary target) To tolerance if symptomatic	Intermittent bouts lasting 3–5 minutes Rest periods at patient's discretion lasting 1–2 minutes shorter than exercise bout duration Total duration of up to 20 minutes	Early mobilization: 3–4 times per day (days 1–3) Later mobilization: 2 times per day (beginning on day 3)	Initially increase duration to 10–15 minutes of continuous exercise, then increase intensity

RPE = rating of perceived exertion
HR = heart rate
bpm = beats per minute
From American College of Sports Medicine: ACSM's Guidelines for Exercise Testing and Prescription. Baltimore, Williams & Wilkins, 1995, with permission.

and joint mobility.[2] Duration of activity is about 10–15 minutes, with a frequency of at least twice per day, and may gradually increase to 20–30 minutes up to four times per week.[22] Intensity of activity can be prescribed for MI or CABG patients as resting heart rate plus 20.[47] In cardiac transplant patients, intensity may be based on ratings of perceived exertion, specifically Borg scale ratings in the range of 11–13 due to the denervated heart.[22]

Modes of activity will include range of motion, intermittent sitting or standing, and walking.[1] Exercises usually will be active, with passive range of motion occasionally prescribed for patients with significant myocardial damage.[22] Patients having undergone CABG or percutaneous transluminal coronary angioplasty are usually exercised more aggressively because there is no permanent myocardial damage.[22] In surgical patients, ambulation may begin on the first treatment day; progression and duration of ambulation is more accelerated; and upper extremity range of motion activities are emphasized more.[47] Contraindications for exercise programs include:[2]

- Unstable angina
- Resting systolic blood pressure > 200 mm Hg or resting diastolic blood pressure > 110 mm Hg should be evaluated on a case-by-case basis
- Orthostatic blood pressure drop of > 20 mm Hg with symptoms
- Critical aortic stenosis (peak systolic pressure gradient > 50 mm Hg with aortic valve orifice area, 0.75 cm$_2$ in average-size adult
- Acute systemic illness or fever
- Uncontrolled atrial or ventricular arrhythmias
- Uncontrolled sinus tachycardia (> 120 beats/min)
- Uncompensated congestive heart failure
- Third-degree AV block (without pacemaker)
- Active pericarditis or myocarditis
- Recent embolism
- Thrombophlebitis
- Resting ST segment displacement (> 2 mm)
- Uncontrolled diabetes (resting blood glucose > 400 mg/dl)
- Severe orthopedic problems that would prohibit exercise
- Other metabolic problems, such as acute thyroiditis, hypo- or hyperkalemia, hypovolemia

Immediately before and after exercise, heart rate and blood pressure are taken and recorded.[22] ECG monitoring can usually be done with telemetry[22] and should be done through much of early phase 1 rehabilitation.[47] Criteria for terminating exercise are as follows:[22]

- Fatigue

- Light-headedness, confusion, ataxia, pallor, cyanosis, dyspnea, nausea, or peripheral circulatory insufficiency

- Onset of angina with exercise

- Symptomatic supraventricular tachycardia

- ST displacement $\geq$ 3 mm from rest

- Ventricular tachycardia

- Exercise-induced left bundle branch block

- Onset of second- or third-degree A–V block

- R on T PVCs.

- Frequent multifocal premature ventricular contractions ($>$ 30% of the complexes)

- Exercise hypotension ($>$ 20 mm Hg drop in systolic blood pressure)

- Excessive blood pressure risk: systolic $>$ 220 or diastolic $>$ 110 mm Hg

- Inappropriate bradycardia (drop in heart rate greater than 10 beats/min) with increase or no change in workload

Specific exercises, advanced in a step-wise fashion, have been described in detail, and consultation of these sources are highly recommended prior to setting up an inpatient cardiac rehabilitation program.[22,47] The rate of progression depends on the individual, but the patients usually are progressed one to two steps per day.[22,47] Early treatment may result in hypotension, a major medical problem in cardiac rehabilitation patients.[47] Table 7 lists guidelines that have been suggested and may be implemented in a cardiac rehabilitation program to avoid complications associated with hypotension. Table 8 gives examples of specific exercises that may be used for a phase 1 cardiac rehabilitation program.

Proper breathing instruction should be done by a trained member of the cardiac rehabilitation team, such as a respiratory therapist, trained nurse, or physical therapist. Instruction should include a description of diaphragmatic or "belly" breathing to avoid atelectasis of the lower lobes of the lung.[47] Patients also should be taught proper leg dangling technique, with the feet supported on a stool as the patient sits on the side of the bed, with thighs not resting on the edge of the mattress. This is to avoid decreased venous return to the heart and increased potential for blood clotting, which may occur if the thighs rest on the edge of the mattress.[47] Patients should have blood pressure monitored before and after climbing stairs. If the patient's systolic blood pressure drops more than 20 mm Hg after climbing stairs, this activity should be stopped for the day.[47]

TABLE 7. Guidelines Regarding Hypotension in Cardiac Rehabilitation

All patients will have orthostatic blood pressure measurements sitting, and 30 seconds after standing, prior to starting exercise. If a significant drop occurs, results should be verified in the other arm or by another staff member.

Symptomatic patients will not be exercised.

Systolic blood pressure should be at least 90 mm Hg prior to exercise.

If systolic blood pressure is less than 90 mm Hg, the patient will not be exercised until consulting with the attending physician or medical director of the cardiac rehabilitation program.

If the systolic blood pressure drops 10–20 mm Hg with standing and the patient is asymptomatic, the medical director will be notified before the patient exercises.

If the systolic blood pressure drops greater than 20 mm Hg with standing and the patient is asymptomatic, the attending physician will be notified prior to exercise. If the attending physician approves exercise, the medical director will be consulted prior to exercise.

Adapted from Pollock ML, Wilmore JH, Fox SM III: Exercise in Health and Disease: Evaluation and Prescription for Prevention and Rehabilitation. Philadelphia, WB Saunders, 1984.

Cardiac rehabilitation in patients who have had surgery is beneficial[51] and should include upper extremity range of motion activities. Chest wall surgery entails significant soft tissue and bony damage, and sequelae include adhesions and muscle contraction, leading to decreased strength and range of motion.[47] Range of motion exercises for the upper extremities should be designed to strengthen and stretch muscles of the shoulder girdle and the chest. Table 9 describes upper extremity exercises that may be used postoperatively. Patients should be taught proper form and technique for these exercises by a therapist prior to starting, and they initially should be supervised to ensure that they are doing the exercises correctly.

In cardiac transplant patients, passive range of motion activities may begin immediately, with an initial frequency of twice per day. Borg scale intensities of 11–13 are appropriate for transplant patients during phase 1 rehabilitation.[22] An exercise program for patients having had heart transplantations is outlined in Table 10.

Due to the decreasing length of inpatient phase 1 cardiac rehabilitation programs, step-wise progression of programs may no longer be feasible.[2] The American College of Sports Medicine has published a functional classification system to assist in prescribing activities during inpatient cardiac rehabilitation.[2] The guidelines presented in Table 11 may be useful for upper limits of intensity and patient activities.

Patient education should take place concurrently with exercise periods and nursing care as well as during dedicated education sessions. Topics should cover orientation to the exercise program; explanation of the perceived exertion scale; instruction in self-pulse monitoring; explanation of the benefits of exercise, proper nutrition, and diet; and instruction in proper breathing techniques and body mechanics.[47] A discharge goal of a functional capacity of 5 METs is desirable but may be overambitious in some cases. Patients' functional capacities may be assessed by activity performance or by a graded exercise test. Prior to discharge, the patient should be aware of activities that are appropriate and inappropriate for his or her functional capacity and be aware of what cardiovascular symptoms

---

TABLE 8. Phase 1 Exercise Program for Cardiac Rehabilitation

Five to ten repetitions of each exercise will be performed

Step 1 (1.0–1.5 METs)
Active range of motion to all extremities while lying in bed using proper breathing.
Shoulder: abduction, adduction, flexion, extension, internal and external rotation.
Hip: abduction, adduction, flexion, extension, internal and external rotation.
Knee and elbow: flexion and extension
Active foot: circling at least one time per hour.
Surgical patients: up in chair two times daily, ambulation with assistance in room.

Step 2 (1.0–1.5 METs)
Repeat all exercises as in step 1.
Surgical patients: with bed at 45° angle. Up in chair as desired at least two times daily. Short walks with assistance in room and corridor.

Step 3 (1.0–2.0 METs)
Repeat all exercises as in step 2 with mild resistance.
Surgical patients: exercises done while sitting on bed. Increase walking, chair sitting as in step 2.

Step 4 (1.5–2.0 METs)
Active range of motion to all extremities while sitting using mild resistance and proper breathing.
Shoulder: exercise done with flexed elbow (abduction, adduction, flexion, extension, internal and external rotation).
Surgical patients: up as desired in room without assistance. Longer walks in halls with assistance at least two times daily.

Step 5 (1.5–2.0 METs)
Repeat exercises of step 4 with moderate resistance and proper breathing. Walk to tolerance, not more than 50 feet.
Surgical patients: exercises in standing position with 1–2 pound weights, lateral side bends, trunk twists. Continued walking.

(Continued on facing page)

need to be reported.[2] Patients also should be aware of outpatient cardiac rehabilitation programs and, if possible, enrolled in phase 2 programs prior to discharge.

PHASE 2

Phase 2 of the cardiac rehabilitation program should be instituted within the first 3 weeks after discharge from the hospital.[1] This phase traditionally lasts up to 12 weeks,[2] is usually hospital-based or free-standing,[47] and involves continuous or intermittent ECG monitoring.[22] The amount of supervision and monitoring may be based in part on risk stratification guidelines[1,2] (see Table 1) but also should take into account psychosocial and clinical assessment.[22] A major goal of phase 2 is developing a safe, effective exercise program that can be carried over to the patient's home and lifestyle.[2] However, there are other important goals, including providing appropriate, sufficient

---

TABLE 8.   Phase 1 Exercise Program for Cardiac Rehabilitation (*Continued*)

Five to ten repetitions of each exercise will be performed

Step 6 (1.5–2.0 METs)
Active range of motion activities to all extremities with 1- to 2-pound weights while standing.
  Shoulder: add arm circles, scapular adduction. Walk to tolerance, not more than 100 feet.
  Surgical patients: walking as desired, without assistance.
Step 7 (1.5–2.5 METs)
Repeat exercises in step 6. Walk to tolerance, not more than 200 feet.
  Surgical patients: repeat step 6. Add slight knee bends; continue walking, walk down one flight of stairs
  with assistance (up on elevator).
Step 8 (1.5–2.5 METs)
Repeat exercises in step 7. Walk to tolerance, not more than 300 feet.
  Surgical patients: repeat step 7. Continue walking, walk down two flights of stairs with assistance (up on
  elevator).
Step 9 (2.0–2.5 METs)
Repeat exercises in step 8. Add slight knee bends, four-way body bends. Walk to tolerance, walk down
one flight of stairs with assistance (up the elevator).
  Surgical patients: up one flight of stairs, down one.
Step 10 (2.0–2.5 METs)
Repeat exercises in step 9. Down two flights of stairs with assistance.
  Surgical patients: repeat step 9.
Step 11 (2.5–3.0 METs)
Repeat exercises in step 10. Down one flight of stairs and up with assistance.

From Fardy PS, Yanowitz FG: Cardiac Rehabilitation, Adult Fitness, and Exercise Testing. Baltimore, Williams & Wilkins, 1995, with permission.

patient supervision to detect possible complications of exercise and to effectively manage these problems medically; to return the patient, if possible, to premorbid vocational and recreational activities; and to educate the patient and family on the benefits of secondary prevention of cardiac disease.[2]

Although many types of patients can benefit from a phase 2 cardiac rehabilitation program, not all patients are eligible for reimbursement. The patients who are usually eligible for a phase 2 program as determined by reimbursement guidelines are those with documented MI, CABG surgery or angioplasty, heart transplants, valvular or congenital heart disease surgery, or stable angina pectoris.[22] Patients with elevated risk factors may also benefit from a phase 2 program.[22] If possible, a referral to a phase 2 program is desirable because it will help to expedite the patient's entrance into the program and prevent any delays between phase 1 and phase 2.[47] The referral needs to be done by a physician, usually the primary care physician, cardiologist, or surgeon.[22] An orientation to the program should take place prior to beginning phase 2, and, if possible, may be done while an inpatient.[22] The orientation should be designed to allow the patient to meet the staff, see the facility, explain and demonstrate the exercise equipment, discuss lifestyle modifications, and provide an opportunity for questions.[22] Equipment

---

TABLE 9. Range of Motion Exercises for the Postoperative Patient

---

Patients usually perform 5 repetitions of each exercise and progress to 10–15 repetitions. When patients are able to comfortably progress to 10–15 repetitions, 1- to 3-pound weights can be added to the broomstick or the extremity.

Exercise 1: Behind head press

Standing, feet shoulder-width apart, broomstick or dowel held in front of body at waist level. With arms extended, raise stick over head. From this position, bend elbows and lower stick behind head to touch back of neck, then extend arms and raise stick over head. Lower stick with arms extended to waist level.

Exercise 2: Swinging stick

Standing, feet shoulder-width apart, stick held in front of body at waist level. Swing arms up to the side at approximately the ear level, lower to waist, and repeat to other side.

Exercise 3: Stick behind back

Standing, feet shoulder-width apart, stick behind the back at waist level with hands shoulder-width apart and arms extended. Extend shoulders and raise stick as high as possible without leaning forward or bending the elbows. Lower stick back to starting position.

Exercise 4: Stick sliding up back

Standing, feet shoulder-width apart, stick held behind the back at waist level with hands together and elbows extended. Slide the stick up the back as high as possible while bending the elbows. Lower back to starting position.

Exercise 5: Arm circles

Standing, with hands on shoulders and arms abducted. Rotate elbows in large circles backward.

Exercise 6: Advanced arm circles

Standing, arms extended and abducted at the shoulder, parallel to the floor. Rotate the arms backward in large circles. When first starting, do one arm at a time, advance to both arms and 1- to 3-pound wrist weights.

Adapted from Pollock ML, Wilmore JH, Fox SM III: Exercise in Health and Disease: Evaluation and Prescription for Prevention and Rehabilitation. Philadelphia, WB Saunders, 1984.

---

needs are discussed in other sources[1,22] and, in addition to exercise machines, should include ECG monitoring (telemetry and/or hard-wire systems) and emergency equipment such as defibrillators, code carts, and airway supplies.[22]

Exercise prescription guidelines for phase 2 are similar to those for phase 1. The mode of exercise will involve continuous, aerobic activities using large muscle groups. The mode will include multiple activities such as treadmills, bicycle and rowing ergometers, stair-climbing machines, and resistance exercises to carry over the beneficial training effects to real-life activities.[2] Usually, phase 2 programs involve walking, jogging, or biking, which can be done in supervised situations on treadmills or calibrated bicycle ergometers. Swimming is continuous, uses large muscle groups, minimizes musculoskeletal injury, and keeps the heart rate lower but is not recommended until after the 6–8 weeks exercise tolerance test.[47] Duration is eventually 1 hour for each session, which includes a warm-up and a cool-down period.[22] Overall duration of the phase 2 period is usually about 12 weeks.[1,22] The recommended frequency of exercise is three times per week in an organized outpatient facility and four days per week in a

TABLE 10.   Activity Levels for Inpatient Physical Therapy after Cardiac Transplantation

Level 1
   Reeducation of neuromuscular relaxation to counteract muscle tension
   Reeducation of thoracic and diaphragmatic breathing
   Review of posture principles, body mechanics, and transfer techniques
   Exercises (up to 10 repetitions, supine, performed with a wand):
      Shoulder flexion
      Shoulder abduction
      Shoulder horizontal abduction
      Hip/knee flexion and extension
      Hip abduction
      Ankle pumps
   Up in chair 20–30 minutes
Level 2
   Breathing and relaxation techniques
   Exercises (up to 10 repetitions, seated):
      Wand exercises per level 1
      Shoulder circling
      Trunk rotation
      Hip/knee flexion (seated marching)
      Knee extension
      Ankle pumps
   Gait: standing pregait activities (dips, weight shifting)
   Up in chair 30–60 minutes
Level 3
   Exercises (up to 10 repetitions, standing):
      Head circles
      Arm circles
      Trunk rotation
      Trunk lateral flexion
      Dips
      Toe raises
      Wand exercises
   Gait: short walks in the room as tolerated
   Up in chair as desired
Level 4
   Exercises (up to 10 repetitions, standing):
      Head circles
      Arm circles
      Trunk rotation
      Trunk lateral flexion
      Toe raises
      Wand exercises: progress to wrist weights (begin at 1 pound)
      When patient has full shoulder range of motion, elbow flexion/extension with wrist weights

(Continued on following page)

TABLE 10. Activity Levels for Inpatient Physical Therapy after Cardiac Transplantation *(Continued)*

Gait: walk in room as desired
Stationary cycle: 5 minutes at minimal resistance
Level 5
  Exercise and walking as per level 4
  Stationary cycle: 10 minutes at minimal resistance
  Add cool-down stretches for quadriceps and heel cords
Level 6
  Exercise and walking as per level 4
  Stationary cycle: 15 minutes at minimal resistance
  Cool-down stretches as per level 5 plus hamstring stretch
Level 7
  Exercise and walking as per level 4
  Stationary cycle: 20 minutes at mild resistance (RPE 11–13) (include 2–3 minute slower warm-up and
    cool-down)
  Cool-down stretches as per level 6

RPE = rating of perceived exertion
Adapted from Fardy PS, Yanowitz FG: Cardiac Rehabilitation, Adult Fitness, and Exercise Testing. Baltimore, Williams & Wilkins, 1995.

home program.[47] One study suggests that an exercise frequency of two times per week is as effective as three times per week for cardiorespiratory conditioning in early phase 2 programs.[17]

High-risk or unstable patients should be in supervised programs and, therefore, not home programs.[47] Intensity should be kept low initially, and increases in the duration of training will increase the workload.[47] Initial target heart rates in phase 2 can be set at less than 120 bpm or resting heart rate plus 20 bpm for MI patients and resting heart rate plus 30 bpm for postoperative patients.[2,47] If the patient has exertional angina or myocardial ischemia, the target heart rate should be set at 10 bpm below the anginal or ischemic threshold.[2,47] About 6–8 weeks after the event, the patient should have a symptom-limited graded exercise test, and the target heart rate can then be set at about 60–85% of maximum heart rate or 70–75% of the heart rate reserve.[47] An upper limit for exercise intensity that the patient should not exceed should be set at about 10 bpm below the heart rate associated with certain clinical situations (Table 12).

Progression of the phase 2 exercise program may be done initially by keeping exercise intensity low (about 40–60% of functional capacity) until a duration of 10–15 minutes of continuous activity is achieved.[2] At this point, mild to moderate intensities of exercise (about 50–70% of functional capacity) may be prescribed, with the goal of increasing duration approximately every 1–3 weeks until the patient is exercising continuously for 20–30 minutes.[2] Increasing intensity should be dictated by the patient's medical status, and it may be best not to accelerate the exercise program for the first 6–8 weeks to allow healing to occur.[47]

TABLE 11.   Functional Classification Guide for Inpatient Activities

---

Functional Class I
  Sits up in bed with assistance
  Does own self-care activities—seated or may need assistance
  Stands at bedside with assistance
  Sits up in chair 15–30 minutes, 2–3 times per day
Functional Class II
  Sits up in bed independently
  Stands independently
  Does self-care activities in bathroom, seated
  Walks in room and to bathroom (may need assistance)
Functional Class III
  Sits and stands independently
  Does own self-care activities in bathroom, seated or standing
  Walks in halls with assistance short distances (50–100 feet) as tolerated, up to 3 times per day
Functional Class IV
  Does own self-care and bathes
  Walks in halls short distances (150–200 feet) with minimal assistance, 3–4 times per day
Functional Class V
  Walks in halls independently, moderate distances (250–500 feet), 3–4 times per day
Functional Class VI
  Independent ambulation on unit 3–6 times per day

Adapted from American College of Sports Medicine: ACSM's Guidelines for Exercise Testing and Prescription. Baltimore, Williams & Wilkins, 1995.

TABLE 12.   Signs and Symptoms Below Which an Upper Limit for Exercise Intensity Should Be Set

---

1. Onset of angina or other symptoms of cardiovascular insufficiency
2. Plateau or decrease in systolic blood pressure, systolic blood pressure > 240 mm Hg or diastolic blood pressure > 110 mm Hg
3. > 1 mm ST segment depression, horizontal or downsloping
4. Radionuclide evidence of left ventricular dysfunction or onset of moderate to severe wall motion abnormalities during exertion
5. Increased frequency of ventricular arrhythmias
6. Other significant electrocardiographic disturbances (e.g., second- or third-degree AV block, atrial fibrillation, SVT, complex ventricular ectopy)
7. Other signs/symptoms of intolerance to exercise

From American College of Sports Medicine: ACSM's Guidelines for Exercise Testing and Prescription. Baltimore, Williams & Wilkins, 1995, with permission.

Table 13 shows an example of a recommended walking program. Patients may be progressed from one step to the next if they are stable at one level for at least 1–2 weeks.[47] The walking program may be used for most patients prior to the 6–8 week exercise tolerance test.

After 6–8 weeks, patients who have above average fitness levels and who have no complications may progress to a jog-walk program[47] (Table 14). When patients are capable of walking on a 5% grade at 3.5 mph, they are capable of jogging.[47] Patients may progress to a community-based program upon reaching step 8 of the walking program or after several weeks on the walk-jog program.[47]

TABLE 13. Twelve-Step Walking Program for Outpatients

Step	Speed (mph)	Elevation (%)	Duration (min)	METs
1	1.5	0	20–30	2.0
2	2.0	0	20–30	2.0
3	2.0	0	5	2.0
	2.5	0	40–60	2.5
4	2.5	0	5	2.5
	3.0	0	40–60	3.0
5	3.0	0	5	3.0
	3.5	0	40–60	3.5
6	3.0	0	5	3.0
	3.5	0 (1 min),	40–60	3.5
	3.5	2.5 (4 min), repeat		4.2
7	3.0	0	5	3.0
	3.5	0 (1 min),	40–60	3.5
	3.5	2.5 (6 min), repeat		4.2
8	3.0	0	5	3.0
	3.5	0 (1 min),	40–60	3.5
	3.5	2.5 (10 min), repeat		4.2
9	3.0	0	5	3.0
	3.5	0 (1 min),	40–60	3.5
	3.5	2.5 (14 min), repeat		4.2
10	3.0	0	5	3.0
	3.5	2.5	40–60	4.2
11	3.0	0	5	3.0
	3.5	0 (1 min),	40–60	3.5
	3.5	5.0 (1 min), repeat		6.9
12	3.0	0	5	3.0
	3.5	0 (1 min),	40–60	3.5
	3.5	5.0 (2 min), repeat		6.9

Adapted from Pollock ML, Wilmore JH, Fox SM III: Exercise in Health and Disease: Evaluation and Prescription for Prevention and Rehabilitation. Philadelphia, WB Saunders, 1984.

TABLE 14. Five-Step Walk-Jog Program for Outpatients

Step	Speed* (mph)	Elevation (%)	Duration (min)	METs
1	3.0	0	5	
	3.0 (1 min),	0	30–40	3.0
	5.5 (1 min), repeat	0		8.3
2	3.0	0	5	
	3.0 (1 min),	0	30–40	3.0
	5.5 (2 min), repeat	0		8.3
3	3.0	0	5	
	3.0 (1 min),	0	30–40	3.0
	5.5 (4 min), repeat	0		8.3
4	3.0	0	5	
	3.0 (1 min),	0	30–40	3.0
	5.5 (7 min), repeat	0		8.3
5	3.0	0	5	
	3.0 (1 min),	0	30–40	3.0
	5.5 (10 min), repeat	0		8.3

*patient will walk at 3.0 mph and jog at 5.5 mph

Adapted from Pollock ML, Wilmore JH, Fox SM III: Exercise in Health and Disease: Evaluation and Prescription for Prevention and Rehabilitation. Philadelphia, WB Saunders, 1984.

Monitoring of patients in phase 2 cardiac rehabilitation should include blood pressure measurements and evaluation of heart rate to ensure that patients are exercising within their target heart range.[1] Continuous ECG monitoring in phase 2 is not widely agreed upon. A set of guidelines has been recommended by the American College of Cardiology and the American Heart Association Subcommittee on Cardiac Rehabilitation (Table 15). Other methods of monitoring outside the traditional phase 2 setting include transtelephonic transmission of ECG monitoring from home-based exercise programs.[49]

PHASE 3

Phase 3 cardiac rehabilitation programs usually consist of a supervised community-based program or an unsupervised home program.[47] Some sources divide this period into two phases, phase 3 and phase 4.[1,22] When this distinction is made, the phase 3 program is usually considered the supervised outpatient exercise program, which generally lasts 4–24 months, is directed by an exercise professional or nurse, and includes intermittent ECG monitoring.[1,22] Phase 4 is considered to be the ongoing maintenance program of indeterminate length that generally does not include ECG monitoring or clinical supervision.[1,22] We refer to this stage of cardiac rehabilitation as phase 3 only. Patients generally begin phase 3 programs when they are felt to have stable cardiovascular responses to exercise and when the physiologic gains from the exercise program

---

TABLE 15. Characteristics of Patients Most Likely to Benefit from Continuous Electrocardiogram Monitoring During Cardiac Rehabilitation

1. Severely depressed left ventricular function (ejection fraction below 30%)
2. Resting complex ventricular arrhythmia
3. Ventricular arrhythmias appearing or increasing with exercise
4. Decrease in systolic blood pressure with exercise
5. Survivors of sudden cardiac death
6. Survivors of myocardial infarction complicated by congestive heart failure, cardiogenic shock, and/or serious ventricular arrhythmias
7. Severe coronary artery disease and marked exercise-induced ischemia (ST segment depression $\geq$ 2 mm)
8. Inability to self-monitor heart rate because of physical or intellectual impairment

From American Association of Cardiovascular and Pulmonary Rehabilitation: Guidelines for Cardiac Rehabilitation Programs. Champaign, IL, Human Kinetics, 1995, with permission.

TABLE 16. Guidelines for Progression to Independent Exercise with Minimal or No Supervision

1. Functional capacity $\geq$ 8 METs or twice the level of occupational demand
2. Appropriate hemodynamic response to exercise (increase in blood pressure with increasing workload) and recovery
3. Appropriate electrocardiogram response at peak exercise with normal or unchanged conduction, stable or absent arrhythmias, and stable and acceptable (i.e., < 1 mm ST segment depression) ischemic response
4. Cardiac symptoms stable or absent
5. Stable and/or controlled baseline heart rate and blood pressure
6. Adequate management of risk factor intervention strategy and safe exercise participation such that the patient demonstrates independent and effective management of risk factors with associated positive changes in those risk factors
7. Demonstrated knowledge of the disease process, signs and symptoms, medication use, and side effects
8. Demonstrated compliance and success with a program of risk intervention

From American College of Sports Medicine: ACSM's Guidelines for Exercise Testing and Prescription. Baltimore, Williams & Wilkins, 1995, with permission.

---

have been achieved.[1] The objectives of long-term programs include maintaining fitness, providing professional supervision, introducing new exercise activities, teaching skills for self-monitoring and self-awareness, and continuing with educational and behavioral goals.[22]

Phase 3 rehabilitation programs may be directed not only toward secondary prevention of coronary artery disease but also toward primary prevention. Patients who are eligible for phase 3 rehabilitation programs include those with coronary artery disease or risk factors and healthy subjects interested in improving fitness levels.[22]

Progression to a phase 3 program that is self-managed is a desirable goal, although certain patients who have a high risk for complications or who are unable to self-monitor may need to remain in a clinically supervised program.[2] The disease process and the ECG should remain stable, and there should be no evidence of worsening ischemia or congestive heart failure prior to progressing to a long-term maintenance phase.[29] Monitoring of patients during phase 3 can include heart rate, blood pressure, and rhythm checks before, halfway through, and after exercise, as well as 10–15 minutes before leaving the exercise area.[47] Continuous ECG monitoring should be phased out as soon as is medically feasible and may be accomplished at the attending physician's discretion by shifting to intermittent ECG monitoring and then heart rate self-monitoring.[2] Guidelines for progression to independent exercise are listed in Table 16.

Exercise prescription guidelines for phase 3 include a frequency of three to five times per week for 20–60 minutes. The intensity should be 60–85% of maximal heart rate. Activities include walking, biking, jogging, swimming, calisthenics, weight training, and endurance sports.[46] A fatigue-limited exercise test should be the source of maximal heart rate. Another method of prescribing heart rate intensity is to estimate the target heart rate at one half of the interval between the resting heart rate and the peak heart rate as determined by a fatigue-limited exercise test: THR = [(PHR − RHR) × 0.5] + RHR.[29] Walking or walk-jog prescriptions have been described,[28] and an example of a walk-jog exercise program for phase 3 is given in Table 17. A patient should be considered stable at a step level for 1–2 weeks before progressing to the next step level.[45]

WEIGHT/RESISTANCE TRAINING IN CARDIAC REHABILITATION

Cardiac rehabilitation has traditionally emphasized aerobic, continuous, and rhythmic activities to increase cardiorespiratory endurance. Resistance exercises such as weight lifting have been avoided because concerns exist about increased blood pressure response, ischemia, and arrhythmias.[53] However, properly prescribed resistance training in conjunction with aerobic exercise has been shown to have a beneficial effect on strength, cardiovascular endurance, hypertension, and hyperlipidemia.[24] Cardiac patients require a certain minimal level of strength to carry out daily activities, similar to noncardiac patients.[50] Isodynamic or nonsustained isometric activities are now recommended for many cardiac patients to help gain strength and facilitate returning to work.[55] Resistance training may not be appropriate for patients with congestive heart failure (CHF), severe valvular disease, uncontrolled arrhythmias, or significant left ventricular dysfunction and should be deferred until 4–6 weeks of supervised cardiorespiratory endurance activities have been completed.[2] Indications for resistance exercise training for outpatients include 4–6 weeks have passed since patient's MI or CABG, patient has been in supervised aerobic program for 4–6 weeks or completed phase 2, patient's blood pressure is less than 105 mm Hg, patient's peak exercise capacity is greater than 5 METs, and patient is not compromised by CHF, unstable symptoms, or arrhythmias.[2]

Circuit weight training (CWT) has been recommended for cardiac patients because they have the added benefit of increased cardiovascular fitness. CWT has been shown

TABLE 17. Sixteen-Step Walk, Walk-Jog Program for Cardiac Patients in Phase 3 Exercise Programs

Step	Speed (mph)	Duration (min)	METs	Total METs (per workout)
1	2.5	30–60	2.5	2.5
2	3.0	30–60	3.0	3.0
3	3.25	30–60	3.25	3.25
4	3.5	30–60	3.5	3.5
5	3.75	30–60	4.0	4.0
6	4.0	30–60	4.6	4.6
7	3.75 (2 min)	30–45	4.0	4.6
	5.0 (30 sec), repeat		6.9	
8	3.75 (2 min)	30–45	4.0	5.0
	5.0 (1 min), repeat		6.9	
9	3.75 (2 min)	30–45	4.0	5.5
	5.0 (2 min), repeat		6.9	
10	3.75 (1 min)	30–45	4.0	6.0
	5.0 (2 min), repeat		6.9	
11	3.75 (1 min)	30–45	4.0	6.3
	5.0 (4 min), repeat		6.9	
12	3.75 (1 min)	30–45	4.0	6.5
	5.0 (6 min), repeat		6.9	
13	3.75 (1 min)	30–45	4.0	6.6
	5.0 (8 min), repeat		6.9	
14	3.75 (1 min)	30–45	4.0	6.6
	5.0 (10 min), repeat		6.9	
15	3.75 (1 min)	30–45	4.0	7.9
	5.5 (10 min), repeat		8.3	
16	3.75 (1 min)	30–45	4.0	8.0
	5.5 (12 min), repeat		8.3	

Adapted from Pollock ML, Pels AE: Exercise prescription for the cardiac patient: An update. Clin Sports Med 3:425–443, 1984.

not only to increase strength and endurance but also to have beneficial effects on body composition, bone density, and self-confidence.[56] CWT has been shown to not elevate blood pressure above clinically acceptable levels.[13] Guidelines for CWT are listed in Table 18.

Components of a CWT prescription include amount of resistance and number of repetitions at each station, time for completion of each station, rest interval between stations, number of stations, and number of circuits to be completed.[22] General recommendations for these parameters are made in Table 19.

The specific resistance activities in CWT should include strengthening of all the major muscle groups. Different exercises at different stations may be varied from circuit to circuit or from day to day to avoid monotony. However, over the course of a week,

---

TABLE 18. Weight Training Guidelines for Low-Risk* Cardiac Patients

---

1. To prevent soreness and injury, initially choose a weight that will allow the performance of 12–15 repetitions comfortably, corresponding to approximately 30–50% of the maximum weight load that can be lifted in one repetition. (Note: Selected stable, aerobically trained cardiac patients may eventually use loads corresponding to a more traditional program of weight training, i.e., 60–80% of 1RM.)
2. Perform one to three sets of each exercise.
3. Avoid straining. Ratings of perceived exertion (6–20 scale) should not exceed fairly light to somewhat hard during lifting.
4. Exhale (blow out) during the exertion phase of the lift. For example, exhale when pushing a weight stack overhead and inhale when lowering it.
5. Increase weight loads by 5–10 pounds when 12–15 repetitions can be comfortably accomplished.
6. Raise weights with slow controlled movements; emphasize complete extension of the limbs when lifting.
7. Exercise large muscle groups before small muscle groups. Include devices (exercises) for the upper and lower extremities.
8. Weight train at least 2–3 times per week.
9. Loosely hold hand grips when possible; sustained, tight gripping may evoke an excessive blood pressure response to lifting.
10. Stop exercises in the event of warning signs or symptoms, especially dizziness, arrhythmias, unusual shortness of breath, and/or angina pectoris.
11. Allow minimal rest periods between exercises (e.g., 30–60 seconds) to maximize muscular endurance and aerobic training benefits.

---

*Low risk is arbitrarily defined as individuals with good left ventricular function (i.e., ejection fraction ≥ 45%) and reasonable cardiorespiratory fitness (≥ 7 METs) without ischemic ST segment depression, hypotensive or hypertensive blood pressure responses, serious ventricular arrhythmias, or symptoms.
From Franklin BA, Bonzheim K, Gordon S, Timmis GC: Resistance training in cardiac rehabilitation. J Cardiopulm Rehabil 11:99–107, 1991, with permission.

all muscle groups should be exercised; larger muscle groups should be exercised before smaller muscle groups. Table 20 gives examples of modes of activities for different muscle groups.

CARDIAC REHABILITATION IN SPECIAL POPULATIONS

PATIENTS WHO HAVE NOT HAD AN EXERCISE STRESS TEST

Some patients may not have an exercise stress test prior to beginning a cardiac rehabilitation program. Some of these patients include extremely deconditioned patients; patients with musculoskeletal limitations that may not have an adequate maximal exercise test, such as severe arthritis, stroke, or amputation; patients with severe left ventricular systolic dysfunction; or patients with stable coronary artery disease in whom a repeat entry exercise test may not offer any new information.[36] These patients should initially have close or one-to-one supervision; ECG, blood pressure and perceived exertion monitoring; and

TABLE 19. Circuit Weight Training Parameters for Cardiac Patients

Resistance	30–60% of 1 RM (repetition maximum) or low to moderate weight loads
Repetitions	8–20 (10–15 most often recommended)
Exercise duration	20–30 minutes
Number of stations	5–18
Number of circuits	1–3 (depends on patient fitness level and time allotment for resistive exercise)
Rest interval between stations	≥ 30 seconds (potential for greater improvement in cardiovascular endurance with shorter rest intervals; Greater heart rate, blood pressure recovery with longer rest intervals and less risk of cardiovascular complications)
Speed of muscle contraction	Lift to a count of 2, lower to a count of 4. Complete limb flexion/extension
Place of circuit weight training session	After the cardiac rehabilitation program aerobic phase; ensures adequate warm-up, less risk of musculoskeletal injury, and prioritizes aerobic phase
Frequency	Alternating 2–3 days per week
Progression	Increased resistance once 10–15 repetitions can be performed comfortably (RPE 11–13). Increase sets depending on time allotment for session, fitness level, and fatigability of the participant.
Specificity	All major muscle groups. Exercise large muscles before small muscles.

RPE = rating of perceived exertion
From Verrill DE, Ribisl PM: Resistive training in cardiac rehabilitation: An update. Sports Med 21:347–383, 1996, with permission.

should exercise within their physical limitations and below their symptomatic threshold.[36] Exercise intensity can be estimated at an initial intensity of resting heart rate plus 20 bpm. As the patient progresses asymptomatically, the exercise intensity can be gradually increased to an RPE of 12–13, and the heart rate at this level may be used to monitor intensity. Exercise duration may be started at 5 minutes per episode, working up to a cumulative duration of 30–45 minutes.[36]

HEART TRANSPLANTATION

In the transplanted heart catecholamines such as epinephrine and norepinephrine are the primary mediator of hemodynamic responses. The surgically denervated transplanted heart becomes supersensitive to catecholamines, and the resting heart rate increases. At the same time, the transplant patient has lower cardiac output, oxygen consumption, and physical work capacity.[41] Immunosuppressive medications may cause additional morbidity. Patients taking cyclosporine often develop hypertension. Prednisone therapy may cause a variety of problems, including sodium and fluid retention, increased potassium excretion, and loss of muscle mass.[9] Heart rate range is significantly affected in cardiac transplant patients, being approximately half that of normal patients.[9] Transplant patients also tend to go into anaerobic exercise earlier than normal subjects.[9]

Table 20. Resistance Activities by Muscle Groups

Muscle Group	Resistance Exercises
Rhomboids, teres, latissimus dorsi, posterior deltoids, elbow flexors	Seated rows
Deltoids and triceps	Overhead press
Latissimus dorsi and elbow flexors	Lateral pulls
Gluteal, quadriceps, and hamstrings	Knee flexion/extension or leg press
Anterior thigh and leg	Toe raises, leg raises
Biceps	Biceps curls
Triceps and pectorals	Push-ups and bench press
Abdominals	Partial curl-ups, crunches

Adapted from Verrill DE, Ribisl PM: Resistive training in cardiac rehabilitation: An update. Sports Med 21:347–383, 1996.

Exercise prescription is similar to what has been discussed previously and is recommended at frequencies of three to five times per week for durations of 30–45 minutes of continuous or interval activities such as walking, walk-jogging, and cycling. Intensity may be at an RPE of 12–14 or a MET level slightly below the ventilatory threshold. Patients should have longer warm-up and cool-down periods to compensate for the longer amount of time needed for the physiologic response to exercise.[9]

VALVULAR HEART DISEASE

Cardiac rehabilitation postoperatively in patients with valvular heart disease is similar to that of post-CABG patients.[37] Care should be taken to avoid high-impact exercises or exercises with a risk of trauma in patients who are on anticoagulation medications to avoid hemarthrosis and bruising.[41]

LEFT VENTRICULAR DYSFUNCTION

Patients with an ejection fraction of < 30% may be included in the group of patients with left ventricular dysfunction. These patients are at a higher risk of sudden death and show an inconsistent response to exercise. The normal peripheral and central effects of exercise may not occur in these patients, and at rest or minimal exertion they may have elevated heart rate, dyspnea, and fatigue. Exercise may cause a further decrease in ejection fraction. Exercise should be done gradually, with carefully monitored increases in heart rate, not to exceed 10 bpm below any significant endpoint such as hypotension, dyspnea, or arrhythmia. Because these patients can tolerate only limited workloads, total exercise can be increased by increasing the duration. This may be done by prolonging the warm-up and cool-down. If resistance training is to be part of the program, it should be dynamic and not isometric. Monitoring should include continuous telemetry throughout the exercise period, including warm-up and cool-down, as well as routine blood pressure and heart rate response to exercise monitoring. Patients who also have unstable angina, decompensated heart failure, or hemodynamic instability as a result of arrhythmia are not candidates for exercise rehabilitation.[41] Exercise should be aerobic in nature and performed three to five times per week.[31]

REFERENCES

1. American Association of Cardiovascular and Pulmonary Rehabilitation: Guidelines for Cardiac Rehabilitation Programs. Champaign, IL, Human Kinetics, 1995.
2. American College of Sports Medicine: ACSM's Guidelines for Exercise Testing and Prescription. Baltimore, Williams & Wilkins, 1995.
3. American College of Sports Medicine: Essentials of Sports Medicine. St. Louis, Mosby, 1996.
4. American College of Sports Medicine: Exercise for patients with coronary artery disease. Med Sci Sports Exerc 26(3):i–iv, 1994.
5. American College of Sports Medicine: Proper and improper weight loss programs. Med Sci Sports Exerc 15(1):ix–xiii, 1983.
6. American College of Sports Medicine: The recommended quantity and quality of exercise for developing and maintaining cardiorespiratory and muscular fitness in healthy adults. Med Sci Sports Exerc 22:265–274, 1990.
7. American Heart Association: Cardiac Rehabilitation Programs: A statement for healthcare professionals from the American Heart Association. Circulation 90:1602–1610, 1994.
8. American Heart Association: Exercise Standards: A statement for healthcare professionals from the American Heart Association. Circulation 91:580–618, 1995.
9. Badenhop DT: The therapeutic role of exercise in patients with orthotopic heart transplant. Med Sci Sports Exerc 27:975–985, 1995.
10. Barnard RJ, Gardner GW, Diaco NV, et al: Cardiovascular responses to sudden strenuous exercise: Heart rate, blood pressure, and electrocardiogram. J Appl Physiol 34:152–157, 1973.
11. Barnard RJ, MacAlpin R, Kattus AA, et al: Ischemic response to sudden strenuous exercise in healthy men. Circulation 48:936–942, 1973.
12. Borg GA: Psychosocial basis of perceived exertion. Med Sci Sports Exerc 14:337–381, 1982.
13. Butler RM, Palmer G, Rogers FJ: Circuit weight training in early cardiac rehabilitation. J Am Osteopath Assoc 92:77–85, 1992.
14. Debusk RF: American College of Physicians position paper. Evaluation of patients after recent acute myocardial infarction. Ann Intern Med 110:485–488, 1989.
15. DeBusk RF, Blomqvist G, Kouchoukos NT, et al: Identification and treatment of low risk patients after acute myocardial infarction and coronary artery bypass graft surgery. N Engl J Med 314:161–166, 1986.
16. Dishman RK: Prescribing exercise intensity for healthy adults using perceived exertion. Med Sci Sports Exerc 26:1087–1094, 1994.
17. Dressendorfer RH, Franklin BA, Cameron JL, et al: Exercise training in early post-infarction cardiac rehabilitation: Influence on aerobic conditioning. J Cardiopulm Rehabil 15:269–276, 1995.
18. Dunbar CC, Glickman-Weiss EL, Edwards WW, et al: Three-point method of prescribing exercise with ratings of perceived exertion is valid for cardiac patients. Percept Mot Skills 82:139–146, 1996.
19. Dunbar CC, Kalinski MI, Robertson RJ: A new method of prescribing exercise: Three point ratings of perceived exertion. Percept Mot Skills 83:384–386, 1996.
20. Ewart CK: Psychological effects of resistive weight training: Implications for cardiac patients. Med Sci Sports Exerc 21:683–688, 1989.
21. Fardy PS: Isometric exercise and the cardiovascular system. Phys Sports Med 9:43, 1981.
22. Fardy PS, Yanowitz FG: Cardiac Rehabilitation, Adult Fitness, and Exercise Testing. Baltimore, Williams & Wilkins, 1995.

23. Foster C, Anholm JD, Hellman CK, et al: Left ventricular function during sudden strenuous exercise. Circulation 63:592–596, 1981.
24. Franklin BA, Bonzheim K, Gordon S, Timmis GC: Resistance training in cardiac rehabilitation. J Cardiopulm Rehabil 11:99–107, 1991.
25. Goldberg AP: Aerobic and resistive exercises modify risk factors for coronary heart disease. Med Sci Sports Exerc 21:669–674, 1989.
26. Goldberg L, Elliot DL: Exercise for Prevention and Treatment of Illness. Philadelphia, FA Davis, 1994.
27. Graves JE, Pollock ML: Exercise testing in cardiac rehabilitation: Role in prescribing exercise. Cardiol Clin 11:253–266, 1993.
28. Harrison P: Walk-jog prescription introduced by Toronto centre now a mainstay of cardiac rehabilitation. Can Med Assoc J 149:470–472, 1993.
29. Hartley HL: Exercise for the cardiac patient: Long-term maintenance phase. Cardiol Clin 11(2): 277–284, 1993.
30. Harvey AM, Johns RJ, McKusick VA, et al: The Principles and Practice of Medicine. 22nd ed. East Norwalk, CT, Appleton and Lange, 1988.
31. Hiatt RH, Regensteiner JG, Wolfel EE: Special populations in cardiac rehabilitation: Peripheral arterial disease, non-insulin-dependent diabetes mellitus, and heart failure. Cardiol Clin 11:309–321, 1993.
32. Karvonen MJ, Kentala E, Mustula O: The effects of training on heart rate. A "longitudinal" study. Ann Med Exp Biol Fenn 35:307, 1957.
33. Laslett L, Paumer L, Amsterdam EA: Exercise training in coronary artery disease. Cardiol Clin 5:211–225, 1987.
34. Londerbee B, Moeschberger ML: Effect of age and other factors on maximal heart rate. Res Q Exerc Sport 53:297–304, 1982.
35. Mahler DA, Fronco MJ: Clinical applications of cardiopulmonary exercise testing. J Cardiopulm Rehabil 16:357–365, 1996.
36. McConnell TR: Exercise prescription: When the guidelines do not work. J Cardiopulm Rehabil 16:34–37, 1996.
37. Moldover JR, Bartels MN: Cardiac rehabilitation. In Braddom RL (ed): Physical Medicine and Rehabilitation. Philadelphia, WB Saunders, 1996.
38. Moore GE: Primary care management of cardiac rehabilitation. Phys Sports Med 25:96i–aa, 1997.
39. Narloch JA, Brandstater ME: Influence of breathing technique on arterial blood pressure during heavy weight lifting. Arch Phys Med Rehabil 76:457–462, 1995.
40. Noble BJ, Borg GA, Jacobs I, et al: A category-ratio perceived exertion scale: Relationship to blood and muscle lactates and heart rate. Med Sci Sports Exerc 15:523–528, 1983.
41. Pashkow FJ: Rehabilitation strategies for the complex cardiac patient. Cleve Clin J Med 58:70–75, 1991.
42. Pina IL, Madonna DW, Sinnamon EA: Exercise test interpretation. Cardiol Clin 11:215–227, 1993.
43. Pollock ML, Gettman LR, Milesis CA, et al: Effects of frequency and duration of training on attrition and incidence of injury. Med Sci Sports Exerc 9:31–36, 1977.
44. Pollock ML, Miller HS, Linnerud AC, et al: Frequency of training as a determinant for improvement in cardiovascular function and body composition of middle-aged men. Arch Phys Med Rehabil 58: 141–145, 1975.
45. Pollock ML, Pels AE: Exercise prescription for the cardiac patient: An update. Clin Sports Med 3:425–443, 1984.
46. Pollock ML, Schmidt DH: Heart Disease and Rehabilitation. Champaign, IL, Human Kinetics, 1995.
47. Pollock ML, Wilmore JH, Fox SM III: Exercise in Health and Disease: Evaluation and Prescription for Prevention and Rehabilitation. Philadelphia, WB Saunders, 1984.
48. Robbins SL, Cotran RS, Kumar V: Pocket Companion to Robbins Pathologic Basis of Disease. Philadelphia, WB Saunders, 1991.
49. Sparks KE, Shaw DK, Eddy D, et al: Alternatives for cardiac rehabilitation patients unable to return to a hospital-based program. Heart Lung 22:298–303, 1993.
50. Sparling PB, Cantwell JD, Dolan CM, Niederman RK: Strength training in a cardiac rehabilitation program: A six-month follow-up. Arch Phys Med Rehabil 71:148–152, 1990.

51. Squires RW: Cardiac rehabilitation issues for heart transplantation patients. J Cardiopulm Rehabil 10:159, 1990.
52. Stewart KJ: Introduction to the symposium. Resistive weight training: A new approach to exercise for cardiac and coronary disease prone populations. Med Sci Sports Exerc 21:667–668, 1989.
53. Sword DO: Resistance training in cardiac rehabilitation: Risks, benefits and recommendations. J S C Med Assoc 88:69–74, 1992.
54. U.S. Department of Health and Human Resources: Physical Activity and Health: A Report of the Surgeon General. Atlanta, Centers for Disease Control and Prevention, National Center for Chronic Disease Prevention and Health Promotion, 1996.
55. Verrill DE: Resistive exercise training in cardiac rehabilitation. Am Coll Sports Med Cert News 6:1–7, 1996.
56. Verrill DE, Ribisl PM: Resistive training in cardiac rehabilitation: An update. Sports Med 21:347–383, 1996.
57. Wade OL, Bishop JM: Cardiac Output and Regional Blood Flow. Philadelphia, FA Davis, 1962.
58. Ward A, Malloy P, Rippe J: Exercise prescription guidelines for normal and cardiac populations. Cardiol Clin 5:197–210, 1987.
59. Wenger NK: Cardiac rehabilitation implications of the AHCPR guideline. Hosp Med April 31–38, 1997.
60. Wenger NK: The physiologic basis for early ambulation after myocardial infarction. In Wenger NK (ed): Exercise and the Heart. Philadelphia, FA Davis, 1978.

STUART J. GLASSMAN, MD

6

Pulmonary Dysfunction

WHAT IS PULMONARY REHABILITATION?

Exercise prescription for patients with pulmonary dysfunction is part of the larger topic of pulmonary rehabilitation, which is the focus of this chapter. Pulmonary rehabilitation has been defined by a number of organizations, including the American College of Chest Physicians' Committee on Pulmonary Rehabilitation and the American Thoracic Society.[2] It is felt to be an individually tailored, multidisciplinary program that is formulated through diagnosis, therapy, emotional support, and education to stabilize or reverse pulmonary disease.[23] It is also designed to help return patients to the highest possible function. The components of pulmonary rehabilitation/pulmonary exercise include overall team assessment in a multidisciplinary fashion, exercise training, patient education, psychosocial intervention, and follow-up.[11] The multidisciplinary team consists of several members, including pulmonologists, internists, and physiatrists, all of whom should be familiar with pulmonary disease and pulmonary rehabilitation, and therapists, nurses, nutritionists, social workers, case managers, and psychologists. Respiratory therapy is a hallmark of pulmonary rehabilitation.[1,4] All the team members work together to individualize the patient's treatment plan and to help improve the patient's functional status. The exercise itself consists of conditioning activities, upper and lower extremity strengthening, and respiratory muscle strengthening.[5]

Training focuses on breathing techniques, bronchial hygiene, activities of daily living, relaxation, energy conservation, and medications management.[11] Counseling, support systems, and anger and depression management are also key psychosocial issues that must be addressed during this treatment program.[12] Follow-up after pulmonary rehabilitation and exercise has been completed in the supervised setting will focus on patient outcomes, exercise maintenance in the community, and support group meetings for the patient and the family. It is of utmost importance that each program is individually tailored for the patient's specific needs.

INDICATIONS FOR PULMONARY REHABILITATION

Clearly, patients with chronic obstructive pulmonary diseases (COPD) represent a major group of patients who will benefit from pulmonary rehabilitation,[8,17,32] but patients with other conditions also may benefit from comprehensive pulmonary exercise and rehabilitation programs.[4,5] For this discussion, COPD shall refer to patients who have emphysema or chronic bronchitis. Asthma is considered separate from COPD but definitely responds quite well to pulmonary rehabilitation and overall exercise management. Children with cystic fibrosis also can benefit from exercise pulmonary rehabilitation programs.[1,21] Secretion mobilization and management and, also, overall exercise improvement have been shown to occur through focused, formal exercise programs.

Patients who have restrictive lung diseases, such as neuromuscular disease, muscular dystrophy, amyotrophic lateral sclerosis, and polio, have been shown to benefit from enhanced pulmonary exercise programs.[4,5] Such patients are often not included in typical outpatient pulmonary rehabilitation programs, but there is much support in the literature demonstrating that exercise prescription and individualized pulmonary rehabilitation programs are of utmost importance for these patients.

Lastly, surgical patients, specifically those undergoing lung volume reduction surgery or possibly lung transplant, are felt to be eligible for and benefit tremendously from pulmonary rehabilitation and exercise training.

LOCATION OF THE PROGRAM

Pulmonary rehabilitation often begins in the acute care facility, sometimes even in the emergency room as the patient is being treated for an acute exacerbation. Oral and aerosolized medications and oxygen therapy are often the hallmarks of the early interventions. After becoming stabilized, patients may move to the acute care medical floor, where therapy and psychosocial interventions are indicated. Patients who have COPD or exacerbations of asthma may subsequently be referred to an acute inpatient rehabilitation hospital for comprehensive pulmonary rehabilitation (Fig. 1). Because the length of stay in acute care hospitals has decreased over the past decade, many acute rehabilitation hospitals have formalized pulmonary rehabilitation programs to handle patients who have left the acute care hospital early. The pulmonary rehabilitation program in the acute inpatient rehabilitation facility will allow for more extensive exercise and team management. Often, the goal during acute rehabilitation is to increase exercise tolerance, improve activities of daily living, allow the patient to gain insight into his or her disease management, and facilitate discharge to home.[25] Patients at this level of care are often expected to tolerate about 3 hours of therapy daily. A recent study of a short-stay comprehensive inpatient pulmonary rehabilitation program showed that the 12-minute walk test was improved during a hospitalization of about ten days.[30] During this ten-day stay, all patients were discharged home, and 50% were discharged off of oxygen. Overall pulmonary function status, based on a 56-item questionnaire, was found to have improved by 40%.

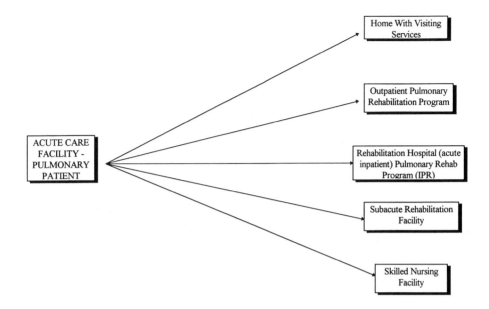

FIGURE 1. Postacute discharge planning for the pulmonary rehabilitation patient.

If patients are more severely involved and not able to tolerate 3 hours of therapy a day, referral to a subacute or skilled nursing facility may be more appropriate. In this location, exercise training is often held for 1–2 hours a day, but patients are able to receive 3 hours of therapy if indicated. This may be appropriate for longstanding COPD patients, who are quite deconditioned and are in the early phases of exercise training. In the subacute and/or skilled nursing facility, the pulmonary rehabilitation program is still multidisciplinary in nature: patients are seen by therapists, case managers, physicians, dietitians, and psychologists. It is possible for patients to go from the acute care hospital to a subacute facility and then be upgraded into the acute rehabilitation hospital, depending on their progress. It is really the ability to participate in the program that determines what level of postacute care will be selected for the patient. Certainly, the ultimate goal of the pulmonary rehabilitation programs is to improve exercise condition and get the patient home. Some studies have shown that a comprehensive home-based pulmonary rehabilitation program can give good results in cases in which the patient is being seen in the home and at an outpatient therapy center.[29]

Lastly, many patients who leave the acute care hospital and go home directly are often enrolled in comprehensive outpatient pulmonary rehabilitation programs, either community- or hospital-based.[7,31] The programs usually last 3 days a week for 6–12 weeks, depending on the severity of the case. Any of the facilities described above can provide the necessary pulmonary exercise and rehabilitation program for the appropriate patients.

ASSESSING THE PULMONARY REHABILITATION PATIENT

One of the baseline tests that is needed for assessing the pulmonary patient for exercise is pulmonary function testing (PFT).[16] PFT will allow for evaluating future changes in pulmonary status and lung disease, help determine possible impairments, and identify whether a patient has a restrictive or obstructive disease. During PFT, the functional vital capacity (FVC), residual volume (RV), and total lung capacity (TLC) are parameters that are evaluated to give an indication of the patient's functional and pulmonary status. A baseline chest radiograph will help identify the possible coexistence of pneumonia or atelectasis. Clearly, these are objective tools to measure lung status.

Quality-of-life indicators such as the Medical Short Forms-36 Questionnaire, the Baseline Dyspnea Index, and the Sickness Impact Profile are important questionnaires to determine the patient's overall status.[20] A comprehensive history and physical is mandatory at the beginning of any pulmonary rehabilitation program. Oxygen saturation, via pulse oximetry at rest and with exercise, both on room air and with oxygen, may help to establish the need for oxygen supplementation. Clearly, exercise testing is important for accurate measurement of exercise tolerance and to prove changes over time. Exercise testing can be done using the simple 6- or 12-minute walk test or more complex cardiopulmonary exercise stress testing, which may help identify coexisting cardiac disease in a pulmonary patient.[6,16] Treadmill and bicycle ergometry testing are acceptable methods of pulmonary stress testing.[6,26] Depending on the level of the facility, expired gas analyses and determination of maximum minute ventilation can give more specific data concerning cardiopulmonary status.

After the exercise test assessment has been made, exercise training for pulmonary rehabilitation patients is important.[6,26-28] This is often carried out by starting with a comfortable exercise level for the patient, which should allay the patient's fears of worsening dyspnea and hypoxemia. Exercise training parameters can look at target heart rates, use the Borg Scale of Perceived Exertion, and use the Rate of Perceived Dyspnea (RPD) scale.[32] These indicators are usually scaled on a 0–10 basis, with 0 indicating no discomfort or restlessness and 10 indicating extremely severe exertion or dyspnea. The exercise sessions will often include 20–30 minutes of continuous activity at the predicted target heart rate and a warm-up and cool-down phase. Thrice weekly exercise training sessions is the goal for most pulmonary training programs. Monitoring of heart rate, blood pressure, and pulse oximetry is important during any kind of exercise testing program. Equipment that can be used for exercise training can include the treadmill, bicycle, and rowing ergometer. Walking and arm/leg combined exercise can be prescribed. Arm-only activity can be done but may not be as effective as using leg-only or arm/leg combinations.[13]

In addition to assessing exercise training and testing for the extremities, respiratory muscle training is a vital part of a pulmonary exercise program.[4] Pursed lip breathing is important because it will prevent airway collapse upon exhalation, which may actually improve oxygen saturation.[4] Diaphragmatic breathing during inspiration will improve air exchange and facilitate muscle relaxation to help improve breathing efficiency.

MEDICATIONS FOR PULMONARY REHABILITATION PATIENTS

Categories of medications that are often used in combination with exercise programs for pulmonary rehabilitation patients include oral medications, aerosolized medications, and oxygen/nebulizer delivery systems. Oral medications, such as theophylline, metered dose inhalers, nebulizer treatments, mucolytics, corticosteroid and antiinflammatory medications, and antibiotics can all play a role in the treatment of various pulmonary rehabilitation patients.[4] Bronchodilators, often first-line treatment for asthma and COPD patients, are split into two categories: (1) sympathomimetics, which include the beta-agonists, and (2) the anticholinergics, which work by blocking reflex bronchoconstriction. Combination therapy is also felt to be more effective than single-agent therapy. Expectorant medications, such as guaifenesin, also can improve cough secretions. Oxygen can ease breathing. Proper use of the above medications will help improve overall breathing ability and increase exercise tolerance and ability.

BREATHING TECHNIQUES

Exercise for the arms and legs is not the only type of exercise required for pulmonary rehabilitation/pulmonary dysfunction patients. Proper diaphragmatic and respiratory muscle exercises are part of any pulmonary rehabilitation program. As mentioned, pursed lip breathing and diaphragmatic breathing will help ease the work of breathing and improve overall oxygenation.[1] Incentive spirometry, which is often done by the patient in a self-supervised setting, can be effective in improving airway exchange. Other breathing techniques include chest physical therapy to help mobilize secretions and to improve cough expectoration and postural drainage. Positioning of the patient is often important for improving ventilation. Segmental breathing exercises, which are also known as lateral costal breathing, can use manual counterpressure and chest wall compliance to help improve ventilation. All of these breathing exercises will help to improve airway and oxygen exchange, which should result in improved exercise capacity. Physical therapists, occupational therapists, and respiratory therapists can be involved in the teaching and training for breathing exercises and techniques.[11]

NUTRITION AND SMOKING

No discussion about exercise training and prescription can be complete without addressing nutrition. The adage, "We are what we eat," is applicable. Many pulmonary rehabilitation patients have a higher resting energy requirement for eating properly, and nutrition becomes a large focus of pulmonary rehabilitation programs.[3,19] Many COPD patients have a less than ideal body weight and have a reduced fat-free mass. Since COPD patients have increased energy requirements to breath, their caloric needs are actually higher. Almost 50% of pulmonary patients cannot maintain adequate nutrition. Malnourished patients will have a higher likelihood of infection, worse ventilation, and higher morbidity. Proper ratios of carbohydrates, proteins, and fat intake must be determined. Improving nutritional status and getting patients closer to ideal body weight should be an important goal of a pulmonary exercise program.

Clearly, smoking has a large effect on the development of COPD.[11] It may take 10 years for a smoker to develop traumatic airway disease even though PFT may not change significantly. The important point is that stopping smoking protects the patient from worsening pulmonary disease and may help to reverse changes. Often, when patients see that their pulmonary function tests have become altered, they may be more likely to quit smoking. There are a number of ways of managing smoking cessation, including patient and family education, group counseling, nicotine gums and nicotine patches, and possible hypnosis. Regardless of the method, if smoking stops, nutrition will improve and energy abilities and exercises tolerances will most likely increase.

EXTREMITY CONDITIONING EXERCISES

Exercise conditioning has been shown to improve maximum oxygen uptake, strength and endurance, and coordination.[6,26,28] Increased muscle mass and a better vascular-hemodynamic system will help improve peripheral extraction of oxygen, which will lead to better physical activity. Exercise performance will improve, and the patients will have a better sense of well being. The type of exercise that is indicated for most pulmonary dysfunction patients are conditioning exercises of low resistance and high repetition. These exercises will provide better endurance and may be more easily tolerated by a pulmonary rehabilitation patient. It is important to set target heart rates, usually at 70–85% of the age-predicted maximum. Some patients may be able to work at a training heart rate of 50–65%. The exercise session—30 minutes of sustained aerobic activity three times per week with additional time for warming up and cooling down—can provide the desired training effect if followed closely. In the inpatient setting, patients often exercise 5–7 days per week to increase their functional abilities.

Leg exercises can provide a better training effect than arm exercises alone. Twelve-minute walk distances have been shown to improve, and dyspnea and blood lactate levels actually decrease.[9] The patient's cough and secretion management also can improve. Both mild and severe cases of pulmonary disease can improve as a result of exercise training. Arm and leg combination exercises, such as those carried out using a rowing machine, cross-country ski machine, and combination arm/leg bicycle ergometer, can provide even larger improvements in exercise tolerance. Arm exercises alone can actually hamper diaphragmatic function due to the loss of the stabilizing effect of the shoulder girdle. However, the arm exercises that are done often on a UBE ergometer can improve endurance and aerobic capacity in patients who cannot perform walking or leg function training.

PSYCHOSOCIAL ISSUES

As exercise capacity improves in pulmonary rehabilitation patients, motivation will increase, dyspnea will eventually decrease, and an overall improved sense of well being will occur. This can help decrease anxiety and stress, improve coping skills, and allow patients to focus on items such as increasing their exercise ability, improving their nutrition, and stopping smoking.[3,12] Activities of daily living may be performed more easily.[10,25] Depression and overall somatic complaints have been shown to decrease. Exercise can be a useful psychosocial intervention when combined with other stress reduction techniques and, of course, smoking cessation education. Exercise alone is not a cure-all but can be beneficial when combined with the other facets of a multidisciplinary team approach.

OUTCOMES

Under managed health care, the measurement of outcomes has become important. Should the outcomes be physiologic, psychological, or financial? Improved 12-minute walk distances, better aerobic capacity, and improved oxygen saturations all occur in successful pulmonary rehabilitation programs.[14,22] Another physiologic outcomes tool that can measure success for pulmonary rehabilitation programs is the Functional Independence Measure (FIM), which examines improved activity in 18 categories of self-care, mobility, and function. It is often used in rehabilitation medicine for measuring improvement with therapy treatments, and it certainly has a role in outcomes assessment for pulmonary rehabilitation.[25] Smoking cessation, decreased depressive indices, improved quality of life indicators, and stress reduction are measured easily and provide good psychosocial outcomes for a pulmonary rehabilitation program. Lower morbidity and mortality rates, with lower health care costs, have been demonstrated in multiple studies of pulmonary rehabilitation programs.[18,24] These programs have been shown to be cost-effective, showing decreased hospital days and decreased emergency visits for the patients who graduate from a pulmonary rehabilitation program.

Return to work in and of itself may not be a good indicator of the success of pulmonary rehabilitation programs, because many pulmonary rehabilitation patients are older than 55. Studies have shown that pulmonary rehabilitation can help return patients to gainful employment, but teaching new vocations to older patients is sometimes difficult.

In terms of surgical outcomes, a National Institutes of Health multicenter trial for lung volume reduction surgery is in process. A key component of the study is the fact that both the surgical and control patients will receive pulmonary rehabilitation. This sends the message that pulmonary rehabilitation is felt to provide a health-related benefit and may help to improve surgical outcomes.

Whether inpatient- or outpatient-based, pulmonary rehabilitation has demonstrated good outcomes on various levels and is cost-effective for hospitals and patients alike.[11,18] Each program can determine which parameters it wants to follow for outcomes, and outcomes should be examined in the areas of physiologic functioning, psychosocial/quality-of-life indicators, and cost-related entities.

EXERCISE PRESCRIPTION FOR NON-COPD PATIENTS

This section examines exercise and treatment issues for patients with pulmonary conditions other than COPD, including neuromuscular diseases such as amyotrophic lateral sclerosis, polio and post-polio syndrome, muscular dystrophy, and cystic fibrosis. Ventilator-assisted patients can be included in any one of these diseases. Although not typically seen in most outpatient pulmonary rehabilitation programs, these patients are often inpatients, especially in acute and long-term rehabilitation hospitals.[1,4] In the early stages of these diseases, patients are often diagnosed while still ambulatory. They can participate in active exercise programs similar to traditional COPD patients, but they require some adaptive equipment. Studies have shown improved aerobic capacity in patients with slowly progressive neuromuscular disease who are undergoing exercise conditioning.

As these progressive diseases worsen, patients may cease being ambulatory and become more sedentary. Depending on which areas are affected, patients can still work on upper extremity conditioning and strengthening exercises such as with a UBE arm ergometer or with a wheelchair ergometer system. Eventually, as arm and leg weakness prevents use of exercise equipment, patients can still focus on ventilatory muscle training to help maintain breathing capacity.[4,15] This is often accomplished by maximal inspiratory efforts or via resistive inspiratory loading, which is usually given two to three times a day for about 5–10 minutes. Respiratory muscle endurance can improve more than muscle strength. Vital capacity and minute ventilatory volume can improve, while better oxygenation can improve the quality of life and overall sense of well being. As respiratory muscles fatigue, noninvasive ventilator aids can be used to help maintain oxygenation and cough capabilities.[5] These devices can be used for 1–2 years. Eventually, patients may require tracheostomy and become dependent on a ventilator to sustain function.[15] Glossopharyngeal breathing is a technique that can help provide sustained time off the ventilator.

Cystic fibrosis and muscular dystrophy often afflict children.[1,21] Many patients with muscular dystrophy have rib cage deformities and impaired oxygenation and restrictive lung disease as seen on PFT. In these cases, the patients may not even be ambulatory, but pulmonary exercise and rehabilitation is important for them to maintain oxygenation. Cystic fibrosis is a common respiratory disease of young adults that is inherited as an autosomal recessive trait.[21] Epithelial cells are resistant to chloride permeability, and respiratory infections and pulmonary inflammation of the bronchials can occur. Thick secretions plug airways, and breathing becomes more difficult. The exercise treatment plan for cystic fibrosis will focus on secretion mobilization using chest percussion and postural drainage, deep breathing, and exercise techniques. Steroids are often indicated, as is aerosolized human recombinant DNAase. Upper extremity exercises in cystic fibrosis patients can improve respiratory muscle endurance. Regular aerobic exercise, such as swimming, walking, or jogging, can improve exercise tolerance and airflows. Exercising in a hot environment is contraindicated for patients with cystic fibrosis, because they have a defect in sweat excretion. Chest physical therapy and postural drainage should be done along with the exercise program.

Another childhood disease of importance is asthma. Exercise conditioning and training is indicated for patients with asthma.[21] Exercise will help the medication regimen for asthma treatment, and exercise testing can confirm the diagnosis of exercise-induced asthma. Expiratory flow rates will drop after vigorous exercise testing, and this drop will return to baseline after 30–60 minutes. Patients who exercise regularly and continue with their regular asthma medications do improve exercise tolerance. The exercise program itself need not worsen their daily asthma symptoms or likelihood of developing exercise-induced asthma in a laboratory. Improved cardiopulmonary fitness has been demonstrated in asthma patients who underwent exercise training. Most studies have shown that exercise is not harmful for asthma patients and can actually improve their functional status. Asthmatics have even competed and won gold medals in Olympic competition. It is felt that inspired air during exercise should be warmed and possibly humidified. This would explain why many patients who have been competitors may have had clinical asthma and were not aware of it. Patients who exercise in cold, dry climates may want to have a scarf around their mouth to help humidify the incoming air. A few minutes before undergoing exercise training, the asthmatic patient will most likely want to use inhaled medications, including albuterol, cromolyn sodium inhalers, or possibly long-term steroid treatments.

CASE STUDY

The patient is a 56-year-old white man who had been admitted through a local hospital emergency room after having been found at home by his grandchildren, when he was determined to be unresponsive. He had been having worsening shortness of breath over a number of days and, when questioned in the emergency room, stated that he had not taken his pulmonary medications for about a week. The patient had a medical history of severe COPD and had been on oxygen for about 5 years. He also had a history of congestive heart failure and hypertension and was morbidly obese—about 150 pounds over ideal body weight. He also had a history of gastric ulcers and a right lower lobe pneumonia. When admitted to the emergency room, the patient was found to have had severe worsening leg edema, and congestive heart failure was suspected. He was emergently intubated. He required machine-assisted ventilation for 2 days and then was able to be extubated and placed on a 50% Venti-mask. His pCO_2 was at a level of 60, and his oxygen partial pressure was 60 with an oxygen saturation of 90%.

The patient received intravenous antibiotics for his right lower lobe pneumonia. He had been given intravenous steroids and then oral steroids for his severe exacerbation of COPD. He then was switched over to oral antibiotics for his pneumonia. He began ambulating approximately 5 feet with the moderate assist of two people and was transferred to the rehabilitation hospital for the comprehensive inpatient pulmonary rehabilitation program.

The patient's medications upon admission had included Augmentin, prednisone, Habitrol nicotine skin patch, Pepcid, albuterol nebulizers, Atrovent inhalers, heparin subcutaneous injections for deep vein thrombosis prophylaxis, and Lasix; 3–4 L of oxygen were required to keep the oxygen saturation at or above 91%.

The patient had been depressed over the past 4–5 months because his wife had separated from him during that time. He had resumed smoking over the past 4 months. He was not working and said his basic activities included sitting around the home, watching television, and eating. He had not been driving for a number of months. He required ambulation with a walker and minimal to moderate assistance of two people.

His physical examination on admission to the rehabilitation hospital showed that he had distant breath sounds bilaterally; they were coarse, and no rales were heard. He had 2+ edema bilaterally in his feet.

His progress in the rehabilitation hospital was based on working on physical therapy, occupational therapy, respiratory therapy, and psychosocial involvement for issues of addressing possible depression and adjustment to his pulmonary disease. He continued to use the nicotine patch. During the rehabilitation hospital stay, he improved in all areas. His right lower lobe pneumonia improved. He had gone through exercise training in the pulmonary rehabilitation program daily. He initially had been consulted by the pulmonologist, and the attending physician was the physiatrist. His oxygen requirements improved to the point where he only required 1½ L with activity. His edema progressed from 2+ down to 0–1+ edema. He was able to tolerate walking over 300 feet with oxygen at 1½ L and was able to do full activities of daily living and dressing in the morning without oxygen. The patient did not require the use of the walker at the time of discharge. He had gone through the exercise program at the rehabilitation hospital focusing on increasing his endurance to 30 minutes of continuous activity and had 3 hours of therapy daily about six times per week. He remained in the hospital for 18 days. He had required minimal to moderate assistance for activities and walking and progressed to becoming completely independent in all areas of dressing, walking, bathing, grooming, and eating. He became able to walk again, independent of any device. He had received dietary and nutrition teaching to encourage him to lose weight. The patient was discharged to home under his own supervision and was connected with an outpatient pulmonary rehabilitation program. The patient had been taken off the prednisone by the time of discharge.

Follow-up conducted 1 month after discharge from the rehabilitation hospital showed that the patient had enrolled in the outpatient pulmonary rehabilitation program at his local community hospital. He had progressed in outpatient therapy to using the treadmill for 10 consecutive minutes at 1.5 miles per hour. He also had been using the bicycle odometer and had maintained his 1½ L of oxygen with activity. His adjustment and depression issues resolved. The patient was eating better and had not smoked since being admitted to the rehabilitation hospital. He had gone out into the community with his portable oxygen tank, had been driving, and had participated in activities with his grandchildren. He lost approximately 15 pounds.

This case demonstrates that the patient with severe COPD who is in a socially isolated environment and is admitted emergently to an acute care hospital can progress through the health care system from the acute care facility, to the rehabilitation hospital, and back to the community while receiving comprehensive pulmonary rehabilitation to increase his or her exercise tolerance and quality of life.

In summary, treatment plans for patients with pulmonary dysfunction require much more than simple exercise prescription. The overall rehabilitation and quality-of-life improvement for patients with COPD, other pulmonary conditions, and neuromuscular disease involves a multidisciplinary team, the use of exercise, medication, breathing techniques, nutritional assessment, and smoking cessation. Outcomes have demonstrated good results in improved health care utilization and cost savings, with better exercise capacity and quality-of-life indicators for the patient. As physicians work together to manage the pulmonary patient's rehabilitation program, even more improvements and more scientific data should emerge in this exciting and evolving area of medical treatment.

REFERENCES

1. Alba A: Concepts in pulmonary rehabilitation. In Braddom RL (ed): Physical Medicine and Rehabilitation. Philadelphia, WB Saunders, 1996, pp 324–345.

2. American Thoracic Society: Position statement on pulmonary rehabilitation. Am Rev Respir Dis 124:663, 1981.
3. Angelillo VA: Nutrition and the pulmonary patient. In Hodgkin JE, Connors GL, Bell W (eds): Pulmonary Rehabilitation: Guidelines to Success, 2nd ed. Philadelphia, JB Lippincott, 1993.
4. Bach JR: Pulmonary Rehabilitation: The Obstructive and Paralytic Conditions. Philadelphia, Hanley & Belfus, 1996.
5. Bach JR, Moldover JR: Cardiovascular, pulmonary and cancer rehabilitation. 2. Pulmonary rehabilitation. Arch Phys Med Rehabil 77:S45–S51, 1996.
6. Belman MJ: Exercise with patients will chronic obstructive pulmonary disease. Thorax 458:936–46, 1993.
7. Bickford LS, Hodgkin JE, McInturff SL: National pulmonary rehabilitation survey update. J Cardiopulm Rehabil 15:406–411, 1995.
8. Brannon FJ, et al: Cardiopulmonary Rehabilitation: Basic Theory and Application. Philadelphia, FA Davis, 1993.
9. Casaburi R, Patessio A, Ioli F, et al: Reductions in exercise lactic acidosis and ventilation as a result of exercise training in patients with obstructive lung disease. Am Rev Respir Dis 143:9–18, 1991.
10. Christiansen CH, et al: Self care: Evaluation and management. In DeLisa JA (ed): Rehabilitation Medicine: Principles and Practice, 2nd ed. Philadelphia, JB Lippincott, 1993.
11. Connors G, Hilling L (eds): Guidelines for Pulmonary Rehabilitation Programs. American Association of Cardiovascular and Pulmonary Rehabilitation. Champaign, IL, Human Kinetics, 1993.
12. Czajkowski SM, et al: The role of psychosocial factors in chronic obstructive pulmonary disease. Phys Med Rehabil Clin North Am 7:353–365, 1996.
13. Epstein SK, Celli BR, Martinez FJ, et al: Arm training reduces the VO_2 and VE cost of unsupported arm exercise and elevation in chronic obstructive pulmonary disease. J Cardiopulm Rehabil 17:171–177, 1997.
14. Goldstein RS, Avendano AM: Model program development and outcomes in chronic obstructive pulmonary disease. Phys Med Rehabil Clin North Am 7:353–365, 1996.
15. Gracey DR, Hardy DC, Naessens JM, et al: The Mayo Ventilator-dependent Rehabilitation Unit: A 5-year experience. Mayo Clin Proc 72:13–19, 1997.
16. Haas F, et al: Cardiopulmonary exercise evaluation. Phys Med Rehabil Clin North Am 7:241–251, 1996.
17. Hemholz HF: Rehabilitation for respiratory dysfunction. In Kottke FJ (ed): Krusen's Handbook of Physical Medicine and Rehabilitation, 4th ed. Philadelphia, WB Saunders, 1990.
18. Hodgkin JE: Benefits and the future of pulmonary rehabilitation. In Hodgkin JE, Connors GL, Bell W (eds): Pulmonary Rehabilitation: Guidelines to Success, 2nd ed. Philadelphia, JB Lippincott, 1993.
19. Jardim JR, et al: Nutrition, anabolic steroids and growth hormone. Phys Med Rehabil Clin North Am 7:253–275, 1996.
20. Make BJ, Glenn K: Outcomes of pulmonary rehabilitation. In Bach JR (ed): Pulmonary Rehabilitation: The Obstructive and Paralytic Conditions. Philadelphia, Hanley & Belfus, 1996, pp 173–191.
21. Orenstein DM: Rehabilitation for the pediatric patient with pulmonary disease. In Hodgkin JE, Connors GL, Bell W (eds): Pulmonary Rehabilitation: Guidelines to Success, 2nd ed. Philadelphia, JB Lippincott, 1993.
22. Pashkow P, Ades PA, Emery CF, et al. Outcome measurement in cardiac and pulmonary rehabilitation. J Cardiopulm Rehabil 15:394–405, 1995.
23. Petty TL: Pulmonary Rehabilitation. Basics of RD. New York, American Thoracic Society, 1975.
24. Radovich JL, et al: Cost effectiveness of pulmonary rehabilitation programs. In Hodgkin JE, Connors GL, Bell W (eds): Pulmonary Rehabilitation: Guidelines to Success, 2nd ed. Philadelphia, JB Lippincott, 1993.
25. Rashbaum I, Whyte N: Occupational therapy in pulmonary rehabilitation: Energy conservation and work simplification techniques. Phys Med Rehabil Clin North Am 7:325–340, 1996.
26. Ries AL: The importance of exercise in pulmonary rehabilitation. Clin Chest Med 15:327–337, 1994.
27. Rodrigues JC, Ilowite JS: Pulmonary rehabilitation in the elderly patient. Clin Chest Med 14:429–436, 1993.

28. Siebens H: The role of exercise in the rehabilitation of patients with chronic obstructive pulmonary disease. Phys Med Rehabil Clin North Am 7:299–314, 1996.
29. Strijbos JH, Postma DS, van Altena R, et al: Feasibility and effects of a home-care rehabilitation program in patients with chronic obstructive pulmonary disease. J Cardiopulm Rehabil 16:386–393, 1996.
30. Votto J, Bowen J, Scalise P, et al: Short-stay comprehensive inpatient pulmonary rehabilitation for advanced chronic obstructive pulmonary disease. Arch Phys Med Rehabil 77:1115–1118, 1996.
31. Weiser PC, Ryan KP: Tri-state region pulmonary rehabilitation survey: Delivery of exercise conditioning services. J Cardiopulm Rehabil 16:175–182, 1996.
32. Zadai CC: Therapeutic exercise in pulmonary disease and disability. In Basmajian JV, Wolf SL (eds): Therapeutic Exercise, 5th ed. Baltimore, Williams & Wilkins, 1990.

GEOFFREY E. MOORE, MD

7

Exercise Prescription in Renal Failure

Exercise intolerance is a serious barrier to rehabilitation for persons with renal failure. Functional capacity in dialysis patients is typically more than two standard deviations below the age- and gender-predicted norm, and often it is far lower and barely enough to meet needs for self-care activities of daily living (ADL).[7,13] Severe exercise intolerance is probably related to quality of life for most dialysis patients, but this is not the only contributing factor.[3] Renal transplant recipients fare somewhat better, having near normal exercise tolerance and quality of life.[3,15] Historically, caregivers and patients have accepted this predicament as part of being a dialysis patient, but this need not be so. Such problems can often be solved with regular physical activity.

Most efforts to improve exercise tolerance in dialysis patients and transplant recipients have been through aerobic exercise training.[4,5,9,14,17,21] Most of these studies show that exercise training increases peak aerobic exercise tolerance by an average of about 15–20%, but some data suggest that heterogeneity exists in the response to exercise training and that some patients do not improve in an expected fashion.[9] What leads a person to become a non-responder is not known, but suspicions are that the problem may be related to extensive overall disease burden (i.e., multiple and severe concomitant chronic illness). One major difference between the studies is that the studies that did not show an improvement after exercise training enrolled any willing participant, but the studies that did show an improvement were more restrictive in their entry criteria. No controlled trials have assessed the impact of disease burden on adaptability to training.

A major factor that limits exercise tolerance in renal failure patients is that the patients are weak.[2] Indeed, muscle strength is a better predictor of aerobic capacity in dialysis patients than hematocrit, even in anemic patients.[2] There has not, however, been a study of strength training in dialysis patients. In addition to weakness, many renal failure patients have arthritis and subsequently a limited range of motion. Thus, while it is logical to include flexibility and strength components in a comprehensive exercise training rehabilitation program for renal failure patients, no objective data support or refute the idea.

TABLE 1. Complications Related to Exercise in Patients with Renal Disease

Common Complications	Rare Complications
Joint pain / arthritis exacerbation	Hypoglycemia
Exaggerated pressor response	Stress fracture / tendon avulsion
Hypotension	Myocardial infarction
Anhydrosis (prickly heat)	
Angina	

Many renal failure patients have other medical problems. In the United States, for example, about one third of dialysis patients have diabetes, and cardiovascular disease is the largest cause of death in dialysis patients.[20] Any exercise program for such a patient must compensate for these comorbid conditions. At first attempt, this is a daunting task, and many efforts have failed. However, the application of problem-oriented techniques to the exercise domain can yield successful exercise interventions, even in extremely complex patients.[8]

For patients with renal disease, most of the risks of exercise (Table 1) are related to exacerbation of comorbid conditions. Because many patients are advanced in age, arthritis is relatively common. Also common are persons with diabetes and high blood pressure (about 34% and 29% of patients, respectively). Because of renal neuropathy and autonomic dysfunction, many patients are at risk for hemodynamic instabilities. Patients with severe and longstanding hyperparathyroidism are at risk for orthopedic injury due to renal osteodystrophy. Despite the high prevalence of cardiovascular disease, cardiovascular complications are uncommon, which may be due to the fact that much of the exercise program is no more intense than most patient's normal ADLs.

EXERCISE PROGRAMMING

The main purpose of exercise programs for renal disease patients is improved functional capacity and the ability to carry out ADLs; important secondary goals of exercise should be to increase quality of life, functional capacity/ADLs, and mental and emotional status.[19] Although studies show that exercise is safe, some minor special considerations must be made to minimize the risk of complications. These considerations are specific to the type of renal replacement therapy: hemodialysis (Table 2), peritoneal dialysis, and renal transplant (Table 3).

Exercise is most effective for many **hemodialysis patients** during the dialysis treatment,[16] because the duration of dialysis is usually otherwise spent reading, watching television, or sleeping. Further, medical personnel are in attendance should there be any complications. Minor technical problems include (1) how to position the exercise bicycle, (2) how to avoid pulling out the blood access lines, (3) helping the patient use the bicycle while in their dialysis chair, (4) hypotensive episodes, (5) exaggerated pres-

TABLE 2. Exercise Program for Hemodialysis Patients

Stationary Cycling on Dialysis	Aerobic Activities off Dialysis	Strength Training
5-min warm-up, 20–50 min cycling @ effort rating 5–6, 5-min cool-down 3 sessions each week	5-min warm-up, 20–50 min activity @ effort rating 5–6, 5-min cool-down 1–2 sessions each week	6–12 repetitions each lift 1–3 sessions each week

TABLE 3. Program for Peritoneal Dialysis Patients or Transplant Recipients

Aerobic Activities	Calisthenics/Strength Training
5-min warm-up, 20–50 min cycling @ effort rating 5–6, 5-min cool-down 4–6 sessions each week	6–12 repetitions each lift 1–3 sessions each week

sor responses to exercise and sometimes alarmingly high blood pressure, and (6) hypoglycemia in patients with diabetes.

Peritoneal dialysis patients find it easiest to exercise with an empty abdomen, simply for mechanical reasons. Minor technical problems include (1) avoiding contamination of the catheter during profuse sweating or even swimming, (2) exaggerated pressor responses to exercise, which can be alarmingly high, and (3) hypoglycemia in patients with diabetes.

Transplant recipients function nearly normally but do have some minor considerations in their exercise programming. First, because the transplanted kidney is placed in the anterior abdomen and is somewhat vulnerable to blunt trauma, athletes with transplants should be careful about playing contact sports.

The other problem is risk of bone fracture. Many patients have had longstanding hyperparathyroidism prior to transplantation, and almost all transplant recipients take corticosteroids for immunosuppression. Such patients are at risk for stress and avulsion fractures,[1,18] which are most likely to occur in forms of exercise that use forceful contractions (e.g., jumping, running, contact sports, weight lifting). Therefore, low-impact activities are best. Because diabetic renal transplant recipients usually do not receive a pancreas as well, most such patients remain diabetic with the attendant risks of blood sugar abnormalities. Furthermore, about a third of patients will develop diabetes as a result of taking corticosteroids.[10]

GENERAL PROGRAM CHARACTERISTICS

Most patients undertaking an exercise program should start low and go slow. Experience proves that this is safe, and there is little to be gained by aggressive increases in activity level. One should start with intensities that are at the level of normal ADL (or slightly higher) and try for a duration of 5–10 minutes and a minimum frequency of three times per week. Each week, the duration of exercise can be increased by 5 minutes per session. Frequency of sessions can be gradually increased to every day to emphasize the importance of exercise in cardiovascular health and overall fitness.

The intensity of exercise can vary quite a bit, and variations in the exercise routine help maintain motivation. Intensity should be guided by perceived exertion, using the standard Rating of Perceived Exertion (RPE) scale, particularly for hemodialysis patients exercising during the dialysis treatment. Use of target heart rates is also acceptable but requires more sophistication and education, and heart rates will vary with the excess fluid volume. For these reasons, subjective assessments of intensity are preferred. Ultimately, an ideal program would include the following:

- Daily aerobic exercise: 30–60 minutes total activity each day; 30 minutes at RPE 4–7

- 2 or 3 days per week of resistance (strength) training, emphasis on legs and arms

- Daily stretching as warm-up and cool-down

The kind of aerobic exercise is probably not especially important but should be walking, cycling, or other low-intensity activity (Table 4).

SPECIFIC PROGRAM CHARACTERISTICS

Establishing a Goal

Like other medical therapies, exercise programs have a therapeutic goal. Carefully chosen goals of each patient's program will improve the likelihood of success. Examples of appropriate goals are specific activity levels, ability to do 7 METs of peak exer-

TABLE 4. Scale to Gauge Effort during Exercise

Rating	Effort	Sensation
1	None	Sitting
2	Minimal	Easy stretching
3	Very easy	Warm-up/cool-down
4	Easy workout	Can go as long as you want
5	Usual workout	Breathing fully, heart rate up
6	Moderately hard	Can barely talk in sentences
7	Hard	Cannot talk in sentences
8	Very hard	Games (e.g., baseball)
9	Almost at limit	Hard sports (e.g., basketball, soccer)
10	At physical limit	Very hard sports (e.g., running)

cise tolerance, or strength appropriate for the individual's ADL needs. Reasonably achievable goals that have been demonstrated in research protocols include:

- Increased exercise tolerance / aerobic capacity and endurance

- Improved quality of life

- Reduced very low-density–lipoprotein cholesterol and triglycerides

- Increased high-density–lipoprotein cholesterol

- Improved glucose tolerance

- Lower blood pressure and/or need for medications

An exercise test prior to starting a training program is useful in determining a reasonable goal, but it is not necessary. An exercise test provides data for a specific goal as well as a range of training intensity. In the absence of an exercise test, most patients can start at a low level and gradually increase duration and intensity.[11,12]

Assessing Safety

The condition of patients with renal failure is notoriously unstable, particularly hemodialysis patients with multiple comorbidities. Thus, before doing any exercise, such patients should undergo some form of assessment to make sure it is safe to exercise. The assessment usually does not involve anything more than a simple check of vital signs and musculoskeletal symptoms; in diabetics, it also should include a check of blood glucose and skin on weightbearing surfaces. The patient should not exercise if there are any unstable vital signs (e.g., fever, rapid/irregular pulse) or symptoms (e.g., angina, joint pain, dizziness, dyspnea). In diabetics, blood glucose should be controlled; exercise should be postponed for blood glucose lower than 80 mg/dL, for glucose above 350–400 mg/dL, or for ketosis. This routine safety check can be included in a stretching routine as part of the warm-up. Stretching should include upper and lower extremities, the back, hips, and pelvis.

Determining Degree of Difficulty

Exercise intensity should match the goals of the program. Most patients can achieve satisfactory results with moderate to low-level exercise at or slightly above the intensity of usual ADLs. This generally means a perceived exertion of 4–7 on the RPE scale, the ability to comfortably chat while exercising, and enough intensity to break a sweat. Transplant recipients can use target heart rates as a guide to exercise intensity, but dialysis patients cannot reliably do this because they have wide day-to-day variations in heart rate. Dialysis patient should use subjective guides of intensity, such as RPE.

When doing muscle strengthening exercises, the patient should start with a resistance that can be performed about 10 times, and the weight is gradually increased. There is usually not much point in doing more than 10–20 repetitions, because the main goal is to increase strength. Persons with severe renal osteodystrophy or steroid-induced osteoporosis should not lift weights heavier than they can lift for three repetitions.

Determining When to Stop

In general, the patient should not feel exhausted for hours after exercising, but more advanced exercisers who play sports may be perfectly fine doing so on occasion. The patient should not exercise past the point where he or she becomes unable to maintain a steady pace, which is a sign that severe fatigue is impending. It is far better for the person to quit and come back the next day than to continue to the point of exhaustion. In addition, patients should stop if they are having a new onset of musculoskeletal pain, angina, dizziness, headache, unusual dyspnea, or other symptoms suggesting medical instability.

Evaluating Progress

Depending on the individual and the goals, a reasonable time to achieve the goals is 8–12 weeks. For more challenging goals, it helps to have intermediate objectives to maintain motivation and a sense of progress. It is probably not necessary to evaluate progress more often than every 2–4 weeks.

SOURCES OF INFORMATION

The following are excellent resources for assistance with starting an exercise program for patients with renal failure.

Exercise for the Dialysis Patient
Medical Education Institute, Inc.
University Research Park
585 Science Dr., Suite B
Madison, WI 53711-1060
(608) 232-2336 phone
(608) 238-5046 fax
or call Amgen Customer Service
(800) 28-Amgen

Renal Exercise
730 Welch Road, Suite B
Palo Alto, CA 94304
(415) 723-9837 phone
(415) 723-7018 fax
painter@scrdp.stanford.edu

REFERENCES

1. Bhole R, Flynn JC, Marbury TC: Quadriceps tendon ruptures in uremia. Clin Orthop 195:200–206, 1985.
2. Diesel W, Noakes TD, Swanepoel C, Lambert M: Isokinetic muscle strength predicts maximum exercise tolerance in renal patients on chronic hemodialysis. Am J Kidney Dis 16:109–114, 1990.
3. Evans RW, Manninen DL, Garrison LP, et al: The quality of life of patients with end-stage renal failure. N Engl J Med 312:553–559, 1985.
4. Goldberg AP, Geltman EM, Hagberg JM, et al: Therapeutic benefits of exercise training for hemodialysis patients. Kidney Int 24:S303–S309, 1983.
5. Goldberg AP, Hagberg JM, Delmez JA, et al: Effects of exercise training on coronary risk factors in hemodialysis patients. Proc Dial Transpl Forum 9:39–43, 1979.

6. Kutner N, Brogan D, Fielding B: Employment status and ability to work among working-age chronic dialysis patients. Am J Nephrol 11:334–340, 1991.

7. Moore GE, Brinker KR, Stray-Gundersen J, Mitchell JH: Determinants of VO_{2peak} in patients with end-stage renal disease: On and off dialysis. Med Sci Sports Exerc 25:18–23, 1993.

8. Moore GE, Durstine JL: Framework. In Durstine JL, Bloomquist LE, Figoni SF, et al (eds): ACSM's Exercise Management in Persons with Chronic Diseases and Disabilities. Champaign, IL, Human Kinetics, 1997, pp 6–16.

9. Moore GE, Parsons DB, Painter PL, et al: Uremic myopathy limits aerobic capacity of hemodialysis patients. Am J Kidney Dis 22:277–287, 1993.

10. Painter P: Organ transplant. In Durstine JL, Bloomquist LE, Figoni SF, et al (eds): ACSM's Exercise Management for Persons with Chronic Diseases and Disabilities. Champaign, IL, Human Kinetics, 1997, pp 137–140.

11. Painter P: Renal failure. In Durstine JL, Bloomquist LE, Figoni SF, et al (eds): ACSM's Exercise Management for Persons with Chronic Diseases and Disabilities. Champaign, IL, Human Kinetics, 1997, pp 89–93.

12. Painter P, Blagg CR, Moore GE: Exercise for the Dialysis Patient: A Prescribing Guide. Madison, WI, Medical Education Institute, 1995.

13. Painter P, Moore GE: The impact of recombinant erythropoietin therapy on exercise capacity in hemodialysis patients. Adv Ren Replace Ther 1:55–65, 1994.

14. Painter PL: Exercise training during hemodialysis: Rates of participation. Dial Transpl 17:165–168, 1988.

15. Painter PL, Messer-Rehak D, Hanson P, et al: Exercise capacity in hemodialysis, CAPD, and renal transplant patients. Nephron 42:47–51, 1986.

16. Painter PL, Nelson-Worel JN, Hill MM, et al: Effects of exercise training during hemodialysis. Nephron 43:87–92, 1986.

17. Ross DL, Grabeau GM, Smith S, et al: Efficacy of exercise for end-stage renal disease patients immediately following high-efficiency hemodialysis: A pilot study. Am J Nephrol 9:376–383, 1989.

18. Ryuzaki M, Konischi K, Kasuga TC: Spontaneous rupture of the quadriceps tendon in patients on maintenance dialysis: Report of three cases with clinicopathological observations. Clin Nephrol 32:144–148, 1989.

19. Stewart AL, Greenfield S, Hays RD, et al: Functional status and well-being of patients with chronic conditions: Results from the medical outcomes study. JAMA 262:907–913, 1989.

20. United States Renal Data System: USRDS 1993 Annual Data Report. Bethesda, MD, National Institute of Diabetes and Digestive and Kidney Diseases, 1993.

21. Zabetakis PM, Gleim GW, Pasternak FL, et al: Long-duration submaximal exercise conditioning in hemodialysis patients. Clin Nephrol 18:17–22, 1982.

VINCENT YACYSHYN, MD
KAREN L. ANDREWS, MD

8

Exercise in Peripheral Vascular Disease

Rehabilitation of the patient with vascular disease includes the evaluation, diagnosis, and management of arterial and venous diseases. The goal of optimal management is to decrease the morbidity and mortality associated with these diseases.

ARTERIAL DISEASE

EPIDEMIOLOGY

Peripheral arterial disease is a relatively common manifestation of systemic athero-sclerosis; it affects 5% of persons 50 years of age and 20% of persons older than 70 years.[15,30] The most frequent presentation of arterial occlusive disease is intermittent claudication. Epidemiologic studies have demonstrated that limb-threatening is-chemia develops in as few as 2–5% of patients with intermittent claudication moni-tored for up to 10 years.[43] There is an overall reduction of 10 years in life expectancy among patients with peripheral vascular disease, with mortality primarily due to coro-nary artery disease and diabetes mellitus with its associated complications. The mor-tality rate in patients with peripheral vascular disease is 20–30% 5 years after diag-nosis, 40–72% after 10 years, and 74% after 15 years. About 75% of the deaths are caused by cardiovascular events.[6]

ETIOLOGY

There are many causes of arterial occlusive disease, the most common of which is ath-erosclerosis obliterans (ASO). Other disease processes include thromboangiitis obliter-ans (Buerger's disease), Mönckeberg's medial calcific sclerosis, vasospastic disorders (Raynaud's phenomenon, livedo reticularis, and acrocyanosis), thrombosis, embolism, dissection, vasculitis, and fibromuscular dysplasia.

Atherosclerosis

Atherosclerosis is a systemic disorder involving the coronary, cerebral, pulmonary, renal, and peripheral vessels. The earliest pathologic manifestation of atherosclerosis appears to be the intimal streak, although the eventual progression of streaks to fibrous or complicated plaques remains uncertain.[60] Atherosclerotic lesions develop mainly near branches, bifurcations, and bends, all areas of low shear stress, where there is separation from unidirectional laminar blood flow, reversal of flow, and turbulence.[45] There is an inverse relation between shear stress and rate of lumen narrowing. Although low shear stress is associated with atherogenesis and disease progression, regions of moderate to high shear stress are relatively spared from intimal thickening as long as flow remains unidirectional and axially aligned.[45] Atherosclerosis typically involves multiple levels of the arterial tree; however, it tends to be a segmental disease in which intervening arterial segments can be remarkably free of involvement or minimally involved. Associated conditions can affect the location of disease. In diabetics, atherosclerosis occurs with equal frequency in both femoral and tibial arteries; in nondiabetics, the most common sites of severe disease are the abdominal aorta and iliac and femoral arteries.[36]

Many people younger than 65 who have atherosclerosis have one or more identifiable risk factors. The presence of multiple risk factors further increases the risk of atherosclerosis. Smoking is the single highest risk factor in the etiology of peripheral vascular disease.[37] Other risk factors include diabetes mellitus, hypertension, hyperlipidemia, abnormalities of hemostatic function and hemorrheology, abnormalities of homocysteine metabolism, aging, and genetic predisposition. Smoking acts synergistically with other risk factors such as hypertension or hypercholesterolemia to enhance progression of atherosclerotic lesions. Persons with claudication who continue to smoke not only have a greater likelihood of vascular disease progression but also are at higher risk of other adverse outcomes, such as myocardial infarction, stroke, and death, than those who quit smoking.[35]

CLINICAL EVALUATION

History

Chronic arterial occlusive disease usually can be diagnosed from the history and physical examination findings. Unless complicated by thrombus or embolus, the symptoms and signs associated with ASO rarely have an abrupt onset. The most common symptom is intermittent claudication. Lower extremity claudication has two diagnostic clinical features: (1) it is reproduced with a consistent level of exercise from one occasion to the next and (2) it completely resolves within minutes after the exercise has been discontinued.[28] Patients may adapt their behavior and decrease their level of physical activity such that they do not experience claudication pain.

The differential diagnosis of vascular claudication is neurogenic claudication. The location, nature, and quality of the pain may be very similar. Positional exacerbation and relief of pain may provide clues to the source of the pain.

The site of claudication is of rough value for indicating the level of occlusion.[36] Patients with occlusion at or above the ankle can present with claudication in the arch of the foot. Calf claudication suggests occlusion at or above the calf. Patients with isolated aortoiliac disease generally present with buttock pain or sexual dysfunction.

Clinical Findings

Palpation of lower extremity pulses may confirm a diagnosis of vascular claudication. The femoral, popliteal, dorsalis pedis, and posterior tibial arteries are palpated. Auscultation is performed to evaluate for bruits. Doppler devices may be necessary to detect circulation in limbs with advanced disease.

To determine the severity of ischemia, the clinician should look for elevation pallor and dependent rubor and quantitate the venous filling time. Elevation pallor is determined by raising the leg to a 30° angle: if pallor develops within 60 seconds, the patient has mild ischemia; within 30 seconds, moderate ischemia; and within 15 seconds, severe ischemia.[11] Normal venous filling time is classically described as 20 seconds, but this value is altered with associated congestive heart failure, venous insufficiency, pulmonary hypertension, or tricuspid regurgitation. As the disease process advances, resting blood flow rates are affected, and ischemia at rest and impaired skin metabolism result. Clinical findings of ischemia can include trophic changes, dependent rubor, paresthesias (which may be partially or completely relieved with dependency), cutaneous ulceration, and gangrene (Fig. 1).

VASCULAR TESTING

Noninvasive Studies

If ischemia is noted on clinical examination, noninvasive studies can determine the degree and level of ischemia and the potential for healing and provide a baseline for future comparison. Measurement of resting ankle pressure is the most common non-

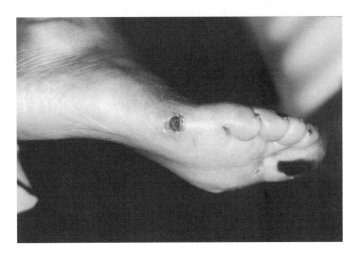

FIGURE 1. Arterial occlusive disease with associated ischemia, ulcerations, and gangrenous changes.

invasive study performed on patients with suspected vascular disease. Variations in systemic pressure between individuals are corrected by expressing the absolute ankle pressure as a ratio relative to the brachial pressure (ankle/brachial index, ABI). The ABI is interpreted as follows: >0.9, normal; 0.8–0.9, mild; 0.5–0.8, moderate; and <0.5, severe.[46]

When patients present with symptoms that occur during exercise, some form of exercise evaluation should be performed. When patients present primarily with symptoms at rest, an evaluation can be performed without exercise testing. The hemodynamic severity of the vascular disease defined by ABI or calf blood flow is not well correlated to treadmill exercise performance. These measures should not be used as the main test of the functional effects of interventions whose primary goal is to improve or relieve claudication.[49] In patients with mild symptoms of claudication, the ABI might be normal at rest but reduced after exercise. At rest, the vascular resistance of the leg is relatively high, and flow through a stenotic lesion can be sufficient to maintain normal distal pressure. After exercise, the vascular resistance is lower and the blood flow through the stenosis may not be sufficient to keep the distal pressure from decreasing.[52] Traditionally, postexercise ABIs are determined by having the patient walk on a treadmill for 5 minutes at 2 miles per hour (mph) at a 10–12% grade. Under these conditions, not all patients achieve maximal exertion. Walking time in repeated tests may vary as much as 50% within the same subject.[29] In contrast, using a progressive increase in workload (a 3.5% increase in grade every 3 minutes until maximum symptoms of claudication are achieved), Hiatt found that the reproducibility of the variables measured at maximum exercise ranged from 7–13%.[29] In addition, the fall in ankle pressure after exercise was greater after walking at 3 mph than at 2 mph despite similar arm pressures at maximal exercise in both protocols. As a result, the 3-mph protocol is recommended when testing patients with mild or questionable arterial disease.[29]

Invasive Studies: Arteriography

Although physiologic testing is excellent for screening and follow-up, arteriography remains the most accurate procedure for the evaluation of infrainguinal arterial occlusive disease. If surgery is anticipated, arteriography is usually needed to determine the length of arterial occlusion, level of distal reconstruction, and patency of the plantar arch. In the presence of inflow vessel disease, special arteriographic techniques such as digital subtraction angiography may be necessary for visualization of distal run-off vessels. Because patients with arterial occlusive disease also can have renal disease, they consequently are at higher risk for renal failure if contrast material is used.

FUNCTIONAL STATUS MEASURES

To evaluate functional status in the patient with arterial occlusive disease, it is important not only to consider laboratory-based measures such as treadmill tests but also to examine the effects of a treatment program on community-based walking ability and quality of life. Questionnaires have been developed and validated to evaluate functional status and provide a valuable adjunct to laboratory-based measures.[49,50] Questionnaires are limited in that self-assessment of physical activity is subject to bias. Monitoring devices such as motion sensors provide a more objective estimate of physical activity. The use of activity monitors requires special equipment that can be costly and places additional demands on the patient. Given the cost and greater complexity of usage, such devices are used primarily in research rather than in the clinical setting.[49]

TESTING FOR ASSOCIATED DISEASES

When evaluating the patient with atherosclerotic occlusive disease, especially if surgical intervention is planned, it is important that the clinical evaluation define and quantify any associated cardiovascular, renal, and pulmonary problems. Because many patients with vascular disease are sedentary and lack symptoms of coronary artery disease, it is easy to overlook asymptomatic but hemodynamically significant coronary arterial disease despite obtaining a thorough history and physical examination. The Framingham study showed an increased incidence of ischemic heart disease in patients with intermittent claudication.[37] Carroll et al. reported that the incidence of electrocardiogram abnormalities at rest was 40% among 81 patients with claudication, and this figure rose to 60% during treadmill walking.[4] The prevalence of serious coronary artery disease ranges from 37–78% in patients undergoing an operation for peripheral vascular disease.[26] Although procedures involving aortic cross-clamping exert a greater acute systemic hemodynamic stress than femoral popliteal surgery, late cardiac morbidity and mortality are significant in all patients with atherosclerotic disease who undergo such procedures.[26] In patients with suspected coronary artery disease who must undergo peripheral vascular surgery, the perioperative mortality rate is about four times higher than for those without coronary artery disease, and the perioperative morbidity is markedly increased.[26]

Exercise testing is recommended for patients with non–insulin-dependent diabetes mellitus before beginning an exercise conditioning program because the prevalence of occult coronary artery disease and silent cardiac ischemia is high. Patients with non–insulin-dependent diabetes mellitus should undergo exercise testing if they are sedentary, older than 35, or have had diabetes for more than 10 years.[30] Clearly, exercise testing is limited in patients who have severe claudication, rest ischemia, or prior amputation. The primary advantage of exercise testing is its wide availability and modest cost. Although electrocardiogram-monitored stress testing is being replaced by pharmacologic infusions, stress testing is still a useful way to obtain objective information regarding the relative degree of impairment imposed by claudication, pulmonary insufficiency, or coronary artery disease.

Dobutamine thallium-201 scintigraphy and echocardiography (or related tests using agents such as adenosine or dipyridamole and uptake agents such as Sestamibi are useful for screening patients with peripheral vascular disease for coronary artery disease because they are minimally invasive and can be performed with the patient at rest. In patients with hemodynamically significant coronary artery disease, the difference in perfusion between myocardium supplied by normal coronary arteries and that supplied by stenotic, nondistensible vessels is accentuated. No uptake is noted in infarcted tissue. Only patients with significant ischemic myocardial territories require further cardiac evaluation. In general, patients with a history of chronic stable angina, with a single uncomplicated myocardial infarction more than 6 months prior to evaluation, or in whom only a small region (single coronary distribution) of myocardial ischemia is detected need no further cardiac evaluation.[19]

TREATMENT

Therapeutic success is most likely to occur with an educated patient and family. It is important to discuss in detail the diffuse and progressive nature of atherosclerosis, the importance of controlling risk factors, and measures to protect the ischemic limb. The ultimate goal is to develop effective therapy that prevents progression of the disease process and possibly promotes regression of existing lesions. The correct diagnosis and cause of the underlying disease process must be identified before proceeding with treatment. Controllable risk factors such as smoking, diabetes, hyperlipidemia, hypertension, and gross obesity as discussed previously should be addressed with appropriate pharmacologic approaches, dietary measures, or behavior modifications. The medical treatment of patients with arterial occlusive disease is directed at intensive risk factor modification to decrease cardiovascular morbidity and mortality. A second treatment goal is to improve exercise performance and functional capacity.[50] Candidates for structured vascular rehabilitation include individuals with documented peripheral arterial insufficiency and (1) intermittent claudication, (2) decreased ability to perform desired activities (secondary to diminished arterial perfusion), or (3) recent surgical revascularization or peripheral angioplasty. (Fig. 2).

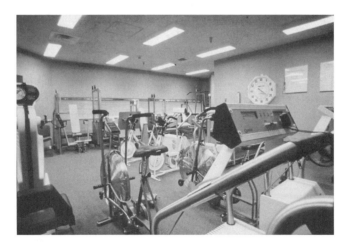

FIGURE 2. Outpatient vascular rehabilitation center.

Exercise

For many years, the main exercises for patients with occlusive arterial disease were the passive movements developed by Buerger, who theorized that blood vessels would accept a greater function in blood transfer if they were alternately emptied and distended.[3] The formation of collaterals was attempted by a series of exercises that consisted of the following sequence: the limbs were supported in an elevated position at an angle of 60–90° for 30–180 seconds or the minimum time required to produce blanching. Following the onset of blanching, the feet were permitted to hang down over the edge of the bed or table for 2–5 minutes or as long as necessary to produce reactive hyperemia or rubor, plus one additional minute (total time not to exceed 5 minutes). Next, the legs were placed in a horizontal position for 3–5 minutes. This cycle was repeated six or seven times at a sitting, and the entire sequence was repeated several times during a day.[3] Oscillating beds were also used to alternately fill the limb with blood and then drain it by positional changes. The angle of depression of the oscillating bed was adjusted to suit the physiologic need. Readjustments were made as circulation improved. The aim on the upswing of the bed was to maintain sufficient elevation long enough for the veins to collapse but not to produce pallor in the capillary bed of the toes.[24] With time, these passive interventions were prescribed less frequently as other therapeutic measures came into vogue. Wisham showed that passive postural movements did not enhance blood flow. Instead, increased flow occurred during and shortly after active exercise and appeared to increase in relation to the intensity of exercise.[61] Foley recommended exercise to stimulate collateral blood flow and improve the metabolic state of the ischemic tissues.[24] The first randomized controlled trial of exercise training in persons with arterial occlusive disease demonstrated a marked improvement in treadmill walking with exercise[39] (Fig. 3).

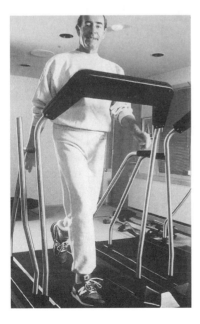

FIGURE 3. Treadmill for graded exercise program.

A successful exercise conditioning program involves an accurate assessment of functional capacity, determination of an effective exercise prescription, and appropriate measurements of outcome.[31] Exercise conditioning programs in arterial occlusive disease follow similar guidelines as more established cardiac programs. Unlike the cardiac patient where some degree of spontaneous recovery occurs and the overall functional capacity can be high (greater than 9 METs), most of the improvement in the patient with arterial occlusive disease is related to the exercise conditioning program and usually occurs at a lower level of initial exercise capacity (5 METs).[31] All studies of exercise conditioning in patients with peripheral arterial occlusive disease report an increase in the treadmill exercise performance and a lessening of claudication pain severity during exercise. This finding demonstrates that exercise training programs can have a clinically important impact on functional capacity in persons for whom other treatment options are limited and spontaneous recovery does not occur.[50]

Effect of Site and Severity of Disease   Although it had been thought that patients with proximal (aortoiliac) occlusive disease may not benefit from exercise training, studies have shown that similar improvement can be achieved in patients with obstruction proximal or distal to the inguinal ligament and in those with combined disease.[5,17,57] Perkins found greater functional improvement in patients with disease confined to the superficial femoral artery treated with exercise training than in patients treated with angioplasty.[47] It was proposed that disease in this arterial segment is often multifocal and less amenable to angioplasty.[47]

Mechanisms of Improvement   The physiologic mechanisms that may be responsible for the observed improvement in walking ability are not clear. Increased collateral circulation had been thought to be the major factor in the functional improvement.[18,58] Ekroth found that maximal calf blood flow did not increase in parallel with increases in walking ability.[17] This finding does not support the earlier belief that physical training is directly associated with the development of collateral circulation. Improved peripheral utilization of oxygen, reduced blood viscosity, and improved glycolytic and oxidative metabolic capacity have been suggested as reasons for the benefits of exercise training.[21,30,38,39,49] More recently, exercise-induced increases in blood flow and shear stress have been observed to enhance vascular function and structure. By increasing the release of nitric oxide and prostacyclin, shear stress augments endothelium-dependent vasodilation and inhibits multiple processes involved in atherogenesis and restenosis.[45] A change in the biomechanics of walking, increased muscle strength, and enhanced resistance to fatigue also may improve exercise performance.

Exercise Protocols   Exercise protocols vary considerably in type, frequency, and duration of exercise. Walking programs must be individualized; however, the usual prescription has a goal of 30–60 minutes, 3–5 days a week at a pace of 2 mph as allowed by cardiac precautions.[14,17] Risk stratification will determine the exercise prescription and level of supervision. The exercise prescription in peripheral arterial occlusive disease is derived from the workload at which moderate claudication occurs and does not correspond to the heart rate minus oxygen consumption relationship used to determine the intensity of exercise in cardiac patients.[31] Upon entry into the conditioning program, the exercise prescription is individualized based on the level of exercise limitation resulting from claudication on an initial graded treadmill exercise test. Appropriate warm-up and cool-down periods along with flexibility exercises are used to decrease the risk of musculoskeletal injury (Fig. 4). The goal of the initial training session is for the patient to spend 35 minutes performing intermittent treadmill exercise, exclusive of the warm-up and cool-down periods, with subsequent increases of 5 minutes each session until a 50-minute exercise session is possible.[49] During the exercise sessions, rest periods (induced by claudication) are interspersed between bouts of walking. The patient walks until a moderate level of pain is reached, rests until the pain abates, and resumes walking until a mild or moderate level of pain recurs. This process is repeated until the 50-minute exercise period has elapsed.[49] A meta-analysis to identify the components of exercise rehabilitation programs that were most effective in improving claudication pain symptoms found that the claudication pain endpoint, the length of exercise program, and the mode of exercise accounted for about 85–90% of the variance in the change in claudication distance.[25] The authors concluded that the optimal exercise program for improving claudication pain distances in patients with peripheral arterial disease uses intermittent walking to near maximal pain during a program of at least 6 months[25] (see Fig. 4).

Protective Footwear

Most amputations in persons with occlusive peripheral arterial disease result from some type of trauma (thermal, chemical, or mechanical) superimposed on the limb with chronic occlusive disease.[59] Thermal injury is prevented by avoiding excessive heat (such as from a heating pad or hot water). Warm outer footwear is recommended in the winter to protect against cold. Keeping an ischemic limb warm attenuates sympathetic tone, avoids vasoconstriction, and improves local cutaneous blood flow and transcutaneous oxygen pressure ($TcPO_2$).[55] Shoes with extra depth and custom inlays should be considered to avoid mechanical trauma.

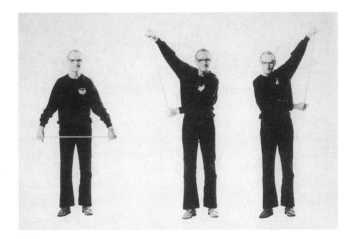

FIGURE 4. Stretching is performed prior to conditioning to avoid musculoskeletal injury.

The use of rocker-sole shoes to lessen the work of the gastrocnemius-soleus muscle groups during ambulation increases walking distance and can be a useful addition to the nonsurgical management of calf claudication.[51] Double-metal upright ankle-foot orthoses to eliminate ankle motion also have been studied. Despite the added weight, fixed ankle, appearance, and change of gait pattern, most patients noted an increase in their walking distance and were pleased with the results they obtained with this orthotic device.[32]

Risk Factor Modification

Peripheral artery disease and coronary artery disease are both manifestations of atherosclerotic disease and have similar risk factors: age, gender (estrogen status), family history, tobacco abuse, hypercholesterolemia, hypertension, diabetes mellitus, and physical inactivity. Patients should be counseled to modify these risk factors into a favorable profile to decrease their risk for further progression of atherosclerotic disease and its sequelae. In addition, if premature atherosclerosis is detected, the patient's first-degree relatives should be screened for heritable risk factors such as homocysteine and possibly familial lipoproteinemia.

Medication

Vasodilators   The general aim of drug therapy for arterial occlusive disease is to increase oxygen delivery. Although vasodilator drugs have been shown to increase blood flow to the limbs and various organs in animal experiments and in humans with vasospastic disorders, their use in peripheral arterial occlusive disease remains questionable.[7] An ideal drug for the treatment of peripheral arterial diseases would dilate blood vessels and increase blood flow only in the areas of deficient blood supply. Such agents do not currently exist. In some circumstances, vasodilation in areas without diseased vessels can actually steal flow from the affected area.[50] Because beta-adrenergic blockade can cause peripheral vasoconstriction, it has been recommended that beta-adrenergic blockers be avoided in patients with arterial occlusive disease.

Anticoagulants and Antiplatelet Agents   Platelet aggregation can exacerbate arterial occlusive disease by causing mechanical occlusion of small arteries or by releasing serotonin and stimulating local vasospasm.[19] There is no evidence that fibrinolytic agents, anticoagulants, or antiplatelet agents are directly effective in the treatment of intermittent claudication. Cyclooxygenase inhibitors such as aspirin decrease both prostacyclin production and thromboxane production. The former effect is proaggregatory and possibly vasoconstrictive, and the latter is antiaggregatory. Although aspirin is widely used for patients with arterial occlusive disease, its best documented effects relate to prevention of coronary and vascular graft thrombosis rather than intermittent claudication.[19,50]

Hemorrheologic Agents   Pentoxifylline (Trental) increases red blood cell deformability, decreases plasma viscosity, and diminishes platelet aggregation by decreasing fibrinogen concentration. It also increases resting and hyperemic extremity blood flow, presumably through its rheologic effects.[48,50] Reports about the degree of clinical improvement in patients taking pentoxifylline for intermittent claudication have been variable.[20,48] In early controlled trials, the drug produced a 22% improvement over placebo in walking distance prior to the onset of claudication and a 12% improvement in the maximal walking distance.[48] Ernst found that the benefit of drug plus physical therapy compared with exercise alone could be observed mainly in the first weeks of treatment and may wear off during long-term therapy.[20] Because pentoxifylline is a methylxanthine derivative, it should not be used in persons intolerant to this class of compounds, which includes caffeine and theophylline.

Antioxidant Agents Oxidation of low-density lipoprotein cholesterol tends to promote atherosclerotic disease development. Free radical injury of endothelial cells is prevented by antioxidant networks. Endogenous systems include glutathionine reductase and nonenzymatic antioxidant free radical scavengers (vitamins E, C, and β-carotene). Although data is preliminary, several animal studies and epidemiologic data suggest vitamins E, C, and β-carotene may retard atherosclerosis.[12] There may be a role for treatment of patients with peripheral arterial occlusive disease with antioxidant medications (vitamins E and C); however, final recommendations await a large-scale study of the effects of antioxidants in patients with peripheral arterial disease.

Revascularization

In patients with ischemic rest pain, ulceration, or gangrene, peripheral bypass surgery or percutaneous transluminal angioplasty may be necessary for relief of symptoms and limb preservation. Patients with incapacitating claudication that is unresponsive to other medical treatments also may be candidates for revascularization.[6,49]

Angioplasty Percutaneous transluminal angioplasty is an established treatment for claudication in patients with arterial occlusive disease. Angioplasty is indicated for focal stenosis or short segmental occlusions in which the adjacent vessels are relatively free of disease. Angioplasty is associated with a low incidence of morbidity. Five-year patency rates of 80–90% have been reported for iliac lesions and 60–70% for superficial femoral artery lesions following angioplasty.[14] A recent study suggested that supervised graduated exercise therapy produces better long-term improvement in mean distance walked before claudication and maximal walking distance in patients suitable for angioplasty than does angioplasty itself.[14] One advantage of angioplasty is that the inpatient stay is only about 48 hours.

Surgery Lundgren conducted a randomized, controlled trial comparing the effects of peripheral bypass surgery, surgery followed by 6 months of supervised exercise training, and 6 months of supervised exercise training alone in 75 patients with claudication. About 13 months after randomization, walking ability was improved in all three groups. The most effective treatment was exercise training plus surgery. The probability of an unlimited symptom-free walking performance was 50% in patients treated with surgery alone but 85% in those who had supplemental training.[42] Vascular reconstruction is indicated in patients with incapacitating claudication, rest pain, gangrene, and tissue loss, especially when the ABI is less than 0.4 or the forefoot TcPO$_2$ is less than 30 mm Hg.

Other Measures

Sympathectomy As reconstructive procedures have extended to distal vessels, sympathectomy has been performed less frequently. Limbs with inoperable arterial disease, ischemic cutaneous ulceration, pain at rest, or pregangrenous changes can be considered for sympathetic denervation. The primary effect of sympathectomy seems to be enhancing pain relief rather than augmenting blood flow to the ischemic limb.

Intermittent Venous Occlusion/Pneumatic Leg Compression Skin blood flow, as reflected by $TcPO_2$, can be augmented acutely in ischemic limbs by intermittent venous occlusion with an externally applied inflatable cuff.[56] Other devices, which apply intermittent circumferential pneumatic compression to the foot or lower limb, show promise as adjunct measures to augment limb perfusion and decrease dependent edema.

Amputation Ideally, all ischemic limbs should be restored to a functional, pain-free state with appropriate management. Unfortunately, extensive vascular disease or underlying medical illness can preclude revascularization. With advances in limb salvage procedures, it is important to review carefully the risk-benefit and cost-benefit ratios with the patient before each intervention. Although in the later stage of disease each patient has a choice between amputation or delay, the choices often are a relatively pain-free comfortable prosthesis or salvage of a painful ulcerated or gangrenous foot.

VENOUS DISEASE

EPIDEMIOLOGY

More than 250,000 new cases of deep venous thrombosis (DVT) occur each year, resulting in approximately 500,000 patients presenting for the treatment of venous stasis ulcers.[13] Lindner found that 80% of patients followed for 5–10 years after venographically documented thrombosis had some symptoms of venous hypertension in association with valvular incompetence. Specifically, 49% had varicosities, 62% edema, 34% hyperpigmentation, and 4% ulceration. The location of the thrombosis influenced the probability of subsequent complications; 100% of iliac, 94% of femoral, and 40% of calf thromboses were symptomatic.[40]

ETIOLOGY

To understand the pathogenesis of venous insufficiency, a basic review of the anatomy and function of leg veins is necessary. The venous system of the lower extremity is divided into three groups: (1) the superficial veins (great and small saphenous veins and their tributaries) (Fig. 5), which are subcutaneous and not well supported by the overlying tissues and skin; (2) the perforating (communicating) veins, which connect the superficial venous system with the deep venous system; and (3) the deep veins, which are supported externally by a strong fascial layer and the surrounding musculature.[41] The communicating pathways are variable from one per-

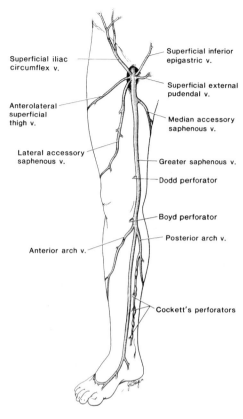

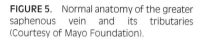

FIGURE 5. Normal anatomy of the greater saphenous vein and its tributaries (Courtesy of Mayo Foundation).

son to another. They are most commonly located on the medial aspect of the calf but may be found at the thigh level.

Many factors can result in the development of venous insufficiency, including heredity, local trauma, thrombosis, and intrinsic defects in the veins or valves themselves. Venous flow is based on a force that pushes the blood proximally (such as gravity or the calf muscle), an adequate outflow, and the presence of competent valves limiting reflux. Any disruption of these components results in chronic venous hypertension.[34] Normally, the pressure in the veins of the leg is equal to the hydrostatic pressure from a vertical column of blood extending to the right atrium of the heart. At the ankle level, the hydrostatic pressure is about 90 mm Hg.[41] During exercise, the pumping action of the calf muscles reduces this venous pressure by two thirds. Even slight muscular movements during normal standing will lower the pressure.[41] Patients with venous insufficiency may fail to reduce ankle pressure, may show a rapid return of venous pressure to resting levels at the end of exercise, or experience a combination of both. The time required for the ankle vein pressure to return to resting levels after exercise is an indicator of the degree of reflux in the limb. Nicolaides found that elevated ambulatory venous pressure is associated with an increased incidence of ulceration. When ambulatory venous pressure is below 30 mm Hg, the incidence of ulceration is zero. The incidence of ulceration increases linearly, reaching 100% when the ambulatory venous pressure is greater than 90 mm Hg.[44] The superficial leg veins carry 10–15% of the venous return. Incompetent valves in the superficial veins alone do not cause serious venous hypertension. Venous insufficiency develops only when the valves in the perforator or deep veins are incompetent.

Ultimately, venous hypertension is the result of valve damage and retrograde venous blood flow to the superficial veins. Retrograde flow can occur with (1) faulty communicating and superficial venous valves; (2) damage to the deep vein valves; (3) deep vein occlusion; and (4) muscle dysfunction and pump failure from fibrosis, neuropathies, and inflammatory disease.

Chronic venous insufficiency is usually the result of congenital or acquired valvular incompetence and less frequently obstruction of the veins.[27] Postthrombotic syndrome (recanalization and valve destruction after thrombosis) develops in 67–80% of patients after DVT.[16] A significant proportion of patients with chronic venous insufficiency have primary valvular incompetence with no history or phlebographic evidence of DVT.[27]

Several theories exist regarding the changes in the subcutaneous tissue of patients with chronic venous insufficiency. One hypothesis is that venous hypertension leads to venular dilatation and increased capillary permeability, with transudation of fibrinogen and hemosiderin from the capillaries into the subcutaneous tissue.[2] This theory proposes that the pericapillary fibrin acts as a diffusion barrier and the overlying dermis becomes hypoxic. There are no in vivo studies to document that pericapillary fibrin cuffs act as a diffusion barrier.[8,22] A second hypothesis relates to the accumulation of white blood cells in the dermal capillaries of patients with venous disease. Trapped white cells release free radicals and inflammatory mediators, which are actively responsible for tissue injury.[9] Polymorphonuclear leukocytes, particularly those attached to capillary endothelium, may become activated, causing release of cytoplasmic granules containing proteolytic enzymes. In addition, a nonmitochondrial respiratory burst permits these cells to release free radicals (most notably the superoxide radical), which have destructive effects on lipid membranes, proteins, and many connective tissue compounds. Chemotactic leukotrienes are also released and attract more polymorphonuclear cells.[8]

The true mechanism by which venous hypertension leads to induration and fibrosis of the skin (lipodermosclerosis) and ulceration remains unclear. However, it is apparent that venous hypertension sets the stage for adverse conditions that eventually lead to skin damage and impaired healing.[33]

CLINICAL EVALUATION

History

A complete history and clinical examination are ordinarily sufficient to diagnose venous insufficiency and to determine whether it involves the superficial, deep, or perforating veins individually or in combination. The clinical examination includes inspection, palpation, and subsequent venous testing. Symptoms of chronic venous insufficiency are highly variable and depend on the degree and duration of insufficiency. In general, patients note aching, edema, skin changes, decreased activity tolerance, and progressive leg pain with prolonged standing. If the patient states that the symptoms are unrelieved by leg elevation, especially overnight, the diagnosis of venous insufficiency should be questioned.[34]

Clinical Findings

The earliest sign of chronic venous insufficiency is edema of the lower legs. Initially, this is associated with an upright posture and is noticeable mainly in the evening. Early in the disease, intermittent soft pitting edema is present, but fibrosis eventually develops and the skin demonstrates firm induration. Pigmentation develops next, especially in the medial perimalleolar areas. Venous hypertension causes transudation of serous fluid and red blood cells into the subcutaneous tissue. Hemoglobin from the red blood cells breaks down to produce the pigment hemosiderin. A weepy puritic dermatitis may develop, and recurrent secondary cellulitis is a fairly common complication. Chronic venous insufficiency results in chronic edema, scarring, obliteration of cutaneous lymphatics, decreased skin integrity, hemosiderin deposition (with brownish discoloration), dermatitis, and ulceration (Fig. 6). Fortunately, not all patients with incompetent valves are symptomatic.

VASCULAR TESTING

Although the evaluation of chronic venous insufficiency is accomplished principally with the history and physical examination, noninvasive testing modalities may complement these examinations.

Impedance Plethysmography

Impedance plethysmography assesses volume changes at rest produced by a proximal, pneumatic, venoocclusive cuff. A normal leg swells when a venoocclusive tourni-

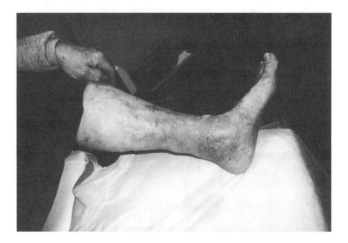

FIGURE 6. Severe manifestations of chronic venous insufficiency with edema, hyperpigmentation, and soft tissue fibrosis.

quet is placed and rapidly returns to its normal size when the tourniquet is released. Venous volume measured by electrical impedance shows a quick return to baseline (within 3–4 seconds) after tourniquet release. In the presence of a proximal lower extremity DVT, the venous system will already be "maximally" filled. When the cuff is inflated, there is little additional increase in venous volume, and after tourniquet release the return to baseline is delayed.[52]

Exercise Venous Plethysmography

Lower limb venous function is tested by performing a plethysmographic evaluation of limb volume before, during, and after exercise. In a normal individual, plethysmography shows a progressive decrease in leg volume during exercise followed by a period after exercise when the volume slowly returns to normal. In venous insufficiency, the exercise-induced decrease in venous volume is less than expected. In addition, when venous incompetence is present, the postexercise return in volume will be more rapid than expected. Exercise venous plethysmography provides a quick and relatively inexpensive way to document or screen for venous incompetence. It also yields quantitative information about the severity of venous insufficiency that is not readily obtained with other noninvasive methods.[53]

Duplex Scanning

Duplex scanning is used to diagnose deep or superficial venous thrombosis, assess venous incompetence, and map the superficial veins before surgical harvest for bypass operations. Duplex scanning also can document the presence of venous incompetence, identify the anatomic sites involved, and quantify the severity.[54]

TREATMENT

Patient education is important in the management of chronic venous insufficiency. Patients must understand the disease process and the correct use of measures to decrease edema. Since venous hypertension is the physiologic cause of the damage in chronic venous insufficiency, the first step of treatment should be to reduce the venous pressure. When elevation is used for edema control, the extremity must be elevated above the level of the heart. This position is not achieved by placing the leg on a foot stool. The pelvis should not be dependent. Patients should lie on a sofa or sit in an orthopedic chair to elevate the legs appropriately above the heart. Periodic elevation of the legs, with the toes about 20 cm above heart level, relieves edema effectively by lowering the hydrostatic pressure to nearly zero.[41] The optimal duration and frequency of leg elevation are not known but should be tailored to the severity of disease.

Compression

Compressive dressings aid venous return by compressing the leg and increasing the interstitial tension. Compression of dilated, engorged superficial and intramuscular veins indirectly increases the efficiency of the calf pump mechanism.[41] With no history of congestive heart failure and no evidence of venous obstruction on noninvasive studies, lower extremity volume can be stabilized with an intermittent pneumatic compression pump. Compressive wraps should be used between pumping sessions. After the volume stabilizes, the patient can be measured for stockings. Elastic stockings should provide a graduated compression, exerting most pressure at the ankle, less at the calf, and least pressure at the thigh. Greatest patient compliance is achieved by prescribing knee-length, graduated compression stockings with a pressure gradient of 30–40 mm Hg. In patients with concomitant arterial disease, lower compression may be required to avoid further compromise of arterial inflow by the extrinsic compression.

Exercise
The value of exercise in the management of chronic venous insufficiency has not been conclusively demonstrated. Exercises involving the leg musculature, such as walking, bicycling, or swimming, promote muscle tone in the calf and enhance venous return (Fig. 7). Exercise, however, produces variable reductions in venous hypertension. In general, patients with chronic venous stasis due to incompetent deep vein valves do not obtain as much reduction in venous pressure as do those in which the primary defect is due to incompetent perforator valves.[23]

Medication
Pentoxifylline has been evaluated in an attempt to alter the leukocyte trapping in tissues. This drug reduces leukocyte adhesiveness and the release of oxygen free radicals and has been shown to be effective in the treatment of venous leg ulcers in early trials.[1,10]

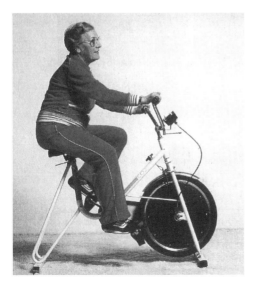

FIGURE 7. Resistance bicycle allows exercise of lower extremity muscles.

Surgery

Surgical intervention for chronic venous insufficiency can include ligation of perforators, direct valve repair, vein segment transposition, or axillary valve autotransplantation.[27]

REFERENCES

1. Barbarino C: Pentoxifylline in the treatment of venous leg ulcers. Curr Med Res Opin 12:547–551, 1992.
2. Browse NL, Burnand KG: The cause of venous ulceration. Lancet 2:243–245, 1982.
3. Buerger L: The Circulatory Disturbances of the Extremities. Philadelphia, WB Saunders, 1924.
4. Carroll RM, Rose HB, Vygen J, et al: Cardiac arrhythmias associated with treadmill claudication testing. Surgery 83:284–287, 1978.
5. Clifford PC, Davis PW, Hayne JA, Baird RN: Intermittent claudication: Is a supervised exercise class worthwhile? BMJ 280:1503–1505, 1980.
6. Coffman JD: Intermittent claudication: Be conservative. N Engl J Med 325:577–578, 1991.
7. Coffman JD: Vasodilator drugs in peripheral vascular disease. N Engl J Med 300:713–717, 1979.
8. Coleridge Smith PD: Pathogenesis of chronic venous insufficiency and possible effects of compression and pentoxifylline. Yale Biol Med 66:47–59, 1993.
9. Coleridge Smith PD, Thomas P, Schurr JH, Dormandy JA: Causes of venous ulceration: A new hypothesis. BMJ 296:1726–1727, 1988.
10. Colgan MP, Dormandy JA, Jones PW, et al: Oxpentifylline treatment of venous ulcers of the leg. BMJ 300:972–975, 1990.
11. Cooke JP, Creager MA: Management of the patient with intermittent claudication. Vasc Med Rev 2:19–31, 1991.
12. Cooke JP, Ma AO: Medical therapy of peripheral arterial occlusive disease. Surg Clin North Am 75:569–79, 1995.
13. Coon WW, Willis PW, Keller JB: Venous thromboembolism and other venous disease in the Tecumseh Community Health Study. Circulation 48:839–847, 1973.
14. Creasy TS, McMillan PJ, Fletcher EW, et al: Is percutaneous transluminal angioplasty better than exercise for claudication? Preliminary results from a prospective randomized trial. Eur J Vasc Surg 4:135–140, 1990.
15. Criqui MH, Fronek A, Barrett-Connor E, et al: The prevalence of peripheral arterial disease in a defined population. Circulation 71:510–515, 1985.
16. Cronan JJ: Venous thromboembolic disease: The role of US. Radiology 186:619–630, 1993.
17. Ekroth R, Dahllöf A, Gundevall B, Holm J: Physical training of patients with intermittent claudication: Indications, methods, and results. Surgery 84:640–643, 1978.
18. Ericsson B, Haeger K, Lindell SE: Effect of physical training on intermittent claudication. Angiology 21:188–192, 1970.
19. Ernst CB, Stanley JC (ed): Current Therapy in Vascular Surgery, 2nd ed. Philadelphia, BC Decker, 1991.
20. Ernst E, Kollár L, Resch KL: Does pentoxifylline prolong the walking distance in exercised claudicants? A placebo-controlled double-blind trial. Angiology 43:121–125, 1992.
21. Ernst EEW, Matray A: Intermittent claudication, exercise, and blood rheology. Circulation 76:1110–1114, 1987.
22. Falanga V: Venous ulceration. J Dermatol Surg Oncol 19:764–771, 1993.
23. Fitzpatrick JE: Stasis ulcers: Update on a common geriatric problem. Geriatrics 44:19–21, 25–26, 31, 1989.
24. Foley WT: Treatment of gangrene of the feet and legs by walking. Circulation 15:689–700, 1957.
25. Gardner AW, Poehlman ET: Exercise rehabilitation programs for the treatment of claudication pain. A meta-analysis. JAMA 274:975–980, 1995.
26. Gersh BJ, Rihal CS, Rooke TW, et al: Evaluation and management of patients with both peripheral vascular and coronary artery disease. J Am Coll Cardiol 18:203–214, 1991.

27. Gloviczki P, Merrell SW: Surgical treatment of venous disease. Cardiovasc Clin 22:81–100, 1992.
28. Hertzer NR: The natural history of peripheral vascular disease: Implications for its management. Circulation 83(suppl):I12–I19, 1991.
29. Hiatt WR, Nawaz D, Regensteiner JG, Hossack KF: Evaluation of exercise performance in patients with peripheral vascular disease. J Cardiopulm Rehabil 12:525–532, 1988.
30. Hiatt WR, Regensteiner JG, Wolfel EE: Special populations in cardiovascular rehabilitation. Cardiol Clin 11:309–321, 1993.
31. Hiatt WR, Wolfel EE, Regensteinter JG: Exercise in the treatment of intermittent claudication due to peripheral arterial disease. Vasc Med Rev 2:61–70, 1991.
32. Honet JC, Strandness DE Jr, Stolov WC, et al: Short-leg bracing for intermittent claudication of the calf. Arch Phys Med Rehabil 49:578–585, 1968.
33. Ibrahim S, MacPherson DR, Goldhaber SZ: Chronic venous insufficiency: Mechanisms and management. Am Heart J 132:856–860, 1996.
34. Jamieson WG: State of the art of venous investigation and treatment. Can J Surg 36:119–128, 1993.
35. Jonason T, Bergstrom R: Cessation of smoking in patients with intermittent claudication. Acta Med Scand 221:253–260, 1987.
36. Jurgens JL, Spittell JA Jr, Fairbairn JF II: Peripheral Vascular Disease, 5th ed. Philadelphia, WB Saunders, 1980.
37. Kannel WB, Shurtleff D: The Framingham Study: Cigarettes and the development of intermittent claudication. Geriatrics 28:61–68, 1973.
38. Kroese A: Physical activity and the peripheral circulation. Scand J Soc Med 29(suppl):47–49, 1982.
39. Larsen OA, Lassen NA: Effect of daily muscular exercise in patients with intermittent claudication. Lancet 2:1093–1095, 1966.
40. Lindner DJ, Edwards JM, Phinney ES, et al: Long-term hemodynamic and clinical sequelae of lower extremity deep venous thrombosis. Vasc Surg 4:436–442, 1986.
41. Löfgren KA: Surgical management of chronic venous insufficiency. Acta Chir Scand Suppl 544:62–68, 1988.
42. Lundgren F, Dahllöf A, Lundholm K, et al: Intermittent claudication-surgical reconstruction or physical training? A prospective randomized trial of treatment efficiency. Ann Surg 209:346–355, 1989.
43. McDaniel MD, Cronenwett JL: Basic data related to the natural history of intermittent claudication. Ann Vasc Surg 3:273–277, 1989.
44. Nicolaides AN, Hussein MK, Szendro G: The relation of venous ulceration with ambulatory venous pressure measurements. J Vasc Surg 17:414–419, 1993.
45. Niebauer J, Cooke JP: Cardiovascular effects of exercise: Role of endothelial shear stress. J Am Coll Cardiol 28:1652–1660, 1996.
46. Orchard TJ, Strandness DE Jr: Assessment of peripheral vascular disease in diabetes: Report and recommendations on an international workshop sponsored by the American Heart Association and the American Diabetes Association. Diabetes Care 16:1199–1209, 1993.
47. Perkins JMT, Collin J, Creasy TS, et al: Exercise training versus angioplasty for stable claudication. Long and medium term results of a prospective, randomized trial. Eur J Vasc Endovasc Surg 11:409–413, 1996.
48. Porter JM, Cutter BS, Lee BY, et al: Pentoxifylline efficacy in the treatment of intermittent claudication: Multi-centered controlled double-blind trial with objective assessment of chronic occlusive arterial disease patients. Am Heart J 104:66–72, 1982.
49. Regensteiner JG, Hiatt WR: Exercise rehabilitation for patients with peripheral arterial disease. Exerc Sports Sci Rev 23:1–24, 1995.
50. Regensteiner JG, Hiatt WR: Medical management of peripheral arterial disease. J Vasc Interv Radiol 5:669–677, 1994.
51. Richardson JK: Rocker-soled shoes and walking distance in patients with calf claudication. Arch Phys Med Rehabil 72:554–558, 1991.
52. Rooke TW: The noninvasive vascular laboratory. Cardiovas Clin 22:27–44, 1992.
53. Rooke TW, Heser JL, Osmundson PJ: Exercise strain-gauge venous plethysmography: Evaluation of a "new" device for assessing lower limb venous incompetence. Angiology 43:219–228, 1992.

54. Rooke TW, Martin RP: Lower extremity venous imaging for the echocardiologist. J Am Soc Echocardiogr 3:158–169, 1990.
55. Rooke TW, Osmundson PJ: The influence of sympathetic nerves on transcutaneous oxygen tension in normal and ischemic lower extremities. Angiology 38:400–410, 1987.
56. Rooke TW, Osmundson PJ: Effect of intermittent venous occlusion on transcutaneous oxygen tension in lower limbs with severe arterial occlusive disease. Int J Cardiol 21:76–78, 1988.
57. Snow CJ, Carter SA: Is exercise therapy beneficial in intermittent claudication? Vasc Diagn Ther 5:20–25, 1984.
58. Skinner JS, Strandness DE Jr: Exercise and intermittent claudication II. Effect of physical training. Circulation 36:23–29, 1967.
59. Spittell JA Jr: Conservative management of occlusive peripheral arterial disease. Cardiovasc Clin 22:209–215, 1992.
60. Strandness DE Jr, Sumner DS: Application of ultrasound to the study of atherosclerosis obliterans. Angiology 26:187–194, 1975.
61. Wisham L, Abramson A, Ebel A: The value of exercise in peripheral arterial disease. JAMA 153:10–12, 1953.

GEOFFREY E. MOORE, MD

9

Exercise Prescription in Persons with Multiple Chronic Diseases

Guidelines on exercise programs in chronic disease typically consider one disease at a time. However, many patients have more than one medical problem, and the persons in greatest need of physical fitness often have multiple medical problems. Exercise research is rarely done with such people because studying two or more chronic conditions is such a formidable undertaking. Therefore, little outcomes-based literature is available on any particular combination of diseases.

However, with good planning and problem management, some of the most chronically burdened and deconditioned of patients can achieve success. The secret lies in having problem-oriented management, a systematic plan that deals with all the problems.

Physicians and nurses have used problem-oriented management techniques for about three decades.[5] In the first half of the 1900s, physician progress notes were commonly long narratives and, in a holistic way, multiple problems were managed as one. But diagnostic and therapeutic tools multiplied from scientific advancement, and clinicians found themselves dealing with problems of increasing complexity. Today's physicians usually outline their care plans, with each section dealing with one small part of the patient's problems. This is most evident in persons with multi-organ failure who are in an intensive care unit. Problem-oriented management has its roots in reductionist modern medicine and specialty- and subspecialty-oriented care.

Exercise specialists do not have much exposure to the problem-oriented approach. However, persons with chronic disease survive longer, patients with an increasing complexity of problems are referred for rehabilitation, and there is an increasing need to adopt problem-oriented management techniques. This chapter discusses how one can implement problem-oriented management. A common combination of diseases—hypertension, hypercholesterolemia, and non–insulin-dependent diabetes—is used as an example.

PROBLEM-ORIENTED MANAGEMENT: THE SOAP NOTE

One issue of complex problem-oriented management is recordkeeping. Clinicians typically use a "SOAP" note format, with SOAP being an acronym for subjective data, objective data, assessment, and plan. Exercise specialists are typically unaccustomed to using SOAP notes, but they are easy to learn and quite handy.

The SOAP format structures the clinician's thinking into four steps:

1. What is the patient experiencing?

2. What physical findings and laboratory data are related to those experiences?

3. What is (are) the explanation(s) for these experiences?

4. What is the plan to either clarify the nature of the problem or to make it better?

The purpose of these steps is to translate the patient's symptoms (step 1) into a detailed description that is specific and measurable. This technical rigor allows the exercise specialist to follow a problem over time and know whether it is getting worse, getting better, or staying the same. The differentiation of a complex set of symptoms into components begins in step 2 and is completed in step 3. Creation of a plan (step 4) creates a benchmark for progress during a follow-up reassessment.

STEP 1: COLLECTING SUBJECTIVE DATA

Subjective data reveal what the patient is experiencing, the patient's perspective, and what the patient is expecting to achieve by seeking exercise therapy. Subjective data are elicited by open-ended questions such as, "What can I do for you?" In terms of lifestyle issues, such as regularly participating in an exercise program, subjective data hint at how ready a patient is to change lifestyle. It also gives a rough notion of whether someone is in average shape or extremely unfit.

Subjective data describe the patient's own goals and desires. The clinician must remember that a good businessperson satisfies the client's goals and must either provide what the customer wants or convince the customer to want something else. For example, a patient who was formerly a 10-km runner developed cardiac ischemia that could not be fixed with surgery or angioplasty. He came to cardiac rehabilitation wanting to participate in a popular race, but no amount of cardiac rehabilitation could return him to his former condition. He had to be convinced to choose a more realistic goal.

STEP 2: COLLECTING OBJECTIVE DATA

Objective data represent the clinician's view of the patient's problems. They are more standardized and quantified than the patient's subjective view. For an exercise specialist, the objective data should include at least a limited physical examination to assess the severity of any pulmonary, cardiovascular, and neuromusculoskeletal diseases. Objective data also include medical records, and patients usually have reams of laboratory reports by the time they arrive at the exercise specialist. It is easy to focus on the severity of the conditions described in the medical test reports, e.g., how high the glycosylated hemoglobin is (reflecting the control of blood sugar in a diabetic) or how severe the coronary artery stenosis is. These are important facts to bear in mind but are more important for medical than exercise management. In an exercise program for a diabetic, for example, none of the training parameters depend on glycosylated hemoglobin.

For our purposes, physical performance is the bottom line for the exercise specialist. The data often will be derived through some form of exercise tests, of which there are seven basic types:

1. Aerobic: treadmill, exercise bike

2. Endurance: 6-minute walk

3. Strength: isokinetic muscle testing, weight lifting

4. Flexibility: goniometry (range of motion)

5. Neuromuscular: reaction times

6. Functional: sit-to-stand

7. Anaerobic: Wingate tests. Anaerobic exercise is more relevant for athletes and thus outside the scope of this chapter.

It is not uncommon for a patient to be referred with no exercise test data and to not be able to afford exercise tests. Although this scenario is not desirable, the therapist can start a particularly conservative exercise program and gradually build the patient's functioning. This takes longer and often requires some extra sessions, but it is safe and it works.

STEP 3: MAKING AN ASSESSMENT

After interviewing the patient, performing a limited physical examination, reviewing the old records, and doing some form of exercise evaluation, the therapist must make an exercise prescription (or program). The two basic approaches one can use with multiple chronic disease are the medical model and the exercise model.

In the medical model, the problems are usually managed by disease, e.g., arthritis, diabetes, and heart failure. This approach has merit because many complications of exercise are likely to be disease-related. In arthritics, the joints will get sore; in diabetics, the blood sugar may go too low; in patients with heart failure, the blood pressure may fall or they may have arterial desaturation.

The exercise model may have more merit, however, because the main goal is to improve exercise tolerance. Orienting the problems on the desired goals helps focus on the main objective. Also, minor complications such as blisters or muscle soreness can be more related to the type of exercise than to the disease. Some exercise-dependent complications can be major, such as closed head and neck injuries when an equestrian rider falls. Therefore, worries about complications do not really favor a disease-based model.

What are the categories of exercise problems? In the main, use the following types of exercise tests: (1) aerobic capacity, (2) strength, and (3) flexibility. An additional category may need to be related to a patient's specific goals, which is really a variant of the "functional" type of tests (e.g., the cardiac rehabilitation patient who wanted to return to running 10-km races). One advantage of using the exercise model for recordkeeping is that the therapist can quantitatively reassess the patient at a later date to determine the degree of success. The disadvantage is that some specific medical problems may require more intensive planning and monitoring.

This latter problem leads to a hybrid model, which is to use a mixture of exercise performance and disease-specific categories. For instance, in a sedentary arthritic, the main objective may be to increase peak functional capacity and endurance, but another objective may be to maintain joint function and not exacerbate joint inflammation. Such a person's problem-oriented management would encompass (1) aerobic capacity, (2) endurance, and (3) arthritis.

On balance, the exercise and hybrid models are preferred, with the choice depending on individual circumstances.

The last part of the assessment step is to concisely summarize the problem. For example:

1. Aerobic capacity: 5 METs due to sedentary lifestyle

2. Endurance: walking limited to 15 minutes due to fatigue

3. Arthritis: moderate degeneation of left knee; not inflamed; ibuprofen 400 mg twice a day for pain, as needed

The assessment needs to state not only the limitation, but why it is a limitation and, in the case of medical management, what is being done to treat the problem. The plan must take these facts into account if it is to be appropriate for the circumstances.

STEP 4: FORMING A PLAN

The main issue in forming a plan is establishing a goal for each problem and an estimated time to reach that goal. Including the estimated time to reach the goal helps maintain realism—people rarely have the perseverance to aim for a goal 3 years hence. One *can* have long-term goals, but they must be able to be broken down into short-term goals that are more immediately achievable and yet clearly demonstrate a successful advance. Part of the art of being a good therapist is judging the patient and choosing an appropriate goal for that individual. Some goals may be motivational more than physical, particularly for persons with low self-efficacy for exercise. These skills are just as important as technical know-how concerning exercise assessment and programming, because to reap the benefits of exercise training takes longer than most people are willing to wait. This is the main reason adherence rates to exercise programs are so low and membership turnover at fitness centers is so high. If a patient is to maintain a lifelong fitness program, exercise must be rewarding.

Medicines are an issue in some cases, such as in patients with diabetes. For example, persons who have insulin-dependent diabetes often need to decrease the insulin dose just prior to exercise. Patients with Parkinson's disease should exercise when their L-dopa levels are at a peak to maximize movement control. In such circumstances, medicines must be included in the plan. The therapist must learn about medicines, how they are used in a given disease, and how they affect exercise capacity.

Any exercise management plan must make some estimation of the risk/benefit ratio. Risks can be disease-dependent or activity-dependent, and both kinds of risks should be included in the plan. For example, for fear of a vertebral fracture, one would not recommend bungee-jumping as an activity to a patient with severe osteoporosis, but the main risk of bungee jumping is trauma from accidents.

Any program must plan for follow-up reassessments. Some of these assessments are frequent, such as daily foot checks in a diabetic; other assessments are made at weekly, monthly, quarterly, or yearly intervals. The time for reassessment depends on the nature of the goal and on the time course of adaptation to exercise training. The expected dose-response relationship is what a therapist really needs to know to plan follow-up reassessments and goals. Unfortunately, the exercise dose-response relationship is poorly understood for most chronic diseases. Perhaps more is known about flexibility, neuromuscular exercise, and functional dose-responses than about aerobic and strength training, because physical therapy and occupational therapy have been using such interventions for a longer time.

When the exercise dose-response relationship is not well known, the therapist may resort to a therapeutic trial. The important thing to remember when performing a therapeutic trial is that there is no real benefit for being aggressive, and some patients may not benefit from a given form of exercise. To be conservative, one should start with intensities at the level of normal activities of daily living or slightly higher for 5-10 minutes at least three times per week. The duration of exercise is gradually increased by 5 minutes per session, and the frequency of sessions is increased as tolerated or needed. Recommending a daily program emphasizes the importance of exercise in health and overall fitness.

HYPERTENSION/HYPERCHOLESTEROLEMIA/DIABETES

One of the most common combinations of medical diseases is hypertension, hypercholesterolemia, and non–insulin-dependent diabetes mellitus (NIDDM). Each of these illnesses is associated with sequelae that limit exercise tolerance, and some patients have multiple complications. The combination of these circumstances can make life (and exercise management) extremely difficult. Table 1 describes a recommended exercise program for these patients.

An important fact about each of these illnesses is that exercise adds to metabolic control, but exercise is not the main line of therapy. Many guidelines and texts recommend exercise and diet as the *first* line of therapy in high blood pressure, hypercholesterolemia, and diabetes, but pharmaceuticals are the *main* line of therapy. Exercise only decreases systolic and diastolic blood pressure about 10 mm Hg, and in only half

TABLE 1. Generic Exercise Program for a Patient with Hypertension, Hypercholesterolemia, and Noninsulin-Dependent Diabetes Mellitus

Mode	Goals	Frequency/Intensity/Time	Time to Goal
Aerobic	Increase aerobic capacity Increase endurance Increase calorie expenditure	Daily Effort scale: 4–7 (see Table 2) 1/2 to 1 hour >700 calories per week	4 months (fitness)
	Reduce body fat Reduce blood pressure Reduce cholesterol Improve glucose control		4–12 months (body fat, blood pressure, lipid and glucose control)
Resistance	Increase strength	2–3 times per week High repetitions, low resistance	2–4 months
Flexibility	Increase/maintain range of motion	3–7 times per week	2–4 months

the patients;[3] cholesterol decreases by about 10% with regular exercise, and low-fat diets give some further reduction; with NIDDM,[2] exercise may decrease the need for hypoglycemic medications by reducing body fat and increasing skeletal muscle insulin receptor activity.[1] Therefore, although exercise has clinically meaningful effects in controlling these illnesses, they are not large effects and do not merit ranking as the main line of therapy.

In medical practice, exercise is underused because physicians are not skilled in lifestyle management, including exercise. Practitioners commonly go directly to drug therapy, which has advantages and disadvantages. An advantage is that immediate use of medications may speed the rapidity with which the illness is under control, but there is no evidence that using drugs first improves outcome. Disadvantages of this approach are that it makes clinicians unaccustomed to using lifestyle interventions and downplays many benefits of exercise. The subliminal message to patients is that exercise is not very important and that it does not modify disease. Although exercise is not a potent tool in controlling these diseases, most patients still need an exercise intervention.

Table 2 outlines a reasonable program and a SOAP note for a patient with hypertension, hypercholesterolemia, NIDDM, and no complications of these diseases.

A patient with some common complications of these illnesses, e.g., coronary artery disease with stable angina, claudication, and peripheral neuropathy in the lower extremities, would need a more complex exercise program to accommodate these complicating factors. Intensity would be limited at (or just below) the angina threshold, and antianginal medications would be accommodated; the exercise intensity, duration, and mode would be chosen to induce mild claudication (prove to improve walking distance); foot inspections would be mandatory before each session; and particular forms

TABLE 2. Example of a Program and SOAP Note for a Patient with Hypertension, Hypercholesterolemia, Noninsulin-Dependent Diabetes Mellitus, and No Complications of Disease

Subjective Data:

Wants to "take better care of myself with diet and exercise."

Objective Data:

- High blood pressure × 10 years; taking metoprolol (β-antagonist) 100 mg once a day
- NIDDM × 5 years: taking Glucophage 1000 mg twice a day
- Hypercholesterolemia: taking simvastatin 40 mg once a day

Resting blood pressure 143/92; pulse 55. Cardiac exam: point of maximal impulse 2 cm lateral to midclavicular line, otherwise normal. No carotid or femoral bruits (flow murmurs). Neurologic exam: normal. Musculoskeletal exam: normal motor and articular findings.

Glycosylated hemoglobin: 6.8
Cholesterol 200, LDL 115, HDL 35, triglycerides 250
Exercise test: peak heart rate 150, peak work rate 7 METs, peak blood pressure 240/110, peak rate-pressure product 36,000; Resting ECG—LVH with resting ST abnormalities; exercise ECG—no significant ECG changes or dysrhythmias during exercise, no cardiac symptoms during exercise.

Assessment:

1) Aerobic: moderate to low fit, at increased risk for cardiovascular mortality based on fitness level
2) Strength: normal for sedentary persons
3) Flexibility: normal for sedentary persons

Plan:

1) Aerobic
   GOALS: Peak exercise tolerance = 9 mets (reduce CV mortality risk / increase fitness); resting blood pressure <140/90 (monitor metoprolol dosing); maintain weight and triglycerides <220 (consider adding fibric acid derivative).
   FIT: Walking / stationary cycling: daily
       Start 10–20 minutes at effort scale of 5; add 3–5 minutes each week up to 40 minutes, then increase intensity to effort scale of 5–7.
   TIME TO GOALS: 3 months (fitness)/6–12 weeks (medical)
2) Strength
   GOALS: Maintain muscle strength and lean mass
   FIT: Twice weekly:
       Biceps curls, side arms: 2–5 kg × 10–20 repetitions, two sets
       Leg press: 20–40 kg × 10 repetitions, two sets
       Toe raises: 20, two sets
   TIME TO GOALS: 3 months
3) Stretching
   GOALS: Maintain range of motion, monitor skin
   FIT: Daily, prior to aerobic exercise:
       Foot and skin check
       Forward bend, hamstring stretch, side bend, calf stretches 15 minutes
   TIME TO GOALS: Indefinite

TABLE 3. Example of a SOAP Note for a Patient with Hypertension, Hypercholesterolemia, Non–insulin-Dependent Diabetes Mellitus, and Complications of These Diseases

Subjective Data:

Is "afraid of losing my independence and being a burden on my family."

Objective Data:

- High blood pressure x 25 years: taking Lopressor (β-antagonist) 50 mg twice a day, lisinopril (angiotensin converting enzyme inhibitor) 20 mg once a day
- NIDDM x 15 years... taking Glucotrol 10 mg twice a day, and Glucophage 1000 mg twice a day
- Hypercholesterolemia: taking simvastatin 40 mg everyday

Resting blood pressure 130/90; pulse 60. Cardiac exam: point of maximal impulse 2 cm lateral to midclavicular line, 2/6 systolic ejection murmur, and soft S4 gallop. Right-sided femoral bruit, minor skin changes below the knee on right. Neurologic exam: diminished sensation to pinprick, light touch and vibration/proprioception below knees, right worse than left; decreased Achilles tendon reflexes. Musculoskeletal exam: grossly normal motor, mild crepitance in left knee, no tenderness or pain; can do forward bend to mid shins.

Glycocylated hemoglobin: 7.4

Cholesterol 220, LDL 130, HDL 35, triglycerides 300

Treadmill test—peak heart rate 140, peak work rate 5 mets, peak blood pressure 190/100, peak rate-pressure product, 26,600; Resting ECG—LVH with resting ST abnormalities; exercise ECG—2 mm inferolateral ST depression during exercise, associated with mild chest discomfort and heart rate of 130 and rate pressure product of 22,000. Mild onset of right calf pain at heart rate of 120, maximal discomfort was 3/4 at peak exercise.

Assessment:

1) Aerobic: low fit, increased risk for cardiovascular mortality; claudication at 2.0 mph; cardiac ischemia as evidenced by symptoms and ST changes at 2.0 mph, 10.5% grade (5 METs).
2) Strength: low
3) Flexibility: reduced forward bend, hip mobility

Plan:

1) Aerobic

GOALS: Peak exercise tolerance = 7–8 METs (reduce CV mortality risk/risk fitness); raise claudication and angina thresholds to 6 and 7 METs, respectively. Lower triglycerides and total cholesterol <220 (consider adding fibric acid derivative).

FIT: Walking/water aerobics: Daily

Start 10–15 minutes at heart rate between 120 and 130; add 3–5 minutes each week up to 40 minutes. Adjust work rate to elicit mild claudication, but avoid angina pectoris. Sublingual nitroglycerin as needed.

TIME TO GOALS: 6–9 months (fitness) / 6–12 weeks (medical)

2) Strength

GOALS: Increase muscle strength

FIT: Twice weekly:

Elastic bands: 10–20 repetitions, two sets; start with yellow, increase as tolerated

Toe raises: 20, two sets

TIME TO GOALS: 3 months

3) Stretching

GOALS: Maintain range of motion, monitor skin and lower extremities

FIT: Daily, prior to aerobic exercise:

Foot and skin check

Forward bend, hamstring stretch, side bend, calf stretches

15 minutes

TIME TO GOALS: Indefinite

of exercise might be excluded to lower the risk of inducing a Charcot's joint. Table 3 outlines a SOAP note for such a patient.

CONCLUSION

Regular exercise is important, not just because being fit extends life but because the ability to do exercise improves one's ability to cope with the physical and other stresses of life. In persons with chronic disease, the main utility of exercise may be to improve ability to perform activities of daily living, increase quality-of-life, and improve psychological status. Any benefits that improve control of chronic diseases such as high blood pressure, high cholesterol, or diabetes are added benefits. Rather than trying to use exercise to achieve outcomes that may be more easily achieved with other means, such as drugs, one should use exercise to do what only exercise can do: improve fitness. In a person with multiple chronic diseases, this can be a formidable task, but problem-oriented exercise management is a valuable tool for the job.

REFERENCES

1. Albright AL: Diabetes. In Durstine JL, Bloomquist LE, Figoni SF, et al (eds): ACSM's Exercise Management for Persons with Chronic Diseases and Disabilities. Champaign, IL, Human Kinetics, 1997, pp 94–100.
2. Durstine JL, Moore GE: Hyperlipidemia. In Durstine JL, Bloomquist LE, Figoni SF, et al (eds): ACSM's Exercise Management in Persons with Chronic Diseases and Disabilities. Champaign, IL, Human Kinetics, 1997, pp 101–105.
3. Gordon NF: Hypertension. In Durstine JL, Bloomquist LE, Figoni SF, et al (eds): ACSM's Exercise Management for Persons with Chronic Diseases and Disabilities. Champaign, IL, Human Kinetics, 1997, pp 59–63.
4. Moore GE, Durstine J: Framework. In Durstine JL, Bloomquist LE, Figoni SF, et al (eds): ACSM's Exercise Management in Persons with Chronic Diseases and Disabilities. Champaign, IL, Human Kinetics, 1997, pp 6–16.
5. Weed LL: Knowledge Coupling: New Premises and New Tools for Medical Care and Education. New York, Springer-Verlag, 1991.

RAJESWARI KUMAR, MD,
SHARON BROADBENT, MD

10

Therapeutic Exercise in Neurologic Disorders

Rehabilitation is an important aspect in the treatment of many neurologic disorders. Rehabilitation combines a medical and a scientific orientation with social service orientation, and, with the help of the rehabilitation team, patients with devastating neurologic disorders can make a successful transition from an acute care hospital setting to the community.

Exercise is an important aspect of rehabilitation. This chapter summarizes the different treatment strategies in commonly seen central nervous system disorders.

CEREBROVASCULAR ACCIDENT

Cerebrovascular accident (CVA), or stroke, is the leading cause of disability in older people and is an important cause of disability in younger people. Approximately 550,000 people suffer from stroke each year. There was a decline of incidence of stroke from 1945 to 1980, mainly due to control of hypertension and other modifiable risk factors. In the early 1980s, there was an increase in the incidence of stroke attributed to the advances in diagnostic technology and ability to detect milder stroke. Prevalence of stroke is the number of stroke survivors at any given time and is determined from the incidence and the average length of survival. In a survey conducted in 1976, the prevalence of stroke was found to be 1.7 million, or 0.8% of the population. The prevalence of stroke has increased slightly due to advances in medical care. Currently there are three million people alive following stroke; all with varying degrees of neurologic impairment.[13,36] Seventy-five percent of strokes occur due to infarction and 15% are secondary to hemorrhage. The remainder are of unknown etiology.[13]

Half to three quarters of stroke patients regain the ability to walk. About 10% of the patients regain complete functional independence, and 10% do not benefit from rehabilitation because their disability is so severe. The remaining 80% of patients (middle band patients) do benefit from rehabilitation. With the help of the rehabilitation team, 80% of the stroke patients can successfully return to their home; thus, the cost of institutionalization can be reduced.[3,9]

Although strict randomized research to prove the effectiveness of rehabilitation may not be feasible at present because so many variables exist and there are ethical considerations involved in the treatment of stroke patients, a few studies do show the importance of stroke rehabilitation. Garraway et al. found that a higher proportion of elderly stroke patients who were rehabilitated in stroke units (50%) regained functional independence compared to those who received therapies on the general medical ward (32%) (p < 0.01). The authors also concluded that the early therapy interventions were more important than the absolute number of therapy sessions. However, this study was not a blind study.[15,46] Other studies showed that patients undergoing intensive rehabilitation (3 or more hours of therapy on 5 or more days per week) showed significant functional improvement compared to those undergoing conventional rehabilitation (rehabilitation provided while the patient is on the medical floor, the number and hours of therapy unstructured).[12,46,48] Smith and coworkers noted that, in addition to the significant benefits to patients undergoing intensive rehabilitation, functional deterioration was noted in the patients who did not receive therapy and who were asked to continue their previously taught exercise program prior to discharge from the hospital.[47] A meta-analysis to compare the effect of a specialized rehabilitation unit and conventional medical care showed that patients in the rehabilitation ward functioned better at the time of discharge, had a better chance of short-term survival, and returned home and remained at home more frequently than those in the medical ward.[12] Gain of activities of daily living and motor function was greatest during the hospitalization and immediately after discharge. This effect was not significant in long-term follow-up. A research synthesis was performed to determine the effect of different intensities of stroke rehabilitation. The analysis included nine controlled studies and 1,051 patients. A statistically significant relationship between intensity and effect was noted. Drawbacks of the various studies included insufficient contrast in the amount of rehabilitation between the experimental and control conditions, organizational setting of rehabilitation management, lack of blinding procedures, and heterogeneity of patients.[27] Comparison of the effect of early, intensive, gait-focused physical therapy showed higher gait velocities in patients who underwent repetitive weightbearing exercises.[33,42]

The Copenhagen and Framingham studies have shown that the neurologic recovery is maximum during the first 11–12 weeks after the onset of stroke. The common practice is to provide intensive rehabilitation in the first few weeks following the stroke because there is functional improvement immediately following rehabilitation.[9,24] However, recent studies have shown that rehabilitation intervention 1 or more years after stroke is also beneficial. Improvement was noted in gait speed, balance, and activities of daily living.[50,52]

The management of stroke patients requires an interdisciplinary approach. Members of the team include the physiatrist, physical and occupational therapist, speech therapist, psychologist, recreation therapist, social worker, dietician, and vocational counselor. A thorough evaluation of patients is important prior to prescribing therapeutic exercise. Mental status is evaluated with the Folstein mini-mental status exam. Presence or absence of aphasia must be determined. Routine manual muscle testing may be difficult in stroke patients because of the synergistic movements in the extremities. Few motor function scales are described in the literature that can be used in such instances. The motor assessment scale is an easily administered score of nine items. Eight of the items involve areas of motor function (supine to sidelying, supine to sitting, sitting to standing, walking, upper arm function, hand movements, and advanced hand activities) and one item involves muscle tone. Each item is rated on a scale of 0–6 in which 6 indicated optimal function.[5]

Brunnstrom staging is another means of assessing motor function in the extremities.[35] Brunnstrom divided the recovery of the arm into six stages. Stage 1 is flaccidity. In stage 2 spasticity is developing. Early synergy patterns are seen. Flexion synergy usually develops before extension synergy. In stage 3 the voluntary movements are developing, but with synergy. Spasticity in the extremity becomes marked. In stage 4 some voluntary movements are possible without synergy. Spasticity is decreased. In stage 5 more movements are possible without synergy. In stage 6 isolated movements are present and spasticity is minimal.[2] Similar staging is available for the lower extremity. The Fugl-Meyer motor assessment score has 155 items, each of which is rated on a three-point scale. Motor function scores are grouped together to get a total score of 100. The motor function is rated as follows: < 50 points = severe motor impairment, 50–84 points = marked motor impairment, and 85–95 points = slight motor impairment.[14]

Therapeutic interventions for impaired mobility and sensorimotor deficit should be started as soon as the patient is medically stable. Practice guidelines for stroke rehabilitation recommend completion of the initial evaluation and institution of therapies within 3 days of admission to the rehabilitation facilities and within 7 days to a lower intensity nursing facility program.[38] Because many of the patients have concomitant coronary artery disease, cardiovascular status should be evaluated prior to prescribing therapy. When indicated, it is important to follow cardiac precautions during therapy.[38]

POSITIONING

Stroke patients should be properly positioned upon admittance to the hospital. This enables the flaccid extremity to overcome certain pathologic forces, such as muscle tone and gravity.[3,9] Patients should be placed on a firm mattress. The upper extremities should be positioned with the shoulder externally rotated and abducted to 90°. The elbow joint should be placed in supination and positioned with 90° of flexion. A rolled towel should be placed in the hand to maintain the wrist in functional extension and fingers in slight flexion. Judicious use of wrist splints is also recommended. This arm position is alternated with internal rotation and partial pronation at the elbow. The arm should be supported by a pillow to prevent edema.

The lower extremity should be positioned in extension at the hip and knee. External rotation of the leg should be avoided. A pillow or a rolled towel should be placed on the lateral aspect of the affected thigh. A multipodus boot can help to maintain dorsiflexion at the ankle as well as prevent pressure sores at the heel. The boot also has a lateral extension to prevent external rotation of the lower extremity.

The preferred sidelying position in hemiplegic patients is lying on the uninvolved side. A pillow should be placed between the legs, and the paretic arm should be supported by a pillow. Sidelying on the involved side is not encouraged. Patients need to be turned every 2 hours to protect the skin.

RANGE OF MOTION EXERCISE

In addition to proper positioning, daily range of motion (ROM) exercise is important to prevent contractures in patients with motor weakness. ROM exercises are prescribed in the early stages to prevent contractures. During the later stages these exercises help to maintain the ROM in each joint. In the early stages, ROM exercises are commonly performed by the nursing staff or therapist. Upon completion of the rehabilitation program, patients or the family members are taught the ROM exercises. The exercises are done several times during the day, usually twice daily.[3,9,35]

In the lower extremity, flexion of the hip and knee and dorsiflexion of the foot are done as a combined movement. In the upper extremity, passive ROM consists of full flexion and extension of the shoulder, full flexion and extension at the elbow, pronation and supination of the forearm, dorsiflexion of the wrist, and flexion and extension of the fingers. These exercises are done slowly to avoid overstretching the soft tissues in flaccid extremities. In spastic hemiplegics, gentle prolonged stretching is recommended, because sudden stretching of the tendons may exaggerate spasticity and may cause pain. Spastic patients may substitute hyperextension of the lumbar spine or sidebending of the whole body during forward flexion and abduction of the shoulder, which should be discouraged. Concomitant use of modalities such as icing may reduce the spasticity and help regain ROM. Ultrasound to the Achilles tendon is a common practice while stretching the tendon in patients with plantar flexion contracture. When limited ROM interferes with function, motor point blocks and nerve blocks with phenol as well as botulinum toxin injections to the spastic muscles may be beneficial. These interventions should be followed by a stretching program. The injections are commonly done in patients with plantar flexion contractures that interfere with gait and in patients with wrist flexion or elbow flexion contractures that interfere with hand function. Use of mechanical devices such as overhead pulleys and skateboards to assist in ROM exercise should be discouraged in stroke patients because these devices are shown to increase the incidence of shoulder pain.[26]

EXERCISES IN BED

Patients are encouraged to turn in bed by themselves as soon as possible. Hooking the involved leg under the uninvolved leg helps the patient to turn easily. Turning toward the affected side is easier, and turning toward the unaffected side may require assistance. Body bridging while in bed helps to strengthen the hip extensors, which are essential for standing balance and walking. Exercises with a Theraband can be used to maintain strength in the uninvolved side.

MOBILIZATION

Prolonged bed rest and passive range of motion is avoided. Stroke patients without significant medical complications should be mobilized in 24–48 hours. The patient should be encouraged to sit on a comfortable chair. Transfers are always performed toward the normal or the stronger side. The wheelchair is placed on the patient's unaffected side; the chair faces the foot of the bed while transferring out of bed and faces the head of the bed while transferring to the bed. The time that the patient sits on a chair is increased as tolerated. Stroke patients have a tendency to lean toward the affected side while sitting. The therapist should work with the patient to improve the sitting balance by encouraging head and trunk flexion toward the uninvolved side to stimulate weight shift.[13] Side-to-side movement of the trunk with the help of the therapist encourages weight shifting. While leaning toward the affected side, the therapist helps to extend the involved arm to support the body weight.[40]

Standing exercises can be done by the bedside or in the parallel bars. The therapist helps in stabilizing the knee on the affected side when the patient stands upright. Weight-shifting exercises are done as soon as the patient is able to stand erect. A limb-load monitor is a device that gives auditory feedback to the patient and helps to increase the weightbearing in the lower extremities. Postural sway biofeedback was found to be more effective in improving balance when compared to traditional therapy.[51] Patients are then taught to step forward and backward with the paretic limb. The paretic limb is initially advanced by the therapist until the patient gains muscular control. When gait becomes stable in the parallel bars, patients should be encouraged to walk outside the bars with the help of an appropriate assistive device.

NEUROMUSCULAR FACILITATION APPROACHES

Over the past few years many neuromuscular re-education programs have developed. Sherrington's concept was that the impulses from the peripheral nerves and receptors influenced the excitability of the spinal alpha motor neurons. A facilitory stimulus from the peripheral nerve can cause discharge from target spinal motor neurons and also from the neurons in close proximity (neurons in the subliminal fringe). An inhibitory peripheral stimulus causes neurons to drop out of the target discharge zone and fall into the subliminal fringe. Neuromuscular facilitation technique uses peripheral impulses to increase the discharge of spinal motor neurons in weak muscles (facilitory stimulus) and, for muscles with abnormal tone, uses peripheral stimulus to reduce the excitability of the spinal motor neuron (inhibitory stimulus).[2] A description of commonly used methods is given below.[2,40]

Neurodevelopmental Technique (Bobath) (NDT) This method was developed in the 1940s. One of the goals of NDT is to retain the muscles for normal functional movement. During the recovery from stroke, patients have a tendency to overuse the uninvolved side to compensate for the loss of motor and sensory function. This leads to less effective patterns of movement. Any movements or activities that increase muscle tone or produce abnormal or compensatory movements of the limb are avoided. One of the principles of NDT is that alignment and symmetry of trunk and pelvis are necessary for good alignment and symmetric use of the extremities. Proper alignment of head to trunk and trunk to pelvis are stressed throughout the therapy sessions. Symmetry is reestablished by incorporating the hemiplegic side in all movements, and postural control is reestablished by helping the patient to orient the head to trunk and the trunk to limbs.

Postural control during functional activities is lost in hemiplegics. For example, in normal humans there is weight shifting to the right side while reaching to the side with the right arm. Hemiplegic patients experience difficulty using the involved arm for functional activities and controlling the trunk for weight shifting to maintain proper posture and balance. Upper extremity weightbearing using the involved upper extremity during sitting is encouraged, and thus flexor synergy movements in the arm are discouraged because the shoulder, elbow, and wrist are in extension. Muscle reeducation is done in individual muscle groups. Shoulder movements with elbow extension are performed first. Grasp activities are included with the wrist in extension.[2,35]

Rood Technique   According to the Rood technique, muscular contraction is first evoked by using cutaneous stimulation. Fast brushing, tendon tapping, or vibration is used for facilitating muscle contraction. Prolonged stretching and icing is used for inhibition of spasticity. The therapist selects the pattern of movement that needs to be reinforced. The desired motor pattern is done passively. The therapist uses sensory stimulation for inhibition or facilitation of the muscles to obtain the desired movement pattern.[2,35]

Brunnstrom Method   Twitchell described synergistic movement of the extremities during recovery of stroke patients.[9] Flexor synergy dominates in the arms, and extension synergy dominates in the lower extremities. Brunnstrom used these motor patterns available for functional activities during the recovery from stroke. The belief is that the mass movement of the extremity helps to facilitate the recovery of voluntary control of the extremity. In addition to synergy patterns, tonic neck reflexes are used to encourage movement of the extremities.[2,35]

The Proprioceptive Neuromuscular Facilitation Technique   In 1951 Kabat found that when topographically aligned groups of muscles were stretched, they produced diagonal movement.[2] The proprioceptive neuromuscular facilitation (PNF) technique uses stronger movement patterns to produce weaker movements. Multiple sensory stimuli are used to facilitate movement. This technique is based on the fact that the normal brain registers total movement of the extremity and not isolated muscle function. The PNF technique uses movements that are spiral and diagonal in nature to resemble movement of the extremities that occurs in functional activities. Goal-directed activities coupled with facilitation technique are used to hasten learning of total patterns of walking and self-care activities. The PNF technique also recommends the rhythmic stabilization technique, which focuses on facilitating alternating contractions of antagonistic muscles of the trunk and extremities.[2,35]

The Carr and Shepard Method   All the above methods focus on the patient as a recipient of facilitation and inhibition techniques provided by the therapist. In the Carr and Shepard method, also known as the motor learning process (MLP), the patient actively participates in learning activities that are functionally important to one's life. Therapy focuses on exercises to gain function rather than involving the patient in a traditional exercise program. Many facilitation and inhibitory strategies are used. Learning includes postural adjustments and limb movements. Compensatory strategies are discouraged. The treatment involves stimulation of weight shifting and normal weightbearing alignment of the body. This method also disagrees with the notion that the intervention should proceed from the proximal to distal direction.[2,35]

None of the above-described sensory neuromuscular training methods have proven to be more advantageous than others. It is now believed that these treatment methods complement each other. However, few studies have compared the effect of different neuromuscular facilitation techniques. One study comparing the effect of the neurodevelopmental technique (NDT) and Brunnstrom method alternated the treatment design (B-N-B-N). Time series analysis showed that only one patient progressed in walking speed during treatment with the Brunnstrom method. There was no difference in the other parameters of gait studied or functional indices.[53] Dickstein et al. studied the effect of conventional physical therapy, PNF technique, and the Bobath (NDT) technique in 131 stroke patients. Outcome measures were the Barthel index, muscle strength, ROM in the ankle and wrist, and ambulatory status as measured using a nominal scale of four categories. There was no statistically significant difference in any of the parameters between the three groups after 6 weeks of treatment.[11] Long-term effects of these neuromuscular retraining methods were studied in two groups of patients, one of which received neuromuscular retraining and the other traditional training. Follow-up after 8 months showed a slight increase in the independence of feeding. No statistically significant differences were noted in all other functional activities. In addition, length of hospitalization was longer in the group that underwent neuromuscular retraining (28.57 versus 68.3 days). The authors, however, did not feel that the type of training alone had an effect on the increased length of stay. The researchers did not explain the reason for this difference.[30] Similar findings were noted even in the short-term outcome when neuromuscular training and traditional training were compared. Both groups improved in function but there was no difference in functional improvement between the two groups.[23,29]

Many of the above studies that tried to determine the effectiveness of different types of therapies included patients with disorders of different causes and locations of neurologic lesions. The heterogeneity of the patient population makes it difficult to determine whether one treatment is more effective than the other. Therapists commonly use many methods to encourage functional improvement.

Electromyographic Feedback Technique The electromyographic (EMG) feedback technique uses multichannel surface EMG for visual and auditory feedback. EMG feedback is used to gain control of muscles or to reduce the muscle activity in the spastic muscles of hemiplegic patients. This requires a well-trained therapist and a motivated patient.[9] Cognitive function and the presence of proprioception are important factors. This technique has been used in the reduction of shoulder subluxation in hemiplegic patients and in the treatment of footdrop, hand and forearm function, and shoulder subluxation.[1,2]

Results of the few studies that have compared the effect of EMG biofeedback techniques are inconclusive. Many of the studies showed that there are no additional benefits to using the biofeedback technique with physical therapy.[22,54] However, a few studies have shown that the biofeedback method is more beneficial in improvement of certain functional outcomes, such as gait parameters and activities of daily living.[4,21] Basmajian found that the effect of EMG biofeedback is more beneficial if started early in treatment.[21] EMG biofeedback has been used in the treatment of dyspahgia after stroke. The treatment includes biofeedback training to improve pharyngeal response during swallowing. Improvement has been noticed after daily sessions of biofeedback training (usually several sessions during the day) to the pharyngeal muscles for about 3 weeks.[6,9] The cost-effectiveness of treatment is still debatable. Availability of the patient, therapist, and equipment for daily treatment sessions is the main difficulty. Further research is warranted into the cost-effectiveness of this modality for the treatment of dysphagia.

Treadmill Training with Partial Body Weight Suspension   Treadmill training with partial body weight suspension is a recently described method to enhance ambulation in hemiplegic patients. The body of the patient is partially suspended by a harness. Patients are encouraged to "walk" on a low-speed treadmill. Therapists help to move the involved extremity. Auditory feedback helps to distribute weight symmetrically. A case-control study on hemiplegic patients showed this method to be a promising adjunct to treatment for regaining ambulatory status. The treadmill training was done on nine stroke patients with a mean poststroke interval of 129 days. The patients had received traditional physical therapy without improvement in their gait pattern. After 25 additional sessions with treadmill training, there was definite improvement in their gait pattern as assessed by functional ambulation category.[17]

Aerobic Training   Recent studies have shown that hemiparetic patients have low endurance to exercise, which may be due to reduced oxidative capacity of the paretic muscles, a decreased number of motor units available for recruitment, and overall reduced endurance. Aerobic exercise has been shown to improve the maximum oxygen consumption in hemiparetic patients. Using a bicycle ergometer for 30 minutes three times a week has been shown to improve aerobic capacity and maximal exercise blood pressure responses in stroke patients.[32,39,40]

Few studies have compared the locations of therapy treatments.[16,20,55] A randomized controlled trial comparing domiciliary and hospital-based rehabilitation for stroke patient after discharge from the hospital showed no difference in outcome, but the domiciliary treatment was less expensive.[16] In another study, 125 elderly stroke patients were randomized into two groups. One group underwent inpatient rehabilitation until maximum benefit of therapies was obtained. Patients in the other group were discharged home as soon as the team felt they were ready, and they continued the therapy as an outpatient. The functional outcome was better in the latter group, but the cost was not significantly different.[61] Comparison of day hospital treatment versus home therapy in a group of stroke patients after discharge noted an increase in cost in the home therapy group.[55] Because these studies were performed outside the United States, no definite conclusion can be made regarding difference in cost.

LONG-TERM EFFECTS OF STROKE REHABILITATION

Many studies have shown that function in stroke patients improves immediately after completion of a supervised therapy program, but long-term follow-up has been discouraging. Patients who have been followed 1 year after the completion of an inpatient rehabilitation program have shown declines in function.[8,27] The clinician must emphasize to both the patient and family that the exercise program should be continued even after discharge from the hospital and that rehabilitation after stroke is a lifelong process.

CASE STUDY

A 71-year-old patient is admitted with a history of acute onset of right-sided weakness. Magnetic resonance imaging showed a lacunar infarct in the internal capsule. The patient was evaluated 4 days after the stroke due to unstable medical conditions. The patient has slightly increased tone and has flexion synergy pattern in the upper extremity and early extension synergy pattern in the lower extremity. The patient also has a history of a three-vessel coronary artery bypass graft a year ago. The patient is cognitively intact. Exercise prescription is as follows: *Precautions*: To follow cardiac precautions while in therapy. Monitor heart rate and blood pressure before and after exercise in therapy. Heart rate not to exceed 20 beats beyond the resting heart rate. Blood pressure (BP) not to exceed 20 points below or above the resting BP.

a. Nursing: Positioning while in bed to keep the involved shoulder in abduction with the elbow in flexion and to keep a rolled towel in the hand. Avoid pillows under the knees. Placement of multipodus boot while in bed or a rolled towel on the lateral aspect of thigh. Turn every 2 hours while in bed.

b. Out of bed in a chair an hour in the morning and an hour in the afternoon. Increase the sitting period gradually until at least 2 hours of sitting in the morning and 2 hours of sitting in the evening can be tolerated.

c. Occupational therapy: Upper extremity range of motion to be done gently to avoid soft tissue stretching. Facilitation technique to improve volitional movement in the extremity. Sitting balance exercises on the mat. Encourage weightbearing on the affected arm. Weightshifting exercises to encourage symmetrical weightbearing. Transfer training to the toilet and tub/shower.

d. Physical therapy: Encourage erect posture and avoid leaning to the affected side. Therapy should progress gradually from standing balance to gait training. Pivot transfer training. Standing balance in the parallel bars. Weight-shifting exercises while standing to increase weightbearing on the affected side. Stepping forward and backward with the right leg. Progress to gait training in the parallel bars. To start bicycle ergometry when the patient can walk one length of the parallel bars with assistance. The patient may participate in 10 minutes of stationary bicycling three times a week. Increase the exercise time with careful monitoring of BP and heart rate until the patient can tolerate 30 minutes of exercise three times a week. EMG biofeedback (if available) daily for 30 minutes to the anterior compartment muscles of the right lower extremity. To use a hemiwalker (or an appropriate assistive device) when walking outside of the parallel bars.

If the patient improves to the point that he is able to walk with an appropriate assistive device, he should be encouraged to continue the aerobic training program at home. If the patient is nonambulatory and has poor motor return in the upper and lower extremities, the patient and family should be instructed in ROM and strengthening exercises. This is to be done preferably twice daily.

MULTIPLE SCLEROSIS

Multiple sclerosis (MS) may be the most commonly diagnosed neurologic disorder of young to middle-aged adults. The disease course is unpredictable yet progressive with periods of exacerbations and remissions. Different patterns of MS have been described, including (1) a *benign* pattern of one or two attacks with mild symptoms and good functional recovery, (2) *relapsing remitting* with nearly full or incomplete remissions followed by long periods of neurologic stability, and (3) *chronic progressive* with an insidious onset and progression of disease. Inflammatory and demyelinating central nervous system lesions are responsible for producing impairments related to motor, sensory, and cognitive deficits. Individuals also may experience coordination disturbances and impaired vision. Other lesions may present as dysarthria, dysphagia, and neurogenic bladder and bowel. Commonly, MS patients will experience fatigability and heat intolerance, both of which may significantly impair their functional abilities.[3,9,10]

Patients with MS can reap many benefits from a therapeutic exercise program, and they can benefit from many of the physiologic responses to exercise as able-bodied people.[37] The cardiac and respiratory response to exercise is modulated by central and reflex neurohumoral interactions among receptors in exercising muscles, the central nervous system, the heart, lungs, and peripheral vasculature. Exercise can improve glucose metabolism as well as reduce levels of cholesterol and triglycerides.[28] Patients also can experience psychological gains, feeling a greater sense of self-esteem and well-being.[36,49] A regular exercise program can maintain general conditioning and prevent disease atrophy in stable to moderately impaired MS patients, and it also helps to maintain optimal functioning to minimize the disabilities associated with MS. Exercise has not been proven to directly affect weakness that results from upper motor neuron lesions.[9]

Because the presentation of MS is variable, the rehabilitation professional needs to tailor the exercise program to each individual. This can be quite challenging because each patient's abilities and symptoms need to be assessed and monitored. When considering the exercise prescription, one needs to take into account the patient's goals, the level of impairment, and the degree of deconditioning. It is also important to ask about a prior history of sports and the degree of participation. During the initial evaluation, it may be useful to determine the extent of disability of the patient.[2] The Kurtzke Disability Status Scale is an impairment scale based on the neurologic examination and scoring of several functional systems involved in MS. The values are scored together with an ambulation index, and the EDSS (Expanded Disability Status Scale) is derived. The scale ranges from zero (normal neurologic examination) to 10 (death due to MS).[3] For example, a grade of 3 indicates moderate disability even though the patient is fully ambulatory. A grade of 6 indicates that assistance is required for walking, and 8 indicates that the patient is restricted to bed but has effective use of the arms. This scoring system is frequently used in clinical trials and is also helpful for monitoring the clinical progress during rehabilitation.

The exercise prescription should include intensity, type, frequency, duration, and time of the day for the fitness program. The patient should be able to perform the program without compromising his or her ability to perform normal activities of daily living. Prior to starting any exercise program, it may be beneficial to obtain a submaximal cardiovascular stress test to determine the appropriate level of exercise. A general conditioning program for the minimally impaired should start with a warm-up period because the body needs to shift from anaerobic to aerobic metabolism. The warm-up should include stretching of the muscles that will be involved in the specific type of exercise. Maximal ROM should be attained, but overexertion could promote fatigue and therefore should be avoided. For patients with a low Kurtzke level, the aerobic program should last 60 minutes. The conditioning portion should last 20–40 minutes at the target heart rate and be followed by 5–10 minutes of cool-down. Patients with heat intolerance may need to increase the cool-down period if the exercise is undertaken in warmer temperatures. One should start the exercise program at a low level, such as 2 METs, and progress the program slowly to decrease the potential for injury to tendons and joints. Hospitalizations for exacerbations will set the program back and will require revision of the program following the exacerbation.

For the patients with Kurtzke ratings of 5–6, the focus of the exercise may be to improve function and gait abnormalities. Patients with MS have shorter stride lengths, slower walking rates, and higher cadence than patients without MS.[2] Ambulation requires strength, endurance, and coordination. Moderately impaired MS patients may be affected by muscle weakness, spasticity, ataxia, and sensory loss. Muscle strength should be maintained, and gait training with appropriate assistive devices may be implemented. Wheelchairs or motorized scooters may help to decrease overexertion and fatigue and should be used for longer distances or more difficult tasks. When prescribing these assistive devices, care should be taken to ensure that the patient does not lose any remaining function by becoming overly dependent on the aids. Daily stretching programs should be implemented for patients with spasticity. Increased spasticity may interfere with functional skills and aggravate fatigue due to movement against constant resistance. For patients with ataxia and tremor, weighted cuffs to the distal extremities may help to dampen the tremor. Balance and coordination retraining may be helpful but are rarely useful due to the progressive nature of the disease.

For the severely impaired patients with a Kurtzke rating of above 7, ROM exercises are essential to prevent joint contractures. Bed mobility and transfer training also may need to be instituted. Wheelchair push-ups should be performed as both exercise and as a means of preventing skin ulcerations. Patients should be positioned properly during exercise; strengthening exercises can be assisted by gravity as weakness ensues. Energy conservation techniques also should be employed to decrease energy expenditure.

Patients with MS may experience fatigue and heat sensitivity with exercise.[37] The cause of the neurogenic fatigue in MS is unknown but may be related to the symptoms of weakness, spasticity, ataxia, depression, and heat intolerance. Both central and peripheral mechanisms may be responsible for fatigue in MS patients.[25,43,44] Exercise to the point of fatigue may not be harmful, but exercising to the point of exhaustion may prolong recovery and temporarily aggravate symptoms. Short rests during exercise at the onset of fatigue (15–30 minutes) may help to minimize fatigue. Patients also should learn to exercise when their energy levels are higher, such as in the morning or after rest periods.

Higher body temperatures aggravate the symptoms of MS. Exercise should be performed in a cooler environment to avoid increasing the core body temperature. The use of air-resistance stationary bicycles and upper extremity ergometers have been helpful with temperature regulation. Cool therapeutic pools not to exceed 84°F (29°C) may be beneficial for conditioning programs.

Therapeutic exercise has many potential benefits in patients with MS. A program of resistive, aerobic, and endurance training can be prescribed safely, but caution needs to be taken when considering the complications of fatigue and hyperthermia with exercise. The exercise programs need to be geared toward the specific limitations and goals of each patient; thus, the exercise prescription may need to be frequently adapted to ongoing changes in the disease process.

CASE STUDY

A 40-year-old woman with a history of relapsing, remitting MS has been discharged from the neurology service after an exacerbation of MS. On neurologic evaluation, spasticity and hyperreflexia are noted in her bilateral lower extremities with a muscle strength of 4/5 in her lower extremities. There was normal strength and no evidence of spasticity noted in the bilateral upper extremities. Her Kurtzke scale was rated as a 4 with relatively severe disability, but she is fully ambulatory and able to be self-sufficient for about 12 hours a day. The exercise prescription would include: *Precautions*: Patient not to do any exercise to the point of exhaustion. Exercise to be done in a cooler environment to avoid an increase in the core temperature. She should be allowed short rest periods if fatigue is experienced during the exercise.

Physical Therapy: Transfer training to include wheelchair to bed, toilet, and shower/tub transfers. Gait training in the parallel bars to progress to ambulation outside the parallel bars with appropriate assistive devices.

A general conditioning program including a stretching program and ROM of the lower extremities should be emphasized. Exercising during the morning hours may be beneficial because her energy levels may be higher. Prior to aerobic conditioning, she should perform a warm-up period of 5–10 minutes of stretching/ROM exercises. ROM exercises should focus on hip extension, knee extension, and ankle dorsiflexion and plantar flexion exercises. She should start at a low exercise intensity level and progress as tolerated to moderate intensity exercise. A stationary bicycle, treadmill, or upper extremity ergometer may be beneficial for aerobic conditioning. The conditioning program should last 20–30 minutes at least three times per week to improve cardiovascular status and prevent disuse muscle atrophy. She should be instructed in a cool-down period of 5–15 minutes.

PARKINSON'S DISEASE

Parkinson's disease (PD) is a degenerative disorder that affects 200,000 people in the United States. The functional deficits are commonly due to bradykinesia, rigidity, and tremor. Bradykinesia is a slowness in initiating movements and is independent of rigidity. Patients have an expressionless face, lack of arm swing during walking, and difficulty initiating and completing simple activities of daily living. Parkinsonian tremor is a slow tremor at 3–5 cycles per second. It is commonly a resting tremor and may affect the limbs or the trunk. It can be unilateral or bilateral and is exaggerated with emotional stress. The frequency of the tremor is reduced by physical activity. Hypertonia, which causes rigidity, is an increase in muscle tone that is felt throughout the range of movement. If superimposed by tremor it causes cogwheeling when passive range is performed. Dementia, dysphagia, hypotonic dysarthria, and autonomic dysfunction are some of the complications that may need attention while treating patients with PD.[3,9] Hoehn and Yahr classified PD into 4 stages. Stage 1 is unilateral involvement only with no functional impairment. Stage 2 has bilateral involvement without impairment of balance. Stage 3 shows first signs of righting reflex; patients have balance problems but still can function independently. Stage 4 has moderate functional impairment but patients can walk unaided. In stage 5 patients are wheelchair-dependent.[18]

Medications to replace dopamine in the central nervous system are the mainstay of treatment in PD. It is important for the clinician to understand how the medication cycle affects the function of an individual. Many rehabilitation interventions are important in the treatment of PD. Physical and occupational therapy helps to improve and maintain higher functional status. Exercises also help in cardiovascular reconditioning.[19,41,51] Problems in movement and posture can cause great impairments in function. Patients develop a fixed posture while sitting and lying. Patients may have difficulty arising from a chair due to lack of initiation to place the legs far under themselves to enable sufficient shifting of the center of gravity to stand. While walking, patients take short shuffling steps. To turn around, patients may take short shuffling steps instead of rotating the whole body. There is also a loss of associated arm swing. Balance is often affected, and patients have difficulty adjusting to even the smallest displacement of center of gravity.

The main focus of therapy in PD is to emphasize proper posture. Patients are encouraged to exercise in front of a mirror. Extension exercises for the trunk are implemented. Patients are instructed to breathe deeply and "feel" the spinal column extending. This exercise is later incorporated into activities such as sitting, standing, and driving. Extension of the hips is emphasized while standing. Stretching of the pectoralis and back extension exercises are often helpful.[9,13,35]

Rhythm and freedom of movement can be encouraged by rhythmically emphasized words or by counting. Arm swing and rotation can be encouraged by the patient holding two sticks and the therapist operating them to simulate arm swing.[35] Large-amplitude movements (PNF) and truncal exercises help patients achieve reciprocal movements in the arms and legs. Use of correct body mechanics during daily activities is important. To overcome rigidity, patients practice slow stretching movements frequently. Frenkel's exercises to improve coordination (repeated movements of the feet in adjacent squares) are recommended.[9] Ambulation through an obstacle course and walking on a balance beam constructed with dotted lines on the floor have been used to improve the gait pattern.[9,35]

Therapists help patients to remain mobile throughout the course of the disease. Patients should participate actively, and therapy should involve functional activities in a structured environment. In stages 1–3 of the disease, postural and endurance exercises are important. In later stages exercises should be tailored to achieve functional goals. Proper positioning to prevent contractures is important in the later stages.

Rehabilitation of PD patients varies from a home-based program to a comprehensive inpatient rehabilitation program depending on the severity of impairment. Studies have shown that any type of exercise program will improve a patient's sense of well-being and functional status. Large-amplitude movements and truncal activities are encouraged. Cueing is used as the major facilitator to obtain rhythmic movements.[19] A randomized single trial cross-over study of patients with advanced PD showed that 4 weeks of an intensive physical rehabilitation program improved the activities of daily living and motor scores compared to a control group that had 4 weeks of normal physical activity. However, the difference was not long-lasting.[7,13] Palmer noticed that two groups of patients involved in a 12-week exercise program that included upper body karate training and an exercise program developed by United Parkinson Foundation were beneficial in improving gait, tremor, grip strength, and motor coordination in both groups, and there was no difference between the two groups.[34]

Magnetotherapy, laser acupuncture, and massage therapy have been tried in PD in other countries, mainly to improve rigidity, but have not shown any promising results.

CASE STUDY

A 58-year-old man was diagnosed with PD 3 years ago. He was started on Sinemet and is referred for an exercise program. On evaluation he is ambulatory without assistive devices but has short shuffling steps and reduced arm swing (Hoehn and Yarr stage 3). He has a stooped posture and bradykinesia. He showed reduced ROM in the hip and shoulders. His breathing is shallow. He is cognitively intact. Exercise prescription is as follows:
Physical therapy three times a week: 45–60 minutes

1. Stretching exercises in supine position to include shoulder abduction, full hip abduction, internal and external rotation for 5–10 minutes.
2. Back extension exercises in prone position.
3. Standing in front of the mirror and thoracic extension exercises with pectoralis stretching. To include lateral bending and spinal rotation.
4. Balance and weight-shifting activities. Example: reaching over while maintaining balance during sitting and standing. The activities to be timed to improve the number of repetitions and to increase the speed of repetition.
5. Gait training: start in the parallel bars to encourage reciprocal movement of the arm and leg. Gait training on a straight line marked on the floor.
6. Low-intensity aerobic exercise on a stationary bicycle or in a pool for 10–15 minutes.

REFERENCES

1. Basmajian JV, Gowland C, Brandstater ME, et al: EMG feedback treatment of upper limb in hemiplegic stroke patients: A pilot study. Arch Phys Med Rehabil 63:613–616, 1982.
2. Basmajian JV, Wolf SL (eds): Therapeutic Exercise, 5th ed. Baltimore, Williams & Wilkins, 1990.
3. Braddom RL (ed): Physical Medicine and Rehabilitation. Philadelphia, WB Saunders, 1996.
4. Burnside IG, Tobias HS, Hurell D: Electromyographic feedback in the remobilization of stroke patients: A controlled trial. Arch Phys Med Rehabil 63:217–222, 1982.
5. Carr JH, Shepherd RB, Nordholm L, Lynne D: Investigation of a new motor assessment scale for stroke patients. Phys Ther 65:175–80, 1985.

6. Crary MA: A direct intervention program for chronic neurogenic dysphagia secondary to stroke. Dysphagia 10:6–18, 1995.
7. Comella CL, Stebbins GT, Brown-Toms N, Goetz CG: Physical therapy and Parkinson's disease: A controlled clinical trial. Neurology 44:376–378, 1994.
8. Davidoff GN, Keren O, Ring H, Solzi P: Acute stroke patients: Long term effects of rehabilitation and maintenance of gains. Arch Phys Med Rehabil 72:869–873, 1991.
9. DeLisa JA, Gans BM (eds): Rehabilitation Medicine: Principles and Practice, 2nd ed. Philadelphia, JB Lippincott, 1993.
10. DeLisa JA, Hammond MC, et al: Multiple sclerosis: Part I. Common physical disabilities and rehabilitation. Am Fam Pract 10:157–163, 1985.
11. Dickstein R, Hocherman S, Pillar T, Shaham R: Stroke rehabilitation. Three exercise therapy approaches. Phy Ther 66:1233–1238, 1986.
12. Evans RL, Connis RT, Hendricks RD, Haselkorn JK: Multidisciplinary rehabilitation versus medical care: A meta-analysis. Soc Sci Med 40:1699–1706, 1995.
13. Formisano R, Pratesi L, Modarelli FT, et al: Rehabilitation and Parkinson's disease. Scand J Rehabil Med 24:157–160, 1992.
14. Fugl-Meyer AR: Assessment of motor function in hemiplegic patients. In Buerger AA, Tobis JS (eds): Neurophysiological Aspects of Rehabilitation Medicine. Springfield, IL, Charles C Thomas, 1976.
15. Garraway WM, Akhtar AJ, Hockey L, Prescott RJ: Management of acute stroke in the elderly: Follow-up of a controlled trial. BMJ 281:827–829, 1980.
16. Gladman J, Whynes D, Lincoln N: The cost comparison of domiciliary and hospital based stroke rehabilitation. DOMINO study group. Age Ageing 23:241–245, 1994.
17. Hesse S, Bertelt C, Schaffrin A, et al: Restoration of gait in non-ambulatory hemiparetic patients by treadmill training with partial body weight support. Arch Phys Med Rehabil 75:1087–1093, 1994.
18. Hoehn MM, Yahr MD: Parkinsonism: Onset, progression and mortality. Neurology 17:427–442, 1967.
19. Hömberg V: Motor training in the therapy of Parkinson's disease. Neurology 43(suppl 6):S45–S46, 1993.
20. Hui E, Lum CM, Woo J, et al: Outcome of elderly stroke patients. Day hospital versus conventional medical management. Stroke 26:1616–1619, 1995.
21. Intiso D, Santilli V, Grasso MG, et al: Rehabilitation of walking with electromyographic feedback in foot-drop after stroke. Stroke 25:1189–1192, 1994.
22. John J: Failure of electrical myofeedback to augment the effects of physiotherapy in stroke. Int J Rehabil Res 9:35–45, 1986.
23. Jongbloed L, Stacey S, Brighton C: Stroke rehabilitation: Sensorimotor integrative treatment versus functional treatment. Am J Occup Their 43:391–397, 1989.
24. Jorgensen HS, Nakayama H, Raaschou HO, et al: Outcome and time course of recovery in stroke. Part II: Time course of recovery. The Copenhagen Stroke Study. Arch Phys Med Rehabil 76:406–412, 1995.
25. Kent-Braun JA, Sharma KR, Weiner MW, Miller RG: Effects of exercise on muscle activation and metabolism in multiple sclerosis. Muscle Nerve 17:1162–1169, 1994.
26. Kumar R, Mettr EJ, Mehta AJ, Cheu T: Shoulder pain in hemiplegia. The role of exercise. Am J Phys Med Rehabil 69:205–208, 1990.
27. Kwakkel G, Wagenaar RC, Koelman TW, et al: Effects of intensity of rehabilitation after stroke. A research synthesis. Stroke 28:1550–1556, 1997.
28. Levine GN, Balady GJ: The benefits and risks of exercise training: The exercise prescription. Ad Intern Med 38:57–79, 1993.
29. Logigian MK, Samuels MA, Falconer J, Zagar R: Clinical exercise trial for stroke patients. Arch Phys Med Rehabil 64:314–317, 1983.
30. Lord JP, Hall K: Neuromuscular reeducation versus traditional programs for stroke rehabilitation. Arch Phys Med Rehabil 67:88–91, 1986.
31. Mayo NE: Epidemiology and recovery. Phys Med Rehabil State Art Rev 7:1–25, 1993.
32. Monga TN, Deforge DA, Williams J, Wolfe LA: Cardiovascular response to acute exercise in patients with cerebrovascular accidents. Arch Phys Med Rehabil 69:937–940, 1988.
33. Nugent JA, Schurr KA, Adams RD: A dose response relationship between amount of weight bearing

exercise and walking outcome following cerebrovascular accident. Arch Phys Med Rehabil 75:399–402, 1994.

34. Palmer SS, Mortimer JA, Webster DD, et al: Exercise therapy for Parkinson's disease. Arch Phys Med Rehabil 67:741–745, 1986.

35. Pedretti LW: Occupational Therapy: Practice Skills for Physical Dysfunction, 4th ed. St. Louis, Mosby Yearbook, 1996.

36. Petajan JH, Gappmaier E, White AT, et al: Impact of aerobic training on fitness and quality of life in multiple sclerosis. Ann Neurol 39:432–441, 1996.

37. Ponichtera-Mulcare JA: Exercise and multiple sclerosis. Med Sci Sports Exerc 25:451–465, 1993.

38. Post-Stroke Rehabilitation Guidelines Panel: Clinical Practice Guidelines. Post-stroke Rehabilitation. Rockville, MD, U.S. Dept. of Health and Human Services,1995, AHCPR publication no. 950662.

39. Potempa K, Braun LT, Tinkell T, Popovich J: Benefits of aerobic exercise after stroke. Sports Medi 21:337–346, 1996.

40. Potempa K, Lopez M, Braun LT, et al: Physiological outcome of aerobic exercise training in hemiparetic stroke patients. Stroke 26:101–105, 1995.

41. Protas EJ, Stanley RK, Jankovic J, MacNeill B: Cardiovascular and metabolic responses to upper and lower extremity exercise in men with idiopathic Parkinson's disease. Phys Ther 76:34–40, 1996.

42. Richards CL, Malouin F, Wood-Dauphinee S, et al: Task-specific physical therapy for optimization of gait recovery in acute stroke patients. Arch Phys Med Rehabil 74:612–620, 1993.

43. Sharma KR, Kent-Braun J, Mynhier MA, et al: Evidence of an abnormal intramuscular component of fatigue in multiple sclerosis. Muscle Nerve 18:1403–1411, 1995.

44. Sheean GL, Murray NMF, Rothwell JC, et al: An electrophysiological study of the mechanism of fatigue in multiple sclerosis. Brain 120:299–315, 1997.

45. Shumway-Cook A, Anson D, Haller S: Postural sway biofeedback: Its effect on reestablishing stance stability in hemiplegic patients. Arch Phys Med Rehabil 69:395–400, 1988.

46. Sivenius J, Pyorala K, Heinonen OP, et al: The significance of intensity of rehabilitation of stroke–A controlled trial. Stroke 16:928–931, 1985.

47. Smith DS, Goldenberg E, Ashburn A, et al: Remedial therapy after stroke: A randomized controlled trial. BMJ 282:517–520, 1981.

48. Smith ME, Garraway WM, Smith DL, Akhthar AJ: Therapy impact on functional outcome in a controlled trial of stroke rehabilitation. Arch Phys Med Rehabil 63:21–24, 1982.

49. Stuifbergen AK: Physical activity and perceived health status in persons with multiple sclerosis. J Neurosci Nurs 29:238–243, 1997.

50. Tangeman PT, Banitis DA, Williams AK: Rehabilitation of chronic stroke patients: Changes in functional performance. Arch Phys Med Rehabil 72:876–880, 1990.

51. Ulm G: The current significance of physiotherapeutic measures in the treatment of Parkinson's disease. Neural Transm Suppl 46:455–460, 1995.

52. Wade DT, Collen FM, Robb GF, Warlow CP: Physiotherapy intervention late after stroke and mobility. BMJ 304:609–613, 1992.

53. Wagenaar RC, Meijer OG, van Wieringen PC, et al: The functional recovery of stroke: A comparison between neurodevelopmental treatment and Brunnstrom method. Scand J Rehabil Med 22:1–8, 1990.

54. Wolf SL, LeCraw DE, Barton LA: Comparison of motor copy and targeted biofeedback training techniques for restitution of upper extremity function among patients with neurologic disorders. Phy Ther 69:719–735, 1989.

55. Young J, Forster A: Day hospital and home physiotherapy for stroke patients: A comparative cost-effectiveness study. J R Coll Physicians Lond 27:252–258, 1993.

DAVID R. GATER, MD, PhD
VIVIANE UGALDE, MD

11

Physiologic Foundations for Exercise Prescription in Tetraplegia

About 230,000 Americans are affected by spinal cord injury (SCI), and approximately 8,000 new cases are reported each year.[123] Of these, about 22% involve complete tetraplegia. Men are affected four times as frequently as women, and 59% are between the ages of 16 and 30. The average lifetime medical costs exceed $1.1 million per individual, and the average lifetime foregone earnings per person exceed $2.1 million. In addressing these tremendous costs, appropriately prescribed exercise intervention may be the most effective and modifiable variable that can be used to improve the longevity, quality of life, and productivity for a person with SCI.

Tetraplegia, a term that is preferred to *quadriplegia,* refers to "the impairment or loss of motor and/or sensory function in the cervical segments of the spinal cord due to damage of neural elements within the spinal canal."[181] It is distinguished from paraplegia in that it includes dysfunction of the arms; both tetraplegia and paraplegia involve impairment of function in the trunk, legs, and pelvic organs. By convention, SCI is classified by the most caudal segment of the spinal cord with normal sensory and motor function on both sides of the body and may be defined as complete (without sensory or motor sparing in the lowest sacral segment) or incomplete (partial preservation of sensory or motor function below the neurologic level and including the lowest sacral segment). The American Spinal Injury Association (ASIA) has defined four degrees of incomplete tetraplegia, ranging from the preservation of sensory, but not motor, function below the neurologic level, to complete sparing of sensory and motor function below the initial injury.[181] Because a tremendous range of abilities and disabilities are associated with different degrees of incomplete SCI, most of the literature investigating exercise in tetraplegia is relegated to individuals with complete lesions. This chapter likewise is limited to exercise responses in complete tetraplegia, and the reader is reminded that responses in incomplete SCI will vary depending on the neurologic level and degree of motor and autonomic function remaining intact below that level.

Although exercise intervention appears beneficial to individuals with SCI, there are no absolute guidelines for its prescription in this population. Essential components of an exercise prescription include mode, frequency, intensity, duration, progression, and goals and should be modified according to the person's fitness level, physical limitations, and stratified risk. Few clinicians are comfortable in prescribing exercise for SCI individuals, because the parameters have not been clearly defined. Inappropriately prescribed exercise may yield minimal or no benefit and may even be dangerous—much the same as with pharmaceutical therapeutics.

This chapter identifies the unique features of tetraplegia that may preclude the use of standard techniques for exercise prescription, reviews the literature regarding exercise and tetraplegia, offers suggestions for exercise prescription based on that review, and explores areas for future investigation in this special population.

PATHOPHYSIOLOGY

The spinal cord is a portion of the central nervous system and is composed of an extremely complex communications network linking conscious and subconscious functions of the brain with portions of the peripheral and autonomic nervous systems. Injury to the spinal cord obstructs the transmission of neural messages through the cord and results in the loss of somatic and autonomic control over trunk, limbs, and viscera distal to the site of the lesion. Appropriate systemic responses to exercise seen in able-bodied individuals are therefore blunted in persons with spinal cord injury and vary inversely with the level of injury. Higher levels of cervical cord injury yield diminishing ability to mount an exercise response, both at a conscious (somatic) and subconscious (autonomic) level (Fig. 1).

SOMATIC NERVOUS SYSTEM DISRUPTION

The somatic nervous system is composed of sensory and motor neural pathways connecting the brain to the body via the spinal cord. Afferent (sensory) fibers convey information of pain, temperature, touch, and position about the body relative to its environment, whereas efferent (motor) fibers allow for voluntary and involuntary (reflex) movement. Efferent pathways are composed of two main components: the upper motor neuron, which arises within the motor cortex and ends in the spinal cord; and the lower motor neuron, which arises within the spinal cord and ends at its designated muscle.

Complete SCI interrupts the transmission of these signals such that sensory information initiated and conveyed by sensory nerves whose cell bodies lie below the lesion is no longer perceived by the brain, and voluntary movement mediated via lower motor neurons below the lesion is no longer possible. Complete tetraplegia may therefore allow no movement of the body below the chin (C1–C3), or may allow shrugging of the shoulders and turning of the head (C4), with abduction/ flexion of the shoulders and elbow flexors (C5), wrist extension (C6), elbow extension/wrist flexion/finger extension (C7), and finger/thumb flexion (C8) depending upon the level of injury. By definition, individuals with complete tetraplegia cannot control the muscles that spread their fingers, nor can they voluntarily control the

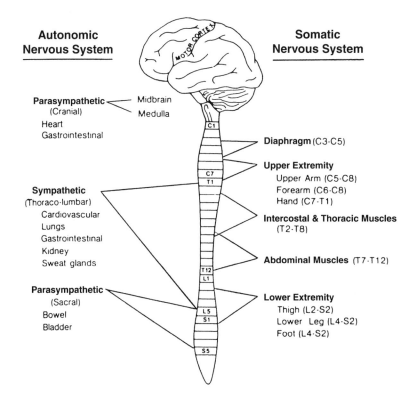

Autonomic Nervous System

Parasympathetic (Cranial)
Heart
Gastrointestinal

Midbrain
Medulla
C1

Sympathetic (Thoraco-lumbar)
Cardiovascular
Lungs
Gastrointestinal
Kidney
Sweat glands

Parasympathetic (Sacral)
Bowel
Bladder

Somatic Nervous System

Diaphragm (C3-C5)

Upper Extremity
Upper Arm (C5-C8)
Forearm (C6-C8)
Hand (C7-T1)

Intercostal & Thoracic Muscles (T2-T8)

Abdominal Muscles (T7-T12)

Lower Extremity
Thigh (L2-S2)
Lower Leg (L4-S2)
Foot (L4-S2)

FIGURE 1. The central nervous system and the neural outflows from the somatic (innervating skeletal muscles) and autonomic (innervating smooth muscle and internal organs) systems. Segmental levels are indicated. (From Glaser RM, Janssen TWJ, Suryaprasad AG, et al: Physical Fitness: A Guide for Individuals with Spinal Cord Injury. Baltimore, Rehabilitation Research and Development Service, Department of Veterans Affairs, 1996, with permission.)

muscles of their trunk or legs. Neurologic classification of SCI is standardized as seen in Figure 2.

THE AUTONOMIC NERVOUS SYSTEM DISRUPTION

The autonomic nervous system (ANS) orchestrates automatic life-sustaining processes and organizes visceral responses to somatic reactions. It is composed of sympathetic and parasympathetic divisions, which regulate the action of smooth muscle and glands. Essential functions of the ANS during exercise include modulating heart rate, stroke volume, blood pressure, blood flow, ventilation, thermoregulation, and metabolism.

The sympathetic nervous system is composed of preganglionic fibers derived from the thoracolumbar spinal cord that synapse on postganglionic fibers near the spinal cord in the sympathetic chain ganglia. The postganglionic fibers innervate smooth muscle, organs, and glands to facilitate the classic "fight or flight" response to sympathetic stimulation—e.g., increased heart rate, stroke volume, ventilation, and sweating,

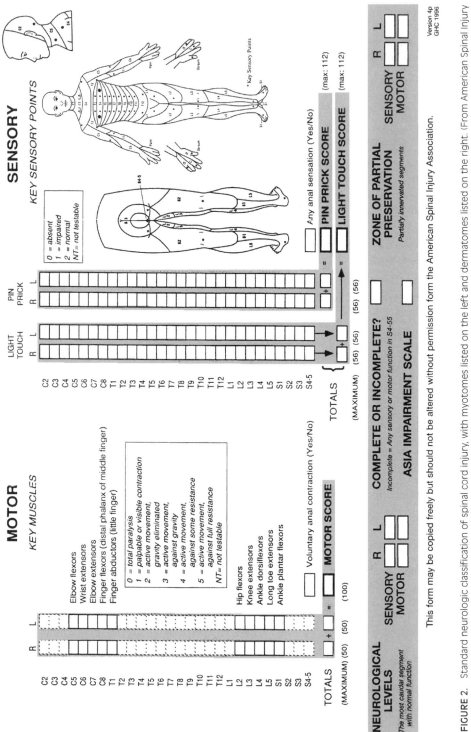

FIGURE 2. Standard neurologic classification of spinal cord injury, with myotomes listed on the left and dermatomes listed on the right. (From American Spinal Injury Association: Standards for Neurological and Functional Classification of Spinal Cord Injury. Chicago, ASIA, 1992, with permission.)

with vasoconstriction of splanchnic vasculature, and vasodilation of skeletal muscle vasculature. Most autonomic reflexes can be stimulated at the level of the spinal cord but are largely modulated by the supraspinal structures of the CNS—namely the medulla, pons, and hypothalamus. In tetraplegia, cortical and subcortical reflexes can be stimulated at the level of the spinal cord, but are largely modulated by the supraspinal structures of the CNS: the medulla, pons, and hypothalamus. In tetraplegia, cortical and subcortical messages relayed along the spinal cord to the thoracic and lumbar sympathetic outflow tracts are interrupted, essentially blocking modulating influences of the CNS. Additionally, sensory information from regions below the injury is conveyed along afferent fibers of the ANS and may synapse with preganglionic efferent fibers in the spinal cord, stimulating reflex sympathetic responses below that level; this sensory information cannot traverse the spinal cord lesion and is therefore not subject to supraspinal modulation.

The parasympathetic nervous system is derived from the craniosacral portions of the CNS and promotes anabolic activity and energy conservation by reducing heart rate, stroke volume, and ventilation and by increasing digestion. The cranial portion of the parasympathetic nervous system is not influenced by spinal cord injury; its effects on cardiac, pulmonary, and upper digestive structures are mediated primarily through the vagus nerve, which exits the CNS at the level of the medulla, above the spinal cord. Conversely, the sacral components of the parasympathetic nervous system arise from the sacral segments of the spinal cord, and while sacral reflex parasympathetic pathways remain intact in tetraplegia, modulating influences from the CNS are blocked.

FEATURES UNIQUE TO SPINAL CORD INJURY

Relative sparing of parasympathetic pathways allows greater CNS modulation of parasympathetic influences over cardiovascular, ventilatory, and metabolic responses in tetraplegia than in able-bodied individuals at rest and during exercise. The combination of blunted sympathetic modulation by the CNS and disrupted somatic control of arms, trunk, and legs yields unique and unusual exercise responses in persons with SCI. Problems peculiar to SCI include blunted cardiovascular, ventilatory, thermoregulatory, and hormonal exercise responses, while associated SCI features of autonomic dysreflexia, osteopenia, upper extremity overuse syndromes, spasticity, and pressure sores make the exercise prescription for this population especially difficult. Additionally, bladder and bowel function are impaired but should not significantly affect the exercise prescription.[254]

CARDIOVASCULAR RESPONSES

In response to acute cervical SCI, bradycardia often ensues due to the disruption of cortical and subcortical influences on the sympathetic nervous system and the preservation of parasympathetic control on cardiac structures.[116,149,172,273] The bradycardia usually resolves in 2–6 weeks, likely due to withdrawal of parasympathetic tone over time as well as to "adaptive" myocardial atrophy.[71,152,196] Normal increases in heart rate and contractility in response to exercise are subject to withdrawal of parasympathetic influences and to increased sympathetic drive. In response to exercise, it appears that complete tetraplegia prevents sufficient sympathetic drive to allow heart rate increases greater than about 130 beats per minute (bpm),[51,93,109,185,186,256] but heart rates above 140 have been reported in rare instances.[268] Heart rate increments in this population are primarily due to parasympathetic withdrawal.[104]

The relative loss of sympathetic tone in tetraplegia results in reduced resting myocardial contractility, reduced peripheral resistance (afterload), and reduced cardiac preload, contributing to adaptive myocardial atrophy[152,196] and subsequently reduced resting stroke volume. Maximal exercise stroke volume, and subsequently cardiac output, is therefore diminished in tetraplegia,[94,130,256] but only a portion of the decrement is directly attributed to impaired sympathetic influences on myocardial contractility. In able-bodied subjects, redistribution of blood flow occurs during exercise in response to increased sympathetic tone, subsequently increasing venous return to the heart, and increasing stroke volume by way of the Frank-Starling mechanism.[10] Conversely, during exercise in tetraplegia, left ventricular end diastolic volume remains largely constant, resulting from unchanged or decreased venous return, ultimately contributing to fairly limited changes in cardiac stroke volume.[93] Inability to shunt blood from the viscera and nonexercising trunk and lower extremity musculature to the working muscles is due to impaired sympathetic responses in SCI; venoconstriction is also impaired, and a large amount of blood remains pooled in the lower extremities and inferior vena cava.[24,26] Further, the inability to voluntarily contract lower extremity musculature eliminates activity of the venous pump system. In circulatory hypokinesis, which has been reported by several investigators,[93,135,256] upper extremity exercise often causes hypotension in tetraplegia, because the increased metabolic demands of exertion are not matched by appropriate hemodynamic responses. McLean et al.[185] reported significantly greater stroke volumes (and cardiac output) in supine compared to upright sitting positions both at rest and during submaximal exercise in tetraplegia. Abdominal binders and stockings,[151,153] lower body positive pressure,[217] and antigravity suits[139] have been used to variably improve venous blood return to the heart during exercise. Additionally, functional electrical stimulation (FES) of lower extremities has been developed in part to enhance venous return, improving left ventricular end diastolic volume and subsequently cardiac output.[87,96,218,221,222]

In a practical sense, community mobility and activities of daily living (ADL) in tetraplegia are performed through upper extremity work, which has unique cardiovascular effects even in the able-bodied population. Heart rate, blood pressure, minute ventilation, oxygen consumption, and respiratory exchange ratios are greater in upper extremity than lower extremity work at the same absolute workload, whereas stroke volume and anaerobic threshold (onset of blood lactate accumulation) are lower.[101,232] Thus, for a given workload, the cardiopulmonary system is stressed to a greater extent when performing upper extremity tasks. The absolute work capacity (and subsequently cardiac output) for upper extremity exercise is about 20–36% less than that of the lower extremity, due to the smaller muscle mass employed,[101] but the maximal heart rate, blood pressure, and rate pressure product is similar.[236] A concern about using upper extremity exercise for cardiovascular conditioning exclusively is that a threshold level of work necessary to yield protective cardiovascular benefits may not be reached.[93,118]

VENTILATORY RESPONSES

Ventilation is significantly impaired in tetraplegia because of paralysis of rib cage and abdominal musculature, reduced pulmonary compliance, and reduced diaphragmatic excursion.[22,65,105,127] The intercostal and abdominal muscles serve as expiratory muscles innervated by thoracic nerve roots from the spinal cord and are therefore no longer subject to voluntary control in tetraplegia. The diaphragm is primarily responsible for inspiration and is innervated by the phrenic nerve, originating from cervical roots C3, C4, and C5. Complete spinal cord lesions above this level separate the breathing centers in the medulla from diaphragmatic control; these patients are ventilator-dependent or require phrenic nerve pacing to the diaphragm to stimulate inspiration.[55,187] Persons with SCI involving the C3, C4, or C5 segments will have impaired ability to stimulate diaphragmatic excursion because of disruption of the phrenic nerve, and they may require assisted ventilation. Tetraplegia below C5 typically spares voluntary control of the diaphragm, although inspiration remains impaired due to paralyzed abdominal muscles, which allow abdominal contents and subsequently the diaphragm to descend. The diaphragm is left at a mechanical disadvantage, allowing less excursion during contraction and subsequently increasing the work of breathing. This effect is partially compensated for with the use of an abdominal binder, which returns the diaphragm to a higher, more functional position.[176]

Hopman et al.[137] demonstrated that tetraplegics have maximal inspiratory pressures of about 70%, maximal expiratory pressures 46%, and inspiratory endurance only 40% of values obtained in able-bodied controls; the ratio of inspiratory endurance to maximal inspiratory pressure was only 0.49 in tetraplegics versus 0.82 in the able-bodied controls. Further, pulmonary function in complete tetraplegia is inversely related to the level of spinal cord injury[2,49] and length of disability[49] but may be improved with aggressive incentive spirometry[126,259] and exercise training.[54,225]

Ventilation during exercise is normally increased by a combination of increased central (sympathetic) drive, local stimulation of chemoreceptors in working muscle, and induced metabolic acidosis sensed by the carotid bodies.[80,81,144,178,207,262,266] All of these control mechanisms may be blunted or absent in tetraplegia, because they require integration at the level of the hypothalamus or medulla. In fact, patients with tetraplegia have abnormally high ventilatory threshold percentages despite having lower peak work capacity than paraplegics or able-bodied athletes, implying blunted responses at each level of ventilatory control.[50,164]

THERMOREGULATION

Heat gains and losses in the human body are dictated by factors of internal metabolism, external work performed, respiratory convective heat exchange, respiratory evaporative heat loss, radiation, convection, conduction of heat exchanged at the skin surface, and evaporation from the skin surface.[5] The ability to thermoregulate in humans is dependent upon peripheral and central temperature sensors, plasma volume and osmolality sensors and autonomic mediated sweating, and vasoconstriction and vasodilation, all of which are integrated and controlled at the level of the hypothalamus.[235] The interruption of autonomic pathways in tetraplegia results in partially poikilothermic responses to thermal stress, providing these individuals much less ability to adapt to environmental and internally generated heat.[73,75,208,235] In complete tetraplegia afferent impulses relaying temperature information from the body are blocked at the spinal cord level, and although volume and osmoreceptors in the hypothalamus remain functional, efferent neural responses mediated via spinal cord pathways are obstructed, severely limiting sweat responses below the SCI. While some investigators demonstrate no significant thermoregulatory activity in complete SCI,[79,261] others have reported at least partial, albeit significantly blunted, sweating responses below the level of SCI during thermal stress, suggesting the presence of thermoregulatory spinal reflexes.[140,223,237] Most sweat responses in tetraplegia, however, are relegated to regions above the level of SCI.

Interestingly, resting heart rates in tetraplegics subjected to 40°C thermal stress for 30 minutes averaged 140 bpm, much higher than that usually achieved during maximal exercise stress testing, and increased disproportionately in response to exercise, suggesting marked fluid shifts between vascular spaces in response to the thermal stress.[208] Tetraplegic subjects in the same study developed aural temperatures of 40.3°C while exercising in the heat, with regional sweat rates above their injury level about six times higher than in able-bodied controls but without significant responses in sweat glands below their spinal cord level. Other investigators have demonstrated an inability of thermally stressed subjects with SCI above the level of T6 to accommodate reductions in stroke volume with appropriate increments in heart rate to sustain cardiac output in prolonged exercise.[99,139,234] Guidelines provided for exercise in the heat have proven beneficial to able-bodied individuals,[7,47] but one must realize that individuals with tetraplegia have special needs and concerns regarding thermal stress and exercise.[183]

ENDOCRINOLOGY

Autonomic dysfunction and somatic paralysis in tetraplegia may significantly affect metabolic and hormonal parameters in SCI patients. As expected, sympathomedullary responses are blunted in tetraplegics at rest[161] and during acute, progressive exercise[103] and sustained exercise,[27] provided autonomic dysreflexia is not induced.[264] Likewise, the adrenocortical-pituitary axis appears to be disrupted in tetraplegia, with flattened circadian rhythms and unregulated corticosteroid responses;[45] however, this may be improved with regular exercise.[253] Coincidentally, immune responses are depressed as indicated by T-cell function or activation but may improve with activity.[57,155,194] Growth hormone release is blunted[16] and chronically depressed in tetraplegia, as evidenced by reduced levels of insulin-like growth factor-1, a convenient indicator of chronic growth hormone secretion.[16,241] As expected, ovulatory menstrual cycles are fairly well preserved in tetraplegia, providing at least some cardioprotective and bone-sparing function in women.[226]

AUTONOMIC DYSREFLEXIA

Autonomic dysreflexia, a significant problem in tetraplegia and SCI above T6, is an uncontrolled outflow of sympathetic activity in response to noxious stimuli below the SCI that can result in life-threatening paroxysmal hypertension.[32,83,191] Information about noxious stimuli (distended bowel or bladder, lacerations, fractures, pressure sores, sunburn) from regions below the SCI is conveyed along afferent fibers of the ANS, which synapse with preganglionic efferent fibers in the spinal cord, stimulating reflex sympathetic responses below that level (Fig. 3). Marked hypertension, mediated primarily by norepinephrine, can result in SCI lesions above T6, due to inability to autoregulate sympathetic outflow to the trunk, lower extremities, and, most importantly, the greater splanchnic nerve, which arises at T7-8 and provides innervation to most of the splanchnic vasculature bed.[58,59,179,180] Pressure receptors in the carotid bodies and aortic arch respond to the abrupt hypertension by stimulating medullary parasympathetic responses, resulting in bradycardia and vasodilation above the SCI, manifested as flushing, headache, hyperhydrosis, piloerection, pupillary dilation, and blurred vision.[32,180,191] Such symptoms herald autonomic crisis, which can lead to intracerebral hemorrhages,[82] seizures,[173] arrhythmias,[100,216] and death if not treated immediately and appropriately.[32,83]

It is conceivable that exercise stressing insensate areas of the body in tetraplegia could provoke autonomic dysreflexia, but only one study has reported such responses.[9] Ashley et al.[9] demonstrated that FES of lower extremities to perform hydraulic resistance training provoked autonomic dysreflexia (reduced heart rate, elevated systolic and mean arterial blood pressure, and headache) in eight of ten SCI subjects with lesions above T6. Conversely, recent reviews report no significant episodes of autonomic dysreflexia in tetraplegic patients training with FES or hybrid (arm crank ergometry plus FES) exercise systems.[92,93,118,221] It may be that the stimulus frequency of 50 Hz used by Ashley et al.[9] was significantly more nociceptive than the frequency of 30–35 Hz used by most other investigators, as all other parameters appeared similar to the protocols used in other studies. It also may be possible that FES systems do stimulate some degree of autonomic dysreflexia but that the increased vascular tone is offset by lower extremity vasodilation stimulated by local metabolites in response to muscular contraction. Additionally, most FES protocols employ a gradually progressive increase in stimulus intensity and duration of exercise bouts, possibly allowing desensitization to the potentially nociceptive properties of FES.

An interesting phenomenon called "boosting" has recently been reported that involves the intentional stimulation of autonomic dysreflexia by SCI athletes to enhance performance.[38,264] To induce a greater sympathetic response for exercise performance, it is estimated that 90–100% of tetraplegic athletes have purposely overdistended their urinary bladder, applied tight leg straps, or sat on sharp objects with variable increases in catecholamine release.[38,264] Such increases in catecholamines would be expected not

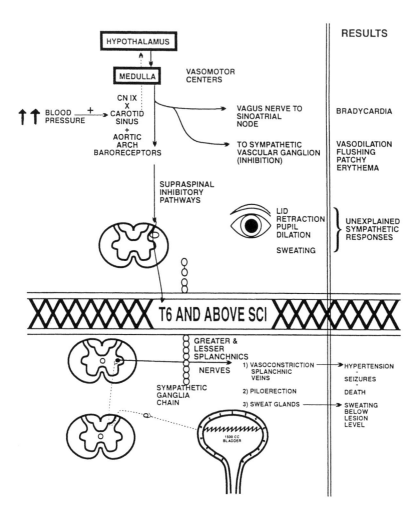

FIGURE 3. Neuroanatomy of autonomic dysreflexia; dashed lines = afferent; solid lines = efferent. (From Ugalde V, Letwiller SE, Gater DR: Bladder and bowel anatomy for the physiatrist. Phys Med Rehabil State Art Rev 10:547–568, 1996, with permission.)

only to enhance lipolysis, glycolysis, and substrate utilization during exercise,[36] but also to reduce lower extremity venous pooling, enhance shunting of blood from viscera to exercising muscles, and enhance sweating in tetraplegic athletes. In addition to the ethical questions posed regarding the use of boosting as an ergogenic aid in sports competition, a significant concern is raised about the inherent dangers and potential fatalities associated with the intentional induction of autonomic dysreflexia to enhance performance.

OSTEOPENIA

Neurogenic osteopenia in complete tetraplegia results from the withdrawal of stress and strain upon bone as modeled by Wolff's law.[274] Paralysis of skeletal muculature below the level of SCI prevents the usual application of external forces (muscle contraction and gravitational loading) required to prevent bone resorption. As a result, urinary excretion of calcium, hydroxyproline, magnesium, and phosphorus are significantly increased, particularly within the first 3 months but remaining so for up to 18 months following acute tetraplegia, indicating an overall trend of bone resorption.[44,46,192] Additionally, plasma parathormone (PTH) and 1,25 $(OH)_2$ vitamin D (calcitriol) levels are reduced acutely and chronically, while calcitonin levels initially increase and remain elevated above control levels and to a greater extent in chronic tetraplegic than in paraplegic subjects.[257] The hypercalcuria can be reduced somewhat with tilt-table weightbearing exercises in incomplete tetraplegia and to a lesser degree with strengthening exercises.[145]

Bone mineral loss as determined by dual-energy x-ray absorptiometry (DEXA) is rapid and linear within the first 4 months of SCI, occurring to a greater extent in the pelvis and lower extremities in tetraplegic and paraplegic individuals.[108] Interestingly, significant bone mineral loss also occurs in the upper extremities, even in paraplegics, without return to baseline. Homeostasis at 67% of original bone mass is achieved at about 16 months after injury, barely above fracture threshold.[108] Even in patients with complete neurologic recovery after SCI, bone mineral content remains below preinjury levels 1 year later.[272] Several studies have attempted to reverse the osteopenic process using FES of the lower extremities,[20,28,128,171,205] but only one has demonstrated significant improvement.[28] BeDell et al.[20] demonstrated a trend toward increasing density of the lumbar spine but not the pelvis after 34 weeks of twice-weekly FES sessions with leg cycle ergometry (LCE). Others failed to demonstrate even a positive trend,[171,205] although Hangartner et al.[128] did report a slowing of the expected rate of bone loss. However, Bloomfield et al.[28] found increased bone mineral density for the lumbar spine after 3 months of training at a threshold power output of 18 watts with FES-LCE. Concurrently, PTH levels rose 75% above baseline after 6 months of training, with similar increases in serum osteocalcin despite unchanged urinary calcium and hydroxyproline levels, suggesting an increase in bone turnover without concomitant resorptive activity.

UPPER EXTREMITY OVERUSE INJURIES

Overuse injuries involving the upper extremities of wheelchair-reliant individuals have been reported by 51–73% of respondents surveyed and occur most frequently at the shoulder.[91,197,243,251,263] About 55% of 136 patients with tetraplegia in one study were noted to have upper extremity pain, 45% of which was attributed to shoulder pathology and an additional 33% to cervical origin.[243] Interestingly, Wylie and Chakera[275] noted a significantly greater incidence in shoulder degenerative changes by radiograph in sedentary (45%) versus active (18%) SCI patients, implying protective effects of moderate activity. Magnetic resonance imaging in another recent study detected rotator cuff tears in 73% of symptomatic paraplegics versus 59% of symptomatic able-bodied subjects; 54% of all paraplegics tested (26 symptomatic, 11 asymptomatic) were found to have rotator cuff tears, most of which were full-thickness.[85] Besides rotator cuff tears, shoulder pathology in another study of 24 tetraplegics included capsular contracture or capsulitis, anterior instability, rotator cuff impingement, osteoarthritis, and osteonecrosis.[39] Recent studies indicate that persons with tetraplegia are especially at risk for shoulder pathology because of muscular limitation, likely rotator cuff, pectoral and latissimus dorsi weakness, truncal instability, and increased functional demand.[177,202,220,228] In a recent review, Apple et al.[6] discussed common causes for upper extremity overuse syndrome in SCI, including rotator cuff tendinitis, subacromial bursitis, bicipital tendinitis, lateral epicondylitis, ulnar neuropathy at the elbow, de Quervain's tenosynovitis, and carpal tunnel syndrome. Uncomfortable and irritating in able-bodied persons, these problems can be disastrous in the tetraplegic who relies heavily on residual function in the upper extremities for ADLs and mobility.

SPASTICITY

Spasticity is velocity-dependent muscle tone associated with hyperactive deep tendon reflexes that occurs in up to 60% of individuals with complete tetraplegia.[182,201] As the result of SCI, central inhibition of spinal reflex arcs is lost, resulting in significant increases in muscle tone, spasms, and hyperreflexia.[280] Some tetraplegics are able to use their spasticity to help them perform mobility and ADL tasks, but many find that the spasticity is painful, disrupts sleep, interferes with function, causes muscle contractures, and can lead to shear- or pressure-induced skin breakdown. Initial steps in managing detrimental spasticity include the removal of noxious stimuli that may be inducing increased tone and the daily prolonged stretch of affected muscle groups;[147] pharmacologic or even surgical intervention may be required.

It is not clear if exercise significantly affects spasticity in tetraplegia. Hjeltnes and Jansen[130] noted a trend toward reduced spasticity with increasing levels of aerobic fitness, but it did not reach significance. Noreau et al.[201] demonstrated no significant relationship between leisure activity levels and spasticity in 50 tetraplegic volunteers, while Douglas et al.[72] noted that FES of the lower extremities in paraplegic subjects actually seemed to increase muscle tone after the training sessions had ceased. Likewise, Glaser[119] cautions that when using FES, sudden unexpected and forceful muscle spasms may occur and that appropriate precautions should be employed to prevent injury. Sipski et al.[245] reported inconsistent changes in spasticity in 28 SCI patients undergoing home FES. In a recent report, however, lower extremity tone was significantly reduced in six SCI subjects immediately following supported standing or aerobic upper body exercise.[89]

PRESSURE ULCERS

Persons with tetraplegia have insensate skin and are unable to detect normal signs of tissue ischemia such as tingling, discomfort, and pain that are noticed by able-bodied individuals. Pressure ulcers occur as the result of unrelieved pressure, usually over a bony prominence, that results in damage of underlying tissue, which may range from nonblanching erythema at the skin to deep open wounds penetrating to the bone. The reported incidence of pressure ulcers in SCI has ranged from 22.8%[267] to 33%,[107] with 31.7% of patients in the Model Spinal Cord Injury Systems reported to have had at least one pressure sore during enrollment in the system.[276] In the latter study, the distribution of pressure ulcers in SCI individuals 1 year after injury included 20.5% at the sacrum, 18.3% at the ischium, 16.6% at the heel, and 12.4% at the trochanter. Curtis and Dillon[60] reported pressure ulcers as only 7% of 291 wheelchair injuries noted by 128 athletes responding to a survey in 1984.

In 1930, Landis determined the average arteriolar pressure preceding the capillary bed in human skin to be about 32 mm Hg. On that basis, it is believed that interface tissue pressures that exceed 32 mm Hg place an individual at risk for pressure sore development.[231] An often quoted study by Kosiak[158] reported tissue breakdown after the application of 60 mm Hg for 60 minutes. Modifying factors for pressure sore development also include duration of pressure application, shear, and friction.[231] For practical application of these principles, Reswick and Rogers[227] developed maximal pressure/time interval guidelines as a deterrent to the development of pressure ulcers. Appropriately prescribed wheelchair seating systems with scheduled pressure relief every 15–30 minutes should reduce the risk of pressure ulcers in the exercising tetraplegic.[90]

PHYSIOLOGIC BENEFITS OF EXERCISE IN TETRAPLEGIA

A recent consensus statement indicated that physical exercise performed on a regular basis has been demonstrated to reduce coronary heart disease risk factors, including blood lipid profiles, glucose intolerance, hypertension, and body composition, and to improve bone density, immune function, and psychologic function in the able-bodied population.[206] The literature regarding exercise in tetraplegia also supports this concept for the SCI population, but the strength of the relationships appears less certain.

CHOLESTEROL PROFILES

Heart disease is the second leading cause of mortality in tetraplegia, accounting for about 22% of all deaths.[123] Silent (unperceived) myocardial ischemia due to disrupted visceral afferent fibers in tetraplegia may prevent recognition of myocardial infarction, as indicated by four of six asymptomatic tetraplegic patients found with abnormal dipyridamole thallium scans in a recent investigation.[15] Likewise, Walker and Khokhar[260] presented a case report of 65-year-old man with C7 tetraplegia who had an asymptomatic large reversible defect at the anterior and anteroseptal walls. Additionally, several studies have demonstrated low levels of high-density lipoproteins (HDL) in SCI individuals,[19,31,33,134,242] which has been strongly linked with the incidence of coronary artery disease (CAD) in able-bodied persons.[42] Tetraplegic men appear to have lower HDL cholesterol than age-matched controls despite desirable total cholesterol levels.[242] Bauman[19] reported that HDL cholesterol was reduced and low-density lipoprotein concentrations were elevated in young SCI subjects compared to able-bodied controls. Likewise, Krum et al.[162] noted more depressed HDL concentrations in 327 patients with SCI than in an able-bodied control group. Bostom et al.[31] noted a direct relationship between HDL cholesterol and peak aerobic power in men with SCI, while Brenes et al.[33] reported significantly higher HDL concentrations in male athletes with SCI than in the control group. Hooker and Wells[134] demonstrated improved cholesterol profiles (total cholesterol/HDL cholesterol from 5.0 to 4.0, HDL from 39 to 47 mg%) in SCI patients who had completed 8 weeks of moderate upper extremity exercise training, and Bauman et al.[14] reported significantly improved (37 to 41 mg%) HDL cholesterol levels after 12 weeks of FES-LCE. These data indicate a positive relationship between activity level and HDL cholesterol, implying reduced risk for CAD in SCI individuals who exercise regularly.

GLUCOSE TOLERANCE

Glucose intolerance, a precursor to diabetes mellitus that has been reported in many SCI patients, is characterized by hyperinsulinemia in response to a glucose challenge.[78,79,281] Similar findings were reported in acutely immobilized spinal trauma patients who had been at bed rest after spine surgery for 3 weeks.[190] Petry et al.[210] found that glycosylated hemoglobin (HbA_{1c}) levels above 6.0 in SCI patients significantly correlated with impaired glucose tolerance or frank diabetes and recommended routine HbA_{1c} screening for patients with SCI. Aksnes et al.[1] noted a dissociation between whole body insulin-mediated glucose uptake and skeletal muscle mass in tetraplegics despite intact glucose transport systems in skeletal muscle, suggesting loss of muscle mass as the primary reason for insulin insensitivity. The hyperinsulinemia in these patients may therefore be related to body composition changes as has been reported in the general population.[252,279] Bauman and Spungen[16] reported that 62% of quadriplegics with a mean duration of injury of 17 years had abnormal glucose tolerance tests, as compared to only 18% of age-matched controls with a similar body mass index. The same study failed to demonstrate a significant correlation between insulin resistance and body composition. This may indicate that lean body mass, particularly skeletal muscle, is not as metabolically active in SCI versus able-bodied individuals. Dearwater et al.[64] compared SCI sedentary controls with SCI athletes and found no significant differences in fasting glucose or insulin concentrations, but they did not conduct glucose tolerance tests. Still, insulin sensitivity has been noted to increase in able-bodied individuals who underwent physical training,[184] possibly reducing the risk for obesity, diabetes, and coronary artery disease.

GLUCOSE METABOLISM

Glucose metabolism has recently been studied in resting T3-4 paraplegics[146] and exercising tetraplegics,[154] demonstrating results consistent with current theories of hormonal control and substrate utilization during exercise. Karlsson et al.[146] found that, despite elevated blood glucose and insulin responses to an oral glucose tolerance test, physically active T3-4 paraplegics had similar rates of glucose production and utilization at rest as their siblings, although catecholamine responses in the paraplegics were blunted during insulin clamping, indicating the lack of centralized nervous activity. Similarly, tetraplegic patients undergoing lower extremity FES to exhaustion were noted to have paradoxic increases in insulin, impaired gluconeogenesis, and impaired lipolysis that were attributed to blunted central sympathetic responses, demonstrating the necessity for neural and hormonal feedback to elicit optimal substrate utilization during exercise.[154] The long-term consequences of these paradoxic exercise responses in the tetraplegia have not been investigated.

HYPERTENSION

Tetraplegia is usually associated with low systolic and diastolic blood pressures,[26] and although one study has demonstrated an increased incidence of hypertension among SCI individuals in comparison to age-matched controls, it did not distinguish tetraplegics from paraplegics or report completeness of SCI lesions.[278] Further, despite greater blood pressure variability in SCI patients recently found with autonomic dysreflexia, no significant difference in blood pressures was noted between those individuals and normals or when compared to SCI subjects without recent autonomic dysreflexia.[163] Although this study specified SCI lesions above T6, it did not indicate the SCI levels, leaving it unclear if most were thoracic-level lesions with relatively preserved sympathetic control of the heart. Most of the exercise literature reports significant problems with hypotension rather than hypertension, although episodic autonomic dysreflexia may pose severe problems in the acute crisis.

BODY COMPOSITION

An additional risk factor for heart disease and glucose intolerance in the SCI population is obesity, as defined by body fat relative to body weight of greater than 25% in men and 32% in women.[174] Obesity is more likely to occur in SCI because of the relative loss of metabolically active muscle tissue, resulting in 12–54% lower basal energy expenditure, depending on the level and completeness of SCI.[53,188,238] Current techniques to determine body composition include skinfold/anthropometric analyses, total body potassium, total body water, bioelectric impedance, air densitometry, DEXA, and hydrodensitometry, long considered the gold standard. Body composition analysis differentiates between fat and lean body mass and until recently has relied on assumed values for bone, muscle, fat, and organ densities derived from cadaver studies performed more than 30 years ago.[34,247] Recent advances in technology have challenged the reliability of those assumptions, and although not entirely validated, the use of DEXA has revolutionized the ability to obtain accurate body composition analyses in persons for whom the previous assumptions were clearly invalid, including those with SCI.[249] Due to the paralyzed trunk and extremities in SCI, fat-free mass density,[40,250] total body water,[224] and bone density[25,98] are significantly reduced compared to that of the normal population.

Despite possible flaws, Olle et al.[204] reported reduced skinfold sums, percentage of body fat, residual lung volumes, and increased fat-free body mass in active versus sedentary SCI individuals. When compared to able-bodied subjects, SCI individuals have been reported to have reduced fat-free body mass and increased percentage of body fat.[30,35,40,109,113,125] Cumulatively, these data indicate that body fat for sedentary persons with SCI ranges from 25–35%, whereas body fat percentages for athletic SCI men and women range between 16–24% and 24–32%, respectively.[156] While the validity of DEXA body composition analysis in the normal population is still being established,[157] most would agree that it is probably the gold standard for body composition analyses in SCI individuals because of its ability to account for marked differences in bone and fat-free mass density apparent in this special population.[156,249] An excellent review of this topic has been completed by Kocina.[156]

SOCIOLOGIC BENEFITS OF EXERCISE

Individuals with acute SCI have many obstacles to overcome during their reintegration into the community, including the need to master community mobility and ADLs, adjust to their disability, and reenter the workforce. Their chances for successful socialization may be significantly enhanced by increasing their physical capacity.

ACTIVITIES OF DAILY LIVING AND COMMUNITY MOBILITY

Functional tasks such as feeding, grooming, hygiene, dressing, bathing, transfers, and toileting are referred to as activities of daily living, and traversing sidewalks, stairs, ramps, paths, and environmental barriers such as curbs and speedbumps are considered tasks of community mobility. According to Noreau et al.,[200,201] about 25% of relatively young patients with paraplegia demonstrated aerobic capacity that is barely sufficient to meet the demands of independent living, and their ability to sustain independence as they age is questionable; the implications toward independence in tetraplegia are concerning. Noreau et al.[201] demonstrated significant associations between habitual physical activity, fitness level, and functional ability in 50 patients with tetraplegia and suggested that greater efforts should be made to provide SCI patients with systematic exercise conditioning programs. Several studies have demonstrated that the strain of performing ADLs and community mobility tasks, determined as a percentage of maximal heart rate or physical capacity, is significantly higher in tetraplegia than in paraplegia and that an inverse relationship exists between physical capacity and physical strain.[62,130,143] Unfortunately, data from Noreau's studies[200,201] were determined from heart rate monitoring and may be somewhat inaccurate, because heart rate is considered a poor measure of physical capacity in tetraplegia due to the impaired sympathetic nervous system and variable relationship with rate of oxygen consumption.[185] Still, it appears that increased physical capacity, when directly measured by oxygen consumption (VO_2), is related to the increased ability to perform ADLs at lower physical strain; only 29% of subjects with $VO_{2Peak} < 15$ ml/kg^{-1}/min^{-1} were able to perform independent ADLs.[143] This has tremendous implications with regard to exercise training, because VO_{2Peak} for untrained tetraplegics reported in the literature ranges from 8.9 ml/kg^{-1}/min^{-1} to 15.2 ml/kg^{-1}/min^{-1}, whereas VO_{2Peak} for trained tetraplegics ranges from 12.4 to 22.4 ml/kg^{-1}/min^{-1}, with most values exceeding 15 ml/kg^{-1}/min^{-1} (Tables 1 and 2.) As expected, exercise responses also vary inversely with the neurologic level of SCI.[77] Further, physical capacity is inversely related to the incidence of medical complications, including osteoporosis and urinary tract infections.[130] Another recent study reported significantly improved physical capacity as determined by absolute peak power output (31.1 W to 37.5 W) in a group of eight untrained tetraplegics monitored over 3 years; although VO_{2Peak} did not significantly change, an inverse relationship was again established between physical strain (monitored by heart rate) and VO_{2Peak}.[142] Of particular note, two patients who demonstrated improved ability to perform ADLs and community mobility had increased their absolute peak power output by only 8 W and 10 W, respectively, demonstrating relatively small increments in physical capacity allowing significant progress toward functionally independent ADLs. Finally, Gerhart et al.[114] reported that 31% of 98 tetraplegics required significantly increased assistance in transfers and 38% with mobility more than 20 years after their injury, with increased reports of shoulder pain, fatigue and weakness, weight gain, and postural changes compared to their less-affected counterparts.

QUALITY OF LIFE

Quality of life is a reflection of well being, happiness, and life satisfaction and makes an individual feel that life is worth living despite physical impairments and associated disabilities.[199] A recent report of a 9-year longitudinal survey for adjustment after SCI indicated a decline in several aspects of subjective well being on the Life Situation Questionnaire, although activity levels were reportedly unchanged.[159] It is suggested that the decline in well being over the past decade reflects the passing of the Americans with Disabilities Act, which may have created unrealistic expectations that life opportunities would immediately improve. Despite these findings, Noreau and Shephard[199] indicate a direct relationship between "quality-adjusted life years" and physical activity in the SCI population. Self-concept in 34 tetraplegics was significantly related to perceived independence, assistance required, living arrangements, and the provision of one's own transportation.[124] Although longitudinal studies are lacking, psychologic testing in wheelchair athletes demonstrates greater self-satisfaction, self-esteem, more independence, greater vigor, and less depression than their inactive SCI counterparts.[199]

VOCATION

A significant goal in rehabilitation following SCI is the return to gainful employment for psychological and financial well being. One year after an SCI, only 8.6% of persons with tetraplegia are employed, but up to 33% are employed 10 years after their injury.[70] Several investigations have attempted to determine significant factors upon which to predict successful return to employment for the SCI individual.[56,66,106]

TABLE 1.   Maximal Exercise Responses to Upper Extremity Ergometry in Untrained Tetraplegics

Study	Mode	Sex	n	Levels of SCI	Age (Yrs)	Mass (Kg)	Peak VO$_2$ (ml/kg^4/min^{-1})	HR (B/min)	P.O. (watts)
Burkett, 1990*	WE	2M 2F	4	C4-7	26.5	60.2	8.9(2.9)	134	N/A
Coutts et al., 1983	WE	M	3	C6-8	29	69.9	14.3	N/A	N/A
Dreisinger et al., 1984	WE	M F	12	C6-8	N/A	N/A	0.873 L/min	121 ± 15	N/A
Erikkson et al., 1988	WE	M	12	C5-8	29 .6 5	63.6 ± 11	13.9 ± 1.9	119	N/A
Hjltues & Janssen, 1990	AC	M	10	C5-8	36	N/A	14.0	N/A	N/A
Hopman et al., 1996	WE	6M 1F	7	C4-8	26.6 ± 6.9	77.6 ± 23.4	8.1	N/A	20.7
Janssen et al., 1993	WE	M	9	C5-8	32.9 ± 14.9	81.2 ± 14.9	13.6 ± 3.1	N/A	33.3
Janssen, 1996	WT	M	8	C4-8	37.3 ± 10	83.1	14.3	N/A	N/A
Lasko-McCarthy & Davis, 1991	WE	M	12	C5-6	29.1 ± 3.4	73.3 ± 9.6	9.4 ± 3.2	112	N/A
	WE	M	10	C7-8	28.9 ± 6.3	70.3 ± 7.7	15.1 ± 4.0	127	N/A
Norea & Shepherd, 1995	WE	M	8	C5-8	31 ± 15	N/A	7.5 ± 1.8	110 ± 12	10 ± 7
Simard et al., 1993	AC	M F	25	C5-6	34.4 ± 8.9	71.8 ± 11.5	WC 10.4 + 3.7 AC 10.8 ± 3.6	N/A	10.1 18.8
	AC	M F	22	C7	33.5 ± 9.5	61.7 ± 10.3	WC 13.9 + 5.3 AC 15.2 ± 4.7	N/A	20.6 28.2
	AC	M F	3	C8	35.0 ± 17.0	56.0 ± 7.0	WC 14.2 ± 2.3 AC 14.4 (4.5)	N/A	23
Van Loan et al., 1987	AC	M F	13	C5-8	29.6 ± 2.5	62.2 ± 3.4	12.0 ± 3.3	109	23.5
Wicks et al., 1977-78	AC WE	F	1	C8	34	N/A	WC 1.196/min AC 0.63L/min	158	N/A

n = number of subjects, HR = heart rate, P.O. = power output, WE = wheelchair ergometer, AC = arm crank ergometer.
*=3 of 4 patients had incomplete SCI lesions.

TABLE 2. Maximal Exercise Responses to Upper Extremity Ergometry in Trained Tetraplegics

Study	Mode	Sex	n	Levels of SCI	Age (Yrs)	Mass (kg)	Peak VO$_2$ (ml/kg^1/min^{-1})	HR (B/min)	P.O. (watts)
Bhambhani et al., 1995	WE	M	8	C5-C8	31.8 ± 6.2	72.1 ± 6.4	19.8 (4.0)	N/A	N/A
Coutts & Stogryn, 1987	WE	M	2	C6-C7	25	N/A	17.1	102	28.5
Dicarlo et al., 1983[a]	AC	M	3/2	C5-C7	25.3/26.5	56.7/52.6	22.4/20.2	N/A	105/67.5
Dicarlo, 1982	AC	M	1	C6	24	74	17.0	120	48
Erikkson et al., 1988	WE	M	8	C5-C8	32 ± 11	62.1 ± 11	17.4 ± 5.1	118	μ/A
Gass et al., 1980[b]	WT	M	7º	C5-T4	30.8	83.3 ± 13.8	12.7 ± 5.9	129 ± 19	N/A
Gass & Camp, 1979	WT	M	1	C6-C7	N/A	54.6	19.4	120	N/A
Hopman et al., 1996	WE	M	8	C4-C8	32.7 ± 12.7	73.6 ± 17.2	14.0	N/A	49.9
McLean & Skinner, 1995	AC	M	7	C5-T1	34-3	69.6 ± 18.5	10.6	118	32.1
	AC	M	7	C5-T1	33.3	66.3 ± 17.7	12.4	122	35.6
Ready, 1984	AC	M	5	C6-C8	25.5 ± 1.5	71.7 ± 7.6	15.0 ± 4.1	122 ± 13	43 ± 11
	AC	M	1	C6	19.0	50.8	15.6	113	37.5
Whiting et al., 1983	WE	M	2	C5-C6	33	81.8	14	136	50
				C6-C7	21	90.9	11.5	126	50
Wicks, 1983[c]	AC	M	5	C7	28.8 ± 4.0	63.3 ± 9.7	WC 14.9 ± 4.6	123	N/A
	WE						AC 13.1 ± 2.2	130	
	AC	M	8	C5-C6	28.6 ± 6.0	67.9 ± 14.7	WC 14.7 ± 5.2	146	N/A
	WE						AC 13.7 ± 4.1	143	
	AC	F	1	C5-6	21	43.6	WC 17.2	136	N/A
	WE						AC 14.8	150	
	AC	F	1	C7	35	70.5	WC13.8	125	N/A
	WE						AC 11.7	117	

n = number of subjects. HR = heart rate. P.O. = power output. WE = wheelchair ergometer. AC = arm crank ergometer.
[a]See text.
[b] Subjects with C5-6 lesions, 2 subjects with T1-T4 lesions. [c] Mixed upper and lower motor neuron lesions.

Based on the relationships found between physical capacity and the ability to perform ADLs, it would appear that increased physical activity or capacity in tetraplegia would enhance one's ability to procure and maintain gainful employment, but the literature has demonstrated variable relationships between these parameters.[61,193,198] In Japan, wheelchair athletes have been found to have lower absentee rates and earn higher wages than their less active cohorts.[193] Further, Noreau and Shephard[198] suggested a positive relationship between vocational status, productivity, and physical fitness based on stepwise regression analysis involving four fitness variables among 74 paraplegic individuals; similar relationships have not been established for tetraplegia. However, Curtis et al.[61] found no significant correlation between time spent in sports participation and functional or employment status, although sports participation did not appear to limit vocational pursuits. Further investigations are needed to determine the relationship between fitness levels and vocation outcome in tetraplegia.

EXERCISE TRAINING IN TETRAPLEGIA

Physical activity has been defined as "any bodily movement produced by skeletal muscles that results in energy expenditure and is clearly distinguished from exercise which is characterized as a subset of physical activity that is planned, structured, and repetitive and has as a final or an intermediate objective the improvement or maintenance of physical fitness."[41] Exercise training, therefore, in the strictest sense, should have a measurable, defined goal at its inception and an organized plan to achieve that goal. In approaching the exercise prescription for patients with tetraplegia, one must first determine the purpose of exercise and the most appropriate way to measure progress toward that goal.

In a broad sense, there are only two types of exercise: anaerobic, which can be performed in short bursts without oxygen, and aerobic, which requires oxygen to sustain rhythmical movement. However, at any given time during exercise training both are being employed to a variable extent. Anaerobic exercise such as resistance training and sprinting can significantly improve measurable quantities of peak strength and power, whereas aerobic exercise is primarily employed to improve endurance (time to exhaustion) and total work capacity, as measured by peak oxygen consumption or caloric expenditure. Central and peripheral mechanisms are involved in the adaptation of both types of exercise. Central mechanisms of adaptation include disinhibition of the CNS and ANS and hormonal alterations that affect whole-body metabolism, immune function, and cardiopulmonary dynamics. Peripheral mechanisms of exercise adaptation include enzymatic (affecting substrate storage and utilization) and structural (fiber cross-sectional area and capillary density) changes within skeletal muscle and also, sweat gland density within the skin. Each adaptation will depend on the specific type (specificity) and quantity (overload) of exercise training employed; hence are defined the two main principles of exercise training.[248] An additional principle, that of reversibility, bears mention; when no longer subject to habitual stimulation, the body will revert to its previous level of function.

When testing exercise capacity or when prescribing exercise, it is important to stay focused on the purpose. If a tetraplegic person's main purposes for exercise training are to improve body composition, wheelchair endurance, and ability to perform independent ADLs, the testing and prescription should include wheelchair endurance training and specific resistive exercises appropriate to the completion of the specific ADLs. Conversely, if the same individual is most concerned about cardiopulmonary function, reducing risk factors for CAD, and lower extremity fractures, attempts should be made to include lower extremity exercise in the training and testing regimen. If an exercise test is indicated, it should include components pertinent to the individual's goals.

TESTING

Graded exercise testing is performed in the able-bodied population to assess aerobic fitness or training effects in asymptomatic or athletic populations, screen individuals at risk for heart disease, determine progress in rehabilitation, demonstrate maximal strength and power capacities, and assist with the exercise prescription.[239] A review by Davis[63] noted that SCI patient care might be improved by performing exercise tests to assess physical fitness components, establish relationships between fitness and posttraumatic return to gainful employment, screen for cardiopulmonary risks, and determine how fitness parameters change over time.

The American College of Sports Medicine (ACSM) has established guidelines for medical testing and exercise testing in the able-bodied population,[150] but the guidelines may not apply to those with tetraplegia, who have unique risks and responses to exercise. It appears prudent, therefore, for persons with tetraplegia to obtain medical clearance, including a 12-lead electrocardiogram and risk profile assessment, prior to participation in a strenuous exercise program. Should an exercise test be indicated or desired, the next step is to determine the most appropriate testing mode and protocol.

Davis[63] described three common methods of exercise stress testing for the SCI population: field testing, arm crank ergometry (ACE), and wheelchair ergometry (WCE) (Fig. 4). Field testing is perhaps the easiest, least expensive, and most mobility-specific and has been demonstrated to provide a good estimate of VO_{2max} in selected wheelchair users,[102,229] although recent data have failed significantly to correlate with actual VO_2.[258] ACE is the most established and widely validated upper extremity test system,[12,29,170,233] but it lacks mobility specificity.[63] Conversely, WCE is very mobility-specific to tetraplegics who perform community mobility with a manual wheelchair. Several systems have been developed and tested, including wheelchairs mounted on a motorized treadmill,[109,255] low friction rollers,[175] and specialized devices to simulate overground propulsion.[120,167,271] WCE has been found to induce similar[218] or greater[110] VO_{2peak} responses than ACE but with peak lower power output.[122]

Continuous incremental graded protocols and discontinuous multilevel protocols have been established for use with ACE or WCE.[121,167] Continuous protocols are progressive with increasing levels of exercise intensity and have well-defined submaximal or maximal endpoint criteria. The disadvantage to the standard continuous protocol is

TABLE 3. American College of Sports Medicine Recommendations for Medical Examination and Exercise Testing Prior to Participation and Physician Supervision of Exercise Tests

A. Medical examination and clinical exercise test recommended prior to:

	Apparently Healthy		Increased Risk*		Known Disease†
	Younger‡	Older	No Symptoms	Symptoms	
Moderate exercise§	No‖	No	No	Yes	Yes
Vigorous exercise¶	No	Yes#	Yes	Yes	Yes

B. Physician supervision recommended during exercise test:

	Apparently Healthy/Increased Risk*		No Symptoms	Symptoms	Known Disease†
	Younger‡	Older			
Submaximal testing	No‖	No	No	Yes	Yes
Maximal testing	No	Yes#	Yes	Yes	Yes

*Persons with two or more risk factors or one or more signs of symptoms.

†Persons with known cardiac, pulmonary, or metabolic disease.

‡Younger implies ≤ 40 years for men, ≤ 50 years for women.

§Moderate exercise as defined by an intensity of 40% to 60% $\dot{V}o_{2max}$; if intensity is uncertain, moderate exercise may alternately be defined as an intensity well within the individual's current capacity, one which can be comfortably sustained for a prolonged period of time, that is, 60 minutes, which has a gradual initiation and progression, and is generally noncompetitive.

‖A "No" response means that an item is deemed "not necessary." The "No" response does **not** mean that the item should not be done.

¶Vigorous exercise is defined by an exercise intensity > 60% $\dot{V}o_{2max}$; if intensity is uncertain, vigorous exercise may alternately be defined as exercise intense enough to represent a substantial cardiorespiratory challenge or if it results in fatigue within 20 minutes.

#A "Yes" response means that an item is recommended. For physician supervision, this suggests that a physician is in close proximity and readily available should there be an emergent need.

From Kenney WL (ed): ACSM's Guidelines for Exercise Testing and Prescription, 5th ed. Baltimore, Williams & Wilkins, 1995, with permission.

"Field" Testing

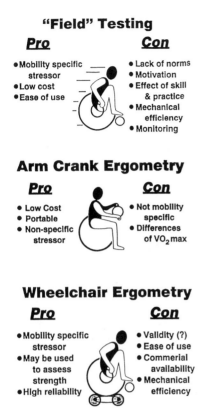

Pro
- Mobility specific stressor
- Low cost
- Ease of use

Con
- Lack of norms
- Motivation
- Effect of skill & practice
- Mechanical efficiency
- Monitoring

Arm Crank Ergometry

Pro
- Low Cost
- Portable
- Non-specific stressor

Con
- Not mobility specific
- Differences of VO_2max

FIGURE 4. Advantages and disadvantages of the three primary modes of upper extremity ergometry: field testing, arm crank ergometry, and wheelchair ergometry. (From Davis GM: Exercise capacity of individuals with paraplegia. Med Sci Sport Exerc 25:423–432, 1993, with permission).

Wheelchair Ergometry

Pro
- Mobility specific stressor
- May be used to assess strength
- High reliability

Con
- Validity (?)
- Ease of use
- Commerial availability
- Mechanical efficiency

that it requires too much time for practical completion, with the subject fatiguing at less than maximal capacity.[121] Glaser et al.[121] prefer discontinuous, submaximal protocols for stress testing wheelchair users, because they are comfortable, safe, and relatively easy to administer. A recommended protocol would use a constant speed (3 km/hr^{-1}) with a metronome-guided crank rate of 50 revolutions per minute and an initial resistance of 5 W. Each stage would last 4–6 minutes with 5-minute rest intervals and progressive 5–10 W increments employed with each new stage; most tetraplegic patients will have a peak power output of 25–85 W (see Tables 1 and 2). To measure VO_{2Peak} and power output, a continuous, shortened protocol can be employed, allowing an initial intensity level of 50% of the predicted maximal power output as determined from submaximal testing, shortening each stage of testing to 2 minutes, and allowing no rest between stages. A similar protocol has been described by Langbein et al.[167] using the Wheelchair Aerobic Fitness Trainer, a wheelchair ergometer developed by the Veterans Administration that can accommodate the user's own wheelchair. They employ a continuous protocol with a fixed speed of 2 miles/hr^{-1}, initial intensity of 6 W, and 5- to 7-W increments between 3-minute stages; 20 seconds of rest between stages allows for blood pressure determination. In addition to oxygen consumption and power output, blood pressure, electrocardiogram, and perceived exertion (Table 4) should be monitored at the end of each exercise stage. For individuals undergoing testing to rule out ischemic heart disease, 1–4 scaled angina ratings[150] and postexercise echocardiography[166] or thallium imaging[15] may significantly improve the sensitivity and specificity of the exercise stress test. Termination of the test should be consistent with ACSM guidelines.[150]

Additional testing that may be appropriate includes pulmonary function tests; quantified strength, anthropometric, and flexibility measures; DEXA scan to determine body composition and bone mineral density; radiographs of paralyzed extremities; lipid profiles; and HbA_{1c} to rule out glucose intolerance.

EXERCISE MODES

Upper Extremity Training

Upper extremity exercise can be prescribed specifically to increase strength and endurance or to minimally improve cardiopulmonary dynamics in the tetraplegic individual. There is a surprising paucity of literature regarding strength training in tetraplegia, considering the importance of upper body strength for certain ADLs and community mobility. An extensive MEDLINE search by the authors covering the last 30 years yielded only four (non–FES-related) resistive exercise studies involving the upper extremities of SCI subjects.[43,48,86,203] Chawla et al.[43] suggested a weight training program based on a review of animal and human studies and reported that it had improved ADL function in ten

TABLE 4. Original and Revised Scales for Ratings of Perceived Exertion (RPE)

Original Scale		Revised Scale	
6		0	Nothing at all
7	Very, very light	0.5	Very, very weak
8		1	Very weak
9	Very light	2	Weak
10		3	Moderate
11	Fairly light	4	Somewhat strong
12		5	Strong
13	Somewhat hard	6	
14			Very strong
15	Hard	8	
16		9	
17	Very hard	10	Very, very strong
18		■	Maximal
19	Very, very hard		
20			

From Kenney WL (ed): ACSM's Guidelines for Exercise Testing and Prescription, 5th ed. Baltimore, Williams & Wilkins, 1995, with permission.

patients; specific ADLs were not described, and quantitative measures of strength were not performed. Cooney et al.[48] assessed the effects of a 9-week hydraulic resistance exercise circuit-training program on cardiovascular fitness parameters in a mixed group of tetraplegic and paraplegic subjects. Estennne et al.[86] employed a prospective, controlled, serially assigned isometric training program specifically designed to strengthen the pectoralis major in C5-8 tetraplegic patients undergoing inpatient rehabilitation. A series of ten isometric pectoral contractions held 6 seconds, with 6 seconds of relaxation between repetitions, was performed daily for 6 weeks; significant gains in pectoral isometric strength and expiratory reserve volumes were noted compared to controls. Finally, Olenik et al.[203] demonstrated that rowing exercises and standard scapular stabilization exercises created greater needle electromyographic activity in scapular muscles than did backward wheeling, and, on that basis, recommended rowing as a more appropriate form of scapular strengthening exercise because of its value as a cardiovascular exercise. It seems inherent from the large number of shoulder and upper extremity musculoskeletal problems encountered by tetraplegics that a prophylactic, structured, and progressively resistive strengthening program focusing on scapular, rotator cuff, and pectoral muscles would place them at reduced risk for overuse injury and may improve their ability to perform functional tasks. To date, however, it appears that resistance training in tetraplegics is, as noted almost 20 years ago, "empirically controlled, rather than scientifically based."[43]

Upper extremity aerobic conditioning in tetraplegics has received a more extensive evaluation, as indicated by the number of investigations listed in Tables 1 and 2. However, only five of the listed studies represent training studies, and a critical review of these studies demonstrates significant variability in exercise prescription and results.[68,69,112,186,268] In 1982 DiCarlo[68] reported a case study in which he prescribed ACE at an intensity of 80% maximal heart rate (HR_{max}) three times a week for 8 weeks to a man with C6 tetraplegia, progressively advancing the exercise duration from 15 minutes initially to a maximum of 35 minutes. The subject's VO_{2Peak} increased from 11 ml/kg^{-1}/min^{-1} to 17 ml/kg^{-1}/min^{-1}, and his peak power output (PO_{Peak}) increased from 35 W to 48 W, representing significant changes in work capacity in only 2 months. In 1983, DiCarlo's group[69] reported an additional investigation in which four untrained SCI subjects performed 30 minutes of ACE at 60–80% of HR_{max} three times per week for 5 weeks with similar results. One must note that one subject had a spinal cord injury at T7-8, and another had a "congenital" C6-7 lesion that was likely incomplete based on the subject's training PO_{Peak} and VO_{2Peak}. Even if these two subjects are ignored to meet the criteria for reviewing complete tetraplegia, the remaining two subjects still had notable increases in VO_{2Peak} (14.1 ml/kg^{-2}/min^{-1} to 20.2 ml/kg^{-1}/min^{-1}) and PO_{Peak} (52.5 W to 67.5 W), especially considering the short length of the study. Gass et al.[112] trained seven subjects (four with C5-6 lesions, three with T1-4 lesions) five times weekly to exhaustion on a graded exercise test protocol using a wheelchair on a treadmill ergometer. After 7 weeks of training, the mean VO_{2Peak} had increased from 9.5 ml/kg^{-1}/min^{-1} to 12.7 ml/kg^{-1}/min^{-1}, and endurance time increased by 4.4 minutes, suggesting considerable change in functional capacity.[112]

An exercise training study reported by McLean and Skinner[186] matched 14 tetraplegic subjects on PO_{Peak} to either a supine or sitting exercise training regimen to assess for changes in postural position on stroke volume, cardiac output, and exercise capacity. Having their subjects perform ACE in a sitting or supine position at 60% of their PO_{Peak} three times a week for 10 weeks with progressive increments in either duration or resistance yielded no significant differences in stroke volume or cardiac output, although absolute VO_{2Peak} increased from 720 L/min^{-1} to 780 L/min^{-1}, suggesting peripheral adaptations.[186] A possible flaw in the study design, common to many investigations of exercising tetraplegics, was not matching individuals according to the level of their SCI; five of seven subjects in the supine group had C5 tetraplegia, compared to only two of seven in the sitting group. Recall from the earlier discussion that C5 tetraplegics cannot voluntarily exercise wrist extensors or triceps, and C6 subjects cannot voluntarily use triceps, whereas C7-8 SCI persons can use all of the upper extremity musculature except finger abductors and adductors. Because significantly less muscle mass is being exercised, C5 tetraplegics therefore have significantly less potential to change VO_{2Peak} than C6 tetraplegics, who in turn have less capacity to change than subjects with C7-8 tetraplegia; these principles must be considered in assigning matched groups exercise training investigations. The final training study assessed change in VO_{2Peak} and PO_{Peak} in two tetraplegics who trained with a wheelchair on an indoor track 20 minutes a day, three times a week for 8 weeks.[268] Intensity of training was initially set at 75% HR_{max} and arbitrarily changed to 85% HR_{max} at 5 weeks for subject A (C6-7 tetraplegia) and at 6 weeks for subject B (C5-6 tetraplegia). Subject A subsequently improved PO_{Peak} but not VO_{2Peak}, and subject B improved both VO_{2Peak} and PO_{Peak}. In critically reviewing these studies, it appears that individuals with tetraplegia can benefit from upper extremity exercise, but the most appropriate dosing with regard to intensity, duration, and frequency remains unclear.

Functional Electrical Stimulation

Computerized FES has been developed as a neuromuscular aid to restore purposeful movement of limbs paralyzed by upper motor neuron lesions. In use for over 35 years, it has been refined with computer technology to be used as an exercise enhancement tool for patients with SCI. Phillips in 1987 proposed medical guidelines for patient participation in FES rehabilitation, including medical criteria for inclusion and exclusion.[211] Numerous reviews have been devoted to FES and its potential to stimulate beneficial exercise adaptations in patients with tetraplegia and paraplegia.[92,117,118,121,209,214,215,277] Briefly, FES of the lower extremities can be used to stimulate strength[88,222,230] and endurance[88,133,219,222] training of those limbs and has the potential to improve energy expenditure; increase stroke volume;[97,133] increase total body PO_{Peak}, VO_{2Peak}, and ventilatory rate;[8,13,13a,133] reverse myocardial disuse atrophy;[195,196] increase HDL levels and improve body composition;[14] improve self-perception;[246] and possibly increase lower extremity bone mineral density.[28,128] Despite these remarkable findings, functional gains in upper extremity strength, aerobic capacity, community mobility, and ADLs have not been demonstrated in response to FES lower extremity training. A major disadvantage of the FES system is that many individuals and medical facilities cannot afford it and do not have the time to use it appropriately.

Combined Arm Crank Ergometry and FES-Leg Cycle Ergometry

A logical and intuitive progression in the development of FES lower extremity exercise training has been the combined use of concurrent ACE and FES-LCE, termed HYBRID exercise.[92,118] As expected from the combination of upper and lower extremity exercise,[21] PO_{Peak}, VO_{2Peak}, stroke volume, and cardiac output significantly increase during HYBRID exercise bouts with tetraplegic subjects[95,133,160,189,212] and for combined upper extremity rowing plus lower extremity FES;[168] however, circulatory factors may limit arm exercise performance. As with FES-LCE, no studies have demonstrated the translation of functional gains in upper extremity aerobic capacity, community mobility, or ADLs (beyond that seen by upper extremity exercise alone) for the teraplegic individual in response to HYBRID exercise training.

EXERCISE PRESCRIPTION

The most important consideration in creating an exercise prescription is patient compliance, and the prescription must be individualized to the patient's goals, current fitness level, physical limitations, stratified risk, and financial limitations to maximize chances for successful outcome. As with the prescription of medications, the exercise prescription in tetraplegia should address the person's diagnosis, indications, contraindications, mode, intensity and duration of dose, frequency, progression, and length of intervention. Ideally, the prescription would be generated by a team composed of an exercise physiologist, physical therapist, and physician knowledgeable about SCI.

Goals

Succinct, precise, and quantifiable goals will optimize chances for a successful outcome. Goals must be individualized to the person and can incorporate several intermediate goals to allow continued feedback and motivation. Functional and physical goals are usually easier to measure quantifiably than psychological goals, which may be somewhat abstract. Examples of appropriate goals include a 10-pound weight loss in 6 months, independent car transfers, or the completion of a 10-kilometer wheelchair race in less than 60 minutes. John Hockenberry, a paraplegic journalist for National Public Radio, made a goal of independently riding the rapid transit trains in Chicago and was able to achieve that goal despite several intervening years of being sidetracked.[131] A clearly written, quantifiable goal is an essential component of the exercise prescription.

Fitness Level

Most tetraplegics will have aerobic fitness levels well below that of the sedentary able-bodied population, whose VO_{2Peak} may be < 28 ml/kg/min.[115] Peak exercise capacity is most easily quantified by determining peak oxygen consumption and power output on a maximal graded exercise test, but this may not be practical for all individuals. One must remember that peak heart rates for tetraplegics performing a graded exercise test do not necessarily correlate with peak capacity. Field tests have been used in some settings to determine fitness level, with distance traversed in 12 minutes being a practical example. Other measurable components of fitness include muscle strength and endurance, flexibility, pulmonary function, and body composition. Assessment of fitness level is essential to appropriately prescribe initial levels of intensity and duration of exercise.

Stratified Risk

Coronary artery disease risk factors include age, family history, cigarette smoking, hypertension, hypercholesterolemia, diabetes mellitus, and physical inactivity in the able-bodied population (Tables 5 and 6). It appears that tetraplegia conveys additional risk for heart disease than is present in the able-bodied population. The standardized mortality ratios (compared to 1.0 in the able-bodied population) for ischemic heart disease and arterial disease are 5.8 to 20.0, respectively, in SCI individuals younger than

---

TABLE 5. Stratified Risk

Absolute Indications

1. Acute myocardial infarction or suspicion of a myocardial infarction
2. Onset of moderate-to-severe angina
3. Drop in SBP with increasing workload accompanied by signs or symptoms or drop below standing resting pressure
4. Serious arrhythmias (e.g., second- or third-degree atrioventricular block, sustained ventricular tachycardia or increasing premature ventricular contractions, atrial fibrillation with fast ventricular response)
5. Signs of poor perfusion, including pallor, cyanosis, or cold and clammy skin
6. Unusual or severe shortness of breath
7. Central nervous system symptoms, including ataxia, vertigo, visual or gait problems, or confusion
8. Technical inability to monitor the ECG
9. Patient's request

Relative Indications

1. Pronounced ECG changes from baseline [>2mm of horizontal or downsloping ST-segment depression, or > 2mm of ST-segment elevation (except in a VR)]
2. Any chest pain that is increasing
3. Physical or verbal manifestations of severe fatigue or shortness of breath
4. Wheezing
5. Leg cramps or intermittent claudication (grade 3 on 4-point scale)
6. Hypertensive response (SBP >260 mm Hg; DBP >115 mm Hg)
7. Less serious arrhythmias such as supraventricular tachycardia
8. Exercise-induced bundle branch block that cannot be distinguished from ventricular tachycardia

---

From Kenney WL (ed): ACSM's Guidelines for Exercise Testing and Prescription, 5th ed. Baltimore, Williams & Wilkins, 1995, with permission.

TABLE 6. Coronary Artery Disease Risk Factors

Positive Risk Factors	Defining Criteria
1. Age	Men > 45 years; women > 55 or premature menopause without estrogen replacement therapy
2. Family history	MI or sudden death before 55 years of age in father or other male first-degree relative, or before 65 years of age in mother or other female first-degree relative
3. Current cigarette smoking	
4. Hypertension	Blood pressure ≥ 140/90 mm Hg, confirmed by measurements on at least 2 separate occasions, or on antihypertensive medication
5. Hypercholesterolemia	Total serum cholesterol > 200 mg/dL (5.2 mmol/L) (if lipoprotein profile is unavailable) or HDL < 35 mg/dL (0.9 mmol/L)
6. Diabetes mellitus	Persons with insulin-dependent diabetes mellitus (IDDM) who are > 30 years of age, or have had IDDM for > 15 years, and persons with non–insulin-dependent diabetes mellitus (NIDDM) who are > 35 years of age should be classified as patients with known disease
7. Sedentary lifestyle/physical activity	Persons comprising the least active 25% of the population, as defined by the combination of sedentary jobs involving sitting for a large part of the day and no regular exercise or active recreational pursuits

Negative Risk Factor	Defining Criteria
1. High serum HDL cholesterol	< 60 mg/dL (1.6 mmol/L)

Notes: (1) It is common to sum risk factors in making clinical judgments. If HDL is high, subtract one risk factor from the sum of positive risk factors, since high HDL decreases CAD risk; (2) Obesity is not listed as an independent positive risk factor because its effects are exerted through other risk factors (e.g., hypertension, hyperlipidemia, diabetes). Obesity should be considered as an independent target for intervention.

* Adapted in part from Summary of the second report of the National Cholesterol Education Program (NCEP) Expert Panel on Detection, Evaluation, and Treatment of High Blood Cholesterol in Adults. J Am Med Assoc 269:3015–3023, 1993.

From Kenney WL (ed): ACSM's Guidelines for Exercise Testing and Prescription. 5th ed. Williams & Wilkins, Baltimore, 1995 with permission.

30, but they fall to 1.3 and 3.1 for SCI persons between the ages of 31 and 60.[67] It is not clear to what relative extent factors of age, family history, cigarette smoking, hypertension, hypercholesterolemia, diabetes, and physical activity contribute to the overall risk for heart disease in tetraplegia.

In addition to cardiac risk profiles, the person prescribing exercise must recognize and address the unique risks associated with exercise in tetraplegia, including the incidence, pattern, and medical management of autonomic dysreflexia; bladder medications, which can affect sweat and blood pressure responses; bladder and bowel management, which can affect timing of exercise or lead to autonomic dysreflexia; areas of skin breakdown; upper extremity musculoskeletal dysfunction; peripheral neuropathies, including carpal tunnel or cubital tunnel syndrome; spasticity and its medical management; heat and cold intolerance; and osteopenia.

Resources

To successfully participate in an exercise program, the tetraplegic must have access to a mildly temperate climate or thermally controlled environment (to avoid the risk of hypo- and hyperthermia), appropriate seating and positioning (to reduce the risk of pressure sores, autonomic dysreflexia, spasticity, and musculoskeletal trauma), and adapted equipment for resistance or aerobic training. Because exercise is associated with significant risks in this population, the initial stages of exercise training should be performed under the supervision of an exercise physiologist or physical therapist well-versed in tetraplegic exercise. Heart rate and blood pressure responses should be monitored during the initial stages to assess for possible episodes of exercise-induced autonomic dysreflexia or hypotension. For upper extremity aerobic exercise, the arm crank or wheelchair ergometer should be adjusted appropriately to allow optimal efficiency and to reduce musculoskeletal injuries at the shoulder, elbow, and wrist, and straps should be applied to the torso to prevent truncal instability. Wheelchair gloves or flexion mitts are important to prevent blisters, lacerations, and abrasions, especially for tetraplegics whose hands and fingers are insensate. Upper arm bands or Co-Ban tape may be used to prevent abrasions at the medial upper arm with wheelchair propulsion. Velcro straps and cuffed weights are commonly used for resistance-training equipment modifications. Abdominal binders and leg wraps may be used to promote improved pulmonary dynamics and greater venous return, allowing improved cardiac output via the Frank-Starling mechanism. FES-LCE and HYBRID systems are commercially available but are more expensive to purchase and maintain than ACE. The individual's time constraints, transportation availability, required assistance, and financial constraints should also be discussed, because these factors will significantly affect compliance with the exercise program.

Diagnosis

Establishing the level of neurologic injury and the completeness of the lesion has tremendous implications in exercise prescription. Tetraplegics with complete lesions at or above C4 will be relegated to FES-LCE or HYBRID exercise equipment. C5 tetraplegics will require exercises that do not require active wrist extension, elbow extension, or grasp. Tetraplegics with C6 lesions have active wrist extension but little or no elbow extension or grasp. C7 tetraplegics can actively extend their elbows but still cannot grasp, and individuals with C8 lesions have function of the upper extremities except finger abduction and adduction. The prescription must be modified to allow accommodation of these differences. Furthermore, a complete lesion precludes automatic control of sympathetic responses below that level, whereas incomplete SCI may allow varying degrees of sympathetic response. Additionally, incomplete tetraplegics who have relative sparing of sensation in the lower extremities may not be able to tolerate FES-LCE or HYBRID exercise modes because of pain.

Indications

Indications for exercise training include, but are not limited to, deconditioning, neurologically intact muscular atrophy, obesity, reduced ability to perform community mobility and ADLs, impaired glucose tolerance, and improvement of cardiac risk profile.

Contraindications

In addition to the absolute and relative contraindications for exercise suggested by ACSM for the able-bodied population,[150] tetraplegics with uncontrolled autonomic dysreflexia, grade III or IV pressure sores, or recent deep vein thrombosis should refrain from exercise until medical clearance is obtained. Tetraplegics should not exercise in temperature extremes without close medical supervision.

Exercise Mode

Allowing the patient to make an informed choice of the exercise mode will dictate, to a large degree, patient compliance. The person prescribing the exercise should be aware of the available options, including manual wheelchair propulsion, ACE, WCE, FES-LCE, HYBRID, and resistance training equipment, and the advantages and disadvantages of each.

Intensity

The most appropriate way to monitor and prescribe intensity of aerobic exercise for the individual with tetraplegia remains somewhat controversial. The ACSM recommendations for the able-bodied population indicate that exercise intensity should be within 60–90% of maximal heart rate or 50–85% of maximal VO_2 to significantly improve cardiovascular fitness parameters.[4] Recall, however, that heart rate response in tetraplegia is largely degree-dependent on parasympathetic withdrawal rather than sympathetic stimulation, providing the basis for significantly lower maximal heart rates seen in tetraplegia (130 versus 180–200 bpm in the able-bodied) and contributing to the great variability noted between VO_{2Peak} and heart rate in this population.[186] Janssen et al.[143] developed regression equations predicting heart rate reserve values of 30–80%, corresponding to 50–85% VO_{2Peak} in high paraplegics and tetraplegics, but, again, variability seemed large. Although improvements have been demonstrated while using exercise intensity of 60–85% HR_{max} in this population, it is not clear that this is the best way to monitor intensity. McLean and Skinner recommended prescribing intensity as a percentage of PO_{Peak}, but this would require constant reevaluation to maintain optimal training intensity, because PO_{Peak} would be expected to increase linearly with training. Rate of perceived exertion (RPE) may be the most appropriate scale on which to base prescribed intensity of exercise for tetraplegics (see Table 4); it has been used with good success in cardiac transplant patients who have denervated hearts,[148] although this too has limitations.[240]

Most recently, a consensus statement generated by the Centers for Disease Control and Prevention and the ACSM recommended that "every US adult should accumulate 30 minutes or more of moderate-intensity physical activity on most, preferably all, days of the week."[206] Moderate activity was defined by the panel as activity performed at

3–6 METs (1 MET = oxygen consumption of 3.5 ml/kg^{-1}/min^{-1}) i.e., 10.5 ml/kg^{-1}/min^{-1} to 21 ml/kg^{-1}/min^{-1}, which is near VO$_{2Peak}$ for most tetraplegics and thus not a realistic guideline for tetraplegics (see Table 3).

If the prescription is preceded by a graded exercise test, one may use the RPE values corresponding to 50–85% VO$_{2Peak}$ to assign an exercise range; this should correspond to about 12–13 (somewhat hard) on the Borg RPE scale (see Table 4). Alternatively, 60–90% of HR$_{max}$ may be assigned as the target heart rate zone if a person has a heart rate monitor—recall that tetraplegics would be otherwise unable to self-check their pulse. Without exercise testing, the ability to accurately assign exercise intensity will be markedly impaired. A final consideration would be to have an individual use the "3–5 word sentence rule;" if they are able to speak in three-to-five word sentences during exercise, they should be within an appropriate intensity range.

When using FES-LCE or HYBRID exercise systems, a detailed protocol should be employed to avoid complications such as autonomic dysreflexia or lower extremity fractures. Commercial systems will have the manufacturer's recommendations for initial settings, duration, frequency, and precautions, which should be closely followed. Initial intensity levels will necessarily be less than those employed in upper extremity protocols.

Duration

The duration of a single aerobic exercise bout will vary depending on fitness levels but should be preceded and followed by a 10-minute warm-up and last 20–60 minutes.[4] Prolonged exercise tolerance in tetraplegia has received little attention, and it is therefore recommended that progression of exercise duration be monitored closely and that individuals replenish with small amounts of fluids frequently while exercising. However, tetraplegic patients have neurogenic bladders that may distend with fluid replenishment and elicit autonomic dysreflexia. If prolonged exercise is anticipated, intermittent catheterization should be performed on a scheduled basis or, alternatively, an indwelling Foley catheter is recommended.

Frequency

Aerobic exercise should be performed at least 2 days a week to maintain fitness but may occur up to 5 days a week for optimal gains without negative consequences.[150] Persons with tetraplegia who have VO$_{2Peak}$ < 15.5 mg/kg^{-1}/min^{-1} (< 3 METs), however, may require multiple bouts of exercise lasting 5–10 minutes each day if they are unable to tolerate 20- to 30-minute sessions.

Progression

The initial stages of an aerobic exercise program for tetraplegics should focus more on developing the *habit* of exercise than on the intensity and duration of exercise because exercise adherence may decrease if the program is initiated too rigorously. The duration of the early exercise bouts may be limited by the individual's muscular endurance; upper extremity work often is. Short sessions of 5–10 minutes two to four times daily may be appropriate early in the course of an exercise training program. Individuals should be told to expect delayed-onset muscle soreness, which may persist during the first 2 weeks of the exercise program but should then subside despite increasing intensity or duration. This conditioning stage should last 6–8 weeks.

The improvement stage is marked by more rapid improvement and progression of intensity and frequency of exercise.[150] Once duration of exercise is extended to 30 minutes, intensity may be increased if the individual feels time constraints become a limiting factor. As duration and intensity of exercise are increased, however, frequency should be decreased to prevent overtraining.

Length of Intervention

Maintenance of exercise conditioning is required once an individual has achieved his or her goals or benefits will be lost. The most important factors in extended exercise compliance is that the activity be enjoyable and employable.

Resistance Training

Little research exists in the area of resistance training for neurologically intact muscle in tetraplegia; it is unclear if tetraplegics have different responses to resistance training than do the able-bodied population. It would inherently seem that muscle groups that remain neurologically intact and under voluntary control should respond in similar fashion, but this has not been demonstrated to date. Hormonal responses may not be adequate to elicit similar hypertrophy as seen in the able-bodied population.

We recommend as minimal intervention that scapular stabilization and rotator cuff exercises be employed in all tetraplegic patients capable of voluntary control of these muscles. Initial intervention should include two sets of ten-repetition, 6-second isometric contraction for shoulder protractors, retractors, elevators, depressors, and for internal and external shoulder rotators, progressing to dynamic exercises as static strength plateaus. As per the ACSM guidelines for muscular strength and endurance, we offer a prescription of one set to exhaustion of eight to ten repetitions for each of the major muscle groups of the upper extremity that remain neurologically intact, minimally twice a week.[4]

Application

Example   A 23-year-old woman with C7 ASIA A tetraplegia resulting from a diving accident 12 months ago is referred for an exercise prescription. She underwent anterior and posterior fusion of the 5th, 6th, and 7th vertebral bodies 2 days after her injury without complications and she was placed in a halo brace for 12 weeks, 8 of which she was also involved in inpatient rehabilitation. Her course since then was notable for two or three episodes of autonomic dysreflexia resulting from bladder spasms, which were subsequently treated with oxybutynin, an anticholinergic medication, which she continues to use three times a day. Bladder management is performed with intermittent catheterization four times daily, and she is on a regular bowel care program every other day. She has had one ischial pressure sore, approximately 2 months ago, which is now resolved and which she attributes to "poor memory and weak arms." She now performs depression (lifting her body by extending her arms against the wheelchair) pressure relief every 20–30 minutes and is able to independently transfer using a slide board and modified depression transfer technique. Spasticity became more of a problem about 4 months ago, and she was placed on Lioresal, a GABA-agonist, with significant improvement. She has a power wheelchair that she uses about 80% of the time because "it's easier to get around," and she also has a modified, light-weight sports wheelchair. She uses a bladder inflatable cushion with her power chair and a molded gel cushion in her sports chair. She was previously a gymnast, is 5′3″ tall, and weighs 115 pounds; she weighed 98 pounds after the halo was removed 9 months ago. She is single, has normal menses, and has no family history of osteoporosis. She acknowledges she would love to become independent for community mobility in her manual chair "to feel more normal" and to help with weight control. Her physical exam is consistent with C7 ASIA A (complete) tetraplegia, triceps normal strength but easily fatigued (only two depression lifts completed on test), 12-lead electrocardiogram is normal, and she recently underwent DEXA analyses, which reported 25% body fat and with "slightly reduced bone mineral density at upper and lower extremities."

She underwent an ACE maximal stress test, which demonstrated VO_{2Peak} of 12 ml/kg^{-1}/min^{-1}, HR_{max} of 120 bpm, and total time of 6 minutes 37 seconds. RPE of 13 was noted with heart rate of 84 bpm during the exercise test.

Prescription   Name, date, height, weight, ACE results, DEXA results, CAD risk profile, and electrocardiogram tracing are included in the prescription packet.

Goal:	Lift body weight ten consecutive times from wheelchair in less than 30 seconds and propel manual wheelchair from parking lot through shopping mall to movie theater and back at same pace as walking friends.
Fitness Level:	As above.
Stratified Risk:	No family history of CAD, non-smoker, resting blood pressure 100/60, total cholesterol 180, HDL 40, hemoglobin$_{lac}$ 5.2 mg%. Significant risk factor: inactivity due to SCI. Low-moderate risk for CAD. Discussed additional risks of autonomic dysreflexia, hyperthermia (also an anticholinergic agent that reduces sweat response), pressure sores, skin integrity of hands and arms, bladder/bowel management, risk for shoulder dysfunction, carpal tunnel syndrome, and osteopenia.
Resources:	As above. Intrigued by FES-LCE but not enough to go to nearest training facility 1 hour away. May consider FES-LCE or HYBRID if motivated by current program. Has access to indoor track at university, clearance to use sports chair during cardiac rehabilitation sessions and director of cardiac rehabilitation program willing to monitor exercise during initial 2 weeks. Can obtain abdominal binder, flexion mitts. Sister is motivated and committed to train with her 3 days a week; can borrow heart rate monitor.

Indications:	Deconditioning, upper extremity weakness, requests exercise for weight control.
Contraindications:	None.
Exercise Mode:	Sports wheelchair propulsion on indoor track.
Intensity:	RPE= 11–13 (moderate) initially; check if corresponds with heart rate 84
Duration:	1. Start with sister push-assisting for 5 minutes @ RPE 7, progress to RPE 11–13 for 10 minutes, then 5-minute cool-down @ RPE 7, followed by 10–15 minutes of rest. 2. Repeat with 5-minute warm-up @ RPE 7, 10 minutes @ RPE 11–13, 5-minute cool-down.
Frequency:	5 days/week initially
Progression:	Same protocol for 2 weeks. Change frequency to 4 days/week and progress duration by 1-minute intervals for first portion of exercise, decrease second portion by 1 minute, maintaining total time constant at 20 minutes until entire 20 minutes in first portion. Reduce frequency to 3 days/week and progress duration by 1-minute increments each session, up to 30-minute total. From that point, have sister progressively decrease assistance until independently propelling wheelchair for 30 minutes. Maintain 3 days/week at that pace and duration. Can try outdoor track on temperate (70–75°F) days with appropriate hydration. Consider "mall-wheeling."
Strengthening:	Employ program described above. Use wide Velcro straps at wrist with cable weights for shoulder abduction, elbow flexion, elbow extension starting with light resistance 5–10 pounds, increasing by 1-pound increments every other work-out, which is scheduled twice a week on alternate days of her aerobic training.

FUTURE INVESTIGATIONS

Despite tremendous progress in the understanding of exercise responses in tetraplegia in recent years, there is still much to learn from and about this very special population. Exercise needs to be investigated in a dose-response format to appropriately weigh the relative risks and benefits and to establish relative and absolute contraindications for its use in tetraplegia. Different levels of tetraplegia respond differently to exercise intervention because of differences in available muscle mass and different levels of neck, scapular, and humeral stability. It remains unclear whether parasympathetic withdrawal during exercise is sufficient in degree or consistency to warrant heart rate monitoring for exercise intensity. It is also unclear to what extent respiratory dynamics can be changed in response to exercise intervention and to the degree with which this may affect cardiac venous return. Mortality statistics indicate that heart disease is much more prevalent in SCI than in able-bodied individuals, but it is not clear to what extent known risk factors may influence those statistics, nor the degree to which they are amenable to exercise intervention with reduced work capacity. Does FES-LCE or HYBRID exercise offer cardiovascular risk benefits significant enough to warrant the expenditure, and are those modes of exercise superior to upper extremity training alone in doing so? Is prophylactic external cooling appropriate for tetraplegics exercising in the heat? Can exercise training improve thermoregulation in SCI? Are secondary complications of SCI reduced as a result of exercise intervention? Perhaps most importantly, does exercise intervention improve functional ability, quality of life, vocational outcome, and productivity? These and many other questions remain unanswered and warrant pursuit.

REFERENCES

1. Aksnes AK, Hjeltnes N, Wahlstrom EO, et al: Intact glucose transport in morphologically altered denervated skeletal muscle from quadriplegic patients. Am J Physiol 271(3 Pt 1):E593–600, 1996.
2. Almenoff PL, Spungen AM, Lesser M, Bauman WA: Pulmonary function survey in spinal cord injury: Influences of smoking and level and completeness of injury. Lung 173:297–306, 1995.
3. Altus P, Hickman JW, Nord HJ: Accidental hypothermia in a healthy quadriplegic patient. Neurology 35:427–428, 1985.
4. American College of Sports Medicine: The recommended quantity and quality of exercise for developing and maintaining cardiorespiratory and muscular fitness in healthy adults. Med Sci Sports Exerc 22:265–274, 1990.
5. Aoyagi Y, McLellan TM, Shephard RJ: Interactions of physical training and heat acclimation. The thermophysiology of exercising in a hot climate. Sports Med 23:173–210, 1997.
6. Apple DF, Cody R, Allen A: Overuse syndrome of the upper limb in people with spinal cord injury. In Apple DF (ed): Physical Fitness: A Guide for Individuals with Spinal Cord Injury. Baltimore, Department of Veterans Affairs, Veterans Health Administration, Rehabilitation Research & Development Service, Scientific and Technical Publications Section, 1996.
7. Armstrong LE, Epstein Y, Greenleaf JE, et al: ACSM position stand on heat and cold illnesses during distance running. Med Sci Sports Exerc 28(12):i–x, 1996.
8. Arnold PB, McVey PP, Farrell WJ, et al: Functional electric stimulation: Its efficacy and safety in improving pulmonary function and musculoskeletal fitness. Arch Phys Med Rehabil 73:665–668, 1992.
9. Ashley FA, Laskin JJ, Olenik LM, et al: Evidence of autonomic dysreflexia during functional electrical stimulation in individuals with spinal cord injuries. Paraplegia 31:593–605, 1993.
10. Åstrand P-O, Cuddy TE, Saltin B, Stenberg J: Cardiac output during submaximal and maximal work. J Appl Physiol 19:268–274, 1964.
11. Balady G, Weaver D, Rose L, Ryan T: Arm exercise-thallium imaging testing for the detection of coronary artery disease. J Am Coll Cardiol 9:84–88, 1987.
12. Bar-Or O, Zwiren LD. Maximal oxygen consumption test during arm exercise-reliability and validity. J Appl Physiol 38:424–426, 1975.
13. Barstow TJ, Scremin AM, Mutton DL, et al: Changes in gas exchange kinetics with training in patients with spinal cord injury. Med Sci Sports Exerc 28:1221–1228, 1996.
13a. Barstow TJ, Scremin AM, Mutton DL, et al: Gas exchange kinetics during functional electrical stimulation in subjects with spinal cord injury. Med Sci Sports Exerc 27:1284–1291, 1995.
14. Bauman WA, Alexander LR, Zhong Y-G, Spungen AM: Stimulated leg ergometry training improves body composition and HDL-cholesterol values. J Am Paraplegia Soc 17:201, 1994.
15. Bauman WA, Raza M, Chayes Z, Machac J: Tomographic thallium-201 myocardial perfusion imaging after intravenous dipyridamole in asymptomatic subjects with quadriplegia. Arch Phys Med Rehabil 74:740–744, 1993.

16. Bauman WA, Spungen AM: Disorders of carbohydrate and lipid metabolism in veterans with paraplegia or quadriplegia: A model of premature aging. Metabolism 43:749–756, 1994.
17. Bauman WA, Spungen AM, Flanagan S, et al: Blunted growth hormone response to intravenous arginine in subjects with a spinal cord injury. Horm Metab Res 26:152–156, 1994.
18. Bauman WA, Spungen AM, Raza M, et al: Coronary artery disease: Metabolic risk factors and latent disease in individuals with paraplegia. Mt Sinai J Med 59:163–168, 1992.
19. Bauman WA, Spungen AM, Zhong YG, et al: Depressed serum high density lipoprotein cholesterol levels in veterans with spinal cord injury. Paraplegia 30:697–703, 1992.
20. BeDell KK, Scremin AME, Perell KL, Kunkel CF: Effects of functional electrical stimulation-induced lower extremity cycling on bone density of spinal cord-injured patients. Am J Phys Med Rehabil 75:29–34, 1996.
21. Bergh U, Kanstrup I-L, Ekblom B: Maximal oxygen uptake during exercise with various combinations of arm and leg work. J Appl Physiol 41:191–196, 1976.
22. Bergofsky EH: Mechanism of respiratory insufficiency after cervical cord injury (a source of alveolar hypoventilation). Ann Intern Med 61:435–437, 1964.
23. Bhambhani YN, Burnham RS, Wheeler GD, et al: Physiological correlates of simulated wheelchair racing in trained quadriplegics. Can J Appl Physiol 20:65–77, 1995.
24. Bidart Y, Maury M: The circulatory behavior in complete chronic paraplegia. Paraplegia 11:1–24, 1973.
25. Biering-Sorenssen F, Bohr H, Schaadt O: Bone mineral content of the lumbar spine and lower extremities years after spinal cord lesion. Paraplegia 26:293–301, 1988.
26. Blackmer J: Orthostatic hypotension in spinal cord injured patients. J Spinal Cord Med 20:212–217, 1997.
27. Bloomfield SA, Jackson RD, Mysiw WJ: Catecholamine response to exercise and training in individuals with spinal cord injury. Med Sci Sports Exerc 26:1213–1219, 1994.
28. Bloomfield SA, Mysiw WJ, Jackson RD: Bone mass and endocrine adaptations to training in spinal cord injured individuals. Bone 19:61–68, 1996.
29. Bobbert AC: Physiologic comparison of three types of ergometer. J Appli Physiol 15:1007–1014, 1960.
30. Bosch PR, Wells CL: Effect of immersion on residual volume of able-bodied and spinal cord injured males. Med Sci Sports Exerc 23:384–388, 1991.
31. Bostom AG, Toner MM, McArdle WD, et al: Lipid and lipoprotein profiles related to peak aerobic power in spinal cord injured men. Med Sci Sports Exerc 23:409–414, 1991.
32. Braddom RI, Rocco JF: Autonomic dysreflexia: A survey of current treatment. Am J Phys Med Rehabil 70:234–241, 1991.
33. Brenes G, Dearwater S, Shapera R, et al: High density lipoprotein cholesterol concentrations in physically active and sedentary spinal cord injured patients. Arch Phys Med Rehabil 67:445–450, 1986.
34. Brozek J, Grande F, Andersson JT, et al: Densiometric analysis of body composition: Revision of some quantitative assumptions. Ann N Y Acad Sci 110:113–130, 1963.
35. Bulbulian R, Johnson RE, Gruber JJ, Darabos B: Body composition in paraplegic male athletes. Med Sci Sports Exerc 12:195–201, 1987.
36. Bunt JC: Hormonal alterations due to exercise. Sports Med 3:331–345, 1986.
37. Burkett LN, Chisum J, Stone W, Fernhall B: Exercise capacity of untrained spinal cord injured individuals and the relationship of peak oxygen uptake to level of injury. Paraplegia 28:512–521, 1990.
38. Burnham R, Wheeler GD, Bhambhani Y, et al: Intentional induction of autonomic dysreflexia for performance enhancement in wheelchair athletes. Clin J Sports Med 4:1–10, 1994.
39. Campbell CC, Koris MJ: Etiologies of shoulder pain in cervical spinal cord injury. Clin Orthop 322:140–145, 1996.
40. Cardus D, McTaggart WG: Body composition in spinal cord injury. Arch Phys Med Rehabil 66:257–259, 1985.
41. Casperson CJ, Powell KE, Christenson GM: Physical activity, exercise, and physical fitness: Definitions and distinctions for health-related research. Public Health Rep 100:126–131, 1985.
42. Castelli WP, Garrison RJ, Wilson PWF: Incidence of coronary heart disease and lipoprotein cholesterol levels: The Framingham Study. JAMA 256:2835–2838, 1986.

43. Chawla JC, Bar C, Creber I, et al: Techniques for improving the strength and fitness of spinal cord injured patients. Paraplegia 17:185–189, 1979–80.

44. Claus-Walker JC, Campos RJ, Carter RE, et al: Calcium excretion in quadriplegia. Arch Phys Med Rehabil 53:14–20, 1972.

45. Claus-Walker JC, Halstead LS: Metabolic and endocrine changes in spinal cord injury: II. Partial decentralization of the autonomic nervous system. Arch Phys Med Rehabil 63:576–580, 1982.

46. Claus-Walker J, Spencer WA, Carter RE, et al: Bone metabolism in quadriplegia: Dissociation between calciuria and hydroxyprolinuria. Arch Phys Med Rehabil 56:327–332, 1975.

47. Convertino VA, Armstrong LE, Coyle EF, et al: ACSM position stand on exercise and fluid replacement. Med Sci Sports Exerc 28(1):i–vii, 1996.

48. Cooney MM, Walker JB: Hydraulic resistance exercise benefits cardiovascular fitness of spinal cord injured. Med Sci Sports Exerc 18:522–525, 1986.

49. Cooper RA, Baldini FD, Langbein WE, et al: Prediction of pulmonary function in wheelchair users. Paraplegia 31:560–570, 1993.

50. Coutts KD, McKenzie DC: Ventilatory thresholds during wheelchair exercise in individuals with spinal cord injuries. Paraplegia 33:419–422, 1995.

51. Coutts KD, Rhodes EC, McKenzie DC: Maximal exercise responses of tetraplegics and paraplegics. J Appl Physiol 55:479–482, 1983.

52. Coutts KD, Stogryn JL: Aerobic and anaerobic power of Canadian wheelchair track athletes. Med Sci Sports Exerc 19:62–65, 1987.

53. Cox SR, Weiss SM, Posuniak EA: Energy expenditure after spinal cord injury: An evaluation of stable rehabilitation patients. J Trauma 25:419–423, 1985.

54. Crane L, Klerk K, Ruhl A, et al: The effect of exercise on pulmonary function in persons with quadriplegia. Paraplegia 32:435–441, 1994.

55. Creasey G, Elefteriades J, DiMarco A, et al: Electrical stimulation to restore respiration. J Rehabil Res Dev 33:123–32, 1996.

56. Crisp R: Vocational decision making by sixty spinal cord injury patients. Paraplegia 30:420–424, 1992.

57. Cruse JM, Lewis RE, Bishop GR, et al: Neuroendocrine-immune interactions associated with loss and restoration of immune system function in spinal cord injury and stroke patients. Immunol Res 11:104–116, 1992.

58. Curt A, Nitsche B, Rodic B, et al: Assessment of autonomic dysreflexia in patients with spinal cord injury. N Neurol Neurosurg Psychiatry 62:473–477, 1997.

59. Curt A, Weinhardt C, Dietz V: Significance of sympathetic skin response in the assessment of failure in patients with spinal cord injury. J Auton Nerv Syst 61:175–80, 1996.

60. Curtis KA, Dillon DA: Survey of wheelchair athletic injuries: Common patterns and prevention. Paraplegia 23:170–175, 1985.

61. Curtis KA, McClanahan S, Hall KM, et al: Health, vocational, and functional status in spinal cord injured athletes and nonathletes. Arch Phys Med Rehabil 67:862–865, 1986.

62. Dallmeijer AJ, Hopman MTE, van As HHJ, ver der Woude LHV: Physical capacity and physical strain in persons with tetraplegia, the role of sport activity. Spinal Cord 34:729–735, 1996.

63. Davis GM: Exercise capacity of individuals with paraplegia. Med Sci Sports Exerc 25:423–432, 1993.

64. Dearwater SR, Laporte RE, Robertson RJ, et al: Activity in the spinal cord-injured patient: An epidemiological analysis of metabolic parameters. Med Sci Sports Exerc 18:541–544, 1986.

65. DeTroyer A, Heilporn A: Respiratory mechanics in quadriplegia. The respiratory function of the intercostal muscles. Am Rev Respir Dis 122:591–600, 1980.

66. DeVivo MJ, Rutt RD, Stover SL, Fine PR: Employment after spinal cord injury. Arch Phys Med Rehabil 68:494–498, 1987.

67. DeVivo MJ, Stover SL: Long-term survival and causes of death. In Stover SL, DeLisa JA, Whiteneck GG (eds): Spinal Cord Injury: Clinical Outcomes from the Model Systems. Gaithersburg, MD, Aspen Publishers, 1995, pp 289–316.

68. DiCarlo SE: Improved cardiopulmonary status after a two-month program of graded arm exercise in a patient with C6 quadriplegia. Phys Ther 62:456–459, 1982.

68. DiCarlo SE, Supp MD, Taylor HC: Effect of arm ergometry training on physical work capacity of individuals with spinal cord injuries. Phys Ther 63:1104–1107, 1983.
70. Dijkers MP, Abela MB, Gans BM, Gordon WA: The aftermath of spinal cord injury. In Stover SL, DeLisa JA, Whiteneck GG (eds): Spinal Cord Injury: Clinical Outcomes from the Model Systems. Gaithersburg, MD, Aspen Publishers, 1995, pp 185–212.
71. Dixit S: Bradycardia associated with high cervical spinal cord injury. Surg Neurol 43:514, 1995.
72. Douglas AJ, Walsh EG, Wright GW, et al: The effects of neuromuscular stimulation on muscle tone at the knee in paraplegia. Exp Physiol 76:357–367, 1991.
73. Downey JA, Chiodi HP, Darling RC: Central temperature regulation in the spinal man. J Appl Physiol 22:91–94, 1967.
74. Downey JA, Huckaba CE, Kelley PS, et al: Sweating responses to central and peripheral heating in spinal man. J Appl Physiol 40:701–706, 1976.
75. Downey JA, Huckaba CE, Kelley PS, et al: Thermoregulation in the spinal man. J Appl Physiol 34:790–794, 1973.
76. Dreisinger TE, Dalton RB, Whiting RB: Maximal wheelchair exercise: Comparison of ablebodied and wheelchair bound. Med Sci Sports Exerc 16:147, 1984.
77. Drory Y, Ohry A, Brooks ME, et al: Arm crank ergometry in chronic spinal cord injured patients. Arch Phys Med Rehabil 71:389–392, 1990.
78. Duckworth WC, Jallepalli P, Solomon SS: Glucose intolerance in spinal cord injury. Arch Phys Med Rehabil 64:107–110, 1983.
78. Duckworth WC, Solomon SS, Jallepalli P, et al: Glucose intolerance due to insulin resistance in patients with spinal cord injury. Diabetes 29:906–910, 1980.
80. Duffin J: Neural drives to breathing during exercise. Can J Appl Physiol 19:289–304, 1994.
81. Eldridge FL: Central integration of mechanisms in exercise hyperpnea. Med Sci Sports Exerc 26:319–327, 1994.
82. Eltorai I, Kim R, Vulpe M, et al: Fatal cerebral hemorrhage due to autonomic dysreflexia in a tetraplegic patient: Case report and review. Paraplegia 30:355–360, 1992.
83. Erickson RP: Autonomic hyperreflexia: Pathophysiology and medical management. Arch Phys Med Rehabil 61:431–440, 1980.
84. Eriksson P, Lofstrom L, Ekblom B: Aerobic power during exercise in untrained and well-trained persons with quadriplegia and paraplegia. Scand J Rehabil Med 20:141–147, 1988.
85. Escobedo EM, Hunter JC, Hollister MC, et al: MR imaging of rotator cuff tears in individuals with paraplegia. AJR Am J Roentgenol 168:919–923, 1997.
86. Estenne M, Knoop C, Vanvaerenbergh J, et al: The effect of pectoralis muscle training in tetraplegic subjects. Am Rev Respir Dis 139:1218–1222, 1989.
87. Faghri PD, Glaser RM, Figoni SF: Functional electrical stimulation leg cycle ergometer exercise: Training effects on cardiorespiratory responses of spinal cord injured subjects at rest and during submaximal exercise. Arch Phys Med Rehabil 73:1085–1093, 1992.
88. Faghri PD, Glaser RM, Figoni SF, et al: Feasibility of using two FNS exercise modes for spinal cord injured patients. Clni Kinesiol 43:62–68, 1989.
89. Fehr LS, Fisher MA, Langbein WE: Effect of supported standing and upper body exercise on lower extremity spasticity in persons with spinal cord injury. Rehabil Res Dev Rep 34:275–276, 1997.
90. Ferguson-Pell MW: Technical considerations: Seat cushion selection. J Rehabil Res Dev Clin Suppl 2:47–73, 1992.
91. Ferrara MS, Davis RW: Injuries to elite wheelchair athletes. Paraplegia 28:335–341, 1990.
92. Figoni SF: Exercise responses and quadriplegia. Med Sci Sports Exerc 25:433–441, 1993.
93. Figoni SF: Perspectives on cardiovascular fitness and SCI. J Am Paraplegia Soc 13:63–70, 1990.
94. Figoni SF, Boileau RA, Massey BH, Larsen JR: Physiologic responses of quadriplegic and able-bodied men during exercise at the same VO_2. Adapted Phys Activity Q 5:130–139, 1988.
95. Figoni SF, Glaser RM, Collins SR: Peak physiologic responses of trained quadriplegics during arm, leg and hybrid exercise in two postures [abstract]. Med Sci Sports Exerc 27:S83, 1995.
96. Figoni SF, Glaser RM, Rodgers MM, et al: Acute hemodynamic responses of spinal cord injured indi-

viduals to functional neuromuscular stimulation-induced knee extension exercise. J Rehabil Res Dev 28:9–18, 1991.

97. Figoni SF, Rodgers MM, Glaser RM, et al: Physiologic responses of paraplegics and quadriplegics to passive and active leg cycle ergometry. J Am Paraplegia Soc 13:33–39, 1990.

98. Finsen V, Indredavik B, Fougner KJ: Bone mineral and hormone status in paraplegics. Paraplegia 30:343–347, 1992.

99. Fitzgerald PI, Sedlock DA, Knowlton RG: Circulatory and thermal adjustments to prolonged exercise in paraplegic women. Med Sci Sports Exerc 22:629–635, 1990.

100. Forrest GP: Atrial fibrillation associated with autonomic dysreflexia in patients with tetraplegia. Arch Phys Med Rehabil 72:592–594, 1991.

101. Franklin BA: Exercise training and arm ergometry. Sports Med 2:100–119, 1985.

102. Franklin BA, Swnatek KI, Grais SL, et al: Field test estimation of maximal oxygen consumption in wheelchair users. Arch Phys Med Rehabil 71:574–578, 1990.

103. Frey GC, McCubbin JA, Dunn JM, Mazzeo RS: Plasma catecholamine and lactate relationship during graded exercise in men with spinal cord injury. Med Sci Sports Exerc 29:451–456, 1997.

104. Freyschuss U: Autonomic nervous mediation of the heart rate acceleration on an isometric muscle contraction in tetraplegic men. Acta Physiol Scand 57(suppl 342):28–33, 1970.

105. Fugl-Meyer AR: A model of treatment of impaired ventilatory function in tetraplegic patients. Scand J Rehabil Med 3:167, 1971.

106. Fuhrer MJ, Carter RE, Donovan WH, et al: Postdischarge outcomes for ventilator-dependent quadriplegics. Arch Phys Med Rehabil 68:353–356, 1987.

107. Fuhrer MJ, Garber SL, Rintala DH, et al: Pressure ulcers in community-resident persons with spinal cord injury: Prevalence and risk factors. Arch Phys Med Rehabil 74:1172–1177, 1993.

108. Garland DE, Stewart CA, Adkins RH, et al: Osteoporosis after spinal cord injury. J Orthop Res 10:371–378, 1992.

109. Gass GC, Camp EM: Physiological characteristics of trained Australian paraplegic and tetraplegic subjects. Med Sci Sports Exer 11:256–259, 1979.

110. Gass GC, Camp EM: The maximum physiological responses during incremental wheelchair and arm cranking exercise in male paraplegics. Med Sci Sports Exerc 16:355–359, 1984.

111. Gass GC, Camp EM, Davis HA, et al: The effects of prolonged exercise on spinally injured subjects. Med Sci Sports Exerc 13:277–283, 1981.

112. Gass GC, Watson J, Camp EM, et al: The effects of physical training on high level spinal lesion patients. Scand J Rehabil Med 12:61–65, 1980.

113. George CM, Wells CL, Dugan NL, Hardison R: Hydrostatic weights of patients with spinal cord injury. Phys Ther 67:921–925, 1987.

114. Gerhart KA, Bergstrom E, Charlifue SW, et al: Long-term spinal cord injury: Functional changes over time. Arch Phys Med Rehabil 74:1030–1034, 1993.

115. Gettman LR: Fitness testing. In Durstine JL, King AC, Painter PL, et al. (eds): ACSM's Resource Manual for Guidelines for Exercise Testing and Prescription, 2nd ed. Philadelphia, Lea & Febiger, 1993, pp 229–246.

116. Gilgoff IS, Davidson SL, Hohn AR: Cardiac pacemaker in high spinal cord injury. Arch Phys Med Rehabil 72:601–603, 1991.

117. Glaser RM: Exercise and locomotion for the spinal cord injured. Exerc Sport Sci Rev 13:263–304, 1985.

118. Glaser RM: Functional neuromuscular stimulation. Exercise conditioning of spinal cord injured patients. Int J Sports Med 15:142–148, 1994.

119. Glaser RM: Physiologic aspects of spinal cord injury and functional neuromuscular stimulation. Cent Nerv Syst Trauma 3:49–61, 1986.

120. Glaser RM, Foley DM, Laubach LL, et al: An exercise test to evaluate fitness for wheelchair activity. Paraplegia 16:341–349, 1979.

121. Glaser RM, Janssen TWJ, Suryaprasad AG, et al: The physiology of exercise. In Apple DF (ed): Physical Fitness: A Guide for Individuals with Spinal Cord Injury. Baltimore, Department of Veterans Affairs, Veterans Health Administration, Rehabilitation Research & Development Service, Scientific and Technical Publications Section, 1996.

122. Glaser RM, Sawka MN, Brune MF, Wilde SW: Physiological responses to maximal effort wheelchair ergometry and arm crank ergometry. J Appl Physiol 48:1060–1064, 1980.
123. Go BK, DeVivo MJ, Richards JS: The epidemiology of spinal cord injury. In Stover SL, DeLisa JA, Whiteneck GG (eds): Spinal Cord Injury: Clinical Outcomes from the Mode Systems. Gaithersburg, MD, Aspen Publishers, 1995, pp 21–51.
124. Green BC, Pratt CC, Grigsby TE: Self-concept among persons with long-term spinal cord injury. Arch Phys Med Rehabil 65:751–754, 1984.
125. Greenway RM, Houser HB, Lindan O, Weir DR: Long-term changes in gross body composition of paraplegic and quadriplegic patients. Paraplegia 7:301–317, 1970.
126. Gross D, Ladd HW, Riley EJ, et al: The effect of training on strength and endurance of the diaphragm. Am J Med 68:27–35, 1980.
127. Haas F, Axen K, Pineda H, et al: Temporal pulmonary function changes in cervical cord injury. Arch Phys Med Rehabil 66:139–144, 1985.
128. Hangartner TN, Rodgers MM, Glaser RM, Barre PS: Tibial bone density loss in spinal cord injured patients: Effects of FES exercise. J Rehabil Res Dev 31:50–61, 1994.
129. Hjeltnes N: Capacity for physical work and training after spinal cord injuries and strokes. Scand J Rehabil Med 29:245–251, 1982.
130. Hjeltnes N, Jansen T: Physical endurance capacity, functional status and medical complications in spinal cord injured subjects with long-standing lesions. Paraplegia 28:428–432, 1990.
131. Hockenberry J: Moving Violations: A Memoir: War Zones, Wheelchairs, and Declarations of Independence. New York, Hyperion, 1995.
132. Hooker SP, Figoni SF, Rodgers MM, et al: Metabolic and hemodynamic responses to concurrent voluntary arm crank and electrical stimultion leg cycle exercise in quadriplegics. J Rehabil Res Dev 29:1–11, 1992.
133. Hooker SP, Figoni SF, Rodgers MM, et al: Physiologic effects of electrical stimulation leg cycle exercise training in spinal cord injured persons. Arch Phys Med Rehabil 73:470–476, 1992.
134. Hooker SP, Wells CL: Effects of low- and moderate-intensity training in spinal cord-injured persons. Med Sci Sports Exerc 21:18–22, 1989.
135. Hopman MT: Circulatory responses during arm exercise in individuals with paraplegia. Int J Sports Med 15:126–131, 1994.
136. Hopman MT, Dallmeijer AJ, Snoek G, et al: The effect of training on cardiovascular responses to arm exercise in individuals with tetraplegia. Eur J Appl Physiol 74:172–179, 1996.
137. Hopman MT, van der Woude LH, Dallmeijer AJ, et al: Respiratory muscle strength and endurance in individuals with tetraplegia. Spinal Cord 35:104–108, 1997.
138. Hopman MTE, Oeseburg B, Binkhorst RA: Cardiovascular responses in persons with paraplegia to prolonged arm exercise and thermal stress. Med Sci Sports Exerc 25:577–583, 1993.
139. Hopman MTE, Oeseburg B, Binkhorst RA: The effect of an anti-G suit on cardiovascular responses to exercise in persons with paraplegia. Med Sci Sports Exerc 24:984–990, 1992.
140. Huckaba CE, Frewin DB, Downey JA, et al: Sweating responses of normal, paraplegic and anhidrotic subjects. Arch Phys Med Rehabil 57:268–274, 1976.
141. Janssen TW, van Oers CA, Hollander AP, et al: Isometric strength, sprint power, and aerobic power in individuals with a spinal cord injury. Med Sci Sports Exerc 25:863–870, 1993.
142. Janssen TWJ, van Oers CAJM, Rozendaal EP, et al: Changes in physical strain and physical capacity in men with spinal cord injuries. Med Sci Sports Exerc 28:551–559, 1996.
143. Janssen TWJ, van Oers CAJM, van der Woude LHV, Hollander AP: Physical strain in daily life of wheelchair users with spinal cord injuries. Med Sci Sports Exer 26:661–670, 1994.
144. Jennings DB: Respiratory control during exercise: Hormones, osmolality, strong ions, and $PaCO_2$. Can J Appl Physiol 19:334–349, 1994.
145. Kaplan PE, Roden W, Gilbert E, et al: Reduction of hypercalcuria in tetraplegia after weight-bearing and strengthening exercises. Paraplegia 19:289–293, 1981.
146. Karlsson A-K, Attvall S, Jansson P-A, et al: Influence of the sympathetic nervous system on insulin sensitivity and adipose tissue metabolism: A study in spinal cord-injured subjects. Metabolism 44:52–58, 1995.

147. Katz RT: Management of spasticity. Am J Phys Med Rehabil 67:108–116, 1988.
148. Kavanagh T: Physical training in heart transplant recipients. J Cardiovasc Risk 3:154–159, 1996.
149. Kawamoto M, Sakimura S, Takasaki M: Transient increase of parasympathetic one in patients with cervical spinal cord trauma. Anaesth Intensive Care 21:218–221, 1993.
150. Kenney WL (ed): ACSM's Guidelines for Exercise Testing and Prescription, 5th ed. Baltimore, Williams & Wilkins, 1995.
151. Kerk JK, Clifford PS, Snyder AC, et al: Effect of an abdominal binder during wheelchair exercise. Med Sci Sports Exerc 27:913–919, 1995.
152. Kessler KM, Pina I, Green B, et al: Cardiovascular findings in quadriplegic and paraplegic patients and in normal subjects. Am J Cardiol 58:525–530, 1986.
153. King ML, Lichtman SW, Pellicone JT, et al: Exertional hypotension in thoracic spinal cord injury: Case report. Paraplegia 30:261–266, 1992.
154. Kjaer M, Pollack SF, Mohr T, et al: Regulation of glucose turnover and hormonal responses during cycling in tetraplegic humans. Am J Physiol 271(1 Pt 2):R191–R199, 1996.
155. Kliesch WF, Cruse JM, Lewis RE, et al: Restoration of depressed immune function in spinal cord injury patients receiving rehabilitation therapy. Paraplegia 34:82–90, 1996.
156. Kocina P: Body composition of spinal cord injured adults. Sports Med 23:48–60, 1997.
157. Kohrt WM: Body composition by DXA: Tried and true? Med Sci Sports Exerc 27:1349–1353, 1995.
158. Kosiak M: Etiology and pathology of ischemic ulcers. Arch Phys Med Rehabil 40:62–69, 1959.
159. Krause JS: Adjustment after spinal cord injury: A 9-year longitudinal study. Arch Phys Med Rehabil 78:651–657, 1997.
160. Krauss JC, Robergs RA, Depaepe JL, et al: Effects of electrical stimulation and upper body training after spinal cord injury. Med Sci Sports Exerc 25:1054–1061, 1993.
161. Krum H, Brown DJ, Rowe PR, et al: Steady state plasma [3H]-noradrenaline kinetics in quadriplegic chronic spinal cord injury patients. J Auton Pharmacol 10:221–226, 1990.
162. Krum H, Howes LG, Brown DJ, et al: Risk factors for cardiovascular disease in chronic spinal cord injury patients. Paraplegia 30:381–388, 1992.
163. Krum H, Howes LG, Brown DJ, Louis WJ: Blood pressure variability in tetraplegic patients with autonomic hyperreflexia. Paraplegia 27:284–288, 1989.
164. Lakomy HKA, Campbell I, Williams C: Treadmill performance and selected physiological characteristics of wheelchair athletes. Br J Sports Med 21:130–133, 1987.
165. Landis E: Micro-injection studies of capillary blood pressure in human skin. Heart 15:209–228, 1930.
166. Langbein WE, Edwards SC, Louis EK, et al: Wheelchair exercise and digital echocardiography for the detection of heart disease. Rehabil Res Dev Rep 34:324–325, 1996.
167. Langbein WE, Maki KC, Edwards LC, et al: Initial clinical evaluation of a wheelchair ergometer for diagnostic exercise testing: A technical note. J Rehabil Res Dev 31:317–325, 1994.
168. Laskin JJ, Ashley EA, Olenik LM, et al: Electrical stimulation-assisted rowing exercise in spinal cord injured people. A pilot study. Paraplegia 31:534–541, 1993.
169. Lasko-McCarthey P, Davis JA: Effect of work rate increment on peak oxygen uptake during wheelchair ergometry in men with quadriplegia. Eur J Appl Physiol 63:349–353, 1991.
170. Lazarus B, Cullinane E, Thompson PD: Comparison of the results and reproducibility of arm and leg exercise tests in men with angina pectoris. Am J Cardiol 47:1075–1079, 1981.
171. Leeds EM, Klose KJ, Ganz W, et al: Bone mineral density after bicycle ergometry training. Arch Phys Med Rehabil 71:207–209, 1990.
172. Lehman K, Lane J, Piepmeir J, Batsford W: Cardiovascular abnormalities accompanying acute spinal cord injury in humans: Incidence, time course and severity. J Am Coll Cardiol 10:46–52, 1987.
173. Linden R, Leffler EJ, Kedia KR: A comparison of the efficacy of an alpha-I-adrenergic blocker and a slow calcium channel blocker in the control of autonomic dysreflexia. Paraplegia 23:34–38, 1985.
174. Lohman TG: Advances in body composition assessment. In Current Issues in Exercise Science Series, Monograph 3. Champaign, IL, Human Kinetics Publishers, 1992.
175. Lundberg A: Wheelchair driving: Evaluation of a new training outfit. Scand J Rehabil Med 12:67–72, 1987.

176. Maloney F: Pulmonary function in quadriplegia: Effects of a corset. Arch Phys Med Rehabil 60:261–265, 1979.
177. Marciello MA, Herbison GJ, Cohen ME, Schmidt R: Elbow extension using anterior deltoids and upper pectorals in spinal cord-injured subjects. Arch Phys Med Rehabil 76:426–432, 1995.
178. Mateika JH, Duffin J: A review of the control of breathing during exercise. Eur J Appl Physiol 71:1–27, 1995.
179. Mathias CJ, Christensen NJ, Corbett JL, et al: Plasma catecholamines during paroxysmal neurogenic hypertension in quadriplegic man. Circ Res 39:204–208, 1976.
180. Mathias CJ, Frankel HL: Clinical manifestations of malfunctioning sympathetic mechanisms in tetraplegia. J Auton Nerv Sys 7:303–312, 1983.
181. Maynard FM, Bracken MB, Creasey G, et al: International Standards for Neurological and Functional Classification of Spinal Cord Injury. Revised. Chicago, American Spinal Injury Association, 1996.
182. Maynard FM, Karunas RS, Adkins RH, et al: Management of the neuromusculoskeletal systems. In Stover SL, DeLisa JA, Whiteneck GG (eds): Spinal Cord Injury: Clinical Outcomes from the Model Systems. Gaithersburg, MD, Aspen Publishers, 1995, pp 145–169.
183. McCann BC: Thermoregulation in spinal cord injury: The challenge of the Atlanta Paralympics. Spinal Cord 34:433–406, 1996.
184. McLean KP: Training-induced changes in glucose regulation during prolonged exercise in persons with quadriplegia [dissertation]. Tempe, AZ, Arizona State University, 1992.
185. McLean KP, Jones PP, Skinner JS: Exercise prescription for sitting and supine exercise in subjects with quadriplegia. Med Sci Sports Exerc 27:15–21, 1995.
186. McLean KP, Skinner JS: Effect of body training position on outcomes of an aerobic training study on individuals with quadriplegia. Arch Phys Med Rehabil 76:139–150, 1995.
187. Miller JI, Farmer JA, Stuart W, Apple D: Phrenic nerve pacing of the quadriplegic patient. J Thorac Cardiovasc Surg 99:35–40, 1990.
188. Mollinger LA, Sparr GB, El Ghatet AZ, et al: Daily energy expenditure and basal metabolic rates of patients with spinal cord injury. Arch Phys Med Rehabil 66:420–426, 1985.
189. Mutton DL, Scremin AME, Barstow TJ, et al: Physiologic responses during functional electrical stimulation leg cycling and hybrid exercise in spinal cord injured subjects. Arch Phys Med Rehabil 78:712–718, 1997.
190. Myllynen P, Koivisto VA, Nikkila EA: Glucose intolerance and insulin resistance accompany immobilization. Acta Med Scand 222:75–81, 1987.
191. Naftchi NE: Mechanism of autonomic dysreflexia. Contributions of catecholamine and peptide neurotransmitters. Ann N Y Acad Sci 579:133–148, 1990.
192. Naftchi NE, Viau AT, Sell GH, Lowman EW: Mineral metabolism in spinal cord injury. Arch Phys Med Rehabil 61:139–142, 1980.
193. Nakamura Y: Working ability of the paraplegics. Paraplegia 11:182–193, 1973.
194. Nash MS: Immune responses to nervous system decentralization and exercise in quadriplegia. Med Sci Sports Exerc 26:164–171, 1994.
195. Nash MS, Bilsker MS, Kearney HM, et al: Effects of electrically-stimulated exercise and passive motion on echocardiographically-derived wall motion and cardiodynamic function in tetraplegic persons. Paraplegia 33:80–89, 1995.
196. Nash MS, Bilsker S, Marcillo AE, et al: Reversal of adaptive left ventricular atrophy following electrically-stimulated exercise training in human tetraplegics. Paraplegia 29:590–599, 1991.
197. Nichols PJR, Norman PA, Ennis JR: Wheelchair user's shoulder? Shoulder pain in patients with spinal cord lesions. Scand J Rehabil Med 11:29–32, 1979.
198. Noreau L, Shepherd RJ: Physical fitness and productive activity of paraplegics. Sports Med Train Rehabil 3:165–181, 1992.
199. Noreau L, Shephard RJ: Spinal cord injury, exercise and quality of life. Sports Med 20:226–250, 1995.
200. Noreau L, Shephard RJ, Simard C: Cardiorespiratory and muscular fitness in a group of individuals with SCI: A distribution to the classification of ISMGF [abstract]. J Am Paraplegia Soc 17:127, 1994.
201. Noreau L, Shephard RJ, Simard C: Relationship of impairment and functional ability to habitual activity and fitness following spinal cord injury. Int J Rehabil Res 16:265–275, 1993.

202. Nyland J, Robinson K, Caborn D, et al: Shoulder rotator torque and wheelchair dependence differences of National Wheelchair Basketball Association players. Arch Phys Med Rehabil 78:358–363, 1997.
203. Olenik LM, Laskin JJ, Burnham R, et al: Efficacy of rowing, backward wheeling and isolated scapular retractor exercise as remedial strength activities for wheelchair users: Application of electromyography. Paraplegia 33:148–152, 1995.
204. Olle MM, Pivarnik JM, Klish WJ, Morrow JR: Body composition and physically active spinal cord injured individuals estimated from total body electrical conductivity. Arch Phys Med Rehabil 74:706–710, 1993.
205. Pacy PJ, Hesp R, Halliday DA, et al: Muscle and bone in paraplegic patients, and the effect of functional electrical stimulation. Clin Sci 75:481–487, 1988.
206. Pate RR, Pratt M, Blair SN, et al: Physical activity and public health: A recommendation from the Centers for Disease Control and Prevention and the American College of Sports Medicine. JAMA 273:402–407, 1995.
207. Paterson DJ: Potassium and breathing during exercise. Sports Med 23:149–163, 1997.
208. Petrofsky JS: Thermoregulatory stress during rest and exercise in heat in patients with a spinal cord injury. Eur J Appl Physiol 64:503–507, 1992.
209. Petrofsky JS, Phillips CA: The use of functional electrical stimulation for rehabilitation of spinal cord injured patients. Cent Nerv Sys Trauma 1:57–74, 1984.
210. Petry C, Rothstein JL, Bauman WA: Hemoglobin A1c as a predictor of glucose intolerance in spinal cord injury. J Am Paraplegia Soc 16:56, 1993.
211. Phillips CA: Medical criteria for active physical therapy. Physician guidelines for patient participation in a program of functional electrical rehabilitation. Am J Phys Med 66:269–286, 1987.
212. Phillips W, Burkett LN: Arm crank exercise with static leg FNS in persons with spinal cord injury. Med Sci Sports Exerc 27:530–535, 1995.
213. Phillips W, Burkett LN, Munro R, et al: Relative changes in blood flow with functional electrical stimulation during exercise of the paralyzed lower limbs. Paraplegia 33:90–93, 1995.
214. Phillips CA, Hendershot DM: A systems approach to medically prescribed functional electrical stimulation. Ambulation after spinal cord injury. Paraplegia 29:505–513, 1991.
215. Phillips CA, Petrofsky JS, Hendershot DM, Stafford D: Functional electrical exercise: A comprehensive approach for physical conditioning of the spinal cord injured patient. Orthopedics 7:1112–1123, 1984.
216. Pine ZM, Miller SD, Alonso JA: Atrial fibrillation associated with autonomic dysreflexia. Am J Phys Med Rehabil 70:271–273, 1991.
217. Pitetti KH, Barrett PJ, Campbell KD, Malzahn DE: The effect of lower body positive pressure on the exercise capacity of individuals with spinal cord injury. Med Sci Sports Exerc 26:463–468, 1994.
218. Pittetti KH, Snell PG, Stray-Gundersen J: Maximal response wheelchair-confined subjects to four types of arm exercise. Arch Phys Med Rehabil 68:10–13, 1987.
219. Pollack SF, Axen K, Spielholz N, et al: Aerobic training effects of electrically induced lower extremity exercises in spinal cord injured people. Arch Phys Med Rehabil 70:214–219, 1989.
220. Powers CM, Newsam CJ, Gronley JK, et al: Isometric shoulder torque in subjects with spinal cord injury. Arch Phys Med Rehabil 75:761–765, 1994.
221. Ragnarsson KT: Physiologic effects of functional electrical stimulation-induced exercises in spinal cord-injured individuals. Clin Orthop 233:53–63, 1988.
222. Ragnarsson KT, Pollack S, O'Daniel W, et al: Clinical evaluation of computerized functional electrical stimulation after spinal cord injury: A multicenter pilot study. Arch Phys Med Rehabil 69:672–677, 1988.
223. Randall WC, Wurster RD, Lewin RJ: Responses of patients with high spinal transection to high ambient temperatures. J Appl Physiol 21:985–993, 1966.
224. Rasmann Nuhlicek DN, Spurr GB, Barboriak JJ, et al: Body composition of patients with spinal cord injury. Eur J Clin Nutr 42:765–773, 1988.
225. Ready AE: Response of quadriplegic athletes to maximal and submaximal exercise. Physiother Can 36:124–128, 1984.
226. Reame NE: A prospective study of the menstrual cycle and spinal cord injury. Am J Phys Med Rehabil 71:15–21, 1992.
227. Reswick JB, Rogers JE: Experience at Rancho Los Amigos Hospital with devices and techniques to pre-

vent pressure sores. In Kenedi RM, Cowden JM, Scales JT (eds): Bedsore Biomechanics. Baltimore, University Park Press, 1976, pp 301–310.

228. Reyes ML, Gronley JK, Newsam CJ, et al: Electromyographic analysis of shoulder muscles of men with low-level paraplegia during a weight relief raise. Arch Phys Med Rehabil 76:433–439, 1995.

229. Rhodes EC, McKenzie DC, Coutts KD, Rogers AR: A field test for the prediction of aerobic capacity in male paraplegics and quadriplegics. Can J Appl Sport Sci 6:182–186, 1981.

230. Rodgers MM, Glaser RM, Figoni SF, et al: Musculoskeletal responses of spinal cord injured individuals to functional neuromuscular stimulation-induced knee extension exercise training. J Rehabil Res Dev 28:19–26, 1991.

231. Salcido R, Hart D, Smith AM: The prevention and management of pressure ulcers. In Braddom RL (ed): Physical Medicine and Rehabilitation. Philadelphia, WB Saunders, 1996, pp 630–648.

232. Sawka MN: Physiology of upper body exercise. In Pandolf KB (ed): Exercise and Sport Science Reviews. Vol 14. New York, Macmillan, 1986, pp 175–210.

233. Sawka MN, Foley ME, Pimental NA, et al: Determination of maximal aerobic power during upper-body exeircse. J Appl Physiol 54:113–117, 1983.

234. Sawka MN, Latzka WA, Pandolf KB: Temperature regulation during upper body exercise: Able-bodied and spinal cord injured. Med Sci Sports Exerc 21(suppl):S132–S140, 1989.

235. Schmidt KD, Chan CW: Thermoregulation and fever in normal persons and in those with spinal cord injuries. Mayo Clin Proc 67:469–475, 1992.

236. Schwade J, Blomqvist CG, Shapiro W: A comparison of the response to arm and leg work in patients with ischemic heart disease. Am Heart J 93:203–208, 1977.

237. Seckendorf R, Randall WC: Thermal reflex sweating in normal and paraplegic man. J Appl Physiol 16:796–800, 1961.

238. Sedlock DA, Laventure SJ: Body composition and resting energy expenditure in long term spinal cord injury. Paraplegia 28:448–454, 1990.

239. Sharkey BJ, Graetzer DG: Specificity of exercise, training, and testing. In Durstine JL, King AC, Painter PL, et al (eds): ACSM's Resource Manual for Guidelines for Exercise Testing and Prescription. Philadelphia, Lea & Febiger, 1993, pp 82–92.

240. Shephard RJ, Kavanagh T, Mertens DJ, Yacoub M: The place of perceived exertion ratings in exercise prescription for cardiac transplant patients before and after training. Br J Sports Med 30:116–121, 1996.

241. Shetty KR, Sutton CH, Mattson DE, Rudman D: Hyposomatomedinemia in quadriplegic men. Am J Med Sci 305:95–100, 1993.

242. Shetty KR, Sutton CH, Rudman IW, Rudman D: Lipid and lipoprotein abnormalities in young quadriplegic men. Am J Med Sci 303:213–216, 1992.

243. Sie IH, Waters RL, Adkins RH, Gellman H: Upper extremity pain in the postrehabilitation spinal cord injured patient. Arch Phys Med Rehabil 73:44–48, 1992.

244. Simard C, Noreau L, Pare G, Pomerleau P: Maximal physiological response during exertion in quadriplegic subjects. Can J Appl Physiol 18:163–174, 1993.

245. Sipski ML, Alexander CJ, Harris M: Long-term use of computerized bicycle ergometry for spinal cord injured subjects. Arch Phys Med Rehabil 74:238–241, 1993.

246. Sipski ML, DeLisa JA, Schweer SA: Functional electrical stimulation bicycle ergometry: Patient perceptions. Am J Phys Med Rehabil 68:147–149, 1989.

247. Siri WE: Body composition from fluid spaces and density: Analysis of methods. In Brozek J, Henschel A (eds): Techniques for Measuring Body Composition. Washington, DC, National Academy of Sciences, 1961, pp 223–224.

248. Skinner JS: General principles of exercise prescription. In Skinner JS (ed): Exercise Testing and Exercise Prescription for Special Cases: Theoretical Basis and Clinical Application. Philadelphia, Lea & Febiger, 1993, pp. 29–40.

249. Spungen AM, Bauman WA, Wang J, Pierson RN: Measurement of body fat in individuals with tetraplegia: A comparison of eight clinical methods. Paraplegia 33:402–408, 1995.

250. Spungen AM, Bauman WA, Wang J, Pierson RN: Reduced quality of fat free mass in paraplegia. Clin Res 40:280A, 1992.

251. Subbarao JV, Klopfstein J, Turpin R: Prevalence and impact of wrist and shoulder pain in patients with spinal cord injury. J Spinal Cord Med 18:9–13, 1995.
252. Szczypaczewska M, Nazar K, Kaciuba-Uscilko H: Glucose tolerance and insulin response to glucose load in body builders. Int J Sports Med 10:34–47, 1989.
253. Twist DJ, Culpepper-Morgan JA, Ragnarsson KT, et al: Neuroendocrine changes during functional electrical stimulation. Am J Phys Med Rehabil 71:156–163, 1992.
254. Ugalde V, Litwiller SE, Gater DR: Bladder and bowel anatomy for the physiatrist. Phys Med Rehabil State Art Rev 10:547–568, 1996.
255. Van Der Woude LHV, Veger HEJ, Rozendal RH, et al: Wheelchair racing: Effects of rim diameter and speed on physiology and technique. Med Sci Sports Exerc 20:492–500, 1988.
256. Van Loan MD, McCluer S, Loftin JM, Boileau RA: Comparisons of physiological responses to maximal arm exercise among able-bodied, paraplegics, and quadriplegics. Paraplegia 25:397–405, 1987.
257. Vaziri ND, Pandian MR, Segal JL, et al: Vitamin D, parathormone, and calcitonin profiles in persons with long-standing spinal cord injury. Arch Phys Med Rehabil 75:766–769, 1994.
258. Vinet A, Bernard PL, Poulain M, et al: Validation of an incremental field test for the direct assessment of peak oxygen uptake in wheelchair-dependent athletes. Spinal Cord 34:288–293, 1996.
259. Walker J, Cooney M, Norton S: Improved pulmonary function in chronic quadriplegics after pulmonary therapy and arm ergometry. Paraplegia 27:278–283, 1989.
260. Walker WC, Khokhar MS: Silent cardiac ischemia in cervical spinal cord injury: Case study. Arch Phys Med Rehabil 73:91–94, 1992.
261. Wallin BG, Stjernberg L: Sympathetic activity in man after spinal cord injury: Outflow to skin below the lesion. Brain 107:183–198, 1984.
262. Ward SA: Peripheral and central chemoreceptor control of ventilation during exercise in humans. Can J Appl Physiol 19:305–333, 1994.
263. Waring WP, Maynard FM: Shoulder pain in acute traumatic quadriplegia. Paraplegia 29:37–42, 1991.
264. Wheeler G, Cumming D, Burnham R, et al: Testosterone, cortisol and catecholamine responses to exercise stress and autonomic dysreflexia in elite quadriplegic athletes. Paraplegia 32:292–299, 1994.
265. Wheeler GD, Ashley EA, Harber V, et al: Hormonal responses to graded-resistance, FES-assisted strength training in spinal cord-injured. Spinal Cord 34:264–267, 1996.
266. Whipp BJ: Peripheral chemoreceptor control of exercise hyperepnea in humans. Med Sci Sports Exerc 26:337–347, 1994.
267. Whiteneck GG, Carter RE, Charlifue SW, et al: A Collaborative Study of High Quadriplegia. Englewood, CO, Rocky Mountain Regional Spinal Cord Injury System, 1985.
268. Whiting RB, Dreisinger TE, Dalton RB, Londeree BR: Improved physical fitness and work capacity in quadriplegics by wheelchair exercise. J Card Rehabil 3:251–255, 1983.
269. Wicks JR, Lymburner K, Dinsdale SM, Jones NL: The use of multistage exercise testing with wheelchair ergometry and arm cranking in subjects with spinal cord lesions. Paraplegia 15:252–261, 1977–78.
270. Wicks JR, Oldridge NB, Cameron BJ, Jones NL: Arm cranking an wheelchair ergometry in elite spinal cord-injured athletes. Med Sci Sports Exerc 15:224–231, 1983.
271. Wilde SW, Miles DS, Durbin RJ, et al: Evaluation of myocardial performance during wheelchair ergometer exercise. Am J Phys Med 60:277–291, 1981.
272. Wilmet E, Ismail AA, Heilporn A, et al: Longitudinal study of the bone mineral content and of soft tissue composition after spinal cord section. Paraplegia 33:674–677, 1995.
273. Winslow EBJ, Lesch M, Talano JV, Meyer PR: Spinal cord injuries associated with cardiopulmonary complications. Spine 11:809–812, 1986.
274. Wolff J: Das Gesetz der Transformation der Knochen. Berlin, Ahirshwald, 1892.
275. Wylie EJ, Chakera TMH: Degenerative joint abnormalities in patients with paraplegia of duration greater than 20 years. Paraplegia 26:101–106, 1988.
276. Yarkony GM, Heinemann AW: Pressure ulcers. In Stover SL, DeLisa JA, Whiteneck GG (eds): Spinal Cord Injury: Clinical Outcomes from the Model Systems. Gaithersburg, MD, Aspen Publishers, 1995, pp 100–119.

277. Yarkony GM, Roth EJ, Cybulski G, Jaeger RJ: Neuromuscular stimulation in spinal cord injury: I: Restoration of functional movement of the extremities. Arch Phys Med Rehabil 73:78–86, 1992.
278. Yekutiel M, Brooks M, Ohry A, et al: The prevalence of hypertension, ischaemic heart disease and diabetes in traumatic spinal cord injured patients and amputees. Paraplegia 27:58–62, 1989.
279. Yki-Jarvinen H, Koivisto VA, Taskinen M, Nikkila EA: Glucose tolerance, plasma lipoproteins and tissue lipoprotein lipase activities in body builders. Eur J Appl Physiol Occup Med 53:253–259, 1984.
280. Young RR: Spasticity: A review. Neurology 44(suppl 9):S12–S20, 1994.
281. Zhong Y-G, Levy E, Bauman WA: The relationships among serum uric acid, plasma insulin, and serum lipoprotein levels in subjects with spinal cord injury. Horm Metab Res 27:283–286, 1995.

DENISE I. CAMPAGNOLO MD, MS

JOHN A. HORTON III, MD

12

Rehabilitation Prescription for the Paraplegic

Spinal cord injury (SCI) remains among the list of medical conditions that are not curable. Today a person who becomes a paraplegic at age 20 lives to an average age of 62, only 15 years less than the general population.[15] With increased life expectancy, the focus of the rehabilitation process has shifted from increasing survival to improving quality of life and maximizing independence.[32]

Throughout this chapter, the American Spinal Injury Association (ASIA) standards for neurologic classification of spinal cord injury are used.[2] Most recently updated in 1996, these standards provide uniform nomenclature surrounding level and completeness of injury. By definition paraplegia results from injury to the spinal cord in the thoracic, lumbar, or sacral segments, including the conus medullaris and cauda equina. There is involvement of the trunk, legs, and pelvic organs. The paraplegic injured at the highest level, T1, has arm and hand function intact.

Every therapy prescription should include the time and frequency of therapy plus the diagnosis, precautions, and goals. The diagnosis allows the health care team to begin to formulate expectations for recovery and to customize the therapy to the injury. For example, a patient who is a T2 ASIA A paraplegic has significantly different goals and potential medical complications than those of an L5 ASIA C paraplegic.

Precautions (Table 1) ensure that the rehabilitation team is aware of limitations that the patient must follow to ensure safety in the rehabilitation setting. This portion of the prescription also advises the health care team of any significant comorbidity that may have an impact on the rehabilitation stay.

Goals are initially assigned by the physiatrist and are formulated based on numerous factors, including level of injury, completeness of injury, patient age, premorbid level of activity and function, cognitive status, existing comorbidity, preexisting psychiatric dysfunction, patient motivation, social support systems, and other mitigating issues pertinent to the patient. Delineating these goals at the beginning of the prescription allows all of the members of the interdisciplinary team to focus on these objectives. As the team becomes more familiar with the patient and as the patient progresses with therapy, the initial goals will be modified. Patient care/family care

---

TABLE 1. Common Precautions that Need to be Written on the Therapy Prescription for Paraplegic Patients

Orthopedic	Medical	Neurologic

Limb weightbearing status:
  Nonweightbearing
  Partial weightbearing
  Weightbearing as tolerated
Spinal instability/Spinal orthotic
Mobilize within specific range:
  Hip flexion no greater than
    90° to avoid changing
    alignment of lumbosacral
    spine
	Autonomic dysreflexia (T6 and above)
	  (with maximum and minimum
	  systolic and diastolic pressures
	  specified)
	Cardiac (with maximum heart rate
	  or MET level specified)
	Respiratory (minimum O_2 saturation,
	  O_2 requirement specified)
	Diabetes
	Skin
	Bleeding (for patients on anticoagulation)
	One-on-one supervision
		Seizure
		Dysphagia
		Dysarthria
		Ataxia
		Safety

---

interdisciplinary conferences can be held as a way to reassess and communicate any new goals.

ACUTE CARE REHABILITATION PRESCRIPTION

The goal of the acute care rehabilitation prescription is to prevent medical complications and to prepare the patient for the acute rehabilitation or home program. The role of the physiatrist in the acute hospital setting is either one of a consultant or, less commonly, the primary caregiver. One of the roles of the physiatrist in the acute care hospital is educating other health care professionals and physicians as to the unique medical needs of the SCI patient. The physiatrist must make sure that other physicians are aware of the recent advances in the use of methylprednisolone in the first hours of the acute injury[8] as well as the need for deep venous thrombosis prophylaxis.[14] The physiatrist makes recommendations concerning starting a bowel and bladder program at appropriate times in the acute care hospitalization. He or she will orchestrate the maintenance of range of motion and the start of a sitting program for the acutely injured patient. Often the physiatrist spends the most time educating the patient and families about their devastating injury and living with the injury. It is often the physiatrist who recognizes concomitant brain injuries in these patients and how it will affect rehabilitation of the SCI. Table 2 lists problems typically addressed by the physiatrist in the acute care setting.

PHYSICAL THERAPY PRESCRIPTION

The physical therapist (PT) should be involved in the patient's care from the first day of hospitalization. The PT's prescription (Table 3) should include maintenance of joint

TABLE 2. Paraplegia: Acute Care Physiatric Consultation Guidelines

Neurology:	Detailed neurologic exam (American Spinal Injury Association standards)
	Methylprednisolone with 3–8 hours of injury if not contraindicated[8]
	Assess for associated traumatic brain injury
Immobilization:	Clear uninvolved spine as soon as possible; air mattress as soon as possible
	Prophylaxis for heterotopic ossification (hip/knee/shoulder/elbow)
Bowel/GI:	Decompress ileus if present
	NPO until bowel sounds
	Nutrition consult
	H_2 antagonist therapy
	Guaiac stools
	Bowel program when taking PO:
	1 docusate sodium tid; 2 senna tablets AM; 1 bisacodyl suppository after dinner
Bladder:	Foley catheter while in spinal shock
	IC program: when no IVs, PO (<800 ml/shift and if patient is of the level to
	do his own ICs)
	Goal: each IC <400 ml
	Fluid restrict 2 L/day if needed
	Balanced bladder-postvoiding residuals <100ml
Lungs:	Positive pressure ventilation; manual and mechanical assisted cough[4]
	Incentive spirometry, follow vital capacity
Extremities:	Resting splint-flaccid; flexion tone reduction splint with tone; functional hand splint
	Deep vein thrombosis (pneumatic compressive boots and antiembolism stockings;
	enoxaparin 30 mg q12 h)
	Spasticity: baclofen; Contractures: (ranging; dynamic splinting)
	Protective boots for ankle dorsiflexion and heel pressure relief
	Routine toe nail care, examine feet and total body skin each day
Skin:	Air mattress or specialty bed, reposition patient at least every 2h
Heart:	Monitor for bradycardia
	Neurogenic hypotension (use vasopressors)
	Monitor for autonomic dysreflexia when out of spinal shock
Metabolism:	Monitor CA^{++} levels. Monitor for anemia
Psychiatry/psy- chology referral:	Adjustment to disability, therapy as appropriate for depression
Temperature:	Monitor temperature each shift
Pain:	Neurogenic pain: low-dose tricyclics; Tegretol; modalities
Discharge planning:	Work with social services; family training, disposition; home aids
Rehabilitation:	Initiate all therapies

range of motion by passive range through full arc at least three repetitions, twice daily (b.i.d.) for paralyzed limbs.[9,20] For joints in which contracture has begun, it is critical to maintain sustained terminal stretch for 20–30 minutes at least b.i.d., concentrating on muscles that cross two joints, such as the gastrocnemius and tensor fascia lata.[26,35] It is important for the patient to lie prone, if possible, to stretch the hip joints. Range

TABLE 3. Example of a Physical Therapy Prescription for Paraplegic Patients

Passive range of motion; maintenance; put paralyzed limbs/joints through full range of motion three times b.i.d.

For contracture, sustained terminal stretch 20–30 min. b.i.d. concentrating on 2-joint muscles; gastroc/soleus heel cord stretching

Active assistive range of motion to active range of motion; progressive resistive exercise to weak muscles

Desensitization for dysesthesias, neurogenic pain

Isokinetic/isometric/isotonic progressive strengthening exercises; progressive resistive exercise to all major muscle groups of upper and lower extremities

Tilt table: progress as needed to improve lower extremity standing tolerance, endurance, and heel cord stretching

Mat mobility: rolling, supine to sit, short and long sitting, static and dynamic sitting balance

Teach pressure-relieving skills, weight shifts in sitting and supine

Transfer training under supervision from mat to chair and chair to all surfaces and floor

Progress to independent transfers as patient improves

Wheelchair mobility skills and parts management: advance to high-level wheelchair skills, including ramps, curbs, safe falling, and arising from fall

Ambulation trial under supervision, beginning with parallel bars for weight shifting; advance to independent ambulation as patient improves with appropriate assistive devices and bracing

Elevations as patient improves

Pulmonary care: chest percussion and postural drainage and manual assisted coughs; progressive resistive exercise to diaphragm with resistive tubing

Deep breathing exercises with 2-lb weight and progress as tolerated

Teach patient to instruct others in care and transfers

Family education and training

Home exercise program

---

of motion is best followed by serial goniometry testing. Isokinetic, isometric, and isotonic progressive strengthening exercises can be begun for upper extremities and spared muscles in the lower extremities. For patients with neuropathic pain, desensitization techniques such as rubbing can be used to reduce pain. The tilt table can be used acutely and is excellent for heel cord stretching and, for incomplete paraplegics who are ambulatory candidates, to improve standing tolerance and endurance. For complete paraplegics, weightbearing on the tilt table may have the added benefit of preventing bone mineral loss. An orthotic should be provided that keeps the ankle dorsiflexed to avoid plantar flexion contracture. Once the thoracolumbar spine has been stabilized or stability has been confirmed, manual assisted coughing should be performed by all caregivers and taught to family members.[9] Mat mobility, including rolling, going from the supine position to sitting, short and long sitting, and static dynamic sitting balance, should be prescribed as soon as the patient can get out of bed and be transported to the physical therapy gym. Teaching the patient and caregivers pressure-relieving skills, such as weight shifts in sitting and the supine position, is essential for the prevention of pressure ulcer formation.[28] Transfer training under supervision from mat to wheelchair and chair to all surfaces, including the floor, should be begun in the acute care hospital and continued in the rehabilitation setting. Wheelchair mobility skills and parts management should be prescribed. Advancement to high-level wheelchair skills, including negotiating ramps and curbs, safe falling, and arising from fall, should be accomplished as the patient gains strength and proficiency. A trial of ambulation under supervision begins with parallel bars for weight shifting and advances to independent walking as the patient improves with appropriate assistive device(s) and bracing. Elevations such as stairs, curbs, and ramps are usually not mastered in the acute care hospital.

The physical therapist must work on pulmonary care with chest percussion, postural drainage, and manual assisted coughing.[9] This is especially important for paraplegics whose level of injury leaves abdominal muscles, and thus the ability to cough, weakened. Progressive resistive exercise to the inspiratory muscles can be provided with resistive tubing and deep breathing exercises with 2-pound weights on the abdomen and progress with increasing weight as tolerated. It is important for all caregivers to teach the patient to instruct others in his care and proper transfer methods. It is critical, even in the acute care hospital, to begin family education and training.

OCCUPATIONAL THERAPY PRESCRIPTION

As soon as the patient is able to be brought to the occupational therapy area, activities of daily living (ADL) skills such as grooming, dressing, bathing, feeding, and homemaking skills should be practiced. Due to equipment limitations in the acute care hospital, functional transfer training is usually difficult. Wheelchairs with removable armrests typically are not available, necessitating transfer boards. Splinting of the upper extremities is usually only needed for paraplegics with concomitant peripheral nerve injuries or burns. Upper extremity strengthening to all muscle groups should be emphasized, as should activities to improve coordination and fine motor control skills. Evaluation for ADL equipment and proper wheelchair prescription is usually reserved for the inpatient rehabilitation setting unless the paraplegic patient is due to be discharged to home from the acute care hospital. Teaching pressure relief skills, how to instruct others to assist ADLs and transfers, and family training all begin in the acute hospital. Table 4 provides an example of an occupational therapy prescription for paraplegic patients.

SPEECH THERAPY PRESCRIPTION

The speech and language pathologist is usually not needed for paraplegic patients unless there is a concomitant traumatic brain injury or tracheostomy.

NURSING

The nursing staff is instrumental in educating the patient in the practicalities of self care. Specific areas that need nursing support include bowel and bladder management and skin care.

TABLE 4. Example of an Occupational Therapy Prescription for Paraplegic Patients

---

Functional transfers; splinting as appropriate
Upper extremity strengthening to all muscle groups, including hand intrinsics
Improve coordination skills and fine motor control skills
Work on writing and desk skills
Evaluate for equipment needed for activities of daily living (ADLs)
Wheelchair evaluation
Work on self-care skills, including dressing, bathing, feeding, and homemaking skills
As patient improves, home evaluation, driver evaluation and training
Teach pressure relieving skills
Teach patient how to instruct others to assist ADLs and transfers
Family education and training and home exercise program

The ultimate goal of a bowel program is to achieve adequate elimination (once per day or every other day) with intervening continence. The initial prescription can start out with a so-called "3-2-1" regimen of three stool softeners daily, two senna tablet stimulants orally in the morning, and one bisacodyl suppository or digital rectal stimulation in the evening.[17,37] This regimen can then be customized to provide the desired bowel regimen. The paraplegic patient is anticipated to be able to independently manage this regimen and accommodate for changes in diet and circumstances. To achieve this goal, nursing education concerning mechanisms of drug action and the technique of digital rectal stimulation are essential.

The health care team must instruct the paraplegic patient in independent bladder management. Overall goals for bladder management include continence, low postvoid residual urine volumes, and low voiding volumes/pressures. The nursing staff serves an essential role teaching patients about management goals, techniques to achieve these goals, and maintenance of clean techniques for the procedure. This education and the refinement of techniques is essential to the patient's long-term survival.

As an easily preventable cause of significant morbidity, pressure ulcers are foremost on the list of items that the nursing staff addresses.[39] In addition to ensuring that the patient is repositioned every 2 hours while in bed, the nursing staff also ensures that the patient understands the requirement for frequent weight shifts when in a seated position.[24,25] Knowledge of the pathophysiology behind the formation of these lesions is essential for the patient to be able to adequately manage their skin, and the nursing staff is a key source of this information.

MEDICAL SOCIAL WORK

Involvement of the medical social worker is essential during acute hospitalization. Discharge planning is begun as soon as possible with referral to appropriate rehabilitation facilities as needed. The social worker is instrumental in family education and counseling with respect to community resources available to the patient.

PSYCHOLOGY

The services of the psychologist are essential in helping the patient come to grips with living life as a paraplegic. Becoming comfortable in public places, developing confidence that independence can be achieved, role adjustment, family acceptance, and support are topics that the therapist should address in the formalized therapy prescription.

ACUTE INPATIENT AND OUTPATIENT REHABILITATION

THE PHYSIATRIST

The role of the physiatrist in the acute impatient rehabilitation setting is to medically manage the patient, prevent medical complications of the injury (e.g., decubitus ulcer, pneumonia, bowel and bladder dysfunction) and facilitate the patient's recovery and rehabilitation. With allowed lengths of stay in acute care settings and with "uncomplicated" SCIs, it is possible for acute rehabilitation admission to begin as soon as 3–5 days after initial injury. The physiatrist must be well trained in the unique problems and management of the SCI patient and be competent in the management of general medical issues to adequately care for these patients.

Another role of the physiatrist is as the leader of the interdisciplinary team caring for the patient. Upon admission to an acute rehabilitation facility, the physiatrist is responsible for establishing a rehabilitation prescription to ensure that all health professionals are coordinated in their efforts to accomplish the identified goals and to ensure that all providers are aware of medical precautions applicable to the patient.

The physiatrist is the key educator for both the patient and the family. Coordinating team conferences, interpreting test results and progress reports, and providing realistic pictures regarding expected recovery and requirements for future care are essential areas for education. This requires the physician to solicit areas of current concern as well as address issues that will significantly affect life once the acute situation has been addressed (e.g., return to work, sexual activities, fertility). Conveying accurate and timely information to the family and patient should provide a realistic picture of expected recovery while maintaining hope and optimism for future quality of life.

In the outpatient rehabilitation setting, the physiatrist can be the primary care provider. The physiatrist typically monitors bladder management, the bowel program, spasticity control, sexuality, infertility, depression, skin management, equipment prescription, autonomic dysreflexia management, and pain control. The physiatrist is often a referral source for the plastic surgeon, urologist, marriage counselor, psychologist, reproductive endocrinologist, orthopedist, neurosurgeon, and others as required.

MEDICAL SOCIAL WORK

During the inpatient rehabilitation stay, the medical social worker is responsible for the ultimate disposition for the patient. Items such as home modification requirements, need for assistance at home, visiting nursing services, and health insurance coverage are analyzed to provide for a safe discharge plan. As in the acute care setting, patient and family training concerning community resources is critical. The role of the medical social worker begins in the preadmission approval stages and continues until discharge.

PHYSICAL THERAPY

The physical therapy prescription in the acute rehabilitation setting and then in the outpatient setting is a continuum of the program that was used in acute care. More progress and more proficiency is achieved by the patient. Ambulation training should be offered to any interested paraplegic and is generally attempted in the later stages of a therapeutic program. Varying degrees of ambulation can be expected in the paraplegic, and this is directly related to the level of injury. Degrees of ambulation include the following:

1. Therapeutic ambulation for exercise only; generally used at the T1-10 levels, with the differences being in the level of assistance and prosthetic requirement. The T1 paraplegic patient will require assistance from a caregiver to ambulate and will be limited to ambulation within parallel bars. The T2-10 paraplegic may not require assistance and will use a bilateral knee-ankle-foot orthosis (KAFO) and a walker or Lofstrand crutches.[36]

2. Functional ambulation (household distances, but uses wheelchair for outside the home). Paraplegics with levels at T11-L2 should be able to achieve this goal depending on motivation and physical condition. Patients will use KAFOs or a combination of KAFO and ankle-foot orthosis (AFO) with Lofstrand crutches.[36]

3. Community ambulation (independent in ambulation greater than 150 feet and generally does not use a wheelchair). Paraplegics with L3 level and below are anticipated to obtain this high level of function. They will require AFOs generally and will use Lofstrand crutches or canes.[21]

FUNCTIONAL ELECTRICAL STIMULATION AMBULATION THERAPY

Functional electrical stimulation (FES) driven ambulation devices have been available since the introduction of the ParaWalker[30,31] in the early 1980s and the ParaStep in 1989.[13] These systems are used in the T4-12 paraplegic patient who has less than 10° of hip or knee contracture and full range in the ankles.[11] Successful standing can be achieved by most patients (92%), but ambulation without assistance was achieved in only 34% in one study.[12] Patients who achieved functional ambulation were able to ambulate an average of 324 feet.[12] Other patient characteristics include good upper extremity strength, being at least 14 years old, intact skin, upper motor neuron injury only, insensate in the areas of stimulation, and independence in transfers. Contraindications include significant osteoporosis, cardiovascular or pulmonary insufficiency, seizure disorder, morbid obesity, pregnancy, autonomic dysreflexia, and a phrenic or cardiac pacemaker.[11–13] In addition to increased mobility, the benefits of this therapy include an improved self image and increased muscle bulk, which may be more important than the mobility issues for some patients.[13]

COMMON REPETITIVE USE INJURIES IN THE PARAPLEGIC

The use of the upper extremities for weightbearing and propulsion makes paraplegics prone to repetitive use types of injuries. This process is accelerated in wheelchair athletes.[3] Common overuse syndromes and some suggestions for preventive prescriptions are provided below.

1. Carpal tunnel syndrome. This syndrome is quite common in wheelchair users and is attributable to the repetitive trauma sustained in contacting the wrist and push rim. There is a higher incidence in paraplegics than in the general population.[1,19] Preventive measures include the use of padded gloves, modification of propulsion technique to limit wrist hyperextension, and the avoidance of striking of the heel of the hand to effect propulsion.

2. Shoulder impingement. Some studies have cited an incidence of 24–26%.[6,10] Shoulder impingement is caused by the upward migration of the humeral head, causing impingement of the supraspinatus tendon. This phenomenon results from a combination of the shoulder's reliance on soft tissue and muscular stabilization and muscular imbalances, which are prone to occur as a result of the demands of wheelchair propulsion.[3] Preventive measures include a program of strengthening to include rotator cuff musculature as well as scapular stabilizers. It is also important to include stretching of shoulder flexors, internal rotators, and adductors, which tend to hypertrophy with the normal propulsive stroke.

3. Bicipital Tendinitis. This condition is rarely seen in isolation and generally occurs as a result of an impingement syndrome.[29] Therefore, use of the strategies described for impingement should prevent this condition.

4. Lateral epicondylitis. This overuse syndrome is a result of wrist extensor muscle activities causing inflammation in the tendon. It occurs in paraplegics when the push phase is finished in hyperpronation and ulnar deviation. The obvious prevention is to modify the terminal phase of push to ensure that the wrist and forearm are held in neutral or slightly supinated positions.[3]

5. Ulnar neuropathy at the elbow. This is the second most prevalent upper limb entrapment in paraplegics.[10] Different theories exist as to the reason for this syndrome, including possible entrapment between the heads of the flexor carpi ulnaris, increased pressures in the cubital tunnel as a result of repeated flexion and extension of the elbow, or direct pressure to the ulnar nerve due to resting the arm on armrests.[3] Preventive measures include the use of elbow pads, stretching of the elbow joint to ensure full range of motion, and a strengthening program of the forearm flexors and extensors to ensure proper biomechanical balance at the joint.

OCCUPATIONAL THERAPY

In the acute rehabilitation and chronic rehabilitation of paraplegic patients, the role and thus the prescription for the occupational therapist is not appreciably different than that found in the acute care setting. Adaptive equipment, proper wheelchair prescription, and higher level functional transfers are emphasized in this setting. Gaining efficiency and proficiency in these tasks is the desired outcome.

RECREATION AND WHEELCHAIR SPORTS

The demographics of SCI create a significant population of young men and women who classically are involved in competitive and recreational sports activities. Recreational therapists are essential in encouraging these patients to resume their public activities. Activities such as going to the mall, movies, restaurants, sporting events, or concerts all begin the process of community reintegration. As patients become adapted to their new living environment, participation in sporting activities may begin.

The National Wheelchair Athletic Association and the National Wheelchair Basketball Association have established classification systems for persons with spinal cord injuries that allow them to compete against each other equally based on level of injury.[7] At the 1996 Paralympic Games in Atlanta, 3500 elite athletes from 120 countries were involved in 17 events. This is only a small sample of the activities that paraplegic patients can enjoy. Table 5 lists sports and competitions that are available to paraplegics.

DRIVING

The use of an automobile is considered essential in today's society. Paraplegia in itself provides no specific contraindication to driving. About 90–100% of all paraplegics can be expected to pass a driving test in a vehicle that has appropriate modifications.[23,27]

A complete program of driver's training should be used to ensure the safety of the patient as well as fellow drivers. This program consists of three parts, as follow:

1. Predriver evaluation involves evaluating the basic needs for operating a vehicle safely. Items include previous driving history, visual acuity, field of vision, color dis-

---

TABLE 5.   Available Sports and Recreational Activities for Paraplegics

Alpine skiing	Marathon and road racing
Archery	Marksmanship
Automobile road racing	Power lifting
Automobile drag racing	Rowing
Basketball	Rugby
Biking (hand cycling)	Sailing
Billiards	Scuba diving
Bowling	Skydiving
Cross country skiing	Softball
Field events, including discus, javelin, shot put	Swimming
Fishing	Table tennis
Golf	Tennis
Hockey	Track racing
Horseback riding	Trap and skeet shooting
Hunting	Waterskiing
Kayaking	

crimination, depth perception, attention, sequencing, problem solving, reaction time, upper extremity and neck range of motion, transfers in and out of the vehicle with a wheelchair, hand and upper extremity dexterity, and others.[5,33]

2. **Automobile prescription** is essential to obtain the correct car or van. Typical requirements include a roomier vehicle to accommodate a wheelchair, an automatic transmission, and some modification to allow for the use of hand throttle and brake controls.[5,23,27] Table 6 lists needed modifications.

3. **Driver training** may be partly conducted in a simulator, but experience with hand controls in the car itself is essential. Many centers have training vehicles available for patients who have not been able to obtain a vehicle prior to testing. Practice is essential so that the patient can become familiar with the controls, seat belts, transfers, and other components of the vehicle. Only after these items have been mastered can safety be maintained on the road. The in-car testing should include as many driving situations and conditions as possible, including complex grade and terrain challenges. The duration of this training program is unique to the patient and may be as short as 4 hours over two sessions.

VOCATIONAL REHABILITATION

Overall only 13–48% of SCI survivors return to work.[38] The factors affecting return to work are many but have been generalized: paraplegics have higher rates of return to work than do tetraplegics, and patients with incomplete injuries have higher rates than

TABLE 6. Car Characteristics and Modifications for Paraplegics

Car Characteristics	Car Modifications
Automatic transmission	Hand controls for brakes and accelerator
Large enough to accommodate wheelchair behind front seat	(push/pull vs push/twist)
	Spinner knob for steering wheel
Power steering (consider low or zero effort)	Hand dimmer switch (common on today's vehicles)
Power brakes	Emergency brake extension
Accessible seat controls	Extension on turn signal and gear lever
Air conditioning (absolute requirement for SCI patients)	Chest level trunk support for higher thoracic injuries
Power windows, door locks, and mirrors	Transfer board
Cruise control	Additional straps for shutting door, closing trunk
High seat backs	Additional exterior mirrors
Seat no higher than 19 inches above ground	Wheelchair loader (top or inside)—optional
Tilt steering	Cellular phone for emergencies
Seat belts not impeding entry and exit	
Vinyl (leather) rather than cloth seat covers	

those with complete injuries. The younger patients do better, and employment rates increase as years after injury increase. The better educated a person is and the more work experience he or she had preinjury correlates with higher chances of employment. Minorities are less likely to be remployed. Completion of a vocational rehabilitation program makes employment more likely.[16] Referral to a vocational counselor should be made as soon as possible in the rehabilitation hospitalization. The specific areas to be addressed include retraining the SCI survivor, workplace education, recommendations regarding work site modification, and adaptive equipment prescriptions. The vocational counselor often interfaces with insurers or state vocational rehabilitation services.

MAINTENANCE THERAPIES

CARDIOVASCULAR MAINTENANCE

Cardiovascular disease is among a growing list of problems for the long-term survivor of SCI. As a result there is an ever-increasing need for exercise and physical fitness among paraplegics. The symptoms of heart disease may be masked or impaired depending on the level of paraplegia; for example, angina may or may not be perceived or may be misinterpreted and, since exercise is limited, shortness of breath may not be elicited. Lifestyle and activity level leave SCI survivors at high risk, which is often not alterable. The usual means of diagnosing cardiovascular diseases may not be available to the disabled. For example, arm ergometry may not impose enough aerobic exercise challenge due to premature arm fatigue, as is sometimes the case with leg fatigue and a traditional treadmill stress test in an able-bodied person. Also, tests that require varied and rapid body position changes are of limited usefulness in paraplegics.

The goals of the exercise program for paraplegics are to strengthen working musculature, improve cardiovascular capacity, and to prevent fatigue and deconditioning so that ADLs can be performed more efficiently. A full medical evaluation should be done prior to beginning an exercise program. Proper warm-up and cool-down is important to all exercise programs. Stretching and flexibility, especially in the shoulders, is important for wheelchair users. The person should begin the exercise program slowly, and duration should be 20–60 minutes.[3] Paraplegics have shown improvements in fitness levels when engaged in exercise programs using 50–60% of heart rate reserve.[22] Hydration should be maintained with enough oral fluid intake, keeping in mind the limitations the bladder program demands. Variables that should be monitored during the development of an exercise program are heart rate, arterial blood pressure, and, if possible, peak oxygen consumption. Monitoring allows for safe exercise programs and documentation of improvement in fitness.

Handheld or wrist weights can be used for strengthening. The upper limb aerobic exercise modes most commonly used are arm crank ergometry, wheelchair ergometry, and wheelchair propulsion on a treadmill. Arm crank ergometers are commercially available, or a lower limb bicycle can be modified into an arm crank ergometer by mounting it on a table. Wheelchair rollers allow paraplegics to propel long distances indoors for use in inclement weather or where transportation is a problem. If exercise facilities are used, there should be enough padding on the seats of the equipment, and the paraplegic should do frequent skin checks before and after exercise. The aisles in the gym need to be wide enough to accommodate a wheelchair, and a floor covering other than carpet is preferred. Assistants in the gym need to made aware of appropriate action in case of hypotension or autonomic dysreflexia.

Electrical stimulation bicycle ergometry (ESBE) also can be used for exercise and fitness.[34] Oxygen consumption has been noted to increase fourfold in paraplegics with the use of ESBE. The commercially available systems REGYS and ERGYS are manufactured by Therapeutic Technologies Inc. (Fig. 1). In addition, ESBE has the added potential advantages of increasing muscle mass in paralyzed muscles and increasing bone density.[34]

CASE STUDIES

CASE 1

B.J. is a 27-year-old man who was involved in a motor vehicle accident as an unrestrained driver. The accident resulted in a severe comminuted fracture of the T12 vertebral body and T10 level complete paraplegia (ASIA A). Upon admission to an inpatient rehabilitation unit his therapeutic exercise program involved stretching and strengthening all upper extremity muscle groups, with a special emphasis on shoulder girdle stretching (Fig. 2). Isotonic upper extremity strengthening was done using free weights as well as the Universal Gym and Total Gym apparatus. The patient was trained and spent a great deal of time in self range of motion exercise for the lower extremities, especially stretching two-joint muscles such as the rectus femoris, tensor fascia lata, hamstrings, and gastrocnemius. Functional training included mat activities, transfers to all surfaces including floor transfers, and pressure relief skill (Fig. 3). Aerobic exercise was accomplished by upper extremity bicycle ergometry (UBE) (Fig. 4) as well as wheelchair treadmill. As his upper body strength and aerobic conditioning improved, the patient was given a trial of ambulation with bilateral KAFOs within the parallel bars. He was also given a trial of arm crank ergometry.

After discharge to home, the patient continued with an outpatient exercise program with free weights and gym equipment for upper body strength maintenance. He declined continued trials of ambulation due to the expense of the braces and limited function. He continued electrically stimulated bicycle ergometry and UBE for aerobic conditioning. He declined a trial of functional electrical stimulation for ambulation.

CASE 2

T.W. is a 19-year-old man who sustained a gunshot wound to the L3-4 intervertebral space. The bullet went through the spinal canal, leaving bone fragments in the canal, which were removed surgically. This act of violence resulted in T.W. having an incomplete cauda equina syndrome with the following motor profile: his hip flexors bi-

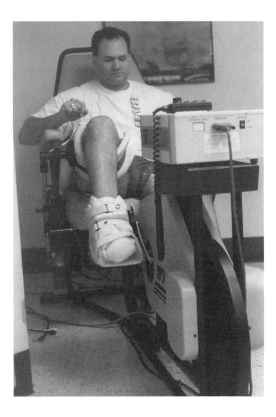

FIGURE 1. *Right and bottom,* Electrical stimulation bicycle ergometry (ESBE) can be used for exercise and fitness, and it has the added potential advantage of increasing muscle mass in paralyzed muscles. The commercially available REGYS and ERGYS systems are manufactured by Therapeutic Technologies Inc. (Tampa, Fla.).

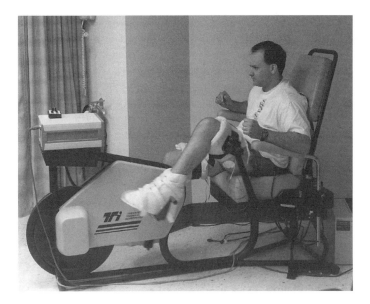

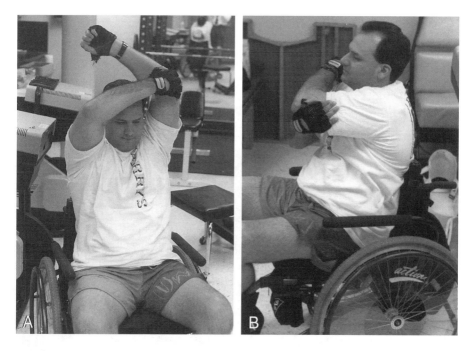

FIGURE 2. Stretching the left latissimus (**A**) and the left posterior deltoid and other shoulder girdle musculature (**B**) prior to exercise.

laterally were 4/5; the right knee extensor was 3/5; the left was 2+/5; the ankle dorsiflexors and plantar flexors were 1/5, as were the knee flexors and hip extensors.

As an inpatient in a rehabilitation hospital initially after his injury, his exercise prescription consisted of stretching and strengthening all upper extremity groups. Special emphasis on shoulder girdle stretching and isotonic upper extremity strengthening was done using free weights as well as the Universal Gym and Total Gym apparatus. He mastered all transfers quickly and became independent in mat activities. Lower limb strengthening was achieved by active full range of motion exercise for the weak muscles (<3/5) as well as a concurrent standing program. Standing was begun in the parallel bars with a KAFO on the left side and an AFO with a solid ankle on the right. Ambulation was progressively worked on for function and conditioning to the point that the patient ambulated independently with bilateral crutches for about 200–250 feet. The patient was discharged to home.

As an outpatient, T.W. continued to work on standing activities and community distance ambulation. He also used swimming for aerobic conditioning. When his left lower extremity strength improved two full grades in all groups, he was instructed on the use of the Universal Gym for quadriceps strengthening. He was given Theraband and strap-on weights for ankle dorsiflexor, plantar flexor, and hamstring strengthening. Hip bridging exercises were used to strengthen his hip extensors. Upon discharge from the out-

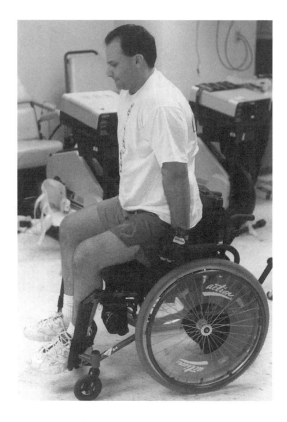

FIGURE 3. A press-up done for ischial pressure relief.

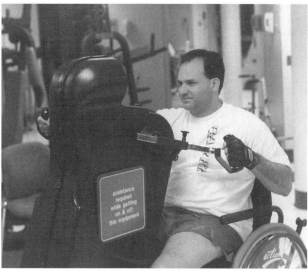

FIGURE 4. Aerobic conditioning with arm crank ergometry.

patient therapy, he no longer required a brace on the right leg for ambulation. His left leg did not improve in strength and still required a KAFO. He was independent in a home exercise program and enjoyed walking long distances for exercise.

CONCLUSION

The rehabilitation prescription for the paraplegic patient starts in the acute care hospital and progresses through the inpatient rehabilitation setting and outpatient/home settings. The various pieces of the prescription are linked to each other and are carried out by the entire rehabilitation team. The goal of the rehabilitation prescription is to avoid the many medical complications of spinal cord injury and provide the SCI survivor with the skills and knowledge needed to attain as much independence as possible. Reintegration into the community and gainful employment is anticipated for every paraplegic who is motivated and has the help of the rehabilitation team.

REFERENCES

1. Aljure J, Eltorai I, Bradley WE, et al: Carpal tunnel syndrome in paraplegic patients. Paraplegia 23:182–186, 1985.
2. American Spinal Injury Association: International Standards for Neurological Classification of Spinal Cord Injury. Chicago, American Spinal Injury Association, 1996.
3. Apple DF, Rayden C, Allen A: Physical Fitness: A Guide for Individuals with Spinal Cord Injury. Baltimore, Veterans Affairs Rehabilitation Research and Development Service, 1996.
4. Bach JR: Rehabilitation of the patient with respiratory dysfunction. In DeLisa JA (ed): Rehabilitation Medicine: Principles and Practice, 2nd ed. Philadelphia, JB Lippincott, 1993, pp 1099–1110.
5. Bartlow S. Driver's ed: A program for the patient with spinal cord injury. Clin Manage 3(2):6–12, 1983.
6. Bayley JC, Cochran TP, Sledge, CB, et al: The weight bearing shoulder: The impingement syndrome in paraplegics. J Bone Joint Surg 69A:676–678, 1987.
7. Botvin Madorsky JG, Curtis KA: Wheelchair sports medicine. Am J Sports Med 12:128–132, 1984.
8. Bracken MB, Shepard MJ, Holford TR, et al: Administration for methylprednisolone for 24 or 48 hours or tirilazad mesylate for 48 hours in the treatment of acute spinal cord injury. JAMA 277:1597–1604, 1997.
9. Bromley I: Tetraplegia and Paraplegia: A Guide for Physiotherapists. New York, Churchill Livingstone, 1985.
10. Burnham RS, Steadward RD: Upper extremity peripheral nerve entrapments among wheelchair athletes: Prevalence, location and risk factors. Arch Phys Med Rehabil 75:519–524, 1994.
11. Butler PB, Major R: The Para Walker. A rational approach to the provision of reciprocal ambulation for the paraplegic patient. Physiotherapy 73:393–397, 1987.
12. Chaplin E: Functional neuromuscular stimulation for mobility in people with spinal cord injuries. The ParaStep system. J Spinal Cord Med 19:99–105, 1996.
13. Clairborne EG, Baxter KK: Introduction to the Parastep System. Neurol Rep 18(2):11–12, 1994.
14. Consortium for Spinal Cord Medicine: Prevention of Thromboembolism in Spinal Cord Injury. Washington, DC, Paralyzed Veterans of America, 1997.
15. DeVivo MJ, Stover SL: Long-term survival and causes of death. In Stover SL (ed): Spinal Cord Injury Clinical Outcomes from the Model Systems. Gaithersburg MD, Aspen Publishers, 1995, pp 289–313.
16. DeVivo MJ, Rutt RD, Stover SL, Fine PR: Employment after spinal cord injury. Arch Phys Med Rehabil 68:494–498, 1987.
17. Ditunno JF, Formal CS: Chronic spinal cord injury. N Engl J Med 330:550–556, 1994.
18. Gallien P, Brissot R, Eyssette M, et al: Restoration of gait by functional electrical stimulation for spinal cord injured patients. Paraplegia 33:660–664, 1995.

19. Gellman H, Chandler DR., Petrasek J, et al: Carpal tunnel syndrome in paraplegic patients. J Bone Joint Surg 70A:517–519, 1988.
20. Halar EM, Bell KR: Contracture and other deleterious effects of immobility. In DeLisa JA (ed): Rehabilitation Medicine: Principles and Practice, 2nd ed. Philadelphia, JB Lippincott, 1993, pp 668–669.
21. Hussey RW, Stauffer ES: Spinal cord injury: Requirements for ambulation. Arch Phys Med Rehabil 54:544–547, 1973.
22. Jocheim KA, Strohkenal H: The value of particular sports of the wheelchair disabled in maintaining health of the paraplegic. Paraplegia 11:173–178, 1973.
23. Kent H, Sheridan J, Wasko E, June C: A driver training program for the disabled. Arch Phys Med Rehabil 60:273–276, 1979.
24. Kosiak M: Etiology of decubitus ulcers. Arch Phys Med Rehabil 42:19–29, 1961.
25. Kosiak M: Etiology and pathology of ischemic ulcers. Arch Phys Med Rehabil 40:62–69, 1959.
26. Kottke FJ, Pauley DL, Potka RA: The rationale for prolonged stretching for correction for shortening of connective tissue. Arch Phys Med Rehabil 47:345–352, 1966.
27. Long C: The handicapped driver - a national symposium. J Rehabil March/April:34–38, 1974.
28. McLean KP, Jones PP, Skinner JS: Exercise prescription for sitting and supine exercise in subjects with quadriplegia. Med Sci Sports Exerc 27:15–21, 1995.
29. Neer CS: Impingement lesions. Clin Orthop 173:70–77, 1983.
30. Nene AV, Patrick JH: Energy cost of paraplegic locomotion using the ParaWalker-electrical stimulation "hybrid" orthosis. Arch Phys Med Rehabil 71:116–120, 1990.
31. Nene AV, Hermens HJ, Zilvold G: Paraplegic locomotion: A review. Spinal Cord 34:507–524, 1996.
32. Noreau L, Shephard RJ: Spinal cord injury, exercise and quality of life. Sports Med 20:226–250, 1995.
33. Simms B: The assessment of the disabled for driving: A preliminary report. Int Rehabil Med 7:187–192, 1985.
34. Sipski ML, DeLisa JA: Functional electrical stimulation in spinal cord injury rehabilitation: A review of the literature. NeuroRehabil 1:46–57, 1991.
35. Spector SA, Simard CP, Fournier SM, et al: Architectural alterations of rat hind limb skeletal muscle immobilized at different lengths. Exp Neurol 76:94–110, 1982.
36. Staas WE, Formal CS, Gershkoff AM, et al: Rehabilitation of the spinal cord injured patient. In DeLisa JA (ed): Rehabilitation Medicine: Principles and Practice, 2nd ed. Philadelphia, JB Lippincott, 1993, pp 886–915.
37. Stiens SA, Bergman SB, Goetz LL: Neurogenic bowel dysfunction after spinal cord injury: Clinical evaluation and rehabilitative management. Arch Phys Med Rehabil 78(3-S):S86–S102, 1997.
38. Trieschmann RB: Spinal Cord Injuries. Psychological, Social and Vocational Rehabilitation, 2nd ed. New York, Demos, 1988.
39. Yarkony GM, Heinemann AW: Pressure ulcers. In Stover SL (ed): Spinal Cord Injury Clinical Outcomes from the Model Systems. Gaithersburg MD, Aspen Publishers, 1995, pp 100–119.

DAVID D. KILMER, MD

13

Case Studies in Neuromuscular Disease Exercise Prescription

The appropriate prescription of exercise in hereditary and acquired neuromuscular diseases (NMD) has been given little attention by clinicians and researchers. Although there have been exciting advances in the understanding of the genetic basis for hereditary NMD, only a handful of clinical trials exist to determine the type, intensity, and frequency of exercise required to potentially benefit this population. Unfortunately, without available research to draw on, clinicians frequently avoid discussing the potential benefits of exercise with their patients or they recommend the avoidance of strenuous exercise fearing accentuation of weakness. The patient may interpret this advice as a recommendation for a sedentary lifestyle.

Through the use of case studies, this chapter provides the clinician with guidelines for exercise prescription for patients with NMD. Both the acute phase of an acquired NMD and a chronic slowly progressive hereditary NMD are considered because they require very different approaches. Recommendations are based on the available research but contain a bias that, as a group, these patients have the potential to lead more productive and fulfilling lives with regular physical exercise as an important component of gaining some control over their disease.

General principles of exercise prescription for patients with NMD are summarized in Table 1 and are described in more detail below:

1. Graded exercise testing is often difficult in NMD patients due to their low exercise tolerance. Because the intensity of prescribed exercise is quite low, unless there are specific cardiac or pulmonary concerns, routine graded exercise testing is not necessary.

2. Adherence to an exercise program is a major problem, and patients are only likely to continue their exercise program if they are obtaining tangible benefits. Thus, the program must be individualized to the patient's goals, interests, abilities, and financial means. For example, a program that only can be effectively performed at a health club may be unreasonable for a patient on a fixed income without access to private transportation.

TABLE 1.   General Principles of Exercise Prescription in Neuromuscular Disease

---

Routine graded exercise testing is not usually required
Adherence to an exercise program is a major issue
Consider the presence of multisystem disease involvement
Components ideally include muscle strengthening, endurance training, and flexibility
Muscles with less than antigravity strength respond poorly to exercise
The program should be started slowly
Overuse weakness is a concern
Disuse weakness may contribute to reduced strength and endurance
Exercise for enjoyment and socialization is preferred over strict protocols

---

3. Consider the presence of multisystem involvement with the particular NMD. For example, persons with myotonic muscular dystrophy frequently have cardiac conduction defects. Other examples include dysautonomia during the acute phase of Guillain-Barré syndrome and cardiomyopathy with inflammatory myopathy, both of which need to be carefully assessed prior to prescribing exercise.

4. The exercise prescription ideally should include the components of warm-up and cool-down and involve aspects of muscular strengthening, endurance training, and flexibility.

5. Because muscles with less than antigravity strength respond poorly to exercise, specific strengthening programs should focus on areas with greater than 3/5 motor strength by manual muscle testing.

6. Patients with NMD may become easily discouraged if the initial exercise prescription is too intense. The prescribing physician should start the patient slowly. Use of a perceived exertion scale is an effective method to monitor the intensity of training.[8]

7. Overuse weakness, the accentuation of muscle weakness or fatigue following physical activity, is a poorly understood phenomenon but a real concern. However, with appropriate precautions provided with the exercise prescription and physician supervision, nearly all patients may benefit from some level of exercise participation.

8. Disuse weakness may be an important component of the patient's reduced muscular endurance and aerobic capacity in both the acute (due to bed rest) and chronic (due to sedentary lifestyle) NMD patient.

9. Exercise for enjoyment and socialization is preferable to a strictly supervised program. In a rapidly progressive disorder such as Duchenne muscular dystrophy or the acute phase of inflammatory myopathy, close supervision is necessary.

CASE 1: POLYMYOSITIS

PRESENTATION OF CASE

A 42-year-old female homemaker has a 6-month history of weakness, particularly in the hip and shoulder girdle, diagnosed as polymyositis (PM) and confirmed by elevation of creatine phosphokinase (CK), myopathic pattern on EMG, and muscle biopsy demonstrating inflammatory cell infiltration and muscle cell destruction. Physical examination demonstrates 4-/5 strength in the proximal muscle groups with 4+/5 strength distally. There are no joint contractures. Her most current CK is 750 U/ml, vital capacity is 75% predicted, with mild dyspnea on exertion. She is receiving prednisone 50 mg/day. The patient was previously an active jogger and swimmer. She wants to start an exercise program but was advised against it by her previous physician, who told her it would exacerbate her weakness. She can walk only short distances before becoming fatigued, and housework causes aching in her shoulders and hips.

CLINICAL ISSUES

Polymyositis is an idiopathic acquired inflammatory myopathy characterized by the acute or subacute onset of proximal-greater-than-distal muscle weakness; systemic complaints of malaise, fever, and anorexia; and muscle pain to a variable extent. Along with dermatomyositis, it may be associated with an underlying malignancy in 10–20% of cases as well as other collagen vascular diseases. Pathologic findings on muscle biopsy include the presence of muscle fiber destruction and mononuclear inflammatory cell infiltration with elevated release of CK into the blood, reflecting disruption of sarcolemmal structure.

Medical management of PM is primarily performed with immunosuppressive medications, including corticosteroids, methotrexate, cyclophosphamide, and azathioprine. The natural history is variable: PM may have no recurrence after an acute episode, have a relapsing and remitting course, or become a chronic disease.

The use of physical exercise in the rehabilitation of PM has received little attention. Many clinicians tend to be extremely cautious about exercise due to the possibility of exacerbating weakness and inflammation.[11] Rest and gentle range of motion are prescribed, particularly when there is elevation of CK. The presence of myocarditis in the acute phase of the illness is also of great concern.[3] Involvement of the respiratory musculature may lead to restrictive lung disease, with or without evidence of pulmonary parenchymal inflammation or fibrosis.[9,38] In a study of 11 patients with PM, most had impaired exercise performance due to peripheral muscle fatigue rather than pulmonary limitations, although asymptomatic pulmonary hypertension was common.[20]

Hicks and colleagues studied a patient with a 4-year history of active stable PM during an isometric strengthening program of the biceps and quadriceps over 4 weeks.[21] The patient increased strength in both muscle groups without significant elevation of CK. In another study of several inpatients with inflammatory myopathy of 3–10 months duration, periods of resistive and nonresistive exercises were alternated.[15] Improvement in muscle strength was noted without significant increases in serum muscle enzymes.

EXERCISE PRESCRIPTION AND PRECAUTIONS

Recommendations regarding exercise prescription cannot be made with scientific justification based on the literature in PM. However, as Escalante notes, recommendations to avoid exercise during periods of active myositis come from extrapolation from patients with active inflammatory arthropathy, not myopathy.[15] The morbidity associated with disuse, including loss of muscle strength, weight gain, and reduced cardiovascular fitness must be balanced with the risk of exacerbating muscle fiber damage. The clinician should have the interest and tools available to monitor effects of an exercise program. Along with serum muscle enzymes, objective strength assessment is the primary method available to monitor the patient with inflammatory myopathy. Handheld dynamometry is an easily available method of serially measuring muscle strength in patients with reduced muscle strength.[23]

This patient is motivated to start an exercise program primarily to improve strength and endurance to more readily perform physical activities such as walking and housework. Adherence to a prescribed program is not likely to be a problem. In fact, she may be overzealous due to her previous athletic background and, therefore, careful monitoring is essential. She has active PM, requiring caution in exercise prescription. Because of these concerns, a supervised exercise program is advised.

A reasonable prescription is for a general upper and lower extremity resistive exercise program to be performed in a physical therapy gym 2–3 days per week, using a weight that can be easily lifted 10–12 times, slowly increased as tolerated but reduced if there is residual muscle tenderness or fatigue from exercising the previous session. Aerobic exercise should be performed on an alternate day, including slow swimming or walking while maintaining exertion in the moderate range, beginning with a 10-minute session and working up to 30 minutes. Physician monitoring should initially consist of weekly strength assessment and measurement of CK, changing to monthly if there are no untoward effects of the exercise program. Gradually, the program may transition away from being therapist-supervised, but the effects of an exercise program in PM is uncertain enough to warrant a cautious approach.

CASE 2: DUCHENNE MUSCULAR DYSTROPHY

PRESENTATION OF CASE

An 8-year-old boy with Duchenne muscular dystrophy (DMD) presents for comprehensive rehabilitation management. He is ambulatory with accentuated lumbar lordosis and mild toe walking. There are no pulmonary or cardiac symptoms. Weight is at the 90th percentile for height. Physical examination reveals mild range of motion loss in hip extension and ankle dorsiflexion, with tight iliotibial bands. There is fair strength of the hip and shoulder girdle musculature and good strength in more distal muscles. On pulmonary testing, forced vital capacity is 75% predicted. His parents remark that he is quite inactive since they have been told by others that exercise can be dangerous in patients with DMD. A stretching program was instituted several years ago but abandoned due to constant complaints by the child.

CLINICAL ISSUES

Duchenne muscular dystrophy is an inherited X-linked recessive disease of muscle characterized by the absence of dystrophin, a structural protein of the muscle cell membrane.[22] This protein seems to be essential for maintaining the cytoskeletal framework of the muscle fiber during muscle contraction.[14] Boys with DMD have a fairly predictable clinical course, with progressive loss of ambulation during the first decade and wheelchair reliance typically between the ages of 9 and 12. Joint contractures, although present early in the heel cords, hip flexors, and ilotibial bands, generally do not become a problem before age 9, with lower extremity contractures and scoliosis both becoming significant issues after the time of wheelchair reliance.[33] Loss of ambulation appears to be due to progressive weakness rather than joint contractures.[33] During the second decade, the disease progresses relentlessly; the primary concerns become cardiopulmonary complications. Death typically occurs between ages 18 and 25.

Because DMD is the most common childhood neuromuscular disease, there have been more studies related to exercise than with other NMDs. However, exercise intervention studies have focused on resistance training through weight lifting, and such exercise programs lack the additional benefits of exercise during childhood: promoting socialization, building self-esteem, and developing motor skills. Because of the progressive nature of the disease, the children have difficulty participating with their peers in the normal physical activities involved in play and exploration of their environment, often leading to social isolation and lack of social development.[25]

Although studies are difficult to compare due to differences in protocols, methods of strength measurement, and lack of control groups, investigations involving muscle strengthening through resistance exercise have generally shown maintenance of strength or mild strength improvement in DMD during the ambulatory phase.[12,39,44] Evidence of overwork weakness has not been shown with any systematic studies using resistance exercise.

Boys with DMD tend to have poor capacity for endurance-type activities, with higher resting heart rates, low cardiorespiratory capacity, and reduced peripheral oxygen utilization compared to controls.[41] Although they seem to fatigue easily, there may be no differences in intramuscular fatigue and excitation-contraction coupling between boys with DMD and controls.[40] The ability to exercise is limited primarily by muscle weakness rather than defects in oxygen transport and mitochondrial function.

Because definitive studies have not been performed in DMD, investigators advocate a submaximal resistance exercise program concentrating on maintaining strength, peak power, and muscle endurance rather than maximal aerobic capacity.[4,18,45] Since it appears that dystrophin's function is to maintain the structure of the muscle fiber during contraction, there is concern that eccentric contractions, which stress the cytoskeletal elements, may cause particular damage to muscle. This was proposed by Edwards and coworkers before the discovery of the gene defect.[13] Thus, there is theoretical rationale to limit eccentric muscle contractions during resistance exercise training in DMD patients; however, in practice this is difficult without the use of isokinetic dynamometers to isolate one type of contraction.

The most effective exercise prescription in DMD uses activities that combine submaximal muscle contractions and gentle stretching in sports and games that may provide social interaction and boost self-esteem. These children should avoid exercising to the point of exhaustion, and rest periods should be encouraged. Formal weightlifting programs should not be the focus of exercise prescription in DMD.

The choice of exercise depends on the age, mobility level, and interests of the child with DMD. One method is to choose among activities based on the functional level of the child.[25] For example, the child with DMD between ages 5 and 8 is generally ambulatory without aids but is prone to easy fatigue with reduced muscle endurance. Swimming and other water games are ideal activities at this stage to provide resistance and flexibility training in an enjoyable manner. This can be continued into later stages as ambulation is lost, although the child may need flotation devices and a nondisabled partner.

Formal exercise treadmill or ergometry testing is rarely necessary in DMD unless there are specific concerns about pulmonary or cardiac symptoms. Predicted forced vital capacity does not undergo a major decline until after 10 years of age,[33] and electrocardiographic abnormalities, although common in DMD, are not associated with complications until later in the disease.

EXERCISE PRESCRIPTION AND PRECAUTIONS

The 8-year-old boy in this case has fairly stereotypic findings at this stage of the disease. The proximal weakness requires the center of gravity to be placed behind the hip joint and in front of the knee joint for stability. Although mild restrictive lung disease is present, he is asymptomatic.

Prior to providing exercise recommendations, the family needs to clearly understand the role of exercise in the overall development of the child. They should be aware that it will not stop progression of the disease but may improve his muscular endurance, maintain range of motion in a less tedious fashion than a strict stretching program, and improve socialization skills.

However, the patient and family also should be cautioned that exercising to exhaustion is counterproductive and may possibly lead to increased weakness. It may be prudent to monitor strength objectively using handheld dynamometry and CK levels during the first several months of an exercise program to ensure that there is no rapid change in strength or muscle enzyme levels.

The ideal exercise program includes the components of stretching, muscle endurance, and submaximal strengthening activities performed at least 3 days per week. Depending on the child's interests and opportunities, this could involve swimming and water games, single or tandem cycling, and canoeing or rowing with friends or family. A stretching program as part of the warm-up and cool-down phases may be incorporated into participation in the game or sport. Finally, because obesity is a major concern, guidance in proper eating habits and nutritional counseling is advised.[33]

CASE 3: GUILLAIN-BARRÉ SYNDROME

PRESENTATION OF CASE

A 35-year-old stockbroker is admitted to the inpatient rehabilitation unit with the diagnosis of Guillain-Barré syndrome (GBS). He was well until 3 days prior to admission, when he began experiencing malaise and progressive difficulty ambulating. Evaluation on admission revealed greater weakness in distal versus proximal muscles, loss of proprioception in the hands and feet, and elevated protein in the cerebrospinal fluid. Nerve conduction studies performed 2 days after admission demonstrated absent F-waves in multiple nerves but otherwise were normal. Over the first week of hospitalization, his negative inspiratory force was diminished but stable, and he was treated with plasmapheresis.

Two weeks following admission, he was able to sit with moderate assistance and stand with maximal assistance blocking the knees, but quickly became light-headed and tachycardic. Strength in the ankle musculature by manual muscle testing was 0/5, knee flexors and extensors 2/5, and hip extensors 3/5. Upper extremity strength was 1/5 in the hand intrinsics, 2/5 at the wrist, and 3/5 in the elbow and shoulder muscles. Proprioception was absent in the hands and feet.

Prior to this acute illness, the patient played golf two or three times per month but was otherwise sedentary.

CLINICAL ISSUES

Guillain-Barré syndrome is an acute idiopathic inflammatory polyneuropathy characterized by fairly symmetric ascending paralysis and sensory loss. Both plasmapheresis and intravenous immunoglobulin have been demonstrated to improve outcome over placebo in large trials,[36,43] but the role of exercise in rehabilitation has been given little attention. Although major residual disability occurs in only 5–10%, up to 65% of patients have some mild residual disability such as footdrop or persistent distal numbness.[37] Time lost from work or school makes an efficient rehabilitation program vital.

In planning a therapeutic exercise program for the patient with GBS, the untoward effects of bed rest must be considered in addition to the denervating disorder. Research in the effects of altered muscle use differentiate between *decreased use* in muscles receiving normal neural input and capable of contraction and *disuse* in functionally denervated muscle.[29] There may be components of each type in a typical case of GBS.

With decreased use from bed rest, there is a progressive loss of strength in the lower-greater-than-upper extremities and extensors-greater-than-flexors.[7] Although peak torque values may diminish around 20% in the knee extensors with 30 days of disuse, muscle endurance may be affected to an even greater extent. In one study, there were still deficits in force output 7 weeks after the restitution of normal weightbearing.[42] Muscle enzyme concentrations affecting oxygen delivery and utilization by the skeletal muscle are deficient following a period of bed rest with a slow recovery. This corresponds to the common clinical finding in the deconditioned patient of minimal one-repetition strength loss but marked inability to perform functional activities requiring endurance.

In normal subjects, high-intensity intermittent exercise regimens during bed rest may attenuate some effects of deconditioning,[19] but effects are unknown in disease states.

Similar to other neuromuscular disorders, clinicians often worry about the possible effects of overwork in patients with GBS, but the literature contains little helpful information. One brief report noted that several patients worsened with vigorous physical exercise, but then improved with reinstitution of bed rest and limited activity.[6] The author recommended activities geared toward function rather than muscle strengthening exercises. No other reports exist regarding overwork weakness in GBS.

Because no systematic studies of therapy regimens exist with GBS, Ropper recommends that until weakness plateaus, passive range of motion and splinting should be done, and active resistance exercise begun during the plateau and recovery phases.[37] In the chronic phase, a patient with mild residual distal weakness 3 years after an acute bout of GBS demonstrated improvement in total work capacity and isokinetic leg strength with an aerobic exercise program.[35]

EXERCISE PRESCRIPTION AND PRECAUTIONS

The patient plateaued in his strength loss but demonstrated the effects of prolonged bed rest upon assuming the upright posture. Dysautonomia is also possible with GBS but less likely in this case without other symptoms. The patient's proximal weakness could result from his neuropathy or the effects of decreased use, but the former is probably the predominant pathology due to the relatively short period of bed rest (2 weeks) compared to the extent of weakness.

The role of exercise in his therapy prescription is to hasten return of muscular strength and endurance while minimizing the possibility of overwork weakness. Although the safest program may be to avoid strengthening exercise altogether and focus on functional activities, the inpatient status with daily careful supervision may allow a more aggressive approach.

The physician should consider including submaximal strengthening exercises during rehabilitation therapy, focusing on improving endurance with functional activities. A low-resistance regimen 3 days per week using elastic resistance bands looped around the extremity may be used initially. The rehabilitation team should monitor closely for evidence of overwork by noting symptoms of muscle aching, increased weakness, or fatigue the morning following therapy. Serial serum CK measurement may be helpful and the intensity of the regimen reduced if any rise is noted.

Although the major focus of his rehabilitation program should be on functional activities such as standing, transfer training, and activities of daily living, gradual inclusion of resistance and aerobic exercise several days per week with careful monitoring can be done as therapy progresses. Resistance training should be in muscle groups with at least 4/5 strength, being careful not to neglect muscle groups with "normal" strength on manual muscle testing due to the known inability to detect significant strength deficits using this measurement approach[5] and reduced muscle endurance from bed rest. An ideal medium for improving both muscular endurance and aerobic capacity is the therapeutic pool, supporting the weakened muscle groups and providing resistance for strengthening.

CASE 4: HEREDITARY MOTOR AND SENSORY NEUROPATHY, TYPE 1

CASE PRESENTATION

A 51-year-old woman with hereditary motor and sensory neuropathy, type 1 (HMSN), also called Charcot-Marie Tooth disease, is evaluated for rehabilitation needs. She first noted difficulty with running and jumping in early adolescence and was diagnosed with HMSN at age 15 due to a strong family history of HMSN. Functionally, the patient is independent with activities of daily living although fine motor tasks are quite difficult and she is having increasing difficulty gripping objects. Ankle-foot orthoses (AFOs) are needed for ambulation due to distal weakness in the lower extremities, and walking beyond the household level causes fatigue. The patient receives disability income and is sedentary most days in her home; in the past she enjoyed gardening and strolling in the neighborhood.

Physical examination reveals a mildly obese woman with normal cardiac and pulmonary examinations. Marked distal atrophy is present in the extremities; no contractures are noted. Motor strength is judged at 2/5 in the ankle dorsi- and plantar flexors, 4/5 at the knees and hips, with 3/5 grip strength and 4+/5 strength in the elbow and shoulder musculature. Sensation is absent to pin up to the midcalf level and to the wrists in the upper extremities. She ambulates using the AFOs without other assistive devices.

CLINICAL ISSUES

Hereditary motor and sensory neuropathy, type 1, is the most common hereditary peripheral neuropathy, inherited in an autosomal-dominant pattern. It is characterized by markedly reduced conduction velocities in both motor and sensory nerves due to demyelination. With advances in molecular genetics, several subtypes have been identified with similar clinical presentation.[10]

Although there is heterogeneous presentation and course, weakness generally progresses slowly in a distal-to-proximal fashion with onset of weakness first usually noted in the second decade. However, quantitative strength testing demonstrates significant weakness in proximal as well as distal musculature, which may not be detected with manual muscle testing.[10,30] This weakness may be due to the disease itself or could be a result of the effects of disuse. Pulmonary and cardiac abnormalities are uncommon, although patients frequently have reduced aerobic capacity.[10] As the patient ages, ambulation may become more difficult. A wheelchair or scooter may be needed for mobility in more severe cases.

Due to the relative rarity of the disease, most exercise intervention studies have combined HMSN with other slowly progressive neuromuscular diseases. A 12-week moderate resistance exercise program including 8 subjects with HMSN that used moderate (<40% one-repetitive maximum knee extension, <20% one-repetitive maximum elbow flexion) weight lifting demonstrated significant strength gains.[2] In a similar population, a higher resistance protocol did not improve strength gains over the lighter resistance program.[24] A recent randomized 24-week proximal lower extremity strengthening trial including 29 HMSN subjects reported moderate improvements in strength and leg-related functional performance.[31] Other strength intervention studies in slowly progressive neuromuscular diseases demonstrated modest improvements in strength, but they did not include subjects with HMSN.[32,34,44] Interestingly, no studies have found evidence of overwork weakness in HMSN patients in both closely supervised and home-based programs.

Limited work has been done regarding the effects of endurance training in HMSN. A 12-week cycle ergometry study including persons with HMSN showed small improvements in maximal oxygen uptake, but the subjects actually increased their heart rate at a submaximal exercise intensity.[17] In a more recent study using a home-based aerobic walking program in slowly progressive NMD subjects, there was modest improvement in aerobic performance without evidence of overwork weakness or excessive fatigue.[46]

Persons with slowly progressive NMD typically lead a sedentary lifestyle, which may compound effects of the disease process on skeletal muscle and the cardiovascular system. Researchers advocate a definite prescription for daily physical activity[45]; however, this is rarely practiced, possibly due to concerns about overuse weakness or excessive fatigue. Along with using methods to objectively and reliably follow progression of strength loss in persons with neuropathic weakness,[23] clinicians should teach their patients energy conservation techniques, which have been shown to be helpful in forestalling fatigue.[1]

EXERCISE PRESCRIPTION AND PRECAUTIONS

In creating an exercise prescription for a patient with HMSN, it is critical to identify her interests and motivations, understand her reasons for not exercising, and formulate realistic goals. Due to progressive fatigue with modest exertion, this patient is likely to be unable to participate in activities she previously found enjoyable. Disuse of her muscles is probably creating a vicious cycle that leads to even less activity.[26]

The risk of coronary artery disease may be reduced by modest physical exertion such as walking and gardening, although maximal oxygen uptake is not altered.[28] If this patient states that her primary goal is to improve endurance and feel more energetic, there is no need for a weight-lifting program that would focus on improving maximal strength. Elastic resistance exercise bands would be the most practical method to provide gentle strength training as an adjunct to other activities.

Because of the low work rates, formal exercise testing is probably not necessary unless there are risk factors for cardiac disease.[16] An exercise program to build muscular endurance should be the primary focus, most likely involving walking in this patient. Initially, prescription would be for 15 minutes 3 days per week, increasing to 30 minutes as tolerated. She should be encouraged to garden or enjoy another activity requiring physical exertion, working toward a goal of exercising each day, which may improve compliance with the program.[27] Obtaining objective strength measurement of major muscle groups using handheld dynamometry at the time of prescription would provide a baseline should there be complaints of increased weakness. If this occurs, the patient should be cautioned to stop exercising and call the physician.

CONCLUSION

Exercise prescription in persons with NMD requires creativity, enthusiasm, and the willingness to accept the possibility of increased progression of weakness. However, we are now probably much too cautious in our recommendations, which unnecessarily adds to the disability already present in our patients. This chapter makes clear the need for further research into the appropriate exercise prescription to help persons with NMD lead more vigorous and fulfilling lives.

This work was supported by Research and Training Grant H133B0026-96 from the National Institute on Disability and Rehabilitation Research, United States Department of Education.

REFERENCES

1. Agre JC, Rodriquez AA: Intermittent isometric activity: Its effect on muscle fatigue in postpolio subjects. Arch Phys Med Rehabil 72:971–975, 1991.
2. Aitkens SG, McCrory MA, Kilmer DD, et al: Moderate resistance exercise program: Its effect in slowly progressive neuromuscular disease. Arch Phys Med Rehabil 74:711–715, 1993.
3. Ansell BM: Juvenile dermatomyositis. J Rheumatol 33suppl:60–62, 1992.
4. Bar-Or O: Role of exercise in the assessment and management of neuromuscular disease in children. Med Sci Sports Exerc 28:421–427, 1996.
5. Beasley WC: Quantitative muscle testing: Principles and applications to research and clinical services. Arch Phys Med Rehabil 42:398–425, 1961.
6. Bensman A: Strenuous exercise may impair function in Guillain-Barré patients. JAMA 214:468–469, 1970.
7. Bloomfield SA: Changes in musculoskeletal structure and function with prolonged bed rest. Med Sci Sports Exerc 29:197–206, 1997.
8. Borg GAV: Perceived exertion: A note on "history" and methods. Med Sci Sports Exerc 5:90–93, 1973.
9. Braun NMT, Arora NS, Rochester DF: Respiratory muscle and pulmonary function in polymyositis and other proximal myopathies. Thorax 38:616–623, 1983.
10. Carter GC, Abresch RT, Fowler WM Jr, et al: Profiles of neuromuscular diseases: Hereditary motor and sensory neuropathy, types I and II. Am J Phys Med Rehabil 749:S140–S149, 1995.
11. Cronin ME: Treatment. In Plotz PH (moderator): Current concepts in the idiopathic inflammatory myopathies: Polymyositis, dermatomyositis, and related disorders. Ann Intern Med 111:143–157, 1989.
12. DeLateur BJ, Giaconi RM: Effect on maximal strength of submaximal exercise in Duchenne muscular dystrophy. Am J Phys Med 58:26–36, 1979.
13. Edwards RHT, Jones DA, Newham DJ, et al: Role of mechanical damage in pathogenesis of proximal myopathy in man. Lancet 8376:548–551, 1984.
14. Ervasti JM, Campbell KP: A role for the dystrophin-glycoprotein complex as a transmembrane linker between laminin and actin. J Cell Biol 122:809–823, 1993.
15. Escalante A, Miller L, Beardmore TD: Resistive exercise in the rehabilitation of polymyositis/dermatomyositis. J Rheumatol 20:1340–1344, 1993.
16. Fletcher GF, Balady G, Froelicher VF, et al: Exercise standards. A statement for healthcare professionals from the American Heart Association. Circulation 91:580–615, 1995.
17. Florence JM, Hagberg JM: Effect of training on the exercise responses of neuromuscular disease patients. Med Sci Sports Exerc 16:460–465, 1984.
18. Fowler WM Jr, Taylor M: Rehabilitation management of muscular dystrophy and related disorders: I. The role of exercise. Arch Phys Med Rehabil 63:319–321, 1982.
19. Greenleaf JE: Intensive exercise training during bed rest attenuates deconditioning. Med Sci Sports Exerc 29:207–215, 1997.
20. Hebert CA, Byrnes TJ, Baethge BA: Exercise limitation in patients with polymyositis. Chest 98:352–357, 1990.

21. Hicks JE, Miller F, Plotz P, et al: Isometric exercise increases strength and does not produce sustained creatine phosphokinase increases in a patient with polymyositis. J Rheumatol 20:1399–1401, 1993.

22. Hoffman EP, Brown RH Jr, Kunkel LM: Dystrophin: The protein product of the Duchenne muscular dystrophy locus. Cell 51:919–928, 1987.

23. Kilmer DD, McCrory MA, Wright NC, et al: Hand-held dynamometry reliability in persons with neuropathic weakness. Arch Phys Med Rehabil 78:1364–1368, 1997..

24. Kilmer DD, McCroy MA, Wright NC, et al: The effect of a high resistance exercise program in slowly progressive neuromuscular disease. Arch Phys Med Rehabil 75:560–563, 1994.

25. Kilmer DD, McDonald CM: Childhood progressive neuromuscular disease. In Goldberg B (ed): Sports and Exercise for Children with Chronic Health Conditions. Champaign, IL, Human Kinetics, 1995, pp 109–121.

26. Kilmer DD: Functional anatomy of skeletal muscle. Phys Med Rehabil State Art Rev 10:413–425, 1996.

27. Lampman RM: Exercise prescription for chronically ill patients. Am Fam Phys 55:2185–2192, 1997.

28. Leon AS, Connet J: Physical activity and 10.5 year mortality in the Multiple Risk Factor Intervention Trial (MRFIT). Int J Epidemiol 20:690–697, 1991.

29. Lieber RJ: Skeletal Muscle Structure and Function: Implications for Rehabilitation and Sports Medicine. Baltimore, Williams & Wilkins, 1992, pp 210–259.

30. Lindeman E, Leffers P, Reulen J, et al: Reduction of knee torques and leg-related functional abilities in hereditary motor and sensory neuropathy. Arch Phys Med Rehabil 75:1201–1205, 1994.

31. Lindeman E, Leffers P, Spaans F, et al: Strength training in patients with myotonic dystrophy and hereditary motor and sensory neuropathy: A randomized clinical trial. Arch Phys Med Rehabil 76:612–620, 1995.

32. McCartney N, Moroz D, Garner SH, McComas AJ: The effects of strength training in patients with selected neuromuscular disorders. Med Sci Sports Exerc 20:362–368, 1988.

33. McDonald CM, Abresch RT, Carter GT, et al: Profiles of neuromuscular diseases: Duchenne muscular dystrophy. Am J Phys Med Rehabil 74:S70–S92, 1995.

34. Milner-Brown HS, Miller RG: Muscle strengthening through high-resistance weight training in patients with neuromuscular disorders. Arch Phys Med Rehabil 69:14–19, 1988.

35. Pitetti KH, Barrett PJ, Abbas D: Endurance exercise training in Guillain-Barré syndrome. Arch Phys Med Rehabil 74:761–765, 1993.

36. Plasma Exchange/Sandoglubulin Guillain-Barré Syndrome Trial Group: Randomized trial of plasma exchange, intravenous immunoglobulin, and combined treatments in Guillain-Barre syndrome. Lancet 349:225–230, 1997.

37. Ropper AH: The Guillian-Barré syndrome. N Engl J Med 326:1130–1136, 1992.

38. Schwarz MI, Matthay RD, Sahn SA, et al: Interstitial lung disease in polymyositis and dermatomyositis: Analysis of six cases and review of the literature. Medicine 55:89–104, 1976.

39. Scott OM, Hyde SA, Goddard C, et al: Effect of exercise in Duchenne muscular dystrophy: Controlled six-month feasibility study of effects of two different regimes of exercises in children with Duchenne dystrophy. Physiotherapy 67:174–176, 1981.

40. Sharma KM, Mynhier MA, Miller RG: Muscular fatigue in Duchenne muscular dystrophy. Neurology 45:306–310, 1995.

41. Sockolov R, Irwin B, Dressendorfer RH, et al: Exercise performance in 6-to-11- year old boys with Duchenne muscular dystrophy. Arch Phys Med Rehabil 58:195–201, 1977.

42. Tesch PA, Berg HE, Haggmark T, et al. Muscle strength and endurance following lower limb suspension in man. Physiologist 34:S104–S106, 1991.

43. Van der Meche FGA, Schmitz PIM, Dutch Guillain-Barré Study Group: A randomized trial comparing intravenous immune globulin and plasma exchange in Guillain-Barré syndrome. N Engl J Med 326:1123–1129, 1992.

44. Vignos PJ Jr, Watkins MP: Effect of exercise in muscular dystrophy. JAMA 197:843–848, 1966.

45. Vignos PJ Jr: Physical models of rehabilitation in neuromuscular disease. Muscle Nerve 6:323–338, 1983.

46. Wright NC, Kilmer DD, McCrory MA, et al: Aerobic walking in slowly progressive neuromuscular disease: Effect of a 12-week program. Arch Phys Med Rehabil 77:64–69, 1996.

JOHN J. NICHOLAS, MD

14

Exercise Prescription for the Arthritic Patient

Exercise prescription for patients with arthritis remains controversial. Exercise and its correlate, hard work, have long been known to affect both inflammatory and degenerative arthritis adversely in many cases. Nevertheless, recent studies have demonstrated that properly selected patients may undergo both strengthening and endurance exercise with successful results. This chapter describes both the adverse influences and benefits of exercise for patients with arthritis.

RHEUMATOID ARTHRITIS

Half a century ago, Piersol and Hollander described "the optimum rest-exercise balance in the treatment of rheumatoid arthritis."[63] They cited an 1889 review that prompted physicians to consider movement, not immobilization alone, for patients with rheumatoid arthritis. They pointed out that "although drug therapy of rheumatoid arthritis had advanced considerably in the past ten years, no agent is as yet available which can be considered specific for the disease. Even enthusiasts admit that physical measures are an essential addition to drug therapy in all cases. Although as yet no means are available for halting the 'storm,' there is much that can be done to help 'the ship' weather the blow, so that when that storm finally subsides, there will be a minimum of wreckage left to clear." Piersol and Hollander discussed at length the dilemma that immobilization causes a decrease in pain and inflammation in arthritic joints but may cause a loss of motion, while use of the joint, and certainly overuse, will cause increased pain. They concluded: "The physician trained in physical medicine can act as consultant, with much to offer in his knowledge of the broad scope of physical management and its place in the rehabilitation of the arthritic patient. His attention to the details of proper support in bed, gradual increase in activity in ambulation and consideration of the body mechanics, covers a part of the treatment program usually forgotten until contractures and deformities have already developed." They also quoted one of their patients, who reported, "The exercise is hard, but the rest is easy."

The dilemma of exercise or rest for patients with rheumatoid arthritis has continued through the years. In a detailed review in 1959, Watkins described the exercise protocol advocated at the Massachusetts General Hospital, then a leading center for the treatment of arthritis.[79] The extensive exercises, probably far beyond the compliance capacity of most patients, was a combination of rest, positioning while asleep, active range of motion, and isometric exercise. The plan seems appropriate today. However, the effect of medical and surgical treatment of rheumatoid arthritis has changed markedly since that paper, and much more data are now available regarding the effect of exercise on patients with arthritis.

A series of data has been collected that describes the effect of exercise on inflamed joints in animals. Glynn et al. reported that rats given inflammatory arthritis suffered much less inflammation if caged than if allowed to run free.[62] Murray described experimental arthritis in rabbits as being much more severe in joints that were allowed full weightbearing and motion.[52] Agudelo caused inflammation of dogs' knees with urate crystals and noted that passive exercise increased the leukocytosis, fluid volume, histologic abnormalities, and xenon clearance from the joints proportionate to the duration of exercise.[1] Merritt similarly described urate-induced synovitis of rabbit joints in which passive range of motion caused a far greater inflammatory response than isometric exercise or simply the joint inflammation alone.[47] Fam et al. induced synovitis in rabbits with calcium pyrophosphate dihydrate crystals and found that, in a 24-hour experiment, passive range of motion increased the inflammation but, after 20–40 days, histologic changes were more adversely effected by immbolization, although synovitis was increased by motion.[14] These experiments suggest that passive motion and weightbearing may be detrimental to inflamed joints.

A further series of "naturally occurring experiments" has similar findings. Thompson et al. described rheumatoid arthritis in patients who had previously had a hemiplegia.[75] The occurrence of erosions, deformities, and subcutaneous nodules was more frequent and severe in the unaffected or nonhemiplegic side. Bland et al. confirmed these findings.[4] Further observations by Stecher et al.,[70] Glyn et al.,[25] Glick,[24] and Glynn[26] suggested that neurologic lesions such as poliomyelitis and trauma diminished the incidence of gout, rheumatoid arthritis, and osteoarthritis in the involved or "unused" extremities. These findings suggested that exercise and use might be detrimental to inflamed joints.

It was, therefore, a landmark event when Machover and Sapecky published a description of 11 hospitalized Veterans Administration patients with rheumatoid arthritis who performed three maximal contractions at 90° of flexion daily five times weekly for 7 weeks and who developed an increase in strength on the exercised side of 23.3% and on the control, or nonexercised, side of 17.6%[44] Two of five wheelchair-bound patients subsequently stood with crutches and were able to walk.

In a series of experiments from Sweden, Ekblom and colleagues described the results of more vigorous exercise in patients with rheumatoid arthritis. Ekblom et al. described 31 female patients with rheumatoid arthritis in remission.[9] The maximum volume of oxygen utilization ($VO_{2\,max}$) was decreased 25% and strength was decreased 33-52% from normal subjects. Ekblom later described 34 patients with rheumatoid arthritis who received muscle strength training and joint mobility training twice a day for 5 weeks, including 20–40 minutes of bicycle ergometry and quadriceps table work as inpatients.[10] They subsequently demonstrated an increase in strength and increase in $VO_{2\,max}$ compared to controls. None of the patients complained that their joints hurt more. In a 7-months' follow-up in 1976, the authors found that the patients had maintained their increase in strength and aerobic capacity and that their joints had not undergone an increase in pain.[54]

Also in 1976, Nordemar et al. performed muscle biopsies before and after an intense exercise program in ten patients with rheumatoid arthritis; the exercise included the use of bicycling, swimming, cycling, skiing, training of the quadriceps muscle, and walking in the park and on stairs 2 hours a day.[55] Each subject showed an increase in the size of both type 1 and type 2 fibers. They also reported no flare-ups of arthritis. In 1981 the authors reported on 4–8 years of follow-up in 23 of these patients.[53] The patients had been bicycling, swimming, skiing, jogging, walking, and participating in other activities, but no exact quantification of the amount of exercise was available. Using a questionnaire response, the authors found a positive correlation between reported activity of daily living (ADL) capacity and the reported amount of physical training and found a negative correlation between ADLs and radiographic findings.

In 1983 Nordesjö et al. found that maximum isometric muscle strength and endurance was 30–45% less than in control patients with rheumatoid arthritis.[56] Another group of researchers, Beals et al., tested eight patients with rheumatoid arthritis, six with osteoarthritis, and six controls on a Cybex machine at 30° per second and isometric exercise at 45° of flexion.[3] They reported that the $VO_{2\,max}$ of the rheumatoid patients was 15.9 and 20.5 ml/kg/min for controls. Maximum strength was decreased, but electromyograms (EMGs) were normal.

Harkcom et al. reported a group of rheumatoid patients who exercised three times a week for 12 weeks and were divided into three groups: groups exercised 15 minutes, 25 minutes, or 35 minutes on a bicycle ergometer.[30] The patients' $VO_{2\,max}$ and duration of exercise increased proportionately to the time of exercise, and the number of painful joints decreased. One of the authors reported in unpublished data that her patients found the exercise on the bicycle ergometer to improve their capacity for exercising, but exercising outdoors on the weekends at home on bicycles, where there was significant resistance from irregular terrain and grades, caused increased knee pain.

A further group of researchers from Denmark reported in 1987 that eight patients with nonacute rheumatoid arthritis increased their maximum isometric strength 38% at four fixed angles and increased their isokinetic strength of the quadriceps muscle 16% at 90°, 60°, and 30° of arc per second after exercising twice weekly for 2 months in water.[8] The $VO_{2\,max}$ also increased. Patients performed walking exercises in all directions under water against the resistance of the water. Others underwent resistance training individually for leg and hip muscles; again, there was no report of an increase in joint pain or inflammation.

Researchers from Columbia, Mo., reported in 1988 that 40 patients with rheumatoid arthritis and 80 patients with osteoarthritis of weightbearing joints had decreased aerobic capacity and ability to walk 50 feet.[51] Many of the patients were then given an exercise program consisting of walking on ground and jogging waist-high and performing calisthenics in water for 1 hour three times a week.[50] Patients experienced increases in $VO_{2\ max}$ and spontaneous activity and decreases in 50-foot walking time, depression, and anxiety. There was no increase in joint pain. They exercised for 12 weeks; the dropout rate was 17%.

Perlman et al. described a "dance-based" aerobic exercise program for rheumatoid arthritis patients called "Educize."[60] This consisted of 1 hour of weightbearing exercise and 1 hour of discussion, education, and counseling. There was no jumping, and the dance activity was slow. The patients found no increase in pain; several subjective parameters increased; and complaints on the arthritis impact measure scale (AIMS) and the 50-foot walk time decreased. Articular swelling and pain also decreased.

In 1991 Kirsteins et al. reported that 11 patients with rheumatoid arthritis who exercised once or twice a week for 10 weeks with tai-chi exercise developed no deterioration.[35] Ekdahl in 1992 described 67 rheumatoid arthritis patients, class 2, whose isometric hip and knee strength was 25% below normals and whose isokinetic knee strength at 60° and 180°/sec of arc were 35% and 25% below normals.[11] Isokinetic endurance was down 55% and aerobic capacity 80%. Hansen et al. studied 75 rheumatoid arthritis patients divided into four groups: an intensely trained group, a lesser intensely trained group, a group trained weekly, and a group treated in a hot water pool instead of with exercise.[29] Two-year follow-up showed that persons in all groups deteriorated over that time in multiple measures. Muscle strength, however, increased in all joints, and 66% of the patients said they felt better and were able to increase their ADLs as opposed to controls. A progression of joint destruction was even demonstrated on radiographs and measured functional scores. Individual patients were able to take up table tennis or pony riding.

In 1994 Stenström studied 48 patients with rheumatoid arthritis, class 2, with mean duration of disease of 14 ($\pm$12) years, who were given a home exercise program.[73] The intervention group was given goal-setting and cognitive treatment in addition. All patients exercised using rubber strips, and about half improved on maximum walking speed and functional tasks, Ritchie index, and joint mobility. Cognitive intervention did not seem to help.

Also in 1994 Lyngberg studied 24 rheumatoid arthritis patients taking low-dose steroids.[42] The treatment group received training for 3 months, including bicycle exercise, heel lifts, and step climbing twice weekly. There were fewer painful and tender joints in the treated exercise group, and disease activity did not increase. The sedimentation rate did not change. Work capacity doubled, and the number of repetitions increased. The authors believed that their study proved rheumatoid arthritis patients on low-dose steroids could undergo training safely. Lyngberg performed a further study of nine elderly women with rheumatoid arthritis who exercised three times a week for 3 weeks; they performed strengthening exercises at 50% maximum contraction and did not note an increase in synovitis and joint pain.[43] Their strength gain was 21%.

Strenström studied 29 rheumatoid arthritis patients, class 2, for 4 years and found that radiographic progression was no more severe in patients who *reported* exercising twice a week compared to those who exercised only once a week.[72] Häkkinen et al.

in 1994 studied 39 patients with rheumatoid arthritis or psoriatic arthritis for 6 months.[28] Twenty-one of the patients had strength training and 18 acted as controls. The authors found a slight increase in erosions in the control group and less of an increase in the exercise group. Special rubber bands were used on all major muscle groups twice a week for 30 minutes. The patients also performed walking, biking, and other activities. Knee extension increased 31.5%. Trunk flexion increased 14.8% and extension 10.7%.

In 1995 Noreau reported the results of a 12-week, twice-weekly exercise program that included dancing without jumps or sudden movements that was designed to elevate the resting pulse to 50% of maximum.[57] There was a 13% increase in aerobic power, no deterioration of joints, and a decrease in painful joint count. There were positive changes in anxiety, depression, fatigue, and tension.

In 1996 Melton-Rogers described eight patients with rheumatoid arthritis who performed stationary bicycle graded exercise and underwater exercise.[46] They found that perceived exertion and respiratory exchange was higher during water running, but minute ventilation and tidal volume were higher during bicycle riding. They believed that this form of exercise was appropriate for patients with rheumatoid arthritis.

Rall et al. in 1996 compared eight rheumatoid arthritis patients to eight younger patients and eight older patients who exercised with high-intensity resistive training of all major muscle groups, performing three sets of eight repetitions twice weekly for 12 weeks.[64] There was no increase in swollen or painful joints. Pain, fatigue score, and 50-foot walk time diminished. The arthritic patients increased their strength 57%, versus 44% for the young and 36% for the older patients.

Van den Ende studied 100 rheumatoid arthritis patients; 25 were in a full weight-bearing intense exercise group, including stationary bicycle; 25 did range of motion and low-intensity isometric exercises; 25 were given individual range of motion and isometric low-intensity exercise, and 25 were sent home with written instructions.[76] Strength improved, range of motion improved 17%, and $VO_{2\ max}$ improved 16% in the high-intensity group. No increases occurred in the second, third, or fourth groups. When studied 12 weeks later, the gains were gone.

These studies, as well as several review articles,[31,49,65,68,71] support the belief that patients with rheumatoid arthritis can undergo aerobic training, underwater exercise, and isokinetic, isometric, and active strengthening exercises, at least in the short term, without detrimental effects. All of the studies have shown increases in strength, aerobic capacity, and, when measured, functional activities without increases in erosions, joint pain, or swelling. Although few, the long-term studies fail to show a detrimental effect on patients with rheumatoid arthritis, but they do not always show sustained gains.

These data allow the physician, therefore, to select patients who have quiescent joints and probably not severe radiologic evidence of joint destruction for prescription of isometric and perhaps active or isokinetic exercise as tolerated. If increased pain or swelling occurs, the exercise should be curtailed or stopped. Aerobic exercise also should be performed at subcapacity without strenuous weightbearing, but many authors have described jogging, bicycling, skiing, and other strenuous weightbearing activities. The suppression of inflammation by methotrexate and other drugs is much more successful now than it was 50 years ago, and this may account for some of the success of these exercise programs. Nonetheless, the physician must be careful to discuss with patients the half-century old dilemma of the balance between rest and exercise and advise patients to stop exercising if there is a deterioration of the joint.

There is no evidence that patients who have had arthroplasty can or cannot tolerate aerobic or strengthening exercises. Physical therapists anecdotally report that patients tolerate isometric exercise following these procedures. Patients report that their ability to walk, perform ADLs, and otherwise exercise is also improved. Most surgeons, however, warn patients that there is evidence that joints that deteriorate the most rapidly following arthroplasty have performed the most physical activity.

It is quite likely that strengthening shoulder abduction, hip extension, and knee extension and flexion will benefit patients. These exercises can be performed with special rubber bands and can be performed as multiple angle isometric exercises with special equipment. High-repetition range of motion exercises probably are not advisable. Aerobic exercise performed on a low-resistance bicycle ergometer or underwater also has been successful and safe. Surprisingly, vigorous exercises that include skiing, running, and bicycling also have been successful, especially in Scandinavian populations.

The medical and surgical treatment of rheumatoid arthritis and patients' capacity to exercise have improved greatly over the years. Only the future can demonstrate how the long-term results of this increased exercise capacity will affect the involved joints.

HAND EXERCISES FOR PATIENTS WITH RHEUMATOID ARTHRITIS

Patients with rheumatoid arthritis almost universally have involvement of their hands. The onset of synovitis is almost immediately accompanied by atrophy of the hand muscles and weakness. An interesting study by Castillo et al. studied 153 radiographs of patients who had classic or definite rheumatoid arthritis.[6] They found that marked cystic changes occurred in inverse relationship to the presence of osteoporosis and that the most extensive cystic changes occurred in patients who performed the most physical activity. Conversely, patients who performed the most physical activity had the least osteoporosis. This suggested that certain bony integrity persisted in the face of rheumatoid arthritis when patients performed vigorous exercise.

In 1993 Hoenig et al. studied 57 patients with rheumatoid arthritis who were randomized to 12 weeks of home hand exercises for 10–20 minutes twice daily, including range of motion exercises, balanced resistive exercises, and range of motion plus balanced resistive exercises.[34] Range of motion exercises were followed by an improved right-hand joint count; range of motion exercises plus resistive exercises were followed by an increased left-hand dexterity; home hand exercise (all groups) showed significantly increased left grip strength. Although the changes were not large, patients who exercised did not notice deterioration of their hand grip or dexterity. Patients who noted an increase in hand discomfort simply reduced the amount of exercise successfully. No functional activities were monitored.

Brighton et al. studied 44 women with rheumatoid arthritis of the hands; 22 were given a daily exercise regimen of six exercises, and 22 served as a control group and had no exercises.[5] At the end of 48 months, grip strength and pinch strength were improved in the exercise group, and function in the control group had deteriorated. The exercises included fast flexion and extension of the fingers, extending the fingers while the hands were flat on the table, rolling and unrolling bandages and a bath towel, gripping a sheet of paper between the thumb and each finger, and repeatedly flexing and extending the metacarpophalangeal joints with the hands placed over the edge of the table. However, hand function was not studied. While this study does not demonstrate the increased hand function following exercise for patients with rheumatoid arthritis, it does demonstrate that no deterioration will occur following exercises and that, with apparent heavy use of the hands, less osteoporosis exists.

The physiatrist should consider prescribing both range of motion and flexion, extension, and adduction exercises for the hands of patients with rheumatoid arthritis.

OSTEOARTHRITIS

The use of exercise to treat patients with osteoarthritis is controversial. One controversy involves whether patients who exercise or subject their limbs to occupational stresses have more severe osteoarthritis than other patients. Another controversy involves whether the prescription of exercise for patients with osteoarthritis is helpful or harmful. We will address each of these issues.

THE EFFECT OF HEAVY WORK, EXERCISE, STRESS, AND STRAIN

In a 2-year prospective study, Michel studied 51 subjects who regularly practiced weightbearing exercise, which was not clearly defined. Assessment of radiographs did not demonstrate an increase in osteophytes.[48] Fries et al. later reported on 451 members of a runners' club and 330 community controls over 8 years.[21] The disabilities and initial disability level had steadily increased for runners versus controls. Ironically, however, the rate of disability was lower in the runners. In addition, runners had a lower mortality rate: 1.49% vs. 7.09% (P = < 0.001). The mean age of the subjects was 50–72. In 1996 Fries et al. performed a 6-year prospective study of 410 runners' club members and 289 community controls.[22] They analyzed them for the occurrence of pain, and the degree of reported musculoskeletal pain was slightly lower in the exercise group—statistically significant for women, but not for men. Mortality rates and disability rates were lower in the exercise group.

In 1955 Kujala et al. studied 117 former top-level male athletes (mean age 45–68 years), which included 28 long-distance runners, 31 soccer players, 29 weight lifters, and 29 shooters.[38] Radiographic examination revealed osteoarthritis in 3% of shooters, 29% of soccer players, 31% of weight lifters, and 14% of long-distance runners. The risk of knee osteoarthritis also was increased in those who had previous knee injuries, high body mass index at age 20, and previous participation in heavy work or work involving kneeling or squatting. Panush et al. described an 8-year prospective study of 13 nonrunners (10 of whom were reexamined) and 16 runners (12 of whom were reexamined) and found no increase in pain and swelling of the weightbearing joints, diminished range of motion, and evidence of osteoarthritis on radiographic evaluation.[59]

In 1996 Spector et al. reported a retrospective study of 16 middle- and long-distance runners, 14 tennis players, and 977 age-matched controls, all of whom were female athletes, in England.[69] The former athletes had greater rates of osteoarthritis on radiographs at all sites. A subgroup of 22 women who reported long-term vigorous weightbearing exercise had similar rates of osteoarthritis. The findings indicate that elite athletes have a two- to threefold increased risk of radiographic osteoarthritis.

In a review, Cooper et al. described a number of articles that defined the risk of osteoarthritis of the knee from occupational physical loads.[7] They reviewed articles demonstrating that male coal miners from England in the 1950s had a higher prevalence of osteoarthritis of the knee than their more sedentary coworkers. In addition, English dock workers were found to have more arthritis of the knee than civil servants. A Swedish study revealed that shipyard workers had more osteoarthritis of the knee than their colleagues working in offices and teaching. In Finland, concrete reinforcement workers and painters had no differences in disability resulting from knee arthritis. The First National Health and Nutrition Examination Survey in the United States revealed that osteoarthritis of the knee was apparently more likely in persons whose jobs required knee bending. In the Framingham study, again, the risk of osteoarthritis of the knee was doubled for men performing work that required considerable knee bending and at least medium physical demands. A California study demonstrated that persons with osteoarthritis were two to three times more likely than controls to have performed moderate to heavy work. In another English study, both men and women with osteoarthritis of the knee demonstrated that squatting, kneeling, or climbing stairs was associated with an increased incidence of osteoarthritis of the knee.

Lane presented a literature review that concluded that normal joints appeared to tolerate prolonged, vigorous, low-impact exercise without an increased incidence of osteoarthritis.[40] However, participating in sports that subject joints to high levels of impact or torsional loading and participating in sports after having had an injury were followed by an increased incidence of osteoarthritis. In further articles in 1993 and 1995, Lane published extensive literature reviews to support her conclusion that there is some evidence that high-impact and high-intensity exercise at an elite level or an intense level is followed by an increase of osteoarthritis.[39,41] She was quite sure this was true in patients who had previously injured joints. A review by Panush and Brown concluded that reasonable rational exercise for patients who did not have underlying joint disease had not been shown to lead to an increased incidence of osteoarthritis.[58]

DECREASED STRENGTH AND ENDURANCE

Several studies have demonstrated that patients with osteoarthritis have lower endurance and strength than control patients. Minor et al. studied 40 patients with rheumatoid arthritis and 80 with osteoarthritis and found that the $VO_{2\,max}$ was 73% of normal value but higher overall in patients with osteoarthritis than rheumatoid arthritis.[51] Ries et al. studied 16 patients who were about to have a total knee arthroplasty, 17 who were deciding whether to have arthroplasty, and 14 healthy subjects.[66] The $VO_{2\ max}$ was diminished in the pre-total knee arthroplasty groups more than in the group considering arthroplasty, and was normal in the healthy individuals. Tan et al. studied 30 patients with osteoarthritis of the knee, 30 patients with pain in the knee but without radiographic evidence of osteoarthritis, and 30 controls at 60° and 180° of arc/sec on an isokinetic dynamometer and at 30° and 60° of knee flexion for isometric testing.[74] Hamstrings and quadriceps were studied, and both groups of patients with knee pain had weaker hamstrings and quadriceps than the pain-free controls, but the ratio of hamstring strength to quadriceps strength was the same.

Philbin et al. reported on 16 patients about to have a total knee arthroplasty, 17 who had not yet had an arthroplasty, and 14 healthy controls.[61] They found that specific sections of the AIMS were diminished for patients with osteoarthritis, and the $VO_{2\ max}$ was decreased.

Studying 17 women with osteoarthritis of the knee and 17 healthy women, Wessel et al. found in 1996 that the isometric torque of the knee extensors was much lower in women with osteoarthritis than in women with no knee problems across several knee angles.[80]

THE EFFECT OF PRESCRIBED EXERCISE ON OSTEOARTHRITIS PATIENTS

Several studies have demonstrated the effect of physical conditioning exercise on patients with osteoarthritis. Minor and coworkers studied patients with osteoarthritis who exercised 1 hour three times weekly for 12 weeks; they were divided into groups who performed walking, walking underwater, and simple range of motion exercises. The walkers performed at 60–80% of their maximum pulse rate for 30 minutes.[50] The aquatic exercise was calisthenics while in chest-high water. The two exercise groups increased the $VO_{2\ max}$, diminished the number of active joints, increased endurance, and the 50-foot walk time diminished. The pain, anxiety, and depression sections of the AIMS decreased as the physical activity increased. None of the patients reported an increase in joint pain. At 1 year, the $VO_{2\ max}$ was nearly the same as that achieved following the exercise program.

In 1992 Kovar studied 47 patients who exercised and 45 control patients who walked under supervision for 8 weeks on a smooth-surfaced hospital corridor for up to 30 minutes and who also underwent an education session.[36] Exercise patients demonstrated an 18.4% increase in the distance walked, and they used less medication. The physical activities section of the AIMS improved 39%, and the AIMS pain subscale diminished 27%. Interestingly, this was a highly educated group, 35 of 55 exercisers and 32 of 50 controls had completed a high school education or more.

In 1993 Green et al. described an interesting study of 47 patients, 23 of whom were performing a physical therapy program and 24 of whom performed the same physical therapy program but underwent twice-weekly deep pool walking for 6 weeks.[27] The exercise program consisted of mild range of motion and bridging exercise with some isometric exercises. There was no increase in response to the exercise program with the hydrotherapy added.

Fisher, Prendergast, and Calkins published a series of papers regarding the effect of isometric exercise with a special machine on osteoarthritis of the knee in a variety of patients.[16–20] First, they compared 18 patients in a Veterans Administration nursing home who could walk at least five steps to controls.[19] The exercise intervention consisted of a special bench where the patient could sit and exercise the quadriceps muscle at different isometric angles of the both the hip and the knee. They performed exercise three times weekly for 6 weeks. The exercise protocol initially consisted of isometric exercise and slow, low-resistance range of motion exercises, and then isotonic exercise was added with low weights. Finally, high-speed, low-resistance exercises were performed. All of the patients had significant osteoarthritis. The results indicated that at all angles of the knee and hip there was an increase in quadriceps strength on the average, but some individual patients did not improve. Timed endurance increased and, subjectively, many patients became more active. Evaluation 4 months later in nine subjects revealed them to be as strong as initially following their exercise program.

Fisher et al. again studied 15 male volunteers from an osteoarthritis clinic who exercised three times a week for 4 months.[20] Eleven subjects finished the study. Initially, strength, endurance, and muscle contraction speed were 50% less than the control subjects, but following exercise there was a 35% improvement in muscle strength, a 35% improvement in endurance, and 50% improvement in muscle contraction speed. The patients became less dependent, and at 8-month follow-up the improvements had been retained. No patients complained that the joints were worse, and eight stated that nocturnal leg cramps had been relieved by the exercise. A Jette Functional Index revealed improvement.

Fisher's group again studied 20 women and 20 men who had the same exercise program added to a previously prescribed physical therapy protocol.[16] The strength of the quadriceps muscles increased 14%, hamstring muscle strength increased 29%, endurance improved 38%, and pain and difficulties of activities of daily living scores decreased. Walking time decreased, and at 3 months the gains had been maintained. Fisher et al. further studied six female and six male volunteers with osteoarthritis of the knee who exercised three times a week for 3 months. Quadriceps strength increased 29%.[17] Their endurance increased, and the hamstring strength increased 23%. On treadmill testing, $VO_{2\ max}$ was increased and 50-foot walking time diminished. The patients' ADL function was too high to improve their Jette Functional Index. The authors concluded that improvement in muscle strengthening was followed by an increase in aerobic functioning also.

In 1997 Ettinger et al. studied 439 patients (364 of whom finished the study) who performed exercises for 3 months and were followed for 15 more months.[13] They all had disability and osteoarthritis on radiographs of the knee. Ettinger divided his patients into an aerobic exercise group, a resistance exercise group, and a group that received a health education program. The aerobic group walked on the track and at home, and the resistance group performed calisthenics. The radiographs did not change over the 18 months of the study. Ettinger concluded that the aerobic activities and the resistive exercises all were followed by a diminution in pain and disability and an improvement in physical performance. The resistance group decreased their disability scores and pain scores both by 8% and increased their walking distance.

Mangione studied 23 women and four men who ran on a treadmill with an apparatus that lifted them.[45] They thus could run with no body weight or with 20% or 40% of their body weight removed. The $VO_{2\,max}$ improved greatly with lessening body weight, but pain in the knees did not change.

Each of these exercise studies has shown that patients with osteoarthritis of the lower limbs can perform aerobic and resistant exercise without an increase in pain. For patients participating in a strengthening program, there clearly was an increase in muscle strength from preexercise condition, where they were weaker than control subjects. This increase in strength is followed by an increase in functional activities and decrease in disability and pain and, on occasion, by an increase in $VO_{2\,max}$.

In addition, the studies that included walking underwater or on the surface of the ground have shown that patients increased their walking distance, their $VO_{2\,max}$, and many subjective measures of disability. While none of the studies lasted any great length of time, it seems that, at least in the short run, patients with osteoarthritis of the knee can perform exercise activity and benefit from it.

Because of the relationship of knee and hip osteoarthritis to heavy occupational and sporting activity, there is probably some reluctance on the part of physicians to prescribe exercise for patients with osteoarthritis. In a 1996 survey by Hochberg et al., of 1001 rheumatologists, only 41.4% always or frequently prescribed exercise for patients with osteoarthritis of the hip and only 53.8% prescribed exercise always or frequently for patients with osteoarthritis of the knee.[33]

CONCLUSION

Many studies are now available, and it seems fairly certain that the excessive activity of a persistent or elite athlete performing heavy weightbearing exercise will increase the individual's susceptibility to osteoarthritis of the knee. If the patient has undergone injury to the joint, susceptibility probably is enhanced. In addition, the evidence shows that many athletes, especially runners, perform for years without any increased evidence of osteoarthritis. Perhaps these individuals have self-selected for their ability to perform this task, or perhaps low-impact exercise may indeed be beneficial for patients with osteoarthritis. In addition, it has been clearly demonstrated that if strength and aerobic capacity in patients with osteoarthritis of the hip and knee is diminished, exercise will improve both of these parameters.

The physician prescribing exercise for patients with osteoarthritis of the hip and knee, and probably other lower extremity joints, should employ cautious optimism. Walking at a reasonable rate on smooth, level surfaces several times a week may be recommended. The prescription of isometric exercises is probably safer than active or isokinetic exercise, and evidence has demonstrated that it is tolerated by many patients up to three times weekly. Initial resistance and repetitions should be minimal. The resistance may be increased as time passes and the patient tolerates the weight, but active exercise against heavy resistance probably should be avoided. Frequent bending or flexing the joint also should be avoided.

Patients should be cautioned that no long-term studies have verified that there are no ill effects from this form of exercise but that, at least in the short-run, they may feel improvement in function, pain relief, strength, and endurance.

ANKYLOSING SPONDYLITIS

Ankylosing spondylitis is one of several diseases described under the term "seronegative spondyloarthropathies," which include ankylosing spondylitis, psoriatic arthritis, Reiter's syndrome, the arthritis of inflammatory bowel disease, and Whipple's disease. The term "spondylitis" associated with these entities refers to the pathologic lesion in the enthesis, the site where a ligament is attached to the bones of the spine. When these sites in the spine are inflamed, there is progressive stiffness and immobility. The lesions in ankylosing spondylitis are more significant and more severe than in the other conditions, and we therefore discuss the rehabilitation of the patient with ankylosing spondylitis, realizing that the techniques and the goals relate, but less strongly, to the other conditions.

The pathogenesis of ankylosing spondylitis, therefore, is that an inflammatory processes is established at the site of the attachment of ligaments and tendons to bone.[23] As the inflammation becomes more severe, a reactive process is established whereby fibrosis and then reactive bone formation occurs. The progression of the fibrosis to bone causes stiffening and loss of motion at all sites.

The goals of rehabilitation of ankylosing spondylitis are primarily to keep the patient from becoming stiffened or ankylosed in an unfavorable position. Medical treatment ameliorates the pain and inflammation, but it does not stop the unrelenting progression of the replacement of soft tissue by bone. A patient with ankylosing spondylitis who is stiffened in a maximally flexed position has greater subsequent disability from his impairment than a patient who is stiffened in a more or less upright posture. The achievement of this posture, therefore, is the goal of exercise prescription in ankylosing spondylitis. Additional attempts to increase the range of motion of the spine have been shown to be minimally successful and temporary.

In 1990 Fisher, Cawley, and Holgate described 33 patients with ankylosing spondylitis, 22 of whom were smokers.[15] Sixteen of the patients walked or cycled more than 3 miles a day or played golf, tennis, or squash three or more times a week. Seventeen performed no exercise at all. On admission, pulmonary function, including forced expiratory volume (FEV_1), forced vital capacity (FVC), functional capacity (FC), and diffusing capacity of lung carbon dioxide (DLCO) were diminished. Smoking had no effect. Those who could perform more exercise had an increased vital capacity and $VO_{2\ max}$. Chest expansion did not have a significant effect on exercise tolerance. It was pointed out that even a modest amount of exercise allowed these patients to perform at a satisfactory level of activity despite having restricted spinal and chest wall mobility.

In 1990 Kraag et al. studied 53 patients with ankylosing spondylitis, 26 of whom received physical therapy and disease education and 27 of whom received neither.[37] Physical therapy consisted of "standard physical therapy proprioceptive neuromuscular facilitation techniques." After 4 months, the exercised patients improved their finger-to-floor distance by 8.3 cm. Their Schober's test did not change, but their function, as evidenced from a questionnaire, improved (p = < 0.001). This study suggested that exercise improved function in these patients, but the finger-to-floor test improvement was probably due to an improvement in hip flexion rather than an increase in spinal flexion.

Viitanen et al. in 1992 studied 362 men and 143 women who were treated with physical therapy as an inpatient for 3 or 4 weeks.[78] The exercise treatment was not carefully described. It was reported that 4 months following the inpatient treatment there was an improvement in range of motion, chin-to-chest difference of 21.7%, chest expansion 31.3%, cervical rotation 22.6%, finger-to-floor distance 36.6%, occiput-to-wall distance 30.8%, the Schober test 12.4%, and vital capacity 7.4%. Carefully analysis, however, revealed that a small percentage of patients actually became worse, a number remained unchanged, and many improved. The Schober test, for example, improved only in about half of the patients.

In 1995 Viitanen, Liimatainen, Suni, and Kautiainen also reported at 15 months on 141 patients with ankylosing spondylitis who underwent 3 or 4 weeks of inpatient physical therapy.[77] At follow-up, chest expansion and vital capacity had significantly deteriorated while cervical rotation, finger-to-floor distance, and fitness index continued to improve. During the treatment period, hot and cold modalities, gymnastics, jogging or walking, pool exercise, stretching, mobilization exercises, and massage were all applied.

Russell, Unsworth, and Haslock in 1993 published a study involving 43 patients with ankylosing spondylitis who attended a voluntary exercise session for 1½ hours per week for not quite 2 months and 14 patients who did not participate.[67] Exercising patients were divided into a vigorous and moderate exercise group. Only the vigorously exercised patients showed some changes. At the end of the time, cervical spine extension had improved 1°. At 6 months, flexion had deteriorated 5.5% and lateral bending 2% in the vigorously exercised group.

In 1994 Bakker et al. studied 144 patients with ankylosing spondylitis divided into a group who performed unsupervised daily individualized exercise at home for 9 months and a second group who participated in supervised group physical therapy 3 hours a week.[2] The addition of group therapy improved mobility 16% versus 9%, fitness improved 4% versus −1%, and global health improved 34% versus 6%. They calculated in 1994 that the beneficial effects of this group therapy cost an additional $409 per patient annually.

These studies have demonstrated that conditioning exercise for patients with ankylosing spondylitis will improve their fitness, capacity to perform daily activities, and perhaps ability to continue working. There is no evidence, however, that range of motion was improved on a lasting basis. The physiatrist, therefore, must patiently persist in trying to help his patients improve their general physical condition. Although there are no direct data for support, they are strongly urged to perform exercise, including spinal extension exercises such as walking into the corner of a room with their elbows outstretched in an effort to extend their spine, push-up exercises, and other exercises designed to help them maintain the upright posture. One's posture at the end of the day is more flexed than at the beginning, so there seems to be a natural tendency for the flexed posture in many individuals. Unfortunately, for the patient with ankylosing spondylitis who has this tendency, this posture may be made permanent if he is not consistently monitored and urged to maintain the upright posture.

POLYMYOSITIS/DERMATOMYOSITIS

Exercise prescription for patients with polymyositis/dermatomyositis (PM/DM) is especially appropriate because the pathology of the disease, unlike other arthritic conditions, is in the muscle. The joints are usually spared. Patients present with weakness and sometimes with muscle pain, abnormal biopsies, elevated serum muscle enzymes, and abnormal EMGs. Treatment with steroids and anticancer drugs is often successful and causes the patients to develop a remission. At that time, they will regain some strength, but it is generally agreed that unless exercise is provided, they will not regain their previous level of strength. The physiatrist, therefore, should prescribe isometric, isokinetic, or active exercise in moderate amounts and monitor the increase in strength carefully. Monitoring is usually done with serum enzymes, and if a marked increase occurs following the initiation of exercise treatment, the exercise should be stopped and reinstituted at a less vigorous level.

In patients with chronic PM/DM there is often replacement of muscle tissue with fibrosis. This can be determined with magnetic resonance imaging, computed tomography, or EMG. The serum enzymes will be diminished proportionate to the loss of muscle tissue. The patient will be weak, and the EMGs will not show as great a volume of motor unit action potentials. These patients may benefit from mild exercise, but they also may have no potential for doing so.

In chronic cases, contractures may occur. The physiatrist will discover this by careful observation and initiate assisted range of motion exercises immediately. It can be safely concluded that strengthening exercises for patients with PM/DM are appropriate when monitored carefully by serum enzyme levels.

Only a few studies monitor the treatment of PM/DM with exercise.[32] In 1993 Hicks et al. studied one patient who underwent isometric strengthening exercises of the right quadriceps and biceps for 4 weeks. There was an increase in isometric peak torque without a sustained rise in creatine phosphokinase (CPK). CPK levels, which were elevated at the initiation of exercise, gradually fell throughout the exercise program. The exercise program consisted of supervised exercise three times a week for 4 weeks on a Cybex machine.

Escalante et al. studied five patients, four of whom performed resistive exercise alternating with nonresistive exercise.[12] Three of the four patients with resistive exercise improved. The one patient who performed the most severe resistive exercise improved a great deal. The CPK was not significantly elevated following exercise in these patients and was normal by 8 hours. The weakest patient made no improvement. A second patient did not gain much in strength but increased ADL skills. The exercise period was 30 minutes of resistive exercise a day for 2 weeks before the second type of exercise was substituted. Each patient also performed functional exercises.

In addition, a dilemma may occur in that a PM/DM patient may suddenly or gradually become weaker. When this occurs, a decision must be made as to whether the patient has become weakened from steroid myopathy or from a lack of sufficient steroid treatment. If increased myositic activity can be demonstrated by an elevated serum enzyme level or the EMG, more steroids are indicated. If there is no sign of increased activity, a gradual decrease in steroid dose may be followed by an improvement in strength.

CASE EXAMPLES

CASE 1

A 40-year-old woman has had rheumatoid arthritis for 3½ years. Low-dose prednisone, nonsteroidal antiinflammatories, and methotrexate have suppressed the inflammation markedly. Her radiographs show minimal juxtaarticular osteoporosis and few erosions. She wants to know if she may pursue an exercise program. You advise the following:

1. Try underwater gravity-reduced exercise in a heated pool three times a week to increase range of motion, strength, and endurance.

2. If no heated pool is available, perform stretching exercises to increase any lack of normal range of motion. When this has been accomplished to the greatest benefit, perform progressive resistive exercises with increasingly strong Therabands for shoulder abduction, wrist extension, and hip and hip extension three times weekly. If joint pain persists more than 24 hours following these exercises, decrease the interval or force of exercises to a tolerable degree.

3. When she can easily perform Theraband exercises, begin to walk on soft surfaces with padded shoes for minimal distances and then increase the distance, as tolerated, three times weekly.

4. Finally, try swimming, rapid walking, jogging, low impact sports, and "aerobic" exercise only after demonstrating the ability to increase strength and endurance without ill effects for 6 months.

5. Note that the exercise will probably make her feel better but that the long-term effects of even well-tolerated strength and endurance exercises in patients with rheumatoid arthritis have not been clearly defined.

CASE 2

A 60-year-old man with symptomatic and radiographically demonstrated osteoarthritis of the knees asks you if he may undergo an exercise program. You make sure that his drug program is optimal and advise the following:

1. Begin a several-week program of stretching to exercise the extension and flexion limits of the hips and knees.

2. Begin isometric quadriceps and hamstring exercises at 90°, 135°, and 180° of knee extension. Increase the repetitions, as tolerated, while sitting at both full and partial hip extension.

3. Note that pain persisting more than 24 hours after exercise is a reason to decrease the exercise effort.

4. Begin walking with padded shoes on smooth surfaces for increasing distances three times a week, as tolerated, when he has demonstrated his ability to increase his strength and endurance.

5. Note that exercise has been shown to increase muscle strength and endurance in patients with osteoarthritis but that the long-term effects of this form of exercise are not known.

CASE 3

A 25-year-old man with ankylosing spondylitis tells you he thinks he is becoming more stooped and that his back is getting stiffer. You advise the following:

1. Begin stretching exercises in the horizontal hyperextended plane of the shoulders, extension of the cervical and thoracic spine, and deep breathing three times weekly.

2. Place his hands on the occiput, face the corner of the room, and walk toward it so that the cervical and thoracic spine will extend.

3. Perform push-up exercises for shoulder strengthening, as tolerated.

4. Note that he will likely be able to keep his back from becoming more stooped and that he may gain extension of the cervical and thoracic spine but that the stiffness will probably progress.

CONCLUSION

Many research studies and patient publications, including those of the Arthritis Foundation, advocate exercise for patients with inflammatory or degenerative arthritis. Patients will probably feel better and perform better if they comply. The physician must be careful to always assess the effects of exercises on individual joints because some may become increasingly inflamed or painful. This joint-by-joint approach to the prescription of exercise in patients with arthritis will probably be successful; however, the long-term results of such exercise are not clearly known.

REFERENCES

1. Agudelo CA, Schumacher HR, Phelps P: Effect of exercise on urate crystal-induced inflammation in canine joints. Arthritis Rheum 15:609–616, 1972.
2. Bakker C, Hidding A, van der Linden S, van Doorslaer E: Cost effectiveness of group physical therapy compared to individual therapy for ankylosing spondylitis. A randomized controlled trial. J Rheumatol 21:264–268, 1994.
3. Beals CA, Lampman RM, Banwell BF, et al: Measurement of exercise tolerance in patients with rheumatoid arthritis and osteoarthritis. J Rheumatol 12:458–461, 1985.
4. Bland JH, Eddy WM: Hemiplegia and rheumatoid arthritis. Arthritis Rheum 11:72–80, 1968.
5. Brighton SW, Lubbe JE, van der Merwe CA: The effect of a long-term exercise programme on the rheumatoid hand. Br J Rheumatol 32:392–395, 1993.
6. Castillo BA, el Sallab RA, Scott JT: Physical activity, cystic erosions, and osteoporosis in rheumatoid arthritis. Ann Rheum Dis 24:522–527, 1965.
7. Cooper C, Campbell L, Byng P, et al: Occupational activity and the risk of hip osteoarthritis. Ann Rheum Dis 55:680–682, 1996.
8. Danneskiold-Samsøe B, Lyngberg K, Risum R, Telling M: The effect of water exercise therapy given to patients with rheumatoid arthritis. Scand J Rehabil Med 19:31–35, 1987.
9. Ekblom B, Lövgren O, Alderin M, et al: Physical performance in patients with rheumatoid arthritis. Scand J Rheumatol 3:121–125, 1974.
10. Ekblom B, Lövgren O, Alderin M, et al: Effect of short-term physical training on patients with rheumatoid arthritis I. Scand J Rheumatol 4:80–86, 1975.
11. Ekdahl C, Broman G: Muscle strength, endurance, and aerobic capacity in rheumatoid arthritis: A comparative study with healthy subjects. Ann Rheum Dis 51:35–40, 1992.
12. Escalante A, Miller L, Beardmore TD: Resistive exercise in the rehabilitation of polymyositis/dermatomyositis. J Rheumatol 20:1340–1344, 1993.
13. Ettinger WH Jr, Burns R, Messier SP, et al: A randomized trial comparing aerobic exercise with a health education program in older adults with knee osteoarthritis. The fitness arthritis and seniors trial (FAST). JAMA 277:25–31, 1997.
14. Fam AG, Schumacher HR Jr, Clayburne G, et al: Effect of joint motion on experimental calcium pyrophosphate dihydrate crystal induced arthritis. J Rheumatol 17:644–655, 1990.
15. Fisher LR, Cawley MI, Holgate ST: Relation between chest expansion, pulmonary function, and exercise tolerance in patients with ankylosing spondylitis. Ann Rheum Dis 49:921–925, 1990.
16. Fisher NM, Gresham G, Pendergast DR: Effects of a quantitative progressive rehabilitation program applied unilaterally to the osteoarthritic knee. Arch Phys Med Rehabil 74:1319–1326, 1993.
17. Fisher NM, Pendergast DR: Effects of a muscle exercise program on exercise capacity in subjects with osteoarthritis. Arch Phys Med Rehabil 75:792–797, 1994.
18. Fisher NM, Pendergast DR, Calkins EC: Maximal isometric torque of knee extension as a function of muscle length in subjects of advancing age. Arch Phys Med Rehabil 71:729–734, 1990.
19. Fisher NM, Pendergast DR, Calkins E: Muscle rehabilitation in impaired elderly nursing home residents. Arch Phys Med Rehabil 72:181–185, 1991.
20. Fisher NM, Pendergast DR, Gresham GE, Calkins E: Muscle rehabilitation: Its effect on muscular and functional performance of patients with knee osteoarthritis. Arch Phys Med Rehabil 72:367–374, 1991.
21. Fries JF, Singh G, Morfeld D, et al: Running and the development of disability with age. Ann Intern Med 121:502–509, 1994.
22. Fries JF, Singh G, Morfeld D, et al: Relationship of running to musculoskeletal pain with age. Arthritis Rheum 39:64–72, 1996.
23. Gardner DL: The Pathological Basis of the Connective Tissue Diseases. Philadelphia, Lea & Febiger, 1992.

24. Glick IN: Asymmetrical rheumatoid arthritis after poliomyelitis. BMJ 3:26–29, 1967.
25. Glyn JH, Sutherland I, Walker GF, Young AC: Low incidence of osteoarthritis in hip and knee after anterior poliomyelitis: A late review. BMJ 2:739–742, 1966.
26. Glynn JJ, Clayton ML: Sparing effect of hemiplegia on tophaceous gout. Ann Rheum Dis 35:534–535, 1976.
27. Green J, McKenna F, Redfern EJ, Chamberlain MA: Home exercises are as effective as outpatient hydrotherapy for osteoarthritis of the hip. Br J Rheumatol 32:812–815, 1993.
28. Häkkinen A, Häkkinen K, Hannonen P: Effects of strength training on neuromuscular function and disease activity in patients with recent-onset inflammatory arthritis. Scand J Rheumatol 23:237–242, 1994.
29. Hansen TM, Hansen G, Langgaard AM, Rasmussen JO: Long-term physical training in rheumatoid arthritis. A randomized trial with different training programs and blinded observers. Scand J Rheumatol 22:107–112, 1993.
30. Harkcom TM, Lampman RM, Banwell BF, Castor CW: Therapeutic value of graded aerobic exercise training in rheumatoid arthritis. Arthritis Rheum 28:32–39, 1985.
31. Hicks JE: Exercise in patients with inflammatory arthritis and connective tissue disease. Rheum Dis Clin North Am 16:845–870, 1990.
32. Hicks JE, Miller F, Plotz P, et al: Isometric exercise increases strength and does not produce sustained creatinine phosphokinase increases in a patient with polymyositis. J Rheumatol 20:1399–1401, 1993.
33. Hochberg MC, Perlmutter DL, Hudson JI, Altman RD: Preferences in the management of osteoarthritis of the hip and knee: Results of a survey of community-based rheumatologists in the United States. Arthritis Care Res 9:170–176, 1996.
34. Hoenig L, Groff G, Pratt K, et al: Randomized controlled trial of home exercise in the rheumatoid hand. J Rheumatol 20:785–789, 1993.
35. Kirsteins AE, Dietz F, Hwang SM: Evaluating the safety and potential use of a weightbearing exercise, Tai-Chi Chuan, for rheumatoid arthritis patients. Am J Phys Med Rehabil 70:136–141, 1991.
36. Kovar PA, Allegrante JP, MacKenzie CR, et al: Supervised fitness walking in patients with osteoarthritis of the knee. A randomized, controlled study. Ann Intern Med 116:529–534, 1992.
37. Kraag G, Stokes B, Groh J, et al: The effect of comprehensive home physiotherapy and supervision on patients with ankylosing spondylitis—a randomized controlled trial. J Rheumatol 17:228–233, 1990.
38. Kujala UM, Kettunen J, Paananen H, et al: Knee osteoarthritis in former runners, soccer players, weight lifters, and shooters. Arthritis Rheum 38:539–546, 1995.
39. Lane NE: Exercise: A cause of osteoarthritis. J Rheumatol 22:3–6, 1995.
40. Lane NE: Physical activity at leisure and risk of osteoarthritis. Ann Rheum Dis 55:682–684, 1996.
41. Lane NE, Buckwalter JA: Exercise: A cause of osteoarthritis? Rheum Dis Clin North Am 19:617–633, 1993.
42. Lyngberg KK, Harreby M, Bentzen H, et al: Elderly rheumatoid arthritis patients on steroid treatment tolerate physical training without an increase in disease activity. Arch Phys Med Rehabil 75:1189–1195, 1994.
43. Lyngberg KK, Ramsing BU, Nawrock A, et al: Safe and effective isokinetic knee extension training in rheumatoid arthritis. Arthritis Rheum 37:623–628, 1994.
44. Machover S, Sapecky AJ: Effect of isometric exercise on the quadriceps muscle in patients with rheumatoid arthritis. Arch Phys Med Rehabil 47:737–741, 1966.
45. Mangione KK, Axen K, Haas F: Mechanical unweighting effects on treadmill exercise and pain in elderly people with osteoarthritis of the knee. Phys Ther 76:387–394, 1996.
46. Melton-Rogers S, Hunter G, Walter J, Harrison P. Cardiorespiratory responses of patients with rheumatoid arthritis during bicycle riding and running in water. Phys Ther 76:1058–1065, 1996.
47. Merritt JL, Hunder GG: Passive range of motion, not isometric exercise, amplifies acute urate synovitis. Arch Phys Med Rehabil 64:130–131, 1983.
48. Michel BA, Fries JF, Bloch DA, et al: Osteophytosis of the knee: Association with changes in weight-bearing exercise. Clin Rheumatol 11:235–238, 1992.
49. Minor MA: Arthritis and exercise: The times they are a-changin'. Arthritis Care Res 9:79–81, 1996.

50. Minor MA, Hewett JE, Webel RR, et al: Efficacy of physical conditioning exercise in patients with rheumatoid arthritis and osteoarthritis. Arthritis Rheum 32:1396–1405, 1989.
51. Minor MA, Hewett JE, Webel RR, et al: Exercise tolerance and disease related measures in patients with rheumatoid arthritis and osteoarthritis. J Rheumatol 15:905–911, 1988.
52. Murray DG: Modification of experimental arthritis in rabbits by tenotomy. J Surg Res 6:488–492, 1966.
53. Nordemar R: Physical training in rheumatoid arthritis: A controlled long-term study. II. Functional capacity and general attitudes. Scand J Rheumatol 10:25–30, 1981.
54. Nordemar R, Berg U, Ekblom B, Edström L: Changes in muscle fibre size and physical performance in patients with rheumatoid arthritis after 7 months' physical training. Scand J Rheumatol 5:233–238, 1976.
55. Nordemar R, Edström L, Ekblom B: Changes in muscle fibre size and physical performance in patients with rheumatoid arthritis after short-term physical training. Scand J Rheumatol 5:70–76, 1976.
56. Nordesjö LO, Nordgren B, Wigren A, Kolstad K: Isometric strength and endurance in patients with severe rheumatoid arthritis or osteoarthritis in the knee joints. Scand J Rheumatol 12:152–156, 1983.
57. Noreau L, Martineau H, Roy L, Belzile M: Effects of a modified dance-based exercise on cardiospiratory fitness, psychological state and health status of persons with rheumatoid arthritis. Am J Phys Rehabil 74:19–27, 1995.
58. Panush RS, Brown DG: Exercise and arthritis. Sports Med 4:54–64, 1987.
59. Panush RS, Hanson CS, Caldwell JR, et al: Is running associated with osteoarthritis? An eight-year follow-up study. J Clin Rheumatol 1:35–39, 1995.
60. Perlman SG, Connell KJ, Clark A, et al: Dance-based aerobic exercise for rheumatoid arthritis. Arthritis Care Res 3:29–35, 1990.
61. Philbin EF, Groff GD, Ries MD, Miller TE: Cardiovascular fitness and health in patients with end-stage osteoarthritis. Arthritis Rheum 38:799–805, 1995.
62. Glynn LE: The chronicity of inflammation and its significance in rheumatoid arthritis. Ann Rheum Dis 27:105–121, 1968.
63. Piersol GM, Hollander JL: The optimum rest-exercise balance in the treatment of rheumatoid arthritis. Arch Phys Med Rehabil 28:500–506, 1947.
64. Rall LC, Meydani SN, Kehayias JJ, et al: The effect of progressive resistive training in rheumatoid arthritis. Increased strength without changes in energy balance or body composition. Arthritis Rheum 39:415–426, 1996.
65. Rall LC, Roubenoff R: Body composition, metabolism, and resistance exercise in patients with rheumatoid arthritis. Arthritis Care Res 9:151–156, 1996.
66. Ries MD, Philbin EF, Groff GD: Relationship between severity of gonarthrosis and cardiovascular fitness. Clin Orthop 313:169–176, 1995.
67. Russell P, Unsworth A, Haslock I: The effect of exercise on ankylosing spondylitis—a preliminary study. Br J Rheumatol 32:498–506, 1993.
68. Semble EL, Loeser RF, Wise CM: Therapeutic exercise for rheumatoid arthritis and osteoarthritis. Semin Arthritis Rheum 20:32–40, 1990.
69. Spector TD, Harris PA, Hart DJ, et al: Risk of osteoarthritis associated with long-term weight-bearing sports. Arthritis Rheum 39:98–995, 1996.
70. Stecher RM, Karnash LJ: Herberden's nodes VI. The effect of nerve injury upon formation of degenerative joint disease of the fingers. Am J Med Sci 213:181–190, 1947.
71. Stenström CH: Therapeutic exercise in rheumatoid arthritis. Arthritis Care Res 7:190–197, 1994.
72. Stenström CH: Radiologically observed progression of joint destruction and its relationship with demographic factors, disease severity, and exercise frequency in patients with rheumatoid arthritis. Phys Ther 74:32–39, 1994.
73. Stenström CH: Home exercise in rheumatoid arthritis functional class II: Goal setting versus pain attention. J Rheumatol 21:627–634, 1994.
74. Tan J, Balci N, Sepici V, Gener FA: Isokinetic and isometric strength in osteoarthrosis of the knee. A comparative study with healthy women. Am J Phys Med Rehabil 74:364–369, 1995.
75. Thompson M, Bywaters EGL: Unilateral rheumatoid arthritis following hemiplegia. Ann Rheum Dis 21:370–377, 1962.

76. van den Ende CH, Hazes JM, le Cessie S, et al: Comparison of high and low intensity training in well controlled rheumatoid arthritis. Results of a randomised clinical trial. Ann Rheum Dis 55:798–805, 1996.

77. Viitanen JV, Lehtinen K, Suni J, Kautiainen H: Fifteen months' follow-up of intensive inpatient physiotherapy and exercise in ankylosing spondylitis. Clin Rheumatol 14:413–419, 1995.

78. Viitanen JV, Suni J, Kautiainen H, et al: Effect of physiotherapy on spinal mobility in ankylosing spondylitis. Scand J Rheumatol 21:38–41, 1992.

79. Watkins AL: Therapeutic exercise in rheumatoid arthritis. Arthritis Rheum 2:21–26, 1959.

80. Wessel J: Isometric strength measurements of knee extensors in women with osteoarthritis of the knee. J Rheumatol 23:328–331, 1996.

ALBERTO ESQUENAZI, MD
ROBERT DiGIACOMO, PT

15

Exercise Prescription for the Amputee

Exercise is a critical activity for old and young alike. It has a protective effect on the heart and a beneficial effect on the musculoskeletal system. Exercise may be even more valuable in a person with an amputation than in the general population because comorbidities such as hypertension and diabetes are usually present in elderly amputees. Many lower limb amputees became amputees in their 50s or 60s, but the range spans from children with congenital limb deficiencies to the elderly. The most common kind of lower limb amputation is transtibial amputation. In some rehabilitation facilities, upper limb amputation may account for up to 30% of all patients. The most frequent causes of amputation are arteriosclerotic occlusive disease, complications of diabetes mellitus, trauma, and malignancies.[16]

Limb amputation should never be viewed as a failure of surgery but instead as the means to return the patient to a more functional level. The value of approaching amputation with a positive and reconstructive approach cannot be overemphasized. The decision to amputate is an emotional process for surgeons, patients, and their families. The rehabilitation team should be ready to respond and assist them.

The stages of amputation rehabilitation and the type of exercise to be prescribed can be delineated according to specific rehabilitation goals.[16] The phases of limb amputation rehabilitation should be divided into nine discrete periods of rehabilitative evaluations and interventions (Table 1). Each of these phases contains specific evaluation items, treatment goals, and objectives. Optimally, rehabilitation of the amputee begins prior to amputation and should be provided by a specialized treatment team that includes a surgeon, a physiatrist or other physician knowledgeable in amputee rehabilitation and prosthetics, a certified prosthetist, an occupational therapist, physical therapist, recreational therapist, psychologist, and social worker. Communication between the team members and with the patient and family is essential and should provide the team with the necessary information to develop a treatment plan from amputation to discharge to home. The patient should be told of the implications of amputation, including phantom sensation.[21] The team should tell the patient what to expect after surgery and rehabilitation, taking into account the patient's physical sta-

TABLE 1.   Phases of Amputee Rehabilitation

Phase	Hallmarks
1. Preoperative	Assess body condition, patient education, surgical level discussion, postoperative prosthetic plans
2. Amputation surgery/reconstruction	Length, myoplastic closure, soft tissue coverage, nerve, handling, rigid dressing
3. Acute postoperative	Wound healing, pain control, proximal body motion, emotional support
4. Preprosthetic	Shaping, shrinking, increase muscle strength, restore patient locus of control
5. Prosthetic prescription and fabrication	Team consensus on prosthetic prescription
6. Prosthetic training	Increase prosthetic wearing and functional utilization
7. Community integration	Resumption of roles in family and community activities; emotional equilibrium and healthy coping strategies; recreational activities
8. Vocational rehabilitation	Assess and plan vocational activities for future; may need further education, training, or job modification
9. Follow-up	Life-long prosthetic, functional, medical assessment, and emotional support

tus, level of amputation, cognition, premorbid lifestyle, and socioeconomic level, and prepare the patient with realistic short- and long-term expectations.

EXERCISE PRESCRIPTION FOR THE PREPROSTHETIC AMPUTEE

Pain control, maintenance of range of motion and strength, and promotion of wound healing are the goals of this stage, which begins with the surgical closure of the wound and culminates with healing after the sutures are removed. The weeks immediately after amputation are the most critical in terms of implementing a comprehensive exercise program. Whenever possible, patients should be placed in a cardiovascular conditioning program before the amputation. When the patient is medically stable, early mobilization, general endurance and strengthening exercise, with an emphasis on the hip stabilizing muscles and the avoidance of joint contractures, and improvement on balance are initiated. Strengthening of upper limb musculature is essential for wheelchair propulsion, transfers, walker, and crutch ambulation for the lower limb amputee and should be aggressively pursued. It is important to emphasize the strength and function of the remaining limbs, with specificity of training as a preferred type of training.

Clinicians need to expect higher functional levels of their patients, especially if the amputation is viewed as a reconstructive procedure that will remove the burden of pain and open wounds. Based on this concept, young and elderly amputees should be given the advantage of receiving care in a rehabilitation program that offers therapy from a multidisciplinary team.[15,16] Patients with amputations once were provided with artificial limbs, and not much attention was paid to training or other special needs. However, the advent of specialized treatment teams and new prosthetic devices in the last two decades has improved the outlook for the lower limb amputee. The patient who has undergone a lower limb amputation may quickly become deconditioned and most likely depressed. A preprosthetic rehabilitation program must be initiated as soon as possible. Pain control and residual limb maturation should be continued during this phase. An increasingly popular method of wound protection and early shaping and shrinking is the removable rigid dressing as proposed by Burgess[6] and Woo.[47] This dressing is easily changed to accommodate the expected accelerated residual limb shrinkage and protects the residual limb during training for mobility skills. It can be applied to transradial- and transhumeral-level amputations but is more difficult to apply and keep positioned in transfemoral amputees. Soft compressive dressings alone are used in many centers.[15]

A skin desensitization program that includes gentle tapping, massage, and soft tissue and scar mobilization and lubrication is recommended.

When the patient is medically stable, early mobilization, general endurance, and strengthening exercise with specificity of training is a preferred type of training. For the lower limb amputee, devices such as the Universal Below the Knee Bicycle Attachment (UBKBA)[13] or the Versaclimber could be used to assist in strengthening exercises. These devices permit early endurance exercise with controlled weightbearing using a cyclical bipedal motion without direct stresses to the residual limb wound while the healing occurs (Fig. 1).

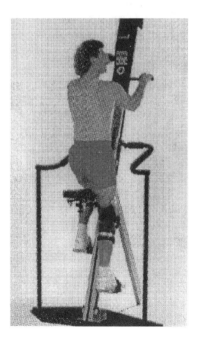

FIGURE 1. Amputee using a Versaclimber for limited weightbearing lower-extremity exercises.

A preparatory prosthesis should be used at this stage to serve as a gait-training tool for a short term and possibly to allow progression in physical fitness and exercise. In most instances, the components of the prosthesis are simple. The prosthetic device should allow for easy adjustability of the socket fit and alignment because increased strength, endurance, weightbearing, and confidence occur with training.

Upper limb support for balance will be necessary for most amputees during fitting of the preparatory prosthesis. A cane or single crutch on the opposite side usually will be sufficient for the unilateral amputee. All unilateral transfemoral amputees should be safe ambulating with bilateral crutches without a prosthesis, because there may be times when the artificial limb may not be used. In some cases, as with a comorbidity, a walker with wheels or a reciprocating system may be used when the device is necessary.

Weight-shifting techniques that include the use of stepping and a balance board should be encouraged. Gait training initially for technique and then for velocity on flat surfaces is essential and then progresses to uneven surfaces and elevations. A review and practice of the use of the prosthesis in transfers, driving, sports, and other activities should always be included in training.

Prosthetic management and gait training are integral to the rehabilitation process. A new amputee or an experienced one who receives a new type of prosthesis should participate in such training.[16] The training program should be a coordinated effect between the physical, occupational, and recreational therapists and the prosthetist with frequent physician input. Each team member will use different techniques to teach and review all of the topics that need to be learned by the amputee. This comprehensive approach has been found to improve functional outcomes. In 1993 in two separate studies, Pinzur et al. and Stewart and Jain concluded that optimal amputee care is provided in specialized well-coordinated multidisciplinary management programs.[16]

In addition to the involved limbs, the remaining limbs must be evaluated in terms of range of motion, strength, sensation, vascularity, coordination, skin integrity, and deformity. In a patient whose amputation is caused by ischemia related to atherosclerosis or diabetes mellitus, similar arterial insufficiency involving the cardiac and cerebral vessels should be suspected. The cardiac and pulmonary status is evaluated to assess the patient's ability to tolerate the rigors of an exercise and rehabilitation program. The patient's willingness and ability to learn new techniques and to participate in a variety of new activities is critical. Thus, cognitive and psychological evaluations are important. Nutritional status, which has a considerable impact on wound healing and strength, must not be neglected. The presence of a variety of other comorbidities such as diabetic retinopathy, peripheral polyneuropathy, nephropathy, and degenerative joint disease also may influence the rehabilitation of the amputee.[19,26,41,46] In short, a thorough medical evaluation of the patient is necessary before an exercise program is initiated.

Patients are often not eager to perform the upper limb exercises that promote the strength and range of motion required for self-care activities. However, most patients with recent amputations are more concerned with mobility than bathing and dressing. Arms provide the power for wheelchair mobility and the use of walking aids. In particular, shoulder stabilizers, adductors, depressors, elbow extensors, wrist stabilizers, and hand grasp strength are of prime importance for supporting the body for transfers and using the more common walking aids. Trunk balance and strength must not be neglected. Sitting balance and bed mobility and transfers are facilitated by strong flexible rotators, flexors, extensors of the back and abdomen, and the extensors of the hips.

The importance of lower limb exercise is obvious. The remaining limb for the unilateral lower limb amputee temporarily becomes the solitary support limb and frequently can develop symptoms consistent with overuse, particularly at the knee and ankle. Stance phase stability requires adequate strength in the hip extensors, abductors, knee extensors, and plantar flexors. Swing phase limb advancement and clearance requires adequate hip flexor and ankle dorsiflexor strength.

Lower limb contractures are common in amputees.[31] Unfortunately, the position of comfort is often the position that can lead to contractures. It is important to continually remind patients that contractures can significantly impair their future mobility and compromise the integrity of the nonamputated limb. The transfemoral amputee often develops contractures of the hip flexors, abductors, and external rotators. The transtibial amputee frequently develops hip and knee flexion contractures. Contractures of the hip flexors, knee flexors, and plantar flexors of the intact limb of the unilateral lower limb amputee will often result from prolonged bed rest in the comfortable posture of semifowler's position. If soft tissue contracture results in an equinus posture, the normal weightbearing posture of the foot is compromised. Pressure distribution to the heel is lost and forces are concentrated on the forefoot. The increased pressure on the forefoot can lead to local pain and tissue breakdown, of particular importance in the presence of peripheral neuropathy. For the upper limb amputee, the elbow, shoulder, and neck musculature are at risk of contracture development.

The "ounce of prevention" maxim certainly applies to limb contractures. Several factors may contribute to contractures, including preoperative positioning, surgical technique, pain, deficient knowledge regarding range of motion, and limited mobility related to ischemia, skin grafts, delayed wound healing, infection, or trauma that led to the amputation. The treatment of contractures may include heating modalities, prolonged passive stretching, spring-loaded orthoses, serial casting, nerve blocks, or further surgery.[31] To avoid contractures, patients are instructed to move the limbs through full range of motion frequently and to avoid postures of comfort for prolonged times. Periods of lying prone should be included in a lower limb amputee's exercise program. A posterior splint may help prevent knee flexion contractures in the transtibial amputee. Frequent reminders and encouragement help the patient comply with these instructions. Contractures are readily prevented through the use of an immediate postoperative rigid dressing.[6,47] The rigid dressing extends proximally to enclose the knee and prevent a flexion contracture.

The lower limb amputee's outlook typically brightens considerably when he learns that he is not confined to bed. Independence in transfers and functional mobilty are of great importance. Bed mobility exercises, including rolling from side to side and sitting, allow the patient to position himself without help. Transfer training allows the patient to expand his world beyond his bed and room. The patient may use sliding board, front-on/back-off, or stand (squat) pivot transfers to move from one surface to another.

Ambulation training without the prosthesis is important to the amputee. Initially, standing balance and standing tolerance are addressed. Once the patient can manage standing, ambulation (hopping) using the parallel bars can begin. As strength and endurance improve, the patient may advance to a walker and to crutches. In addition to allowing greater mobility, the activities improve lower limb strength and range of motion and remind the patient that bipedal walking may soon become a reality.

Return to bipedal ambulation is the stated goal of most lower limb amputees. Amputees often feel that only by returning to ambulation can they resume their previous lives, roles, activities, and socialization.[12] Walking is an enormously important transition for the amputee. Rehabilitation with the preparatory prosthesis begins by introducing the patient to the preparatory prosthesis' components and management. Explanations of how the prosthesis fits, where weight is borne, where and why discomfort may occur, and how adjustments can be made help put the patient at ease. It is useful to remind the patient that walking will be impossible without their weight being supported by some pressure-tolerant portion of the residual limb. Pressure is to be expected and, while uncomfortable at first, should not be painful. Gait training begins with weightbearing and shifting using the parallel bars for upper limb support. The patient gradually progresses to ambulation in the parallel bars. The therapist may find it difficult to focus the patient on proper technique, including equal step length, and appropriate weight-shifting. Gait deviations frequently develop due to the patient's eagerness to begin walking. As the patient establishes a consistent gait pattern and can maintain good form, he advances to a walker, crutches, and unilateral support devices. Once the patient is comfortable with level surfaces, he progresses to stairs, curbs, ramps, and ambulation on uneven terrain. The patient also learns safe techniques for transfers, including to and from the floor.[32]

Stairs are often a source of concern for the amputee. Many individuals use a "bumping" technique to ascend or descend. The patient sits on the steps and uses the arms and remaining lower limb to propel up or down. Of course, the floor transfer at the top or bottom of the stairs also must be addressed. Many amputees use a low box or stool as a step between the floor and the wheelchair or standing posture.

The specific exercise programs and goals are derived from physical, occupational, and recreation therapy with physician guidance. The exercise program for the amputee focuses on four main components of exercise: cardiovascular training, flexibility, muscle strength, and balance.

CARDIOVASCULAR TRAINING

Cardiovascular conditioning must be initiated as early as possible postoperatively. Whenever possible, patients are placed in a cardiovascular conditioning program before the amputation. Amputees must develop improved aerobic fitness levels due to the increased energy demands associated with prosthetic ambulation.[15,44,37] Cardiovascular training should begin with low-impact aerobics for periods of time commensurate with a patient's level of fitness. Using accepted formulas, a target heart range can be established based on the following basic fitness parameters: low to moderate intensity maintains a 50–65% maximum heart rate;[1] and moderate to high intensity maintains a 65–85% maximum heart rate.[26,38] Exercise sessions should begin at no lower than 10 minutes of continual activity, with the goal of working up to 30–40 minutes.[46] If 10 minutes cannot be achieved initially, shorter exercise periods with increased frequency can be used effectively.[39]

Ambulation is a well-known way to improve cardiopulmonary endurance. However, for the recent lower extremity amputee, upper extremity aerobic conditioning may be the only choice.[41] This may be the case when severe postoperative pain, limited functional mobility, and wound protection prohibit lower extremity involvement. One should keep in mind that upper extremity exercises use muscle groups that fatigue easily and increase blood pressure. Also, proof exists that there is no transferability of training from upper extremity exercise to lower extremity exercise, particularly ambulation.

Modalities of alternative exercise include the upper body ergometer (UBE), the Versaclimber, and the UBKBA. The UBE requires the patient to perform clockwise or counterclockwise arm revolutions on a cam-shaft device similar to a bicycle wheel mechanism.[8] The Versaclimber requires an up and down climbing motion on a vertically oriented device that can use one or both lower limbs and one or both upper limbs.

The UBKBA, which was developed in our center, permits early endurance exercise with controlled weightbearing through the amputated limb using a stationary bicycle and a modified adjustable bicycle/residual limb interface. Clinical testing of the device in 12 unilateral below-knee amputees and two bilateral below-knee amputees in the early postoperative period has been reported.[13] The subjects were able to pedal up to an average of 18 minutes (range 13–20 minutes). No residual limb or systemic complications were encountered during the testing. Clinical evidence of cardiac and respiratory responses necessary for conditioning were present. The subjects appeared to derive both physiologic and psychological benefit from training with the device. Stationary biking is less tolling on the cardiovascular system, and stationary bicycles cost less than UBEs.[19] Patients who can perform safe transfers and have an intact, uninvolved lower extremity are good candidates for using a stationary bicycle with or without the UBKBA. These three apparatuses offer variable resistance control, and we recommend working up to at least 30 minutes on the lowest settings before increasing the resistance level.

As the patient's endurance and residual limb tissue tolerance improves, the patient can use a traditional stationary exercise bicycle or a stationary bicycle that allows for upper extremity participation to engage all four extremities during aerobic training.[4,36] These latter bikes usually employ a reciprocating rowing motion for the upper extremities that coincides with lower extremity pedaling. Resistance is gained through an increased pace of performance. Many models are available. A typical low- to moderate-intensity program can begin with 10 minutes of exercise at a pace of 30–40 revolutions per minute (rpm), with the goal of working up to 40 minutes using little or no resistance. For moderate- to high-intensity exercise, a regime begins with a 30-minute session at a pace of 40–90 rpm and progresses to 40 minutes. Subsequent resistance upgrades can be made thereafter. Exercise prescription for all of the described equipment should model that of the stationary bicycle. Chair aerobics is another valuable technique to promote cardiovascular endurance and fitness. Chair aerobics is a continuous 20 to 40-minute group exercise set to music that can involve all four extremities. Patients are grouped according to general fitness levels determined by the formulas highlighted earlier. Resistance may be incorporated to provide additional challenges. This activity is fun and provides a means for socialization with others.

FLEXIBILITY

Following an amputation, adequate lower extremity flexibility is critical to residual limb preparation for prosthetic use, particularly because the incidence of postoperative contracture formation is high.[32,34] Initially, bed mobility exercises should be geared toward independent achievement of the prone position. Prone-lying for extended periods can deliver a prolonged, low-load stretch to the hip extensors.[29] Knee flexion contractures also can be combated in prone by adding resistance to the residual limb. Prone-lying programs should begin with a maximally tolerated period of comfortable stretch and then increase consistently daily.

Positioning programs should be supplemented with self-stretches that the patient can perform in addition to therapy. Traditional Thomas test position hip flexors and long-sitting hamstring self-stretches are easy and effective. Each stretch should be performed bilaterally for 30 seconds with at least five repetitions to each extremity.[2] If a patient's techniques are deemed correct, the stretches should be performed in three to five sessions throughout the day. If self-stretches are not successful, assisted manual stretching must be implemented, with the possible addition of facilitatory techniques. Success has been achieved using proprioceptive neuromuscular facilitatory (PNF) techniques of contract-relax, hold-relax, and slow-reversal-hold-relax with patients demonstrating significant muscle guarding.[45]

MUSCLE STRENGTH

Strengthening exercises to the amputated extremity should immediately focus on neuromuscular reeducation of the musculature that was traumatized by surgery. In addition to functioning as primary movers, these muscle groups play a major role in force distribution at the socket-limb interface. Kegel et al.[23] recommend electromyogram biofeedback for volitional firing of the residual muscles, i.e., the gastrocnemius-soleus group, and of the peroneal and pretibial muscles of the transtibial amputee. For the transfemoral amputee, residual hamstring, quadriceps, adductors, and abductor muscle groups should receive periods of biofeedback training. For the upper limb, the wrist flexors/extensors and the biceps/triceps pairs can be trained in a similar manner. We recommend that the patient be taught how to use the device so that the patient can practice throughout the day. Increased pain or muscular fatigue are the only limitations. When postoperative swelling diminishes, neuromuscular electrical stimulation (NMES) can be considered for persistent problems with residual muscular firing patterns.[11] NMES programs should be patterned to produce tetanic muscle contraction (at least 40 MHz frequency) for an on:off cycle of at least 10:20–30 seconds. Other neuromuscular facilitatory techniques, such as rhythmic initiation of PNF diagonals with manual cues and quick reversals, can be tried as the surgical wound reaches primary intention.[45]

By the end of the first postoperative week, a patient can begin a total body strengthening program designed specifically for proximal stability and distal mobility. Open and closed chain therapeutic exercises can be employed using the overload principle as a goal for strengthening.[20] The DeLorme protocol can be followed with three sets of ten repetitions performed at 50%, 75%, and 100% of a one-repetition maximum.[9,10] The lower extremity regimen should include exercises to the surrounding hip muscles, with particular attention to the hip abductor and hip extensor groups for pelvic stabilization.[16,40] Quadriceps and hamstring strength of the transtibial residual limb plays a crucial role in knee stability for future prosthetic usage.[7,40] Ankle stability for the intact limb is best addressed through weightbearing activities, detailed below in the section on balance. Based on the initial neuromuscular evaluation, cardinal plane isotonic exercises can begin with gravity-eliminated resistance, progressing to antigravity, and finally antigravity plus additional resistance with cuff weights or Theraband. In addition to these traditional open chain exercises, closed chain exercise can be added easily into a mat exercise program. Using simple positioning and a comfortable surface on which to bear weight, all hip and knee muscle groups can perform modified closed chain exercises that are more specific to muscular performance during gait[17] (Fig. 2).

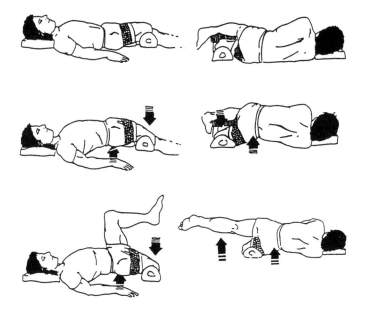

FIGURE 2. Closed chain mat exercises. *Left*, Sample hip extension exercise progression. *Right*, Sample hip abduction progression. (From Gailey RS: One Step Ahead: An Integrated Approach to Lower Extremity Prosthetics and Amputee Rehabilitation. Miami, FL, Advanced Rehab Therapy Inc., 1994, with permission.)

A comprehensive program also should include strengthening of the trunk stabilizers. In particular, exercises should engage the transverse abdominus oblique muscle groups anteriorly and the erector spinae paravertebral muscles posteriorly. Traditional abdominal crunches, crunches with rotation, and back extensions should be performed while the patient is in a pelvic neutral position. This posture usually requires a posterior pelvic tilt to flatten the normal lordotic curve of the lumbrosacral spine. Because these muscles are more postural in function, strengthening should occur through greater numbers of repetitions per set (about 20–40) until fatigue occurs.

Upper extremity strengthening activities are often ignored after the amputee can perform basic bed mobility and transfers. The muscles that stabilize the glenohumeral and scapulothoracic joints play important roles in using an assistive device for gait training and ambulating on all surfaces. Properly balanced muscle group force pairing should include the trapezius/serratus anterior, and rotator cuff/deltoid groups.[27] Seated push-ups, scapular protraction and retraction, and shoulder shrug will help ensure proper scapular positioning for smooth glenohumeral rhythm.[35] Strong internal and external rotators through 90–140°, in the scapular plane, will maintain proper humeral head depression during shoulder elevations.[43] Additionally, elbow stability should be maintained through biceps and triceps strengthening. Upper extremity strengthening should follow the same principles of frequency, intensity, and duration as for the lower extremity musculature. Necessary fine wrist and hand movements are often best strengthened with the occupational therapist's myriad fine motor functional exercises and activities of daily living exercises.

BALANCE

The unilateral lower extremity amputee must develop adequate single-leg stance balance and stability to ensure safe functional mobility without the use of a prosthesis and to prepare for gait training.[42] For the intact limb itself, proper ankle and hip balance strategies can be retrained through simple static standing progressions, which begin with bilateral upper extremity support and progress to unsupported, unilateral standing balance. Dynamic upper extremity movements, within and out of the base of support, are more advanced challenges. Along with the intact limb, trunk stability should be addressed with postural sets that emphasize a balance between the abdominal and paravertebral muscle groups during the above progressions. Trunk stability may be challenged in the quadruped, high-kneeling, and single-leg kneeling positions. These activities also provide weightbearing to a well-healed residual limb. Transtibial amputees should be able to bear weight directly through the knee of their residual limb, and transfemoral amputees can use airsplints for completing these trials. Early weightbearing activities can reduce complaints of residual and limb pain and prepare the residual limb for prosthetic usage.[21,32] Bilateral amputees can gain trunk stability through sitting balance exercises performed on a bolster or therapeutic ball.

EXERCISE PRESCRIPTION FOR PROSTHETIC TRAINING

During the prosthetic training phase of rehabilitation, a prosthesis is prescribed and fabricated. Frequent monitoring of the skin allows for prompt corrections of problems with socket fit and avoids skin breakdown. Skin checks are performed more frequently for first-time prosthetic users and patients with delicate skin. Initially, checking the skin every 10–15 minutes or after every one or two walks may be necessary. Once the patient and clinical staff are comfortable with the socket fit, skin monitoring occurs less frequently.

Tolerance of the prosthesis gradually increases over the first few weeks. Some patients can wear the prosthesis for only 2–3 hours per day during the first week of gait training. The time gradually increases until the prosthesis is worn all day—for 12–16 hours. Throughout the rehabilitation process, the patient should become well versed in skin care. The patient learns to monitor the skin of the residual limb, noting signs of appropriate weightbearing and watching for evidence of skin irritation or breakdown.

When the prosthesis is not worn, the patient wears a stump shrinker or an Ace bandage to prevent residual limb edema and provide volume containment.[15,47]

CARDIOVASCULAR TRAINING

As prosthetic training begins, the variety of cardiovascular conditioning programs available for the amputee increases. Chair aerobics and the primary upper body modalities of the UBE and Versaclimber should continue to be part of a comprehensive conditioning program; however, bilateral lower limb involvement now becomes the focus.

The UBKBA or the stationary bike are logical choices to begin lower extremity conditioning because weightbearing demands on the prosthetic limb are minimized. One special consideration is making sure the socket fits properly. A snug prosthesis will increase the total surface area contact and thus reduce the incidence of skin trauma from shearing forces.[24] Proper adjustment of the height of the seat for the transtibial amputee is important because he or she may not be able to tolerate knee flexion past 90° due to pressure from the posterior socket in the popliteal region. For safety, the prosthetic limb should be secured with toe clips or Velcro. Programs should begin conservatively for 15–20 minutes at low resistance with skin tolerance of the residual limb being the limiting factor. Ensuing sessions should resume the use of the target heart range into a low-resistance, 30- to 40-minute daily routine.[39,46] Resistance should be added only after achieving this time interval consistently. As with aerobic exercise during the preprosthetic stage, a stationary bike that incorporates upper body participation is a better conditioning tool.[4,36]

The treadmill should be considered for cardiovascular conditioning when the patient can maintain a self-selected speed of ambulation around 1 mile per hour (mph). The main advantage of this activity is endurance training in the specific context of ambulation.[5,22] Other features include the ability to modify speed and inclination easily. An effective clinical treadmill must have the ability to start the pace of walking as low as 0.5 mph and have track tread at least 50 cm wide. Parameters of the prescription start with the patients' self-selected speed of gait performed for 8–12 minutes for up to two separate trials. Due to the high requisite force of weightbearing to the residual limb, as well as walking time intervals that are usually much longer than that to which many patients are accustomed, walking programs should start conservatively. After limb tolerance has been achieved, the exercise should progress to maintaining self-selected walking speed for up to 30–40 minutes per session.[38] Most patients exercising at the low to moderate levels of intensity achieve the desired target heart range. If they do not or if a patient can tolerate moderate to high levels of intensity, speeds should be increased 0.2 to 0.4 mph until a more appropriate heart rate is achieved. Another way to raise intensity as well as to change the environmental context is by inclining the platform grading 0.5 degrees at a time until a manageable hill is found. Frequent monitoring of the "sound foot" is imperative because high traction and friction are prime conditions for the development of skin breakdown, particularly in the diabetic insensate foot.[30] One cannot overemphasize the need for selecting appropriate footwear for the amputee.

When the amputee has an intact, matured incision, swimming may become an alternative aerobic training mode.[22] Programs must involve direct therapist guarding and the use of a personal flotation device until aquatic safety has been assured. Sample prescriptions can involve lower extremity emphasis through the use of a kick-board or a modified four-extremity stroke. Beginning times for continuous exercise may range from 5–15 minutes based on the patient's level of amputation and exercising in an unfamiliar environment. Conditioning goals are to achieve 30–40 minutes of continuous exercise while maintaining target heart rate parameters. A complete sequence of instruction along with a specific pool program is described later in this chapter.

FLEXIBILITY

During the prosthetic training phase, the patient should be independent with a self-stretch program that was learned following surgery. The therapist must emphasize strict adherence to this program, because many patients neglect stretching once they begin to reach their goal of walking again. As a consequence, hip and knee flexion contractures can develop. In addition to the recumbent stretches, a weightbearing stretch program incorporating the prosthesis can begin. Techniques for the hip include a lunge stretch with the patient positioned in single-leg kneeling and then leaning forward and allowing the kneeling limb to go into a position of hip extension. An erect hamstring stretch can be accomplished by placing one extremity forward of the other and then bending the trunk toward the limb maintaining lumbar lordosis. Ankle dorsiflexion of the intact limb can be maintained through the traditional heel cord stretch, which has the leg in a position of hip and knee extension with the foot kept flat on the ground. A slight body lean forward stretches the gastrocnemius. Stretching duration and frequencies mimic those outlined in the flexibility section for the preprosthetic amputee (see page 304).

MUSCLE STRENGTH AND ENDURANCE

Muscle strength and endurance take on a more demanding yet very specific mode during prosthetic training. The goal is to achieve sufficient muscular force generation and endurance from the lower extremities to support prolonged periods of gait.[32] The approach begins with pregait activities centered on residual limb weightbearing acceptance and distribution.[17] Bilateral resistance activities and a monitored walking program should immediately follow.

The ability of the residual limb to accept sufficient weight during the single-leg stance phase of gait represents the foundation of effective prosthetic ambulation. A pregait program starts in the safety of the parallel bars and with the close scrutiny of the therapist. After teaching the patient what an equilibrated base of support is, initial weight-shifting skills can begin. Weight shifting anterior to posterior, laterally, and circumducting should all be done with the pelvis remaining at neutral tilt and rotation[17] (Fig. 3). Next, the patient is placed in a normal gait stride position, and the migration of body weight from the toes of the extended limb to the heel of the stridden leg is encouraged. This activity practices the fundamental weight transfer necessary for gait. The therapist should recommend practicing each of these exercises equally within a set, using fairly light to somewhat hard exertion levels common to the ratings of perceived exertion scale (RPE).[3] At least three complete trials should be attempted daily.

The focus shifts from dynamic weight shifting on both lower extremities to activities of prosthetic limb weightbearing. Gailey[17] and others[32] recommend using steps of various heights with the intent of intact limb-stepping. This method encourages pronounced residual limb weightbearing through an exaggerated single-leg support

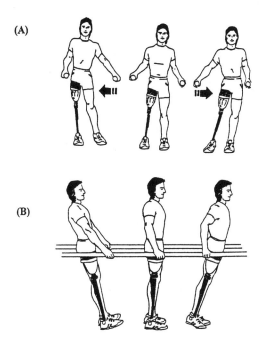

FIGURE 3. Dynamic weight shift exercises. *A*, Medial to lateral weight shifting. *B*, Anterior to posterior weight shifting. (From Gailey RS: One Step Ahead: An Integrated Approach to Lower Extremity Prosthetics and Amputee Rehabilitation. Miami, FL, Advanced Rehab Therapy Inc., 1994, with permission.)

period. The transtibial amputee will benefit from the cocontraction of knee extensors and flexors necessary for maintaining stability during this exercise. This activity allows transfemoral amputees to receive concentrated pelvic stabilization training through the hip abductors firing the residual limb into the lateral wall of the socket. Verbally cueing the patient to maintain an upright posture and a level pelvis helps to strengthen the hip abductor and extensor muscle groups, which is essential to an effective gait pattern for all lower extremity amputees.[16] A height of 2–4 inches can be started using bilateral upper extremity support, with progression to unilateral upper extremity support (intact limb side, then prosthetic side) and, finally, no upper extremity support (Fig. 4). Once mastery occurs at the beginning box height, the subsequent one should be 2 inches higher and be practiced upon through this progression. These exercises must be performed to an RPE level of moderate fatigue for at least three trials daily.

When the patient has gained proficiency in prosthetic limb weight acceptance, as evidenced by a reasonably efficient gait pattern, he or she is ready for some advanced resistance strengthening in standing. With adequate upper extremity support, initial exercises can be open chain movements of the hip and knee groups using gravity as resistance. More challenging exercises can involve Theratubing or an ankle-level cable

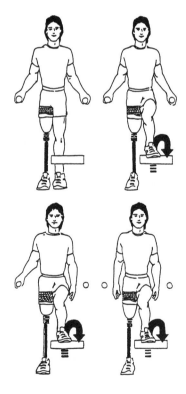

FIGURE 4. Progression series of step-up exercises for unilateral weightbearing.

row set-up. The equipment should be secured to the intact limb first and the patient then instructed in straight plane movements or possible PNF D1/D2 diagonals.[45] In this manner, when one limb is moving against resistance, the stabilizing limb is being strengthened in a closed chain manner. The exercise should be repeated with the prosthetic limb opposing the resistance band or cable. These exercises are executed using the overload principle as a goal for conditioning.[20] The DeLorme protocol can be employed for setting intensity,[9,10] or a therapist can use guidelines set forth by Burgess,[5] who recommends three sets of at least 8–12 repetitions.

BALANCE AND COORDINATION

In the beginning stages of prosthetic training, patients will quickly feel insecure when trying to balance themselves without upper extremity support. They will often flail their arms. The first explanation is the obvious loss of the direct proprioceptive input and sensory feedback the foot had provided. Closer inspection also may reveal an inadequate or improper hip balance reaction on the prosthetic side. An explanation for this occurrence may lie in a person's reliance on ankle balance strategies for correcting most of the typical perturbations to the base of support.[32] If the second line of defense, the hip balance strategy, cannot make up for proprioceptive losses that occur with a lower limb amputation, we do not have a mechanism for stable standing balance. A balance program geared to maximizing available proprioception and the retraining of hip reactions would be a logical approach.

Balance training for new prosthetic users should begin with sharpening of the proprioceptive sense of the trunk over the lower extremities. This may be done by asking patients to repeat some of the earlier weight-shift exercises without the benefit of vision. With patients still using unilateral upper extremity support, the clinician should ask for very slow repetitions of weight shifting with pauses where they perceive midline orientation. The clinician should randomly ask patients to stop at midline and look at their position. Patients often will not be where they had sensed. Patients should be encouraged to practice this exercise often to learn the "feel" of their new body position sense.

Balance training should begin with reeducating patients as to how their hip balance strategy operates. This is accomplished by purposefully perturbing patients out of their base of support and then manually cueing their hips into properly countering this motion. After this concept is learned, standing balance sequences are used that are patterned after motor learning principles, i.e., beginning with the lowest processing tasks and progressing to activities requiring greater coordination demands.[18] Training should begin within the parallel bars, having patients establish standing balance in a statistically unsupported context. Complexity is then added through the following sequence:

1. Lower extremity weight shifting without support.

2. Progressing to upper extremity movements, all within the patient's base of support.

The next level of skills requires reaching and shifting out of the patient's base of support. Add to this more complex manipulation tasks, as follow:

1. Having the patient catch and throw a ball from consistent heights.
2. Progress to catch and throw from random heights.
3. Migrate to the lower extremities and work on unilateral kicking out of a static position.

Locomotion is the next major processing requirement. A therapist can instruct the patient to perform the following activities:

1. Lateral, backward, and crossover stepping patterns.
2. Add a manipulation task of reaching, carrying, catching, and throwing to increase the processing demands, which positively correlates with prompting balance reactions to become more reflexive in nature.[18]

Moving out of the parallel bars into an unsupportive environment represents a major psychological and physical challenge. Once mastery of unsupported standing balance occurs, an extremely advanced progression would be to vary the actual support surface.[18] For example, a patient could perform balance skills going from a concrete surface to a grassy one or to a moving surface such as the treadmill. Retraining balance reactions for bilateral lower extremity amputees actually may be reversed. Attaining a static, unsupported posture may be much harder than performing dynamic reactions, because patients need to use compensatory trunk movements to offset severe sensory and proprioceptive losses. Therefore, these patients may find greater success with learning balance from dynamic postures, because this will train these necessary compensatory movements.

EXERCISE PRESCRIPTION FOR THE ACTIVE AMBULATOR

The active amputee has myriad choices for recreational activity, both in low to moderate and moderate to high preferred levels of exercise intensity. Numerous publications detail recreational activities for the amputee,[5,24,25] and many organizations are devoted to amputee sports at differing levels of involvement (Table 2). The roles of the clinical team members are especially interdependent when attempting to train the patient for recreational activities. The therapeutic recreation therapist interviews the patient to determine his or her recreational interests and conveys the specific physical demands of the chosen sport to the other disciplines. Attainment of the requisite conditioning components falls to the physical and occupational therapists. In addition, the team prosthetist should be consulted concerning possible prosthetic components, adjustments, and adaptations. Once all basic physical and adaptive needs are met, the recreational therapist begins the sport-specific training with other clinicians acting as consultants.

TABLE 2.   Sports Organizations for Amputees

Organization	Telephone number
American Amputee Foundation, Inc.	(501) 666-2523
Amputee Coalition of America	(708) 698-1628
Amputee Sports Association	(912) 927-5406
National Amputee Golf Association	(800) 633-NAGA
National Association of Disabled Swimmers	(813) 775-1078
National Association of Handicapped Outdoorsmen	(618) 532-4565
National Wheelchair Athletic Association	(719) 635-9300
Shake-A-Leg	(401) 849-8898

Low to moderately intense activities popular with amputees include gardening, walking, golfing, biking, and swimming.[24] Swimming, in particular, is an attractive recreational activity[25] due to its relatively low physical demands, accessibility, and no requirement for a specialized prosthesis. Cardiovascular demands vary; the sport can be geared to target ranges as low as 50% of maximum heart rate. Flexibility needs include the maximization of upper and lower extremity passive ranges of motion for stroke efficiency. Strength requirements need only be the ability to complete a full range of motion against mild resistance for low-intensity exercise. Moderate-intensity strength needs can be achieved through sport-specific training in the water.

Swimming instruction begins with the patient learning to achieve the supine float position independently and learning to tread water using a personal flotation device. A kickboard can be an excellent adjunct training tool for lower extremity strengthening prior to stroke training. The format for stroke development begins most easily with the backstroke due to its emphasis on upper extremities and upper body strength.[24] The sidestroke, with the residual limb on the under side, is also quickly learned. The crawl and breast stroke present more of a challenge due to the exhausting compensatory body movements necessary to prevent the tendency to move in a circle.[24] Individuals using a swim prosthesis will have the advantage of involving their residual limb musculature more but will not necessarily improve their swimming proficiency. If a swimming fin can be used as an attachment to the utility prosthesis, there is greater propensity for success with the crawl stroke.[5] Intensity begins with 5- to 15-minute exercise sessions that follow established target heart rate ranges for up to three repetitions daily. Because exposure to the aquatic environment has most likely not occurred since the amputation, conservative accommodation is strongly recommended. Progression to a continuous exercise session lasting 30–40 minutes will guarantee sport-specific aerobic conditioning.[39]

Amputees seeking moderate to high levels of exercise have even greater choices for recreational involvement. In addition to the activities for the low- to moderate-level exerciser, effective participation can be realized in running, aerobic dance, weight lifting, water and downhill skiing, and racquet and team sports.[5,25] Primary wheelchair users and ambulatory amputees can participate in racquet sports, particularly tennis. Those who exercise with their prosthesis must have a proper fit because significant shear forces are encountered.[24] Because special prosthetic devices[14,28,33] and socket interfaces need to be considered prior to sport-specific instruction, consultation with a prosthetist is necessary.

Strength and flexibility requirements for the amputee tennis player involve being able to execute full functional range of motion of the trunk and upper and lower extremities against gravity and being able to maintain a self-selected ambulatory speed without an assistive device. Training should begin with balance and coordination with straight, lateral, and forward/backward movements. Most transtibial and some transfemoral amputees may immediately be able to tolerate one-to-one, residual-to-prosthetic limb movements. Most transfemoral amputees not using a cadence responsive knee will usually need to learn the skip-run technique, skipping once on the intact limb and then swinging the prosthesis.[24] Progression of diagonal movements and random changes of direction then take the forefront. The racquet swing should be introduced in traditional set-up postures statistically, with the focus of achieving adequate trunk rotation on a stable base of support. "Air swinging" added to the previously learned regimen of lower extremity movements occurs next. Finally, hand-eye coordination skills of racquet-to-ball contact completes basic skills development. The intensity of tennis is based on residual limb tolerances, which require frequent skin monitoring during the skill development phase. Skin and aerobic tolerances are then built gradually on an every-other-day basis initially, with the goal of participating in a daily 45- to 60-minute exercise session. An individual advancing beyond this level of exercise intensity should be extremely wary of chronic wear and tear to residual limb tissues.[24]

CONCLUSION

We have reviewed some of the principles of amputee rehabilitation through some of its most important stages. A review of appropriate exercise techniques, their intensity, and modifications to accommodate the amputee were presented based on our clinical experience and substantiated by the literature. We introduce the concept of modified equipment for the specific purpose of exercising while reducing the risk of injury to the residual limb.

REFERENCES

1. Badenhop DT, Cleary PA, Schaal SF, et al: Physiological adjustments to higher- or lower-intensity exercise in elders. Med Sci Sports Exerc 15:496–502, 1983.
2. Beaulien JA: Developing a stretching program. Physician Sports Med 9:59, 1981.
3. Borg GV: Psychophysical basis of perceived exertion. Med Sci Sports Exerc 14:377–387, 1982.
4. Bostom AG, Bates E, Mazzarella N, et al: Ergometer modification for combined arm-leg use by lower extremity amputees in cardiovascular testing and training. Arch Phys Med Rehabil 68:244–247, 1987.
5. Burgess EM, Rappaport A: Physical Fitness: A Guide For Individuals With Lower Limb Loss. Washington, DC, Department of Veteran Affairs-Veterans Health Administration, 1994.
6. Burgess EM, Romano RL, Zettl JH: The Management of Lower-Extremity Amputations. US Government Printing Office, Washington, DC, 1969, publication TR 10-6.

7. Czerniecki JM, Gitter A: Insights into amputee running: A muscle work analysis. Am J Phys Med Rehabil 71:209–218, 1992.

8. Davidoff GN, Lampman RM, Westbury L, et al: Exercise testing and training of persons with dysvascular amputation: Safety and efficacy of arm ergometry. Arch Phys Med Rehabil 73:334–385, 1992.

9. Delorme TL, Watkins A: Progressive Resistance Exercise. New York, Appleton-Century, 1951.

10. Delorme TL, Watkins A: Techniques of progressive resistance exercise. Arch Phys Med Rehabil 29:263–268, 1948.

11. DeVahl J: Neuromuscular electrical stimulation. In Wolf SL (ed): Gersh's Electrotherapy in Rehabilitation. Philadelphia, FA Davis, 1992, pp 218–268.

12. Dise-Lewis J: Psychological adaptation to limb loss. In Atkins JD, Meier HR III (eds): Comprehensive Management of the Upper-Limb Amputee. New York, Springer-Verlag, 1989, pp. 165–172.

13. Esquenazi A, Micheo W, Vachranukunkiet T: Design and construction of a bicycle attachment for conditioning of below knee amputees and its clinical application. Proceedings of the International Society for Prosthetics and Orthotics. Copenhagen, June 29–July 4, 1986.

14. Esquenazi A, Torres M: Prosthetic feet and ankle mechanisms. Phys Med Rehabil Clin North Am 2:299–309, 1991.

15. Esquenazi A: Geriatric amputee rehabilitation. Clin Geriatr Med 9:731–743, 1993.

16. Esquenazi A, Meier R: Rehabilitation in limb deficiency. 4. Limb amputation. Arch Phys Med Rehabil: 77 (Suppl 3): S18–S28, 1996.

17. Gailey RS: One Step Ahead: An Integrated Approach to Lower Extremity Prosthetics and Amputee Rehabilitation. Miami, FL, Advanced Rehab Therapy Inc., 1994.

18. Gentile AM: Skill acquisition: Action, movement, and neuromotor processes. In Carr, JH, Shepherd RB (eds): Movement Science, Foundations for Physical Therapy in Rehabilitation. Gaithersburg, MD, Aspen Publishers, 1987, pp 93–117.

19. Glaser RM, Sawka MN, Laubach LL, Suryaprasad AG: Metabolic and cardiopulmonary responses to wheelchair and bicycle ergometry. J Appl Physiol 46:1066–1070, 1979.

20. Hellebrandt PA, Houtz SJ: Mechanisms of muscle training in man: Experimental demonstration of the overload principle. Phys Ther Rev 36:371–377, 1956.

21. Kamen LB, Chapis GJ: Phantom limb sensation and phantom pain. Phys Med Rehabil State Art Rev 8:73–88, 1994.

22. Karacoloff LA: Lower Extremity Amputations: A Guide to Functional Outcomes in Physical Therapy Management. Gaithersburg, MD, Aspen Publishers, 1985.

23. Kegel B, Burgess EM, Starr TW, Daly WK: Effects of isometric muscle training on residual limb volume, strength, and gait of below-knee amputees. Phys Ther 61:1419–1426, 1981.

24. Kegel B, Webster JC, Burgess EM: Recreational activities of lower extremity amputees: A survey. Arch Phys Med Rehabil 61:258–264, 1980.

25. Kegel B: Sports for the Amputee. Washington, Medic Publishing Co., 1986.

26. Laslett L, Paumer L, Amsterdam EA: Exercise training in coronary artery disease. Cardiol Clin 5:211–225, 1987.

27. Lehmkuhl LD, Smith LK: Brunnstrom's Clinical Kinesiology, 4th ed. Philadelphia, FA Davis, 1983.

28. Leonard JA Jr: Lower limb prosthetic sockets. Phys Med Rehabil State Art Rev 8:129–145, 1994.

29. Light KE, Nuzik S, Personius W, Barstrom A: Low load prolonged stretch versus high load brief stretch in treating knee contractures. Phys Ther 64:330, 1984.

30. Malone JM, Snyder M, Anderson G, et al: Prevention of amputation by diabetic education. Am J Surg 158:520–524. 1989.

31. Mensch G, Ellis P: Contractures. In Banerjee SN (ed): Rehabilitation Management of Amputees. Baltimore, Williams & Wilkins, 1982, pp 213–216.

32. Mensch G, Ellis PM: Physical Therapy Management of Lower Extremity Amputations. Gaithersburg, MD, Aspen Publishers, 1986.

33. Michael J: Prosthetic knee mechanisms. Phys Med Rehabil State Art Rev 8:147–164, 1994.

34. Mital MA, Pierce DS: Contractures. In Amputees and Their Prosthesis. Boston, Little, Brown & Co., 1971, pp 175–176.

35. Mosely JB, Jobe FW, Pinks M: EMG analysis of scapular musculature during a shoulder rehabilitation program. Am J Sports Med 20:128–134, 1992.

36. Mostardi RA, Gandee RN, Norris WA: Exercise training using arms and legs versus legs alone. Arch Phys Med Rehabil 62:332–335, 1981.

37. Pinzur MS, Gold J, Schwartz D, Gross N: Energy demands for walking in dysvascular amputees as related to the level of amputation. Orthopedics 15:1033–1036, 1992.

38. Pitetti KH, Snell PG, Stray-Gunderson J, Gottschalk FA: Aerobic training exercises for individuals who had amputation of the limb. J Bone Joint Surg 69A:914–921, 1987.

39. Pollack M, Geltman L, Milesis C: Effects of frequency/duration of training on attrition and incidence of injury. Med Sci Sports Exerc 9:31–36, 1977.

40. Powers CM, Boyd LA, Fontaine CA, Perry J: The influence of lower extremity muscle force on gait characteristics in individuals with below-knee amputations secondary to vascular disease. Phys Ther 76:367–377, 1996.

41. Priebe M, Davidoff G, Lampman RM: Exercise testing and training in patients with peripheral vascular disease and lower extremity amputation. West J Med 154:598–601, 1991.

42. Serroussi RE, Gitter A, Czerniecki JM, Weaver K: Mechanical work adaptations of above-knee amputee ambulation. Arch Phys Med Rehabil 77:1209–1214, 1996.

43. Townsend H, Jobe F, Pinks M, Perry J: EMG analysis of gleno-humeral muscles during a baseball rehabilitation program. Am J Sports Med 19:264–272, 1991.

44. Traugh GH, Corcoran PJ, Reyes RL: Energy expenditure of ambulation in patients with above knee amputees. Arch Phys Med Rehabil 56:67–71, 1975.

45. Voss DE, Ionta MK, Myers BJ: Proprioceptive Neuromuscular Facilitation-Patterns and Techniques. 3rd ed. Philadelphia, Harper & Row, 1985.

46. Wenger NK, Hallerstein HK: Rehabilitation of the Coronary Patient. New York, Wiley & Sons, 1984.

47. Wu Y, Keagy RD, Krick HJ, et al: An innovative removable rigid dressing technique for below the knee amputation. J Bone Joint Surg 61A:724–729, 1979.

16

Exercise: Spine and Posture

POSTURE

There is probably no single "correct" posture, as Goff postulated in 1951 after study-ing 4000 men.[14] He found four main types of posture, each associated with a body type: fat, muscular, balanced, and thin (elongated or linear). About 34% could not be fitted in any of these categories and were classified as "intermediate." Goff's balanced group (18%) were best adopted to the orthograde posture.

A 1923 study that attempted to correlate posture with health status in students found that poor posture was related to the greatest number of illnesses, nutritional faults, or operations. In this study, however, the classification of posture was not clearly defined but was related to foot and ankle abnormalities, obesity, and poor muscle tone.[20]

Posture has been clarified in terms of its relationship to the center of gravity (CG) and to the degree of curvatures of the lordosis and kyphosis of all spinal curves (Fig. 1). The CG is at the center of the second sacral vertebra. The CG is important because the transverse axes of rotation of all the joints of the vertebral column and the lower limbs tend to fall forward or backward due to gravity dependent on the CG passing be-hind or ahead of the axes.

At the head level, the CG passes in front of the atlantooccipital joint, causing the head to fall forward, but it is dependent on the other curves of the vertebral column (Fig. 2). Posture is dependent on proprioceptive impulses from the spindle systems and the ar-ticular mechanoreceptors (Fig. 3). There is always a degree of sway from the CG both in the sagittal and frontal planes (1.6–41.7 mm sagittal and 1.8–29.7 mm side sway).[1,5,13] In sway the CG always stays in front of the ankle joints as the knee and hips remain "locked" against capsular and ligamentous tension. Only the gastrocnemius-soleus mus-cle contracts in erect static stance.[10]

In the standing posture, the knee can be locked in a hyperextended position and the hip upon the anterior hip joint capsule. The ankle joint cannot be locked but is maintained in a stable position from isometric gastrocnemius-soleus muscle tone. The

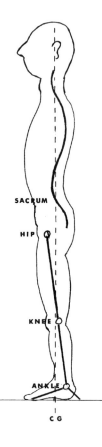

FIGURE 1. Posture as related to the center of gravity (CG).

stability of the entire vertebral column based merely on ligamentous supports is now questioned, because erect posture currently is considered dependent on isometric muscle contraction that relieves ligamentous support. Ligamentous proprioceptive innervation has been considered to elicit appropriate muscular contraction.

Besides being cosmetic, posture is also involved in the evaluation of static low back pain,[7] shoulder tendinitis pain,[9] and cervical discogenic disease.[8] Most pathologic spinal conditions are kinetic, but the static erect postural spine is controlled by isometric muscular contraction.[4] The spine is composed of numerous superincumbent functional units (Fig. 4).

There are four basic curves of the spinal column that are vital in the maintenance of health and function: cervical and lumbar lordosis and thoracic and sacral kyphosis. These curves are interdependent (Fig. 5); an increase is any curvature augments the above and below curves. The degrees of curvature also influence the integrity of the intervertebral discs (Figs. 6 and 7). There remains disagreement as to how to measure the spinal curvature. This is unfortunate, in the author's opinion, because the degree of lordosis is pertinent to spine stability and function (Figs. 8 and 9).

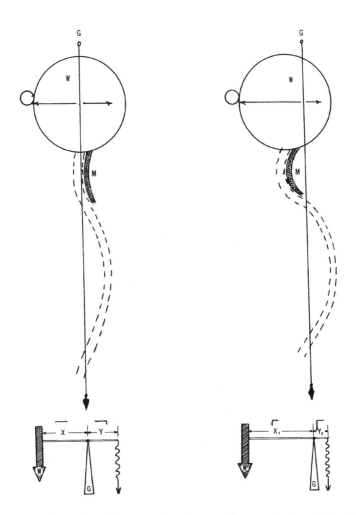

FIGURE 2. Head in relationship to the center of gravity (CG). In the upper drawings, the head is depicted in relationship to the CG. In the bottom drawings, the weight (W) is balanced anterior to the CG (G) and is balanced by the posterior muscles. X is the distance from the CG and Y to that of the extensor muscles.

Posture develops during infancy and childhood,[4,17–19] when bow legs, knock knees, pronated feet, and congenital spinal malformations become apparent. Bone structure is influenced by weight stresses. As is all growth, spinal growth is based on hereditary factors that may be altered by other factors, such as exercise, diet, and even emotions.

Bad postural habits develop in childhood, and the acquired poor posture, which feels normal to the child, becomes accepted. A slumped posture may be a result of peer pressure. Feldenkrais[12a] postulated that "many postures develop from the cringing fear of physical assault by domineering parents or siblings." Emotions also influence posture.

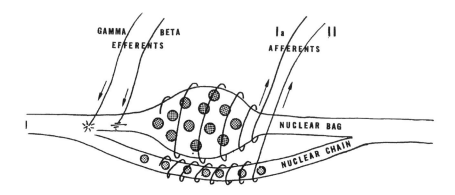

FIGURE 3. Spindle system. The intrafusal muscle fibers (spindle system) determine the length and with the Golgi apparatus Golgi system, the force needed by the extrafusal fibers to accomplish the intended task. The intrafusal spindle system has motor fibers through the gamma and beta efferents that control the length of the spindle. The sensory feedback from the spindle is transmitted by way of the Ia and II fibers.

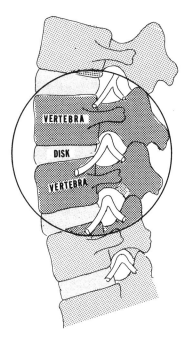

FIGURE 4. Functional unit of the spine. Each functional unit comprises adjacent vertebrae with an interposed disc. In the posterior portion of the unit are facet (zygapophyseal) joints. The ligamentous structures that control stability and motion are the longitudinal ligaments and the posterior interspinous ligaments. The musculature that is involved are the erector spinae and abdominal muscles.

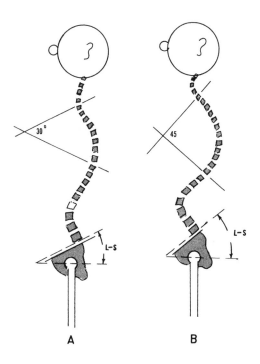

FIGURE 5. Relationship of spinal curvatures. With an increase in cervical lordosis there is a comparable increase in all the other spinal curves.

A   B

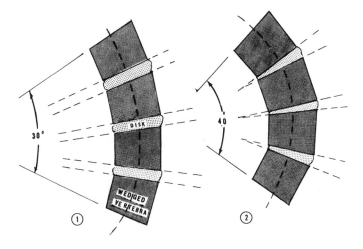

FIGURE 6. Influence of curvature on the intervertebral discs. The degree of curvature influences the extent of disc compression and, to a lesser degree, the shape of the vertebra. In excessive lordosis the nucleus of the disc is also forced toward the convexity.

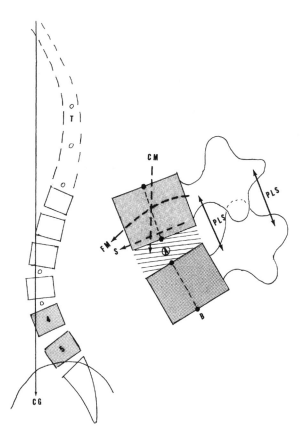

FIGURE 7. Posture related to the center of gravity. *Left,* The lateral view of the spine is related to the CG. *Right,* The CG passes anterior to the lumbar centroids (A) (axis of rotation within the disc). The CG is posterior to the thoracic (T) centroids. This figure depicts a functional unit at the lordotic angulation (CM = compressive moment, FM = flexion moment, and S = shear). These forces rotate (flex) the vertebral bodies, placing the resistance on the posterior ligamentous structures (PLS).

We stand, sit, and walk "as we feel." A person who is depressed, impatient, or angry walks, stands, and sits in a manner that reflects his state of mind.

PRESCRIPTION OF EXERCISE

The following discussion of the prescription of exercise addresses posture (Fig. 10) and kinetic function in regard to all of the above-mentioned factors.

Because exercise is advocated in correcting and maintaining postural muscular strength, endurance and proprioception of the involved muscles must be ascertained. Although muscle "tonus" has been intensively evaluated, disagreement remains. A muscle can maintain tonus yet remain electrically "silent" for long periods.[11,25] Basmajian suggested that tonus should be defined as the general tone of a muscle deter-

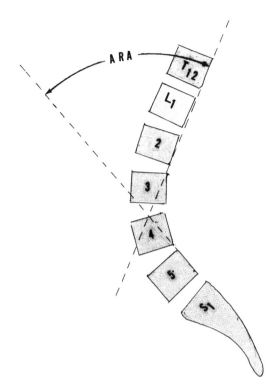

FIGURE 8. Absolute rotation angle: Lordotic angle. A line drawn from the posterior edge of L5 and L1 denotes the absolute rotation angle (ARA), which reflects the lordotic curve.

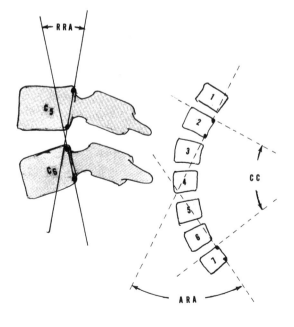

FIGURE 9. Measurement of cervical lordosis. The cervical lordosis (CC) is essentially an aggregate of the individual relative rotational angles (RRA) of two adjacent vertebrae. The total of the RRAs equals the absolute rotational angle (ARA), or the lordosis, assuming that all RRAs are equal.

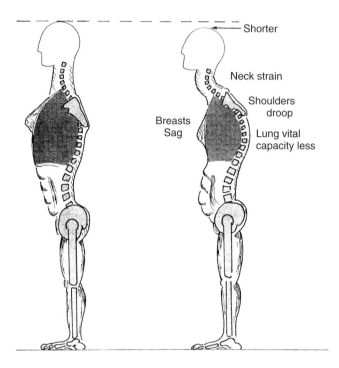

Shorter

Neck strain

Shoulders droop

Breasts Sag

Lung vital capacity less

FIGURE 10. Good and poor, or "forward head," posture.

mined by its passive elasticity or turgor of muscular and fibrous tissues and by continuous contraction of muscle in response to stimulus from the nervous system.[3] The nervous component of general tonus is "probably varying tonic permanent activity of the gamma loop system."[24]

Postural tonus has been accepted as follows: "During easy standing there is no electrical activity in postural muscles until the subject sways sufficiently from the center of gravity,"[23] except from the anterior tibialis and soleus muscles and then only intermittent activity in these.[16] Jacobson, however, found no period of inactivity in the anterior tibialis or soleus during quiet standing. No activity was noted in the quadriceps femoris or erector spinae muscles.[15]

The fact that standing energy requires 30–40% greater energy than does supine energy expenditure belies the fact that "easy stance" relies merely on elastic tissues and not sustained muscular contraction. Whereas sustained musclar activity in the anterior tibialis and some degree of activity in the quadriceps and hamstring muscles has been confirmed, no activity has been demonstrated in the erector spinae muscle groups.

Posture prescription designates that the curvatures be corrected and maintained; the cervical lordosis remains the predominant factor in achieving good posture. The ability of African women to carry heavy objects on their heads while walking for miles with no apparent fatigue appears to defy the laws of physics. Studies of their oxygen consumption to determine the amount of calories burned compared to non-African women of equal size, age, and physical status revealed that the African women could carry a fifth of their body weight without burning extra calories. As the weights that they carried were increased, so were the number of calories burned, but some of the women carried 70% of their body weight. Leaning the entire body against a wall and "pressing" the neck against the wall (Fig. 11) improves spinal posture. Placing a weight on the head and "pushing" upward improves the posture and gives a kinesthetic sensation of good posture (Fig. 12). This exercise decreases the degree of curvatures.

Kinetic spine function demands appropriate flexibility, good muscle tone, and proper body mechanics on how to stand, bend, lift, and push. The best exercise is walking properly (Figs. 13 and 14).

Flexibility exercises done slowly and consistently are necessary for good spinal health and function. Such exercises include flexion in the sagittal plane (Figs. 15 and 16), lateral flexion (Fig. 17) and rotation (Fig. 18). Most daily functional activities demand motion is all planes and a combination of all planes (Fig. 19).

Because the McKenzie[22] concept postulates that extension of the lumbar spine moves the nucleus of the disc anteriorly, thus removing its compressive force away from nociceptive sites, extension exercise often must be prescribed[22] (Fig. 20).

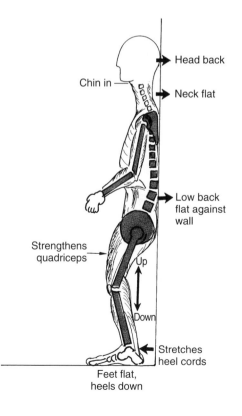

FIGURE 11. Exercise (half squats) for proper posture.

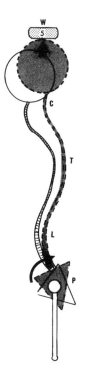

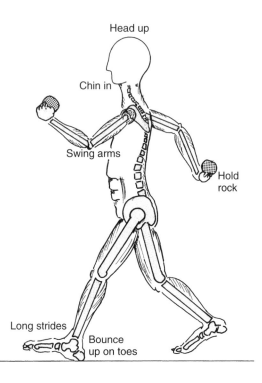

FIGURE 12. Weight-on-head exercise. Placing an acceptable weight on the head initiates proprioceptive impulses and causes the appropriate neck muscle to assume an erect posture within the center of gravity.

FIGURE 13. Walking is the best exercise.

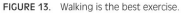

FIGURE 14. Exercises that can be performed while walking.

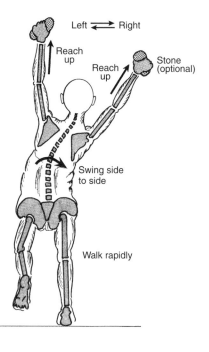

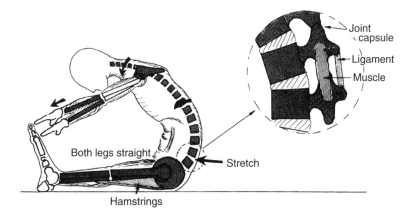

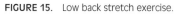

Both legs straight

Stretch

Hamstrings

Joint capsule

Ligament

Muscle

FIGURE 15. Low back stretch exercise.

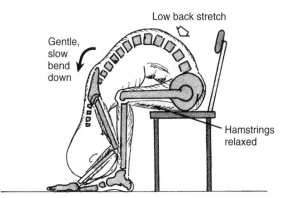

Low back stretch

Gentle, slow bend down

Hamstrings relaxed

FIGURE 16. Low back stretching exercises without hamstring resistance.

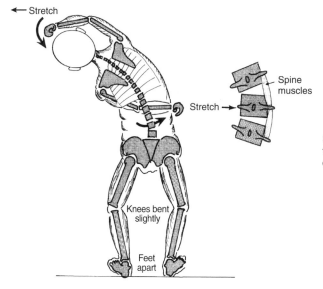

Stretch

Spine muscles

Stretch

Knees bent slightly

Feet apart

FIGURE 17. Side bending exercise to stretch the erector spinae and quadratus muscles.

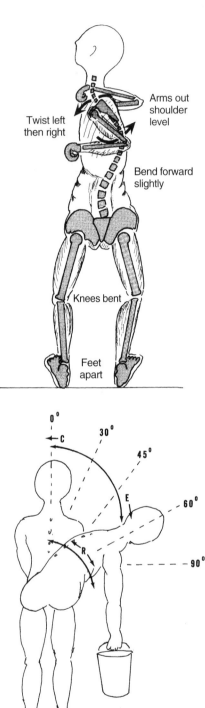

FIGURE 18. Rotational flexibility exercise.

FIGURE 19. All musculoskeletal movements are a combination of flexion, lateral flexion, and rotation.

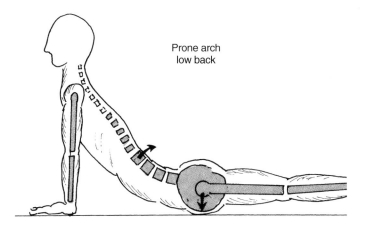

Prone arch
low back

FIGURE 20. Extension exercise for the low back is done in stages. Using arms only, the person extends manually to a bent-arm position on the elbows and then to the extended-arm extension. This position is held for several minutes several times a day.

Muscle strengthening exercises for the abdominal muscles—the flexors and obliques—are accepted as the most important strengthening exercises for the low back and are considered "sit-up" exercises. They must be done properly and in sequence as strength and endurance develop (Figs. 21, 22, and 23).

None of these exercises will be of any value if the person is not skilled and trained in the proper use of his or her body to lift, push, and perform all activities of daily living and vocational activities. These activities are beyond the scope of prescription of exercises, but having normal flexibility and strength will ensure that all daily activities are carried out by a well-conditioned spine.

Proper posture and proper spinal function can be enhanced by appropriate exercises but also must take into consideration the genetic, familial, and psychological aspects of posture. Proper posture and spinal function are mandatory in the performance of activities of daily living but are subservient to proper body mechanics, which can be altered by perturbers and pain (Fig. 24).

There are so many orthopedic spinal problems that may benefit from exercise that a few examples are warranted. Any exercise prescription *must* designate the pathophysiologic basis for exercise and what the exercise attempts to accomplish. A meaningful diagnosis must accompany the prescription as well as specify the accompanying modalities, indications, contraindications, duration, and frequency of the specific exercise.

The Cochrane Collaboration was established in England in 1992 to promote the systematic collection, review, and synthesis of all of the literature regarding a specific orthopedic condition, of which spinal disorders was initially predominant.[6] Of the many spinal disorders and the treatment that were evaluated, exercise is stressed.

For clinically disabling spinal disorders, numerous diagnostic "labels" have become common but have little meaning. Acute, chronic, and recurrent conditions are designated, and each requires a different approach. In the acute cases, "rest" has been the initial ba-

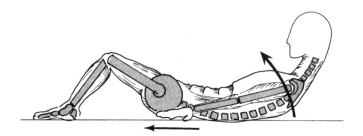

FIGURE 21. The first stage of a sit-up is nuchal flexion with simultaneous abdominal muscle contraction.

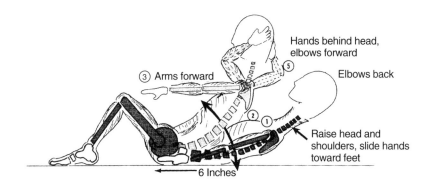

FIGURE 22. Stages of abdominal strengthening exercises.

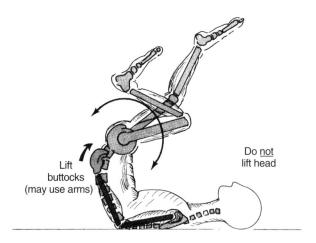

FIGURE 23. General conditioning exercise.

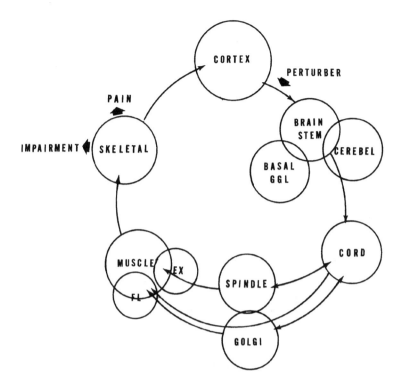

FIGURE 24. A functional model of neuromuscular control.

sis, which implies "no exercise" and essentially no activity. This has been refuted, and now early "activity" is indicated, meaning isometric exercise and gradual kinetic exercise. Regaining flexibility (range of motion) ultimately is indicated, as is strength and endurance.

Discogenic disease is predominant in disabling spinal conditions, and cervical and lumbar disc herniations are the major entities. Exercise has varied from the McKenzie approach, which postulates extension exercise that alters the site of the disc nucleus and "centralizes" the symptoms.[22]

Exercise plays an important role in addressing the "mechanical low back pain" and varies from passive to active,[21] with the active, aerobic approach improving neuromuscular coordination, endurance, and body mechanics. Speed of motion, also termed acceleration, is considered essential[10] and must be incorporated into any exercise program.

In summary, any exercise program must be specific as to the nueromusculoskeletal basis and pathoanatomic dysfunction for which it is prescribed.

ACKNOWLEDGMENT   Several of the illustrations have been adapted or reproduced from Dr. Cailliet's books published by F.A. Davis. Dr. Cailliet and the publisher wish to thank F.A. Davis for this use.

REFERENCES

1. Akerblom B: Standing and Sitting Posture. Stockholm, A-N Nordiska Bokandeln, 1948.
2. Bancroft JH: The Posture of School Children. New York, Macmillan, 1919.
3. Basmajian JV: Muscles Alive: Their Functions Revealed by Electromyography. Baltimore, Williams & Wilkins, 1962.
4. Bell GH, Davidson JN, Scarborough H: Textbook of Physiology and Biochemistry, 4th ed. Edinburgh, Livingstone, 1959.
5. Boman K, Jalavisto F: Standing steadiness in old and young persons. Ann Med Exp Biol Fenniae 31:447–455, 1953.
6. Bombardier C, Esmail R, Nachemson AL: The Cochrane Collaboration Back Review Group for Spinal Disorders. Spine 22:837–840, 1997.
7. Cailliet R: Low Back Pain, 4th ed. Philadelphia, FA Davis, 1988.
8. Cailliet R: Neck and Arm Pain, 3rd ed. Philadelphia, FA Davis, 1991.
9. Cailliet R: Shoulder Pain, 3rd ed. Philadelphia, FA Davis, 1993.
10. Cailliet R: Soft Tissue Pain and Disability, 3rd ed. Philadelphia, FA Davis, 1996.
11. deVries HA: Muscle tonus in postural muscles. Am J Phys Med 44:275–291, 1964.
12. Deyo RA: Historic perspective on conservative treatment for acute back problems. In Mayer TG, Mooney V, Gatchel RJ (eds): Contemporary Conservative Care for Painful Spinal Disorders. Philadelphia, Lea & Febiger, 1191, pp 169–180.
12a. Feldenkrais M: Body and Mature Behavior: A Study of Anxiety, Sex, Gravitation, and Learning. New York, International Universities Press, 1949.
13. Fox MG, Young OG: Placement of gravital line in anteroposterior standing posture. Res Q 25:277–285, 1954.
14. Goff CW: Mean posture patterns with new postural values. Am J Phys Anthrop 9:335–346, 1951.
15. Jacobson E: Innervation and tonus of striated muscle in man. J Nerv Ment Dis 97:197–203, 1943.
16. Kelton IM, Wright RD: The mechanisms of easy standing by man. J Exp Biol Mod Sci 27:505–515, 1949.
17. Lovett RW: Lateral Curvature of the Spine and Shoulder, 5th ed. Philadelphia, Blakiston's Son & Co., 1907.
18. Lowman CL: Posture in early childhood. Calif W Med 41:382–385, 1934.
19. Lowman CL, Colestock C, Cooper H: Corrective Physical Education for Groups. New York, AS Barnes, 1982.
20. Lowman CL, Young CH: Postural Fitness: Significance and Variance. Philadelphia, Lea & Febiger, 1960.
21. Marras WS, Parnianpour M, Ferguson SA, et al. The classification of anatomic- and symptom-based low back disorders using motion measure models. Spine 20:2531–2546, 1995.
22. McKenzie R: A physical therapy perspective on acute spinal disorders. In Mayer TG, Mooney V, Gatchel RJ (eds): Contemporary Conservative Care for Painful Spinal Disorders. Philadelphia, Lea & Febiger, 1991, pp 211–220.
23. Ralston HJ, Lobet B: The question of tonus in skeletal muscle. Am J Phys Med 32:85–92, 1953.
24. Thomas JE: Muscle tone, spasticity. J Nerv Ment Dis 132:505–514, 1961.
25. Zimmer C: No skycaps needed. Biomechanics Watch Discover 1995.

17

Prevention of Athletic Injury

The prevention of athletic injury involves many variables. Equipment, rules, playing surface, ambient conditions, and preseason conditioning are just some of the factors that create a variable milieu for any given sporting event. The safety of the event can be partially modulated by optimizing these factors. The improved protection given by newer football helmets has resulted in a decrease in cervical spine injuries.[23] A ban on spearing in football also has helped to reduce head injuries. The use of the breakaway base has decreased injury patterns in softball and baseball.[10,11] Soft-soled shoes reduce the rate of loading in jumping and landing in volleyball. This simple biomechanical fact helps to reduce the incidence of traumatic overload injury.[26]

This chapter emphasizes that the appropriate implementation of preventive therapeutic exercise now stands as a major tool in the ongoing effort to reduce the incidence of sports-related injuries. Injury prevention is explored in the context of exercise prescription. General principles are presented, and the musculoskeletal kinetic chain is discussed with emphasis on sports-specific injury patterns and exercise.

GENERAL PRINCIPLES OF INJURY PREVENTION

Prior to athletic activity, a warm-up is commonly performed to prepare an athlete to participate in the sport in an optimal physical state to reduce the risk of injury.[16] Many of the benefits of the warm-up are derived from effects on the cardiovascular system; the heart rate increases gradually, also engaging an increased rate of respiration. Vascular resistance in turn decreases, which increases blood flow to the extremities and begins to promote increased availability of oxygen at the tissue level. Studies have shown that active cardiovascular warm-up benefits athletic activity.[9] In one study, men who did not warm up prior to a strenuous cardiovascular activity tended to develop abnormalities on electrocardiogram that did not occur when they did use a warm-up. In fact, higher body temperatures achieved in warm-up may lead to improved muscular performance.[3] This is critical because muscular function stabilizes joints and prevents injury. The warm-up also may increase the elasticity of the musculotendinous anatomic unit, thus decreasing the risk of muscular tear or strain.[21] The warm-up includes submaximal cardiac and kinetic activity that is related to the specific sport that is about to be performed. This may include a low-intensity short-duration jog for mid-distance runners, submaximal sprint starts for sprinters and hurdlers, or low-velocity golf swings for golfers. Warm-ups unrelated to the activity can also be used and are often used in sports that involve sudden activity and of high demand (i.e., sports that would cause significant overload to practice beforehand). Warm-up is generally performed close to the time of the athletic event and usually lasts 15–30 minutes.

The cardiac portion of the warm-up is often incorporated with and followed by a stretching warm-up. This enhances flexibility and allows necessary muscle relaxation. Focused stretching also will better allow a joint to be put through optimal range of motion. It counters the effect of layoffs from activity or the aftermath of previous injury. Appropriate muscle lengthening enhances activity performance by ensuring necessary available range. Before a tennis serve, shoulder flexibility is essential to avoid unnecessary load on static structures such as the anterior capsular restraints. The same is true when considering the golf swing in relation to hip, trunk, and shoulder flexibility. The greater extensibility achieved by stretching will help prevent over-lengthening types of injuries. Stretching should be gentle and performed at the point of tightness, not pain. An effective stretch is generally held for at least 30 seconds.

The cool-down period is an important consideration. During a given athletic event, stroke volume is increased and the leg or arm musculature allows a muscular assist in moving blood back toward the heart. To prevent difficulties with blood pooling in the 10–20 minutes following exercise, a time of low activity occurs. This complements recovery time, allowing the muscular pump to continue working at a lesser intensity. Stretching is optimized after activity and can be done quite effectively given the warmed state of the muscles. Prevention of delayed-onset muscle soreness is another potential benefit of stretching during the cool-down period.

OVERTRAINING

Overtraining predisposes an athlete to injury. Although athletic training involves stressing the body to promote increased strength and fitness, too much training can have negative consequences. The athlete who overtrains will be unable to progress despite continued efforts. Constitutional symptoms such as excessive fatigue, weight loss, and disturbed sleep may occur. The resting pulse rate may increase, and complaints of unusual diffuse pain may occur. There may be an increased risk of stress fractures or other injuries. This underscores the need for rest periods in the course of training, emphasizing that positive adaptations to exercise take place between exercise sessions as opposed to during the actual exercise.

THE PREPARTICIPATION EXAMINATION

Preparticipation examinations of athletes allow for direction of exercise toward athletic injury prevention. Purposes of this examination include detecting medical contraindications, meeting legal and insurance requirements, and evaluating for adequate safe participation in sport. The multiple-station type of examination system lends efficient organization and screening. Having a physician or physicians skilled in examination of the musculoskeletal system is an advantage of using the system, because one of the stations will serve as an area for a specific musculoskeletal screening exam.[5,22] In the optimal setting, the preparticipation examination may be administered for a single sport, allowing more focused attention on typical injury patterns for that sport and focused identification of biomechanical deficit patterns in a given potential athlete. A typical musculoskeletal screening examination is listed in Table 1. Critical focus areas from the history-taking station include reports of previous injury, joint difficulties, head trauma including loss of consciousness, and seizure disorders. Abnormalities necessitating further pursuit can be handled in a sports-specific examination station or by referral. Few athletes require further referral beyond the preparticipation screening examination.[5] Typical focused musculoskeletal examination should clarify difficulties with muscle tightness, malalignment, muscle weakness, and joint instability, often with emphasis on the knee and ankle.[6] For instance, the finding of varus alignment may predispose to stress fractures in basketball.[4] This can be a result of the landing forces that occur after jumping, which often exceed body weight by six to seven times. Greater than 10% asymmetry in side-to-side strength testing, as identified by isometric testing, may predispose to injury. Noting strength deficits during the preparticipation examination may lead to this type of finding in a more specialized setting, again guiding the exercise prescription.

TABLE 1. Musculoskeletal Screening Exam

Athletic Activity (Instructions)	Observation
Stand facing examiner	Acromioclavicular joints; general habits
Look at ceiling, floor, over both shoulders; touch ears to shoulders	Cervical spine motion
Shrug shoulders (examiner resists)	Trapezius strength
Abduct shoulders 90% (examiner resists at 90%)	Deltoid strength
Full external rotation of arms	Shoulder motion
Flex and extend elbows	Elbow motion
Arms at sides, elbows 90% flexed; pronate and supinate wrists	Elbow and wrist motion
Spread fingers; make a fist	Hand or finger motion and deformities
Tighten (contract) quadriceps; relax quadriceps	Symmetry and knee effusion; ankle effusion
"Duck walk" four steps (away from examiner with buttocks on heels)	Hip, knee, and ankle motion
Back to examiner	Shoulder symmetry; scoliosis
Knees straight, touch toes	Scoliosis; hip motion, hamstring tightness
Raise up on toes, raise heels	Calf symmetry, leg strength

Adapted from Smith NJ (ed): Sports Medicine: Health Care for Young Athletes. Evanston, IL, American Academy of Pediatrics, 1983.

STRESS FRACTURES

A stress fracture occurs when bone is unable to accept repetitive subthreshold stress without suffering a partial or complete fracture. Defining the population at risk for stress fractures is far from an exact science. Because this problem has a fairly high incidence in athletic activity, special focus on assessing risk during the preparticipation examination is worthy of mention. Some evidence suggests the prevalence is increased in smokers and those with a family history of osteoporosis and amenorrhea.[2] Running is the sport that is most commonly associated with stress fractures, most often in the tibia but also in the fibula, femur, and pelvis. The metatarsal bones are common sites for stress fractures in ballet dancers,[14] and the coracoid is a site for stress fractures in trapshooters.[15] This underscores the importance of evaluating an athlete based on the specific activity that is to be undertaken. The key historical feature in stress fractures is activity-associated pain that is relieved with unloading. The description of pain may be relatively vague. Clearly an important thrust involves identification of the problem early and relative rest to avoid repeated loading and unloading of the bone, which would lead to increasing fracture. However, exercise prescription in this situation still becomes an important topic. Muscle activity can reduce tensile and shear stress, thus reducing the risk for stress fracture.[19] Muscle action can reduce strain rate and dissipate skeletally generated forces by eccentric contraction.[20] Energy at impact is absorbed by the muscle.[18] Cross-training during injury recovery is important in treating the competitive athlete and paramount to preventing further injury. Athletes recovering from tibia stress fractures may have altered weightbearing status for several months. Prevention of loss of aerobic conditioning, trunk and limb strength, and flexibility is achievable. Nonweightbearing strengthening programs are helpful. Examples include lumbar stabilization exercises and deep water running (see chapter 3).

SPORTS-SPECIFIC CONSIDERATIONS

Sports often involve a series of complex biomechanical functions. One method of focusing on a specific event is to analyze the specific demands of the event. The principles of conditioning and strengthening then can be highlighted in a given region or group of muscles. This section analyzes certain athletic events and identifies the key muscle groups involved. The tables serve as a general guide to each activity, but the concept can be applied to most sports. This is somewhat of a static model, focusing on muscular demand, and other kinetic chain factors, such as related joint restrictions, also need to be addressed. The methods for strength training described in chapter 3 could be used in programming exercise for any of the sample events described below. Essentially, focusing in this way is a form of addressing sport-specific athletic fitness and presumes achievement of general athletic fitness. The next step in preparation for mastery of a given sport is focusing on obtaining sport-specific athletic skill. This concept, in essence, describes a pyramid approach to attaining goals. The concept of periodization is applicable (see chapter 3). By identifying the key muscle groups needed for a given sport (Table 2) one can design a workout of variable volume and intensity

TABLE 2. Key Muscle Groups Used in Specific Sports

Sprint Start Events	Javelin Throw	Freestyle Swimming	Gymnastics- Floor Exercise
Triceps surae muscles	Hip extensors, knee extensors, plantar flexors	Arm flexors, hand flexors, shoulder adductors	All major hip groups
Rectus femoris	Trunk rotators, abdominal muscles	Arm extensors, deltoid	Finger flexors, plantar flexors
Iliopsoas	Hip flexors	Hip flexors, hip extensors	Erector spinae
Tensor fascia lata	Pectoralis major, latissimus dorsi, triceps, brachii	Spine axis stabilizers	Quadriceps, hamstrings

with the cycle of sport-specific competition in mind. This allows "peaking" to occur at the time of athletic competition.

REGIONAL CONSIDERATIONS IN EXERCISE PRESCRIPTION

Prescription of exercise to precondition and prevent athletic injury involves consideration of several general areas. Most programs focus on joint flexibility, muscular strength, muscular endurance, proprioception, and motor coordination or motor control. Often, the application of regional exercise principles involves the coordination of other locations of the locomotor system, called the kinetic chain. The following sections present exercise based on body regions. One must keep in mind, however, that exercising in preparation for a given sport rarely is prescribed for only a single body region. More frequently, consideration of the entire musculoskeletal axis helps define the optimal approach to conditioning and injury prevention. Each section mentions only the most common regional injuries; a much more complex differential exists but is beyond the scope of this chapter.

THE FOOT AND ANKLE

Many popular sports place demand on the ligamentous stability of the foot and ankle, and overuse injury patterns are common in this region. Ligamentous injury to the anterior talofibular ligament and the other ligamentous structures occurs during inversion, eversion, and combination mechanisms. Achilles tendinitis and plantar fasciitis also are common, and they affect athletic performance, training, and playing time. Table 3 lists sports with high rates of foot and ankle injuries.

To ensure excellent coordination, one must be able to perform low-demand isolated exercises prior to progressing to more advanced foot and ankle exercises. Initially, light resistance exercise with the use of resistant bands or cords is used. These bands

---

TABLE 3.   Sports Predisposing to Foot and Ankle Injury

Sport	Injury Patterns
Soccer	Lateral ankle sprains
Basketball	Ankle sprains, Achilles tendon disorders
Handball	Ankle sprains
Rugby	Ankle sprains
Running	Posterior calcaneal problems, plantar fasciitis
Tennis	Achilles tendon disorders, plantar fasciitis
Badminton	Achilles tendinitis
Squash	Ankle sprains, Achilles tendon rupture
Cycling	Achilles tendinitis
Gymnastics	Ankle sprains
Skiing	Retrocalcaneal bursitis

---

have specific resistance characteristics, and the athlete can progress through the varying degrees of resistance. Isolated strengthening of the ankle in plantar flexion, dorsiflexion, eversion, and inversion should all be performed, and combinations of the above directions allow greater variability in strength programming. Standing weight shift exercises, while maintaining neutral spine and hip stability, help develop an overall proprioceptive awareness and are usually performed prior to the introduction of an ankle disk into the balance training program. Closed kinetic chain mobility training is enhanced with the use of an ankle disk. These disks have varying diameters, and some allow changing the relative positions of underlying hemispheres to create greater or lesser challenges to the athlete who is training to stabilize the ankle joint on the board. The use of an unstable surface trains proprioception and strength. In progressing the athlete, demonstration of ankle control in the seated position occurs prior to moving to standing exercise. The athlete must control the ankle disk in multiple directions in a smooth fashion. This is progressed to standing, using both feet and only balancing with one limb on the board. The difficulty factor of the exercise can be increased by taking away the upper extremity support and having the trainee fold his arms across the chest while balancing. In addition, closing the eyes eliminates the visual system as an aid to balancing and controlling ankle disk motion and thus allows greater challenge. Combined functional activities can be added later (Fig. 1).

Lower extremity flexibility cannot be ignored in ankle/foot training, and therefore gentle prolonged stretching of the gastrocnemius-soleus, hamstrings, and rectus femoris (Fig. 2) is performed with the ankle training program. Heel raise exercise bilaterally and unilaterally strengthens the gastrocnemius-soleus complex and trains the ankle in proper subtalar joint alignment. Single-limb stability training is enhanced by having the athlete lean in different directions while supporting himself on one limb, also simultaneously stabilizing the trunk. This can be done in the sagittal, frontal, and transverse planes with the eyes open or closed. Objects such as tennis balls can be

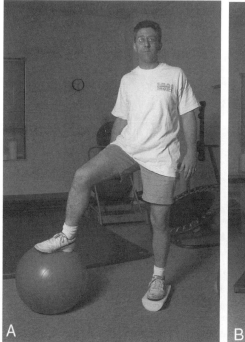

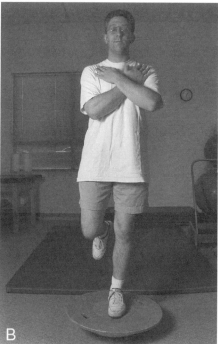

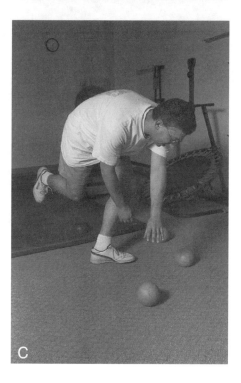

FIGURE 1. Progressive ankle rehabilitation often involves unstable ground surfaces (*A*), eyes-closed proprioceptive challenge (*B*), and demonstration of stable ankle performance in functional challenge activity (*C*).

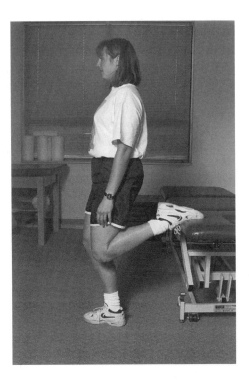

FIGURE 2. One technique for stretching the left rectus femoris. Maintenance of neutral pelvis is necessary for adequate performance.

placed at varying locations away from the body, and the single limb and ankle must be controlled while the athlete leans in the various planes to pick up the objects and return to the standing position. (see Fig. 1C.) Finally, specific jumping exercises to preassigned locations followed by the above-described coordination exercises allow the introduction of plyometric strengthening. The speed at which a designed exercise sequence is performed can be monitored and improved upon with advances in abilities.

Some of the common difficulties encountered in the foot involve the plantar fascia and first metatarsophalangeal (MTP) joint. A stretching program for the fascia can be helpful. Devices exist that stretch the fascia, but they sometimes can overstretch the distal fascial elements between the MTP joints and the phalanges. Since most symptoms arise from the fascia more proximally, this poses a potential problem. Therefore, it is important to mobilize and stretch the portion of the fascia between the calcaneus and midsubstance. This can be done manually with deep soft tissue release techniques or by elevating the MTP joints while stretching the fascia. In addition, efforts to avoid the onset of hallux rigidus are worthwhile and from an exercise standpoint simply involve mobilizing that joint by a combination of manual distraction, rotation, elevation, and depression.

THE KNEE

Typical injury patterns at the knee include meniscal tears, anterior cruciate ligament disruption, medial collateral ligament sprains, patellar tendinitis, and patellofemoral symptoms. Many sports, including football, basketball, and soccer, involve sudden planting and turning of the knee, delivering a high torque that must be absorbed in a short time. Overuse in running events predisposes to overuse injuries at the knee, such as patellar tendinitis or pes anserine bursitis. Sports commonly involving knee injuries are listed in Table 4.

Two significant principles underscore the approach to exercise about the knee: (1) excellent strength and flexibility crossing the knee joint is protective against injury, and (2) there are typical patterns of weakness and tightness about the knee, with exercise being directed to restore and improve flexibility and strength balance. Specifically, the vastus medialis oblique (VMO) muscle tends to be relatively weak compared to the other quadriceps muscles, adding to a potential tendency for lateral patellar tracking. Although isolating the VMO for strengthening is unlikely, selecting it for relatively greater strengthening emphasis is mandatory. This can be done in several ways, including positioning the hip joint in relative external rotation (Fig. 3). In this way, the performance of knee extension strengthening will activate the VMO to a greater degree than would otherwise occur. Inflexibility of the lateral structures, including the retinaculum, iliotibial band, hamstrings, and gastrocnemius, also predispose to poor biomechanics at the knee, and therefore stretching of these structures is helpful in training for athletic participation. The lateral retinaculum can be manually stretched by performing medial patellar glides (Fig. 4). A stretching program for the other three quadriceps groups should be undertaken. Strengthening of the quadriceps and hamstring groups conducted in a closed kinetic chain fashion allows coordinated coactivation, reduction of patellofemoral joint reaction forces, and decreased strain on the anterior cruciate ligaments. This can be carried out using a leg press machine with supine

TABLE 4.   Sports Associated with Knee Injuries

Sport	Injury Patterns
Alpine skiing	MCL, ACL, meniscus
Sailing	Patellofemoral symptoms
Rowing	Chondromalacia, patellofemoral symptoms
Wrestling	Bursitis, meniscus, LCL, MCL
Weight lifting	Chondomalacia, patellar tendinitis meniscus
Gymnastics	Quadriceps tendinitis
Cycling	Medial plicae syndrome, hamstring overload
Swimming	MCL, meniscus
Tennis	MCL, ACL
Basketball	Patellar tendinitis
Soccer	Meniscal tears

MCL = medial collateral ligament
ACL = anterior cruciate ligament
LCL = lateral collateral ligament

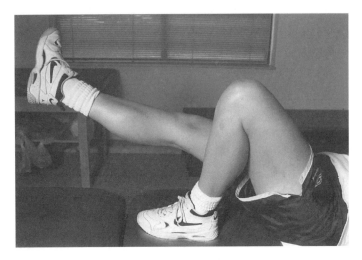

FIGURE 3. Selecting the right VMO for relative strengthening by external rotation at the right hip.

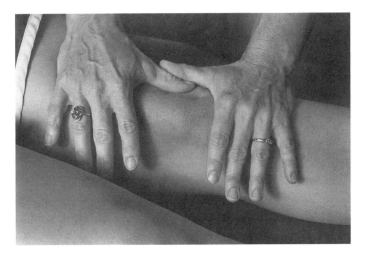

FIGURE 4. Medial patellar glide.

positioning and fixed footplate, a bicycle, or step machine (Fig. 5). Open kinetic chain strengthening of the hamstrings also should be undertaken, with particular emphasis on the eccentric phase (Fig. 6). Achieving a balance between anterior and posterior muscle groups about the knee is a reasonable goal and can be measured isokinetically or by functional testing. Differing sports may be optimally performed at different balances of strength between the hamstring and quadriceps group. For example, cycling may demand greater attention to the hamstrings, because the incidence of hamstring overload injuries is high.[7] Speed-specific training also can be incorporated in the con-

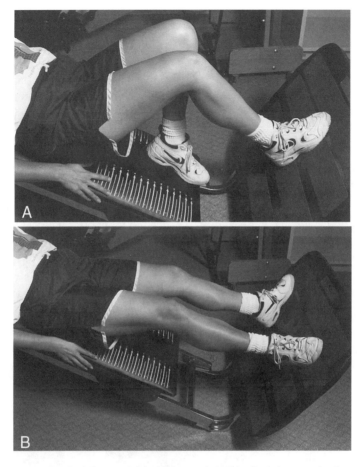

FIGURE 5.   Single leg (*A*) and double leg (*B*) closed kinetic chain strengthening.

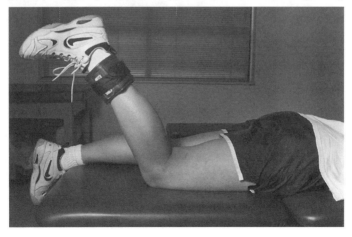

FIGURE 6.   Open kinetic chain strengthening of the hamstring muscles.

trolled preactivity environment, based on the speeds that are anticipated to be obtained during the activity.

Weakness of hip group musculature affects the knee, often by increasing torque at the knee or by promoting stress on the medial aspect of the knee or patellofemoral joint. The critical musculature in need of strengthening usually includes the gluteus medius and hip external rotators. Weakness in these groups leads to increased internal rotation of the femur. Finally, proprioceptive exercise at the knee may help improve coordination (Figs. 7 and 8).

THE LUMBAR SPINE, HIP, AND PELVIS

Adductor strains, thigh contusions, lumbar disc injuries, and ilial and sacral motion restrictions typically affect participants in a wide range of sports. In addition, rotational overload of lumbar spine muscle groups factors into these presentations. Longer distance events such as running may exacerbate prefunctional muscle weakness and motion restrictions, leading to overuse injuries such as iliotibial band syndrome. Table 5 lists additional sports that studies have identified as having a significant rate of injury occurrence. Prevention and exercise routine depend on identifying the potential areas for injury and biomechanical deficit prior to engaging in the activity at the maximal level.

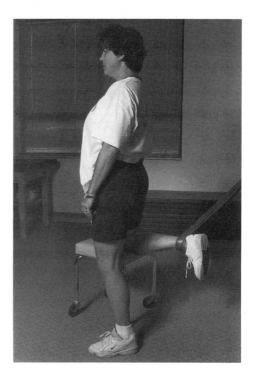

FIGURE 7. Resistive exercise for the right hip external rotators in a single plane.

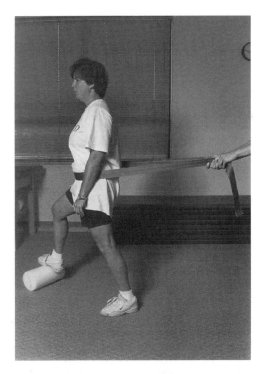

FIGURE 8. Functional activity with resistance incorporating knee proprioception and right gluteus medius function.

The lumbar spine, hip, and pelvis are considered together because of the relative complexity involved. This region acts as the base of the musculoskeletal system and also functions as a key transfer area of forces between the lower extremities, trunk, and upper extremities. In daily activity, these three areas function closely. The lumbar spine transfers weight and bending movements to the pelvis and vice versa. Spine motion is largely guided by function here as well. Compression, torsional, tensile, and vibrational forces all may have a deleterious effect in the unconditioned spine. Disc injury at one motion segment can disturb the kinetics at motion segments above and below the site of injury, placing added stress on these structures, including the hip and pelvis. These changing load characteristics can lead to continued cartilaginous degeneration and

TABLE 5. Sports Commonly Associated with Spine-Based Dysfunctions

Basketball	Gymnastics
Ice hockey	Weight lifting
Rugby	Rowing
Badminton	Archery
Golf	Skating
Squash	

facet arthropathy as increased, potentially asymmetric facet loading occurs. Trunk muscles can have a positive and preventive effect via their forces that can be exerted on the spine, hip, and pelvis region. Several examples serve to highlight this important concept: the gluteus medius muscle stabilizes the pelvis during gait. Weakness of this muscle leads to increased lumbar sidebending and rotation and to functionally destabilizing the pelvis. The psoas is another key muscle that flexes the spine on the pelvis and activates flexion across the hip joint. Inflexibility in this muscle prevents normal hip extension, with a tendency toward lumbar hyperextension and increased facet joint load. If the tightness of the psoas is asymmetric (i.e., the right psoas is tighter than the left), there is potential for a lumbar rotation to the opposite side to also occur. The piriformis muscle laterally rotates the hip and rotates the sacrum. Therefore, tightness can lead to a sacral rotation to the opposite side, and weakness can promote sacral rotation to the same side. This can lead to increased torsional stress at the lumbosacral junction. Finally, the abdominal muscles play a vital role in lumbar stabilization, with weakness leading to a hyperlordotic curve, increasing facet weightbearing and shear forces across the motion segments, which is poorly tolerated by the lumbar discs. This logic can continue to be applied to other muscle groups, such as the quadriceps and gluteus maximus, but the goal is to underscore the importance of mechanical dysfunction and preventive exercise given that most sports will rely significantly on spine function.

Substitution patterns are evident on screening preparticipation examinations. In general, muscle groups attempt to compensate for the lack of function of a weak muscle, such as when hip extensor weakness is compensated by overuse of the lumbar spine extensors. There are general screening tests such as lateral trunk raising and oblique trunk raising that may reveal to the athlete and examiner points of muscular weakness and substitution in the spinal axis that can help direct the exercise program. Overall, lumbopelvic stability describes the ability to maintain symmetry within the lumbosacral spine, pelvis, and hip joint during single limb activities.

Lumbar stabilization exercises increase stability of the trunk and spine, enhance motor control, and allow the athlete to play the major active role in promoting excellence in sports. In general, difficulty levels progress from nonweightbearing to weightbearing activity. There is a gradual reduction in the base of support, with eventual progression to differing postures, functional motions, and then incorporation into the athletic event. The exercises are all done in a functional position, often involving pelvic neutral positioning, which is defined as a painfree midpoint in the lumbopelvic range of motion. This position is maintained during a progression of isometric to dynamic extremity movement done eventually over a mobile base of support.

Lumbar stabilization exercises (Figs. 9–11) are begun in a supine position. Focus is made on pelvic positioning and control, isolated gluteus maximus activation, lumbar spine extension, and lower abdominals, all in the pelvic neutral position. The positioning of the spine and pelvis base is progressed to the prone position and then to sidelying, quadruped, kneeling, and sitting positions. The exercises are then incorporated over an inflated gymnastic ball to challenge the trunk to a mobile unstable base of support. It is important for the athlete to show ability at the lower-level positions prior to progressing to the gymnastic ball.

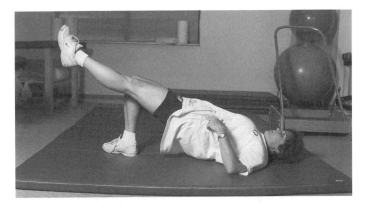

FIGURE 9. Basic bridging exercise challenges multiple lumbar stabilizers simultaneously while maintaining neutral spine.

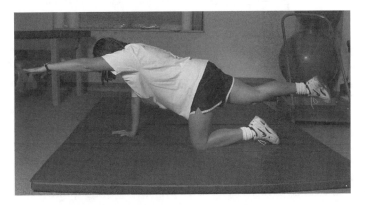

FIGURE 10. Basic quadruped exercise. The goal is to maintain a neutral spine while incorporating limb motions.

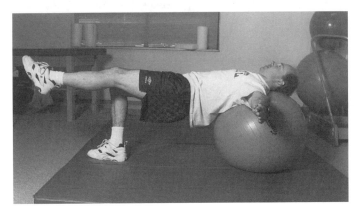

FIGURE 11. Advanced stabilization exercise challenging trunk proprioception, balance, and dynamic trunk control with simultaneous asymmetry in lower extremity and pelvis muscular demands.

The concept of muscles being prone to tightness and prone to weakness (Table 6) has been espoused by Janda.[12,13] Clinical experience often shows these patterns to be true. Stretching of the typically tight groups (Figs. 12–14) makes sense in an injury prevention and fitness maintenance program.

THE THORACIC AND CERVICAL SPINE

Many sports depend heavily on trunk rotation and target acquisition. Golf, for example, requires strength and coordination involving the trunk to effect an optimal swing and prevent overload at other structures such as the shoulder and hip to avoid injury. A baseball pitch demands that the pitcher see the strike zone, home plate, and batter by rotating and maintaining control of the cervical spine during the pitching motion. A tennis serve derives power through force transferred from the legs and through the rotating trunk, shoulder, and arm while rotating the cervical spine to allow the visual system to locate the opponent's service zone. Any deficiencies in the cervical and thoracic region in strength, flexibility, or coordination will cause a decrement in performance or predispose to overload injury at other kinetic chain sites.

The musculature around the cervical and thoracic spine, similar to the lumbar spine and hips, also shows patterns of tightness and weakness (Table 7). There are, however, numerous muscles that comprise the head extensors and flexors, the cervical extensors and flexors, and others that control rotation and sidebending of the cervical spine.[17] From a prevention standpoint, exercise directed at the postural patterns is performed to restore and maintain normal length and flexibility as well as strength (Figs. 15 and 16). The latissimus dorsi muscle is particularly important to adequately stretch, given its ability to influence biomechanics across a large area of the kinetic chain (Fig. 17). As flexibility is obtained, strengthening exercise incorporates the concept of cervicothoracic stabilization, which begins with isometric strengthening of the previously

TABLE 6. Muscles Prone to Tightness and Weakness in the Lumbar Spine, Hip, and Pelvis

Muscles Prone to Tightness	Muscles Prone to Weakness
Gastrocnemius soleus	Peronei
Tibialis posterior	Tibialis anterior
Short hip adductors	Vastus lateralis
Hamstrings	Vastus medialis
Rectus femoris	Gluteus maximus
Iliopsoas	Gluteus medius
Tensor fascia lata	Rectus abdominis
Piriformis	
Erector spinae	
Quadratus lumborum	

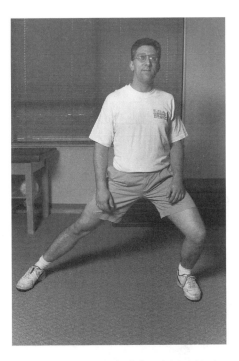

FIGURE 12. One method for right adductor group stretching.

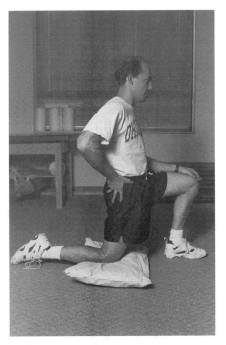

FIGURE 13. Stretching of the right iliopsoas.

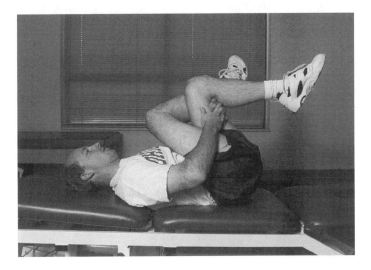

FIGURE 14. Stretching of the right piriformis muscle.

TABLE 7. Muscles Prone to Tightness and Weakness in the Thoracic and Cervical Spine

Muscles Prone to Tightness	Muscles Prone to Weakness
Pectoralis major	Serratus anterior
Upper trapezius	Rhomboids
Levator scapulae	Lower trapezius
Scalenes	Short cervical flexors

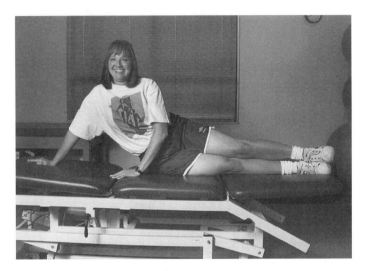

FIGURE 15. Stretching exercise for the right lateral trunk.

tight and weak muscles and then progresses to multiplanar isometrics prior to moving toward resistive exercise (Figs. 18 and 19). This resistive strengthening is often isody-namic and should include the middle and upper trapezius fibers as well as the rhom-boids. This emphasis on scapular stabilization helps decrease a tendency toward tho-racic kyphosis, with all of its postural sequelae, and underscores the important relationship of the cervical and thoracic spine to the shoulder.

THE SHOULDER

Many studies that analyze sports injuries cite rotator cuff impingement and gleno-humeral instability as frequent injury patterns.[1,8] In addition, the acromioclavicular joint is vulnerable if loaded acutely, as in a fall onto the superior aspect of the shoul-der or while checking an opponent in ice hockey using the shoulder to contact the op-ponent. Activities involving external rotation positioning of the shoulder coupled with

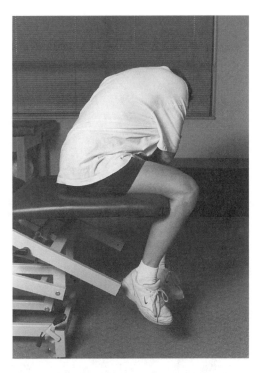

FIGURE 16.   Self-stretching of the upper thoracic rotators.

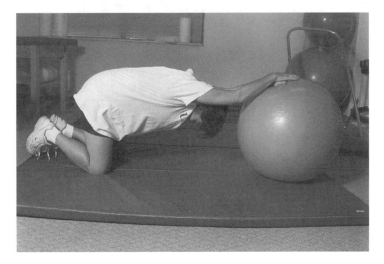

FIGURE 17.   One method of stretching the latissimus dorsi.

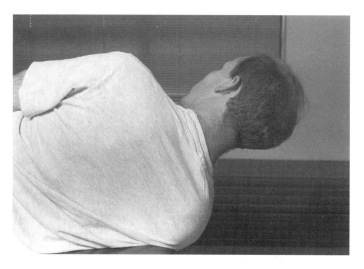

FIGURE 18. Working left cervical rotators and sidebenders in sidelying.

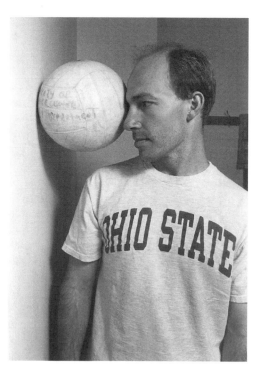

FIGURE 19. Functional cervical strengthening and proprioception.

TABLE 8.   Sports-Specific Shoulder Injury Patterns

Sport	Injury Patterns
Baseball	Rotator cuff impingement
Volleyball	Shoulder instability
Ice hockey	Acromioclavicular injury, anterior shoulder dislocation, rotator cuff tendinitis
Rugby	Shoulder dislocation-anterior
Golf	Rotator cuff impingement
Swimming	Rotator cuff impingement
Gymnastics	Shoulder instability, laxity
Weight lifting	Biceps and triceps tendinitis, rotator cuff impingement
Wrestling	Shoulder dislocation-anterior
Rowing	Rotator cuff impingement
Canoeing/kayaking	Impingement, dislocation, bicipital tendinitis
Archery	Impingement
Cross-country skiing	Scapular and shoulder muscular overload

acceleration can lead to impingement and supraspinatus tendinitis or degenerative injury. Throwing sports in general stress the anterior shoulder and inferior glenohumeral ligament, with potential for anterior instability and frank shoulder dislocation. Many of the injuries are technique-dependent, but biomechanical imbalances in flexibility and strength once again underlie potential problems. Table 8 lists sports in which common shoulder injury patterns are found.

Exercise programming for the shoulder relies on an understanding of the demands of the shoulder during athletic activity and its basic biomechanics. Integral to this is an awareness that the shoulder is a highly mobile unit at the expense of static stability. In essence, shoulder girdle musculature performs a critical stabilizing function beyond that of musculature surrounding many other areas of the kinetic chain. Moreover, exercise for the shoulder is not simply focused on the glenohumeral joint. The acromioclavicular, sternoclavicular, and scapulothoracic joints are all part of the shoulder complex, and preventive exercise should be designed with this in mind. The shoulder, although performing complex combinations of motion and speed, can be thought of in terms of muscular balance in a fairly straightforward fashion. Humeral head depressors, such as the rotator cuff muscles, are required to balance humeral head elevators such as the deltoid. Scapular retraction by the middle trapezius and rhomboids is balanced in concert with scapular protraction, which is performed largely by the serratus anterior. Relative inflexibility is often found in the pectoralis major and minor muscles, predisposing to forward and internally rotated shoulder and glenohumeral posture. This has the potential to increase the incidence of difficulties with shoulder impingement of the supraspinatus tendon. Typical tightness frequently occurs in the posterior capsule of the shoulder, often involving the teres minor and the infraspinatus. With this knowledge in mind, a prefunctional stretching and strengthening preventive program for the shoulder can be designed (Figs. 20 and 21). In addition to isolating and improving potential biomechanical deficits, functional progression of the shoulder program should occur. This involves the use of closed kinetic chain exercise for the shoulder, a form of exercise that offers coactivation of muscle groups, dynamic joint stability, scapular stabilization training, decreased glenohumeral joint reaction forces, and improved proprioception. The importance of proprioception at the shoulder complex cannot be overemphasized. Progression of these exercises includes increasing the amount of weightbearing at the shoulder, changing the exercise surface from a stable one such as a table to an unstable one such a gymnastic ball, increasing the intensity of the exercise, and moving from eyes-open activity to eyes-closed exercise.

Initial exercise may begin by standing and practicing weight shifting into the shoulder complex with the hands on a table, challenging scapular depression. In sidelying, the hand can be positioned to bear weight into the floor, challenging initial scapular mobility. Closed chain exercise for the shoulder also can be performed in the prone position, emphasizing scapular depression and external rotation, and also in the quadruped position. This position allows the introduction of a rocker board under the hands, with or without a gymnastic inflatable ball under the trunk simultaneously, focusing exercise in multiple shoulder planes while controlling the trunk and the shoulder on the unstable surfaces. The use of the ball can be combined with upper body rotation in which the athlete demonstrates functional shoulder control while the body is rotated in different planes. Figures 22–27 show some typical exercises for the shoulder girdle.

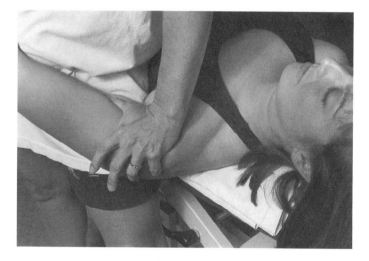

FIGURE 20. Mobilization of the left posterior capsule at the shoulder.

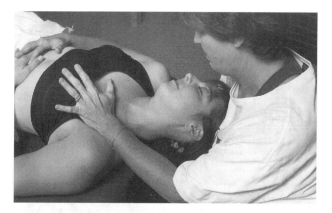

FIGURE 21. Flexibility of the levator scapulae and upper trapezius affects shoulder function.

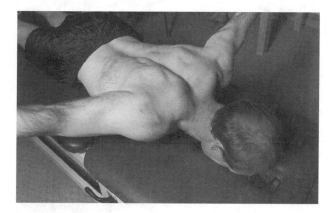

FIGURE 22. Basic scapular stabilizer strengthening for the middle trapezius and rhomboids.

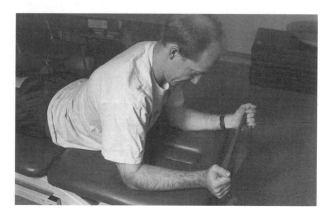

FIGURE 23. Resistive strengthening of the humeral external rotators.

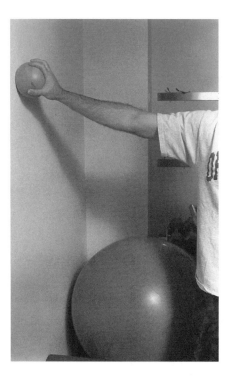

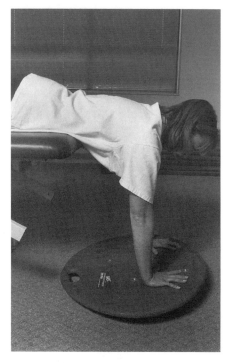

FIGURE 24. Weight into glenohumeral joint against unstable surface is followed by controlled circular motion.

FIGURE 25. Double-arm balance disk training for the shoulder complex.

FIGURE 26. Single-arm balance disk training for the shoulder complex.

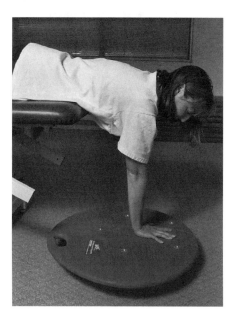

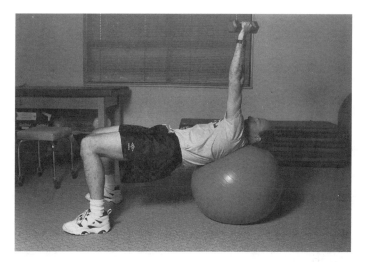

FIGURE 27. Serratus strengthening while balancing on an unstable surface.

THE ELBOW AND WRIST

Typical injuries reported at the elbow fall into consistent categories: medial ligamentous injuries and muscular overuse injuries. Chronic and acute medial collateral ligament strains often are associated with faulty throwing mechanics. This leads to so-called little leaguer's elbow, and the mechanism is that of repetitive valgus stress. Associated paresthesias in an ulnar nerve distribution are often a result of accompanying ulnar neuritis. The medial elbow is the site for flexor and pronator overuse injury called "golfer's elbow." The lateral epicondylar region is the source of symptoms that frequently occur with extensor and supinator overuse injuries; this is called "tennis elbow." The spectrum of injuries at the elbow joint spans a much larger differential than is mentioned here, but the concept of ligamentous and muscular overuse is instructive in introducing preventive exercise in relation to the elbow as a site for clinical symptom presentation. Table 9 depicts sports associated with elbow injuries.

The elbow serves as a key transfer link in the upper extremity kinetic chain. The stresses on this joint site are largely sport-specific but are also largely dependent on shoulder, trunk, and hip function. A given athletic sequence, whether it involves throwing, serving, or hitting a ball or acutely bearing weight, will demand stability and force transfer at the elbow. Faulty biomechanics of a given activity will increase the chance for injury. Some of this may be related to skill, but prefunctional conditioning may help with injury prevention. The critical structures intimately related to the elbow joint of training include the elbow, wrist flexors and extensors, and the intrinsic muscles of the hand and digit. Exercise related to injury prevention involves stretching and strengthening the wrist flexors and extensors (Figs. 28 and 29). Eccentric strengthening should be part of the program, and the use of a wrist rolling device is helpful. Eccentric strengthening increases the probability of functional overload in the

TABLE 9. Elbow Injury Patterns

Sport	Injury Pattern
Tennis	Lateral epicondylitis-osis, medial epicondylitis-osis
Golf	Later epicondylitis-osis, medial epicondylitis-osis
Gymnastics	Triceps overload, biceps and brachialis overload, hyperextension injury
Weight lifting	Triceps overload, biceps and brachialis overload
Bowling	Biceps and brachialis overload
Baseball	Medial epicondylar apophysitis, osteochondritis, medial and lateral epicondylitis-osis, medial collateral ligament injury, ulnar neuritis
Cross-country skiing	Lateral epicondylar overload
Rowing	Lateral epicondylar overload

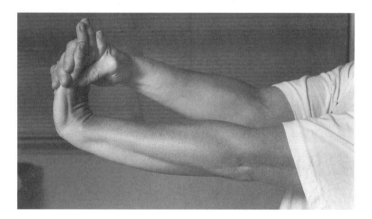

FIGURE 28. Stretching of the wrist flexors.

training setting and, with appropriate relative rest intervals, leads to the greatest strength and endurance gains.

A wrist rolling device is essentially a short wand or pole with a rope or band hanging down from it with a weight attached to it, whether it be a soup can or hand weight. By holding the pole or wand and then wrapping the rope up or down by repetitively rolling the wrists, the wrist flexors and extensors can be concentrically and eccentrically strengthened. An underhand position relative to the pole promotes flexor strengthening, and the overhand position challenges the extensors (Figs. 30 and 31). Resistive bands or tubing also may be used and can involve pronation and supination to strengthen these vital muscle groups (Figs. 32 and 33). Isodynamic strengthening of the biceps and triceps also may be warranted. The biceps are often overloaded in sports, and the triceps stabilize the elbow joint in a high demand fashion in activities such as gymnastic vaulting.

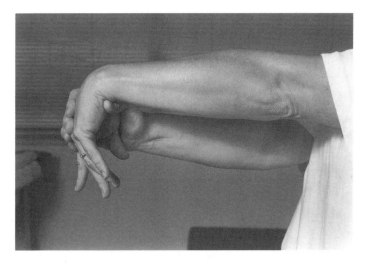

FIGURE 29. Stretching of the wrist extensors.

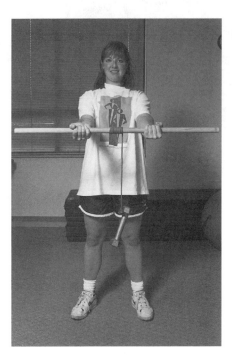

FIGURE 30. Wrist flexor strengthening.

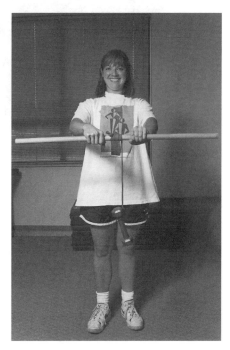

FIGURE 31. Wrist extensor strengthening.

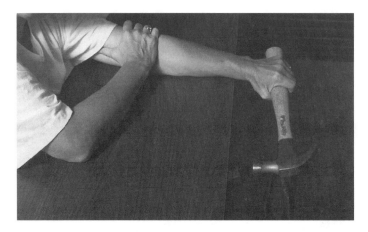

FIGURE 32.   Position for strengthening of supination.

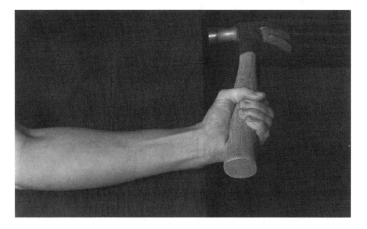

FIGURE 33.   Initial position to begin pronation strengthening exercise.

THE HAND

Preventive hand exercises encompass emphasis on tendon function, strength, and flexibility. Wehbe and Hunter highlighted three hand positions to promote maximum excursion tendon gliding exercises.[24,25] This allows the tendons to move within their sheaths in a free-gliding fashion in the uninjured hand. The three fist positions include hook fist, straight fist, and full fist. Strengthening of the hand intrinsics can be done using common objects. Rubber bands placed around the digits both proximal and then distal to the interphalangeal joints can be opened and closed in a concentric and eccentric fashion (Fig. 34). The grasping and collapsing of a newspaper, page by page, with the wrist kept in anatomic neutral position also promotes excellent hand intrinsic strengthening. Flexibility is maintained by using the opposite hand to isolate and pro-

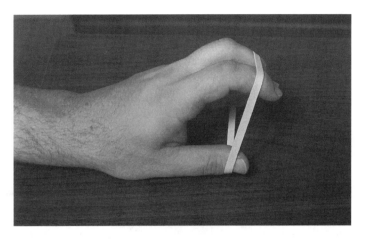

FIGURE 34. Resistive strengthening of hand intrinsics using a rubber band.

mote passive stretch of the digits as well as at the metacarpophalangeal joints into flexion and extension.

CONCLUSION

Exercise accomplishes many goals that help to prevent athletic injury. This chapter has focused on specific anatomic considerations in choosing muscle groups on which to emphasize strengthening and flexibility programs. The approach has looked at overall goals from a sport-specific, regional, and kinetic chain viewpoint. These avenues, in concert with the aerobic exercise and periodization training concepts presented in chapter 3, contain the information necessary to construct an exercise approach that can help lessen the incidence of sports injuries.

REFERENCES

1. Andrews JR, Kupferman SP, Dillan CJ: Labral tears in throwing and racquet sports. Clin Sports Med 10:901–911, 1991.
2. Bennell KL, Malcolm SA, Thomas SA, et al: Risk factors for stress fractures in female track and field athletes: A retrospective analysis. Clin J Sports Med 5:229–235, 1995.
3. Bennett AF: Thermal dependence of muscle function. Am J Physiol 247:217–229, 1984.
4. Cavanaugh PR, Robinson JR: A Biomechanical Perspective on Stress Fractures in NBA Players. A final report to the National Basketball Association. 1989
5. Durant R, Seymore C, Linder CW, et al: The preparticipation examination of athletes: Comparison of single and multiple examiners. Am J Dis Child 139:657–661, 1985.
6. Ekstrand J, Gillquist J: The avoidability of soccer injuries. Int J Sports Med 2:124–128, 1983.
7. Holmes JC, Pruit AL, Whalen NJ: Knee pain in cyclists [abstract]. Presented at the annual meeting of the American Orthopedic Society for Sports Medicine, Sun Valley, ID, 1990.
8. Hovelius L: Shoulder dislocation in Swedish ice hockey players. Am J Sports Med 6:373–377, 1978.
9. Ingjer F, Stromme SB: Effects of active, passive, or no warm-up on the physiological response to heavy exercise. Eur J Appl Physiol 40:273–282, 1979.

10. Janda DH, Hankin FM, Wojtys EM: Softball injuries: Cost, cause, and prevention. Am Fam Physician 33:143–144, 1986.
11. Janda DH, Wojtys EM, Hankin FM, et al: A three phase analysis of the prevention of recreational softball injuries. Am J Sports Med 18:632–635, 1990.
12. Janda V: Muscles, motor regulation and back problems. In Korr IM (ed): The Neurologic Mechanisms in Manipulative Therapy. New York, Plenum, 1978.
13. Janda V: Pain in the locomotor system—a broad approach. In Glascow EF (ed): Aspects of Manipulative Therapy. New York, Churchill Livingstone, 1985.
14. Kadel NJ, Teitz CC, Kronmal RA: Stress fractures in ballet dancers. Am J Sports Med 20:445–449, 1992.
15. McBryde AM: Stress fractures in athletes. J Sports Med 3:212, 1975.
16. van Mechelen W, Hlobil H, Kemper HCG: How Can Sports Injuries be Prevented? NISGZ, Papendal, The Netherlands, 1987, publication 25E.
17. Parke WW, Sherk HH: Normal human anatomy. In Sherk HH, Dunn EJ, Eismon FJ, et al (eds): The Cervical Spine, 2nd ed. Philadelphia, JB Lippincott, 1989.
18. Paul IL, Munro M, Abernethy PJ, et al: Musculoskeletal shock absorption: Relative contribution of bone and soft tissues at various frequencies. J Biomech 11:237–239, 1978.
19. Radin EL, Simon SR, Rose RM, et al: Practical Biomechanics for the Orthopedic Surgeon. New York, Wiley and Sons, 1979.
20. Radin EL: Role of muscles in protecting athletes from injury. Acta Med Scand Suppl 711:143–47, 1986.
21. Safran MR, Seaber AV, Garrett WE: Warm-up and muscular injury prevention. Sprots Med 8:239–249, 1989.
22. Strong WB, Linder CW: Preparticipation health evaluation for competitive sports. Pediatr Rev 4:113–121, 1982.
23. Torg JS: Cervical spine injuries in American football. In Renstrom PAFH (ed): Clinical Practice of Sports Injury Prevention and Care. Oxford, Blackwell Scientific, 1994, pp 13–26.
24. Wehbe MA, Hunter JM: Flexor tendon gliding in the hand. Part 1. In vivo excursions. J Hand Surg 10A:570, 1985.
25. Wehbe MA, Hunter JM: Flexor tendon gliding in the hand. Part 2. In vivo excursions. J Hand Surg 10A:575, 1985.
26. Williams KR: Biomechanics of distance running. In Grabiner MD (ed): Current Issues in Biomechanics. Champaign, IL, Human Kinetics, 1993, pp 3–32.

BARRY GOLDSTEIN, MD, PhD

LANCE GOETZ, MD

JENNIFER YOUNG, MS, PT

STEVEN STIENS, MD

STEPHEN BURNS, MD

18

Treatment of Repetitive Motion Disorders

The number of reported cases of repetitive motion disorders is rapidly growing. Much of the focus on these disorders has been on the public health impact and cost, but there is also considerable controversy as to the pathophysiologic processes involved. Unfortunately, there has been little work on the functional impact and disability as a result of repetitive motion disorders. This chapter reviews the pathophysiology, clinical diagnosis, and treatment—including prescription writing—of four common overuse problems. We discuss problems that commonly affect both disabled and able-bodied individuals.

The first of three sections reviews basic pathophysiologic mechanisms of overuse injuries. Because a treatment plan is derived from an accurate diagnosis and understanding of underlying pathology, this section reviews the current understanding of extrinsic factors, such as biomechanical loads, and the ensuing tissue response to repetitive loading. The second section reviews the impact of repetitive motion disorders on the individual because effective treatment of an overuse syndrome (e.g., impairment) demands that the resultant disability and handicap are recognized. Finally, the last section examines four common overuse problems and the development of a treatment plan for each condition. Case studies are presented to highlight the clinical presentation, assessment, and treatment for each clinical entity.

PATHOPHYSIOLOGY OF REPETITIVE MOTION DISORDERS

Overuse injuries are extremely prevalent. The national surveillance data from the United States Department of Labor Bureau of Labor Statistics (BLS) showed that more than 60% of new occupational illnesses in 1992 were associated with repetitive motion.[99,132] In the BLS system, the highest rates occur in industries with a substantial amount of repetitive work, such as meat packing, automobile manufacturing, and garment construction. Athletes and performing artists also have an extremely high incidence of overuse injuries. Abut 34–50% of sports participants can be expected to be injured, approximately half of whom will have overuse injuries.[73] Musicians and dancers have been reported to experience exceptionally high rates of overuse injuries in both the upper and lower extremities.[36,54]

The evaluation and management of an individual who has suspected repetitive motion disorder is beset with difficulties. Imprecise definitions, a paucity of outcome studies, and a lack of animal models, tissue availability, and analysis of biomechanical loads all contribute to a level of uncertainty in this field that is frustrating for the patient and clinician alike. This insufficiency of data affects all aspects of clinical care, particularly the diagnostic assessment, evaluation of contributory factors, identification of cause-and-effect relationships, and the development of an efficacious treatment program.

Overuse injuries have a diversity of terminology—repetitive motion disorder, repetitive stress syndrome, activity-related musculoskeletal disorders—and have complex multifactorial causes. Further, they can involve many tissues, including muscles, nerves, ligaments, and tendons. Overuse injuries represent several different pathologic entities (e.g., in tendon: tendinitis, tendinosis, peritendinitis) associated with distinct causes, which include repetition, cumulative trauma, and sustained static loading. A useful operational definition is that a repetitive motion disorder is one in which a summation of biomechanical loads is applied beyond the tolerance of the biologic tissues.

It is interesting that many of the terms for repetitive motion disorders imply that the pathology is well understood. In fact, much of this same terminology may be misleading because, in some clinical instances, it is sustained contractions in the absence of motion that appear to be the major causative factor. In considering the basic pathophysiology of repetitive motion disorders, several basic questions arise. Who develops activity-related musculoskeletal disorders? What are the extrinsic and intrinsic factors that contribute to the development of overuse problems? Is the exact cause and diagnosis relevant to treatment?

There is a growing body of basic research that serves as a foundation and basis for clinical care and treatment of activity-related repetitive motion disorders. The overall message is that most tissues, such as connective tissues and muscle, have the capacity to change their structure and composition in response to mechanical stimulation. Under some circumstances this response can be nonadaptive, and pathologic changes occur. In considering the pathophysiology, there are two general areas of consideration: first, the biomechanical loads acting upon a particular body segment and, second, the tissue response to those loads.

BIOMECHANICAL LOADS

Several common physical stressors have been found to be potentiating factors for the development of activity-related repetitive motion disorders: repetition, force, posture, duration, contact stress, vibration, and temperature.[51] A careful examination of these extrinsic risk factors is vital in developing a treatment program because, if the risk factors are not removed or modified, treatment is unlikely to be successful.

Each factor is deserving of careful consideration but beyond the scope of this chapter. For example, repetition refers to the temporal aspect of activity or work. Obviously, more work is performed at a keyboard at 12,000 strokes per hour than at 8,000 strokes per hour. It is less obvious that a closely related factor is relaxation time between activities. Some believe that there is a closer correlation between continuous activity and the development of an overuse disorder than with strict repetition of a task. For example, how frequently does the keyboard operator remove his or her hands from the keys and relax? Is there prolonged, static loading? In the absence of periodic rest, the expected correlation between the number of key strokes and the development of a disorder might be altered.

Vibration is also an important factor. Rather than examining whether vibration is a preexisting potentiating factor, investigators recently have attempted to elucidate the exposure-effect relationship by quantifying properties of frequency, displacement, velocity, and acceleration. For example, Miyashita et al. found that about half of chain saw operators manifested symptoms of repetitive motion disorder after 8,000 hours of total chain saw operating time and that workers with fewer than 2,000 hours of exposure rarely manifested symptoms.[88]

It is important to put these risk factors within some practical, clinical context. Exposure to physical stressors are related to three domains: work (training) requirements, environmental factors, and individual factors. Work or training requirements refer to the quantity and quality of activities. For example, a training program for an athlete involves a specific number of exertions, magnitude of forces, recovery time, type of activities, and other factors. Environmental factors include important aspects such as exposure to cold, vibration, and the physical characteristics of a work station. Individual factors include skill training, posture, physical characteristics, and fitness. To develop an effective treatment program for a repetitive motion disorder, an accurate analysis and subsequent modification of all three of these areas are essential.

In summary, exposure to certain physical stressors appears to be related to the development of activity-related neuromusculoskeletal disorders. Unfortunately, few studies have demonstrated dose-response and cause-and-effect relationships between physical stressors and repetitive motion disorders because methods of measuring these physical stressors are crude and have not been standardized. However, physical stressors are likely directly related to the work environment and work requirements. In general, there is a need for a better understanding of the dynamic effects of activities on neuromuscular function and dysfunction.

TISSUE RESPONSE (ADAPTATION VERSUS INJURY)

In general, compelling evidence exists that significant adaptation occurs in response to mechanical stress in most tissues, particularly in skeletal muscle and most of the connective tissues. Yet several questions must be addressed by the clinician that will have bearing on devising a treatment program. What is it in the loading environment or with internal processes that leads to pathologic rather than adaptive changes? How does a particular tissue change both structurally and biomechanically as a response to a specific type of loading? What factors affect a normal adaptive change to a pathologic process? We will refer to studies on dense connective tissues to illustrate important concepts that can be addressed in answering these questions. Since tendons and ligaments are exposed to large repetitive forces during their role in initiating and guiding joint movements, they offer a good model in studying the biomechanical properties of the normal, injured, and healing stress.

Flint and colleagues made several important clinical and basic observations about connective tissues. In general, they found that tendons and ligaments have the capacity to change their structure, composition, and mechanical properties in response to mechanical stimulation. In other words, Wolff's law, which states that connective tissues orient themselves in form and mass to best resist extrinsic forces, was found to apply to the soft connective tissues as well as bone. Specifically, the basic building blocks for connective tissues were found to change in response to an applied mechanical load. Collagen diameter, orientation, packing, cross-linking, and type were found to adapt to increased mechanical loads, as did the amount and type of glycosaminoglycans. One of the best examples of this phenomenon is found in the region of a tendon that experiences compressional or frictional forces rather than longitudinal (tensile) forces (e.g., the point at which a tendon changes direction as it passes around bone, traverses a narrow tunnel, passes through a pully, or is impinged upon by a neighboring structure). There are several examples in humans, including the tibialis posterior as the tendon lies against the posterior surface of the medial malleolus, supraspinatus as it inserts into the greater tuberosity, flexor hallucis longus as it is in contact with the sustentaculum tali, Achilles tendon as it passes over the calcaneus, and flexor digitorum profundus as the tendons pass through the flexor digitorum superficialis tendons. In each of these examples, the anatomy and composition of the normal tendon changes from that of a regularly arranged dense connective tissue to that of fibrocartilage (fibrocartilage has more and different types of proteoglycan). In other words, when a tendon experiences significant compression and friction, it undergoes adaptive changes from a primary fibrous tissue to one that is more fibrocartilaginous. Further, Flint et al. found that these changes are reversible; they developed animal models to change the mechanical demands across tendons in these compressive areas.

However, although initially adaptive, fibrocartilage is less vascular and less capable of responding to repetitive microinjury than a typical tendon. If the reparative capabilities of the tissue are surpassed, pathologic changes eventually might develop and chronic overuse injuries are thought to be the result. There are numerous clinical examples of this problem in both the lower and upper extremity: Achilles tendinitis in runners and dancers, supraspinatus tears in pitchers, long head of the biceps tendinitis in the bicipital groove, and degenerative changes in the extensor pollicis longus as it changes direction around Lister's tubercle. Indeed, tendon injury within a zone of relatively hypovascular fibrocartilage is probably one of the most important unifying concepts of chronic, overuse injuries.

HEALING

Our consideration of healing and repair also focuses on the dense connective tissues as a model to illustrate important clinical concepts. Most of the basic and clinical science studies have concentrated on the knee even though the occurrence of soft tissue overuse injuries is more common in other joints.[71]

Following *acute injury* to dense connective tissues, there is rapid initiation of a healing cascade. Typically, there are three overlapping phases: inflammatory, proliferative, and remodeling. The healing process is influenced by a variety of factors, including age, drugs, hormones, gender, genetics, and coexisting diseases. From a morphologic point of view, dense connective tissues demonstrate rapid healing following acute injury and are quite normal within 12–16 weeks. However, mechanical properties are much slower to recover; several studies have demonstrated characteristics such as tensile strength to be decreased as late as 1 year after the initial injury.

Woo et al. have conducted further work on healing following acute injuries of ligaments and tendons.[150] A growing body of evidence supports the idea that tension and movement stimulate healing whereas immobilization negatively impacts all structural and biomechanical properties. That has been supported by animal studies, work with the grasping suture technique, studies on the effects of early controlled passive motion, and recent work examining the effects of early active motion following injury. In general, tension and movement have been found to result in increased strength and repair following injury. Conversely, studies in animals and humans have found that immobilization results in decreased collagen synthesis, increased collagen degradation, loss of collagen cross-links, decreased tissue remodeling, and decreased rates of repair.

There is a remarkable lack of similar experimental work on repetitive motion disorders, e.g., chronic injuries. As discussed above, hypotheses about the cause and pathophysiology of these disorders abound and include ischemia-reperfusion, microinjuries surpassing repair capabilities, thermal denaturation, and dysregulation of the epitendon and epiligament. Although there appears to be a close association between repetitive movements and the development of overuse symptomatology, basic questions remain about the injury and subsequent repair processes.[23,28,36] Why are only a subset of individuals affected by repetitive motion disorders? What is the sequence of events that leads to tissue pathology? Although many of these repetitive injuries are referred to as inflammatory disorders, how common is inflammation at the site of injury? Similarly, how common are degenerative rather than inflammatory changes? How do differing treatment strategies affect repair and outcome from repetitive motion disorders? All of these questions have a direct bearing on the development of a treatment plan.

There is a growing body of work that might have a direct bearing on treatment decisions. Although many clinicians approach repetitive motion disorders—lateral epicondylitis, de Quervain's disease, plantar fasciitis—as if there were an inflammatory basis, there is evidence that degenerative changes are often found at the pathologic site. For example, Amadio biopsied tendons and synovium at the anatomic snuffbox of patients diagnosed with de Quervain's disease and found distinct pathologic conditions such as nonspecific tenosynovitis, intersection syndrome, and tendon entrapment. Only one of these conditions demonstrated frank inflammation. Indeed, in nonspecific tenosynovitis, no pathologic changes were usually found. Similar observations have been found with lateral epicondylitis and Achilles tendinitis that lead to questions about the occurrence of inflammatory changes.

Thus, the clinical challenge is to extend these observations and develop hypotheses and treatment protocols. There have been few rigorous longitudinal or interventional studies in the area of repetitive motion disorders. We believe that it is important to bear in mind the relationship between adaptive and pathologic tissue response because it is a dynamic process and many of the changes are thought to be reversible. Yet, it is unclear how to apply this information to chronic injuries even though we know that tendons and ligaments have the capacity to change their structure and composition in an adaptive response to a mechanical challenge. We must question the efficacy of a treatment program for an overuse injury that prescribes inactivity, nonsteroidal antiinflammatory medications (NSAIDs), and corticosteroid injections. Moreover, we propose the following treatment principles for chronic overuse injuries: (1) prevention of further injury—optimize how tissues and joints are used such as by correcting muscle imbalance and reestablishing range of motion and by analysis and modification of biomechanical loads; (2) stimulate healing and repair by prescribing active motion rather than immobilization; (3) avoid or minimize treatments that might cause further injury, e.g., shift equilibrium toward pathologic rather than adaptive response, such as corticosteroid injections and restrictive taping of a joint; and (4) optimize environmental factors, equipment, adaptive aids, and footwear.

THE PERSONAL AND ENVIRONMENTAL CONTEXT

The threshold for seeking medical advice or assistance with a problem often relates to the magnitude of impact it has on the person's performance of perceived life roles. Clearly understanding the chief complaint is essential to addressing why the patient is seeking care. The temporal and situational factors as well as exacerbating and palliating factors should be explored. This evaluation includes the physical world and the societal influences surrounding the patient.

The parts of the environment as they relate to the person have been defined for the purposes of rehabilitation intervention.[124,134] The *immediate environment* can be defined as the space that is in direct contact with the person and includes clothes, braces, jewelry, tools, and wheelchairs or other adaptive equipment that might enable the person to work. The *intermediate environment* is the individual's personal work space and home. Finally, the patient's symptoms must be related to the *community environment,* a space that is open to all others and includes nonexclusive public spaces and those that surround the patient.

The clinician must understand the relationship of the patient's symptoms to characteristics of the environment. There may be personal demands that come through the community environment that define job expectations, cultural norms, and responses to injury and disablement. Efforts are focused on understanding the patient as a unique person with his or her own symptoms and life goals.[134] This assessment includes the person's life activities and relationship with the overuse injury under consideration.

One also must understand the many factions and interactions of the parties that are involved with the person and repetitive motion disorder.[133] Patients may be self-referred, sent by an employer, or referred by a lawyer. Specific interests of other parties are then assessed by asking them who sent them, why, and who will require reports of the visit.

Traditionally, the biomedical approach focuses on the analysis of symptoms, which is confirmed by findings and test results to make a diagnosis. The identification of the pathology due to cumulative trauma only represents an early step in the process of producing a rehabilitative solution for the patient.

The analysis of chief complaints, the patient as a unique person, and the environment provide a background for the specific identification of secondary effects of an overuse injury. This assessment includes the effect of the injury on the person's life activity and life roles.[132] The World Health Organization has devised terminology to describe the various aspects of disablement.[153] *Disablement* is a summary term used to include all secondary effects of pathologic processes or injuries on the person. These effects can be divided into three separate but interrelated domains: (1) organs and systems, (2) the whole person, and (3) society (both physical and psychosocial aspects are included). Problems at the organ level are called *impairments* and refer to structural or functional deficits. Functional limitations experienced at the level of the whole person are called *disabilities* and refer to inability to perform tasks that would otherwise be normal for someone of that age. Task completion requires the participation of the whole person in identification of the tasks and in coordination of multiple organ systems to accomplish completion. Finally, *handicap* refers to the disadvantage experienced by a person as he or she interacts with the physical and psychosocial environment.

A physiatric assessment of the patient's unique constellation of injuries, impairments, disabilities, and handicaps can be organized in the form of a problem list.[133] The first problems listed are the primary diagnosis followed by the secondary effects as a sequence of impairments, disabilities, and handicaps. This formulation can serve as a template for organization of physiatric prescriptions. Although the practice of rehabilitation requires simultaneous interventions to ameliorate pathophysiologic processes as well as disablement, the treatment emphasis changes as patients progress from acute presentation through the chronic phase. The focus of the interventions often progresses down the problem list from diagnoses through impairments, disabilities, and handicaps. As treatment succeeds, prescriptions for treatment should advance to sequentially ameliorate as many barriers to life roles as possible. Initial management of an acute injury often emphasizes treatment to limit the pathophysiologic process. In an overuse injury, this could include prescriptions for NSAIDs, complete rest with splinting, and application of ice. As inflammation subsides, passive and then active exercises can be used to reduce the impairments of limited range and weakness. Reacquisition of effective task performance follows as interventions focus on specific activities that approximate the patient's activity goals. Finally, interventions to minimize handicap are introduced as the patient reenters the work and community environment.

FOUR COMMON OVERUSE PROBLEMS

Four examples of common overuse problems are presented in this section: (a) impingement and rotator cuff disease in an individual with paraplegia, (b) lateral epicondylitis in an able-bodied individual, (c) wrist pain in a person with paraplegia, and (d) knee pain in a basketball player. Each section begins with the presentation of a case, which is followed by a discussion of the epidemiology, etiology, pathophysiology, clinical features, and differential diagnosis. Rehabilitation and prescription writing also are discussed.

CHRONIC SHOULDER PAIN IN INDIVIDUALS WITH PARAPLEGIA: IMPINGEMENT SYNDROME AND ROTATOR CUFF DISEASE

Case Study

Case history.   Mr. A is a 55-year-old left-handed man with complete T8 paraplegia for 30 years who presents with right shoulder pain. The patient has had pain in the affected shoulder "off-and-on again" for several years. He describes the pain "like a toothache" in the lateral and posterior aspect of the right shoulder. Pain is worse with use, particularly when reaching, during transfers, when doing a pressure release, and when he lies on the right side. He denies neck or radiating pain and has not noted any new neurologic symptoms. He denies new skin breakdown. The patient is a farmer and manages 20 acres of land and 50 head of cattle. He is active every day and independent with all activities.

Physical examination.   Remarkable for a middle-aged man, sitting in a wheelchair, with rounded shoulders and a head-forward (protracted head) position. There is no obvious asymmetry of the shoulders or upper extremities except mild atrophy in the right supraspinous fossa. Palpation does not reveal tenderness or anatomic abnormality. Passive and active range of motion are normal (the patient complains of pain during active right shoulder flexion and abduction and when moving from a fully abducted position to the anatomic position. There is give-way weakness and complaints of pain with resisted external rotation, flexion, and abduction at the right shoulder. Impingement sign is negative. There are no signs of shoulder instability. There is no crepitus. Examination of the neck and rest of both upper extremities is normal.

Working diagnosis.   Right supraspinatus tear.

Diagnostic evaluation.   Plain radiographs of the right shoulder reveal a subacromial osteophyte, degenerative changes of the acromioclavicular joint, and a high-riding humerus. Magnetic resonance imaging (MRI) reveals a right partial, full-thickness tear of the supraspinatus muscle.

Introduction and Epidemiology

Shoulder pain is reported in a third to half of patients with spinal cord injury (SCI). Bayley et al.[7] found that 30% of 94 individuals with complete paraplegia had persistent, chronic shoulder pain. Nichols et al.[94] concluded that the prevalence of shoulder pain in the SCI population was approximately 50%. Similarly, Sie et al.[125] reported an incidence of chronic shoulder pain of about 50% in the SCI population. Although the exact relationship is not clear, shoulder pain is thought to be a result of weightbearing and overuse, increasing as a function of age and time since injury in individuals who are primary wheelchair users. A remarkably high prevalence of shoulder and upper extremity pain[8] and rotator cuff tears[6,9] has been reported in individuals who have had a spinal cord injury for 20 years or more.

Etiology and Pathophysiology

Given the estimated prevalence and incidence of shoulder pain in the SCI population, there is a remarkable lack of information about the diagnoses, natural history, and treatment of shoulder problems in these patients. Despite speculation in the literature, the source of shoulder problems in individuals with an SCI remains obscure. Overuse, disuse, impingement, heterotopic ossification, and referred pain (from cervical spondylosis and syringomyelia) have been identified as potential causes. The fact remains that shoulder pain within the SCI population probably includes diverse orthopedic, neurologic, and rheumatologic diagnoses. Therefore, there is no unifying pathophysiologic mechanism to account for most of the problems in this population. Nevertheless, the most frequently cited clinical diagnoses for shoulder pain in the literature are orthopedically related, and there is general acceptance that weightbearing and overuse are the usual causes of shoulder problems.

In the study by Bayley et al.,[7] about two thirds of symptomatic individuals with paraplegia and shoulder pain had chronic impingement syndrome with subacromial bursitis.[3] More than half of the patients with chronic impingement were found to have rotator cuff tears, although, due to Bayley's study design, this is probably an underestimate of the true prevalence of tears. Robinson et al.[118] reported on a case-series of four patients with SCI who had chronic impingement and rotator cuff tears and who subsequently failed conservative therapy and then had successful surgical intervention.[7] Other reports describe characteristics of shoulder pain and functional limitations yet lack diagnostic, treatment, and outcome information.

At our center, we recently compared symptomatic and asymptomatic individuals with paraplegia by MRI.[6] Of the symptomatic individuals with paraplegia, 20 of 28 (71%) symptomatic shoulders demonstrated complete or partial rotator cuff tears. A total of 57% of the individuals had full-thickness supraspinatus tears, 14% had partial-thickness tears, and 29% had no tear. In comparison, investigations of able-bodied patients have reported a much lower prevalence of rotator cuff tears in patients with shoulder pain (surgical or arthroscopic: 17–53%,[10–13] cadaveric studies: 5–17%,[14–18] MRI: 15%[19]).

The pathogenesis of rotator cuff pathology is not clear. Neer proposed that rotator cuff tendinitis and tendinopathy were the result of repeated mechanical impingement.[91] However, others believe the primary factor to be repetitive intrinsic tension overload, named by Nirschl as *angiofibroblastic hyperplasia*.[96–98] Ischemia of the cuff tendons has long been thought to be an important factor in the degenerative changes that occur, but the cause of ischemia remains unknown. Several investigators have reported degenerative changes (tendinosis) and histologic evidence of fibrocartilage within the substance of the supraspinatus tendon.[22,70,147] The latter is a common observation in tendons that are subjected to compressive and frictional forces. Others have reported an inflammatory infiltrate within the subacromial bursa and increased vascularity and hyperemic changes within the rotator cuff tendons, but most studies have not demonstrated inflammatory changes involving the musculotendinous units of the rotator cuff.[22,40,147] How such changes relate to more acute lesions and the beginning of the disease process remains unclear.

Clinical Features and Presentation

The clinical features of musculoskeletal shoulder pain are diverse. Shoulder pain might present unilaterally or bilaterally. Symptoms may begin quite rapidly or gradually over weeks or months. Pain might present as a discrete, self-limiting event or remain as a chronic, persistent problem. Frequently, pain increases with activity in early stages and may become more constant as the disease progresses. Individuals may report no functional limitations or severe limitations with activities such as pressure releases and transfers. Sleep is frequently disrupted, and finding a comfortable position in bed is often a problem.

On physical examination, isometric-resisted tests are particularly helpful and performed with the joint in neutral position. The purposes of these tests are to assess muscular strength and assess whether the test reproduces the person's symptoms. Rotator cuff arthropathies will often manifest during testing of shoulder abduction, external rotation, and internal rotation.

It is essential to first determine if the pain is mechanical. If it is not, other causes must be investigated, such as tumor or referred pain from a radiculopathy or syringomyelia. If the history and physical examination point toward a mechanical problem, using an impairment approach rather than a strict pathologic schema is most helpful in leading to a treatment plan. At the shoulder, four general mechanical impairments are commonly found: weakness, instability, stiffness, and problems with smoothness of movement. Even if one is secure with the diagnosis of rotator cuff tear, one must rule out other mechanical impairments, such as instability or restricted range of motion. Just treating weakness but not treating restricted range of motion will result in further problems. Similarly, if a rotator cuff repair is planned, it is imperative to evaluate stability of the shoulder, because acromioplasty is frequently performed during surgery for the rotator cuff repair. Acromioplasty might result in further loss of shoulder stability. Because the shoulder joint primarily relies on muscular factors for primary stabilization and the coracoacromial arch for secondary stabilization, acromioplasty might eliminate the last remaining structural factor for superior stability in the setting of a large rotator cuff tear.

Differential Diagnosis

In many cases, it is difficult to differentiate between a neck and shoulder problem, and it is important to recall that coexistent disease might occur.

Several principles are helpful in developing a working diagnosis and differentiating between neck and shoulder pathology:[84,87] (1) mechanical shoulder pain is exacerbated by shoulder movement; (2) the symptom pattern in the shoulder frequently involves stiffness and instability; (3) it is not uncommon to have coexisting neck and shoulder problems; (4) mechanical neck pain is aggravated by neck movement; (5) neck problems will often refer to both shoulders; (6) beware if the predominant symptom is not pain, e.g., weakness or sensory change; (7) beware if the predominant symptom is not mechanical pain; and (8) beware of functional problems that are not consistent with the underlying disease process.

The practitioner must recognize that shoulder pain is common among individuals with an SCI and has variable causes, onsets, courses, and outcomes. Because most individuals with shoulder pain have problems of a musculoskeletal nature that involve rotator cuff arthropathies, it is important to develop protection and treatment programs concentrating on impingement and rotator cuff pathology.

Literature Review: Impingement Syndrome and Rotator Cuff Disease in Individuals with Paraplegia

Although investigations into the causes and diagnoses of shoulder problems in this population are limited, there is evidence that impingement and rotator cuff tears are common.[7,35,118] However, there is a remarkable lack of studies on the treatment of rotator cuff arthropathies in these people.

The natural history of rotator cuff arthropathies within the SCI population is not well understood. Treatments of the rotator cuff have not been sufficiently studied in the SCI population to know if any treatment has beneficial long-term effects, particularly the relative success in gaining function by conservative versus surgical approaches. Further, it is difficult to know whether data from the able-bodied population have any relevance to individuals who use their upper extremities for prehension, weightbearing, transfers, and wheelchair propulsion.

We have recently confirmed that surgical repair of rotator cuff tears, although infrequent, has been largely unsuccessful.[49] Robinson et al. report favorable short-term results with surgical decompression of impingement in individuals with paraplegia. However, because both of these studies have serious experimental design limitations, the results must be interpreted cautiously. There is a great need for controlled, prospective studies.

A variety of nonsurgical treatment programs have been used to treat subacromial impingement and rotator cuff arthropathy, most of which involve therapeutic exercises and the use of modalities. Treatments are directed toward managing pain, decreasing inflammation, regaining strength, and regaining motion.

Pain management. Pain is often a significant component of rotator cuff arthropathy, and it interferes with participation in rehabilitation. Relative rest, medications, injections, icing, ultrasound and other heating modalities, transcutaneous electrical nerve stimulation, and acupuncture are all used for pain management. However, little has been done to compare the relative effectiveness of these treatments. Also, many "step" or "phase" programs use one or more of these treatment approaches.

There are many uncontrolled studies using ultrasound for pain management. Several basic studies have shown that ultrasound is the most effective deep-heating modality for larger joints, such as the shoulder and hip.[21,79,80] Other studies have demonstrated the general utility of using ultrasound when stretching tissues.[1,45] Yet, therapeutic effects in managing pain, increasing blood supply, stimulating healing, and increasing tissue management are largely unsubstantiated. Two controlled studies have demonstrated no difference in shoulder pain regardless of whether ultrasound was used.[32,67]

Treatment directed at decreasing inflammation. Although most research does not support an inflammatory cause of rotator cuff arthropathies, the initial phase of many rehabilitation programs is to curtail inflammation. Ice application, oral antiinflammatory medication, electrical stimulation, and corticosteroid injections have all been proposed for this purpose, but little supportive data or clinical studies exist.[16,114] The use of corticosteroid injections and of antiinflammatory medications must be questioned considering the potential negative consequences and long-term effects. Matsen et al. now consider corticosteroid injections as a negative prognostic factor for successful repair of rotator cuff tears.[87] The use of NSAIDs must also be challenged in individuals with an SCI considering their potential nephrotoxocity.

Treatment directed at weakness. Strengthening programs are commonly used in individuals with impingement syndrome and rotator cuff arthropathy. The most common approach has been to study strengthening exercises in the perioperative and postoperative periods,[3,4] particularly isometric exercises prescribed to maintain and recover strength without compromising immobilized, healing tissues. Isotonic exercises are commonly used with certain clinical diagnoses, such as rotator cuff tears and shoulder instability,[48,55,102,140] and some of these programs have been designed to exercise specific muscle groups.[30,69,140] Unfortunately, few rigorous studies have been performed to evaluate the efficacy of these exercise programs. Recently and primarily with athletes, isokinetic exercises have been used to strengthen the shoulder and attempt to improve sports performance.[15,26,34] The advantages of specific types of isotonic, isometric, and isokinetic programs (e.g., concentric versus eccentric training) remain controversial.[26,30,122] Several studies have reported good results of strengthening programs following rotator cuff tears, some of which were reported to be quite large.[14,17,56,119]

Retraining for optimal positioning of the glenohumeral joint during functional activities has been another strategy to promote shoulder strength and stability. Basmajian discussed this concept with regard to frank instability and inferior subluxation, aggravated by a forward lateral slope of the glenoid fossa (e.g., a downward sloping fossa). A common approach has been strengthening scapular stabilizers to correct the position of the scapula.[6] Similar strategies have been recommended for upper extremity positioning during functional activities, and they are particularly important to incorporate during acute rehabilitation as a component of a prevention program.[49]

Treatment directed at loss of motion. Stretching exercises are used to maintain or increase range of motion at the glenohumeral joint of the pectoral girdle. Unfortunately, restricted shoulder motion is quite common; the symptoms may vary from that of intense pain at rest to mild pain that is present when approaching end range. Because the shoulder relies on soft tissues for much of its stability (e.g., positioning and muscular factors for midrange stability and ligament/capsular factors for end range stability) it is imperative that the soft tissues are not overstretched, or instability might result. Restriction of motion may be quite subtle but may compromise certain activities, such as proper technique during wheelchair propulsion or transfers.

Stretching exercises consist of passive, assisted, or active exercises. Passive exercises, as advocated by Codman, Maitland, and Hellebrandt et al.[57,85] have been demonstrated to be effective in maintaining motion during rehabilitation programs and preventing stiffness and adhesions postoperatively.[43,60,92,150,151] As always, prolonged stretching with prior heating of the soft tissues is optimal because the tissues are viscoelastic.[74] Although assistive exercises, in which the uninvolved arm assists the involved shoulder through a range of motion, and active exercises have been widely used and promoted, there have been few controlled, prospective studies.[57,64,149,152]

Regaining full flexibility and balance of strength of the pectoral girdle has been studied even less than the glenohumeral joint. Lack of strength in the pectoral girdle is a common problem for individuals with a disability, particularly for those who use a wheelchair. It is also common in some sports that result in great strength and development of some muscles but not others. Tight, short anterior muscles and lengthened, weak posterior muscles are common in individuals with paraplegia who use a wheelchair. Compensatory movements at the glenohumeral joint commonly occur to offset the abnormal position and loss of motion at the pectoral girdle. Many types of stretching programs have been advocated for regaining full range of motion, but no comparative studies have tested the relative efficacy of one program over another.

There are other conjectural treatments for restricted range of motion. Manual medicine, joint mobilization, and other movement mobilization techniques have all been proposed, but there have been few scientific studies.[78,95,144]

Treatment and Prescription Writing for an Individual with Paraplegia

It is the opinion of the authors that there are three goals for a treatment program for rotator cuff arthropathy: (1) full restoration of shoulder function, (2) partial restoration of shoulder function that is functionally relevant, and (3) pain relief. The MRI data from Escobedo et al. suggest that older persons with an SCI who have been injured for many years will frequently have severe, multiple tears.[6] In such cases, full restoration of the rotator cuff by surgical repair is unlikely, particularly if there are other discouraging prognostic factors. Partial restoration of shoulder function might be a realistic goal in some, but it is not clear that the functional result will be relevant to activities of daily living (ADLs), transfers, pressure releases, or overhead reaching. Most individuals with a rotator cuff tear, including massive tears, are able to perform ADLs, transfers, and pressure releases. Overhead reach might continue to be a problem, but even individuals with full-thickness tears will frequently have significant active total elevation. Bokor et al. found that the results of nonoperative management of full-thickness tears of the rotator cuff included average active total elevation of 149°.[25] Regardless, we encourage all individuals with an SCI to modify their environment and use adaptive aids to avoid repetitive overhead reaching. If someone develops shoulder pain, we vigorously stress the importance of avoiding impingement-prone positions such as forward flexion and abduction.

Acute shoulder pain in individuals with paraplegia. Evaluation and directed treatment of acute shoulder pain are different in individuals with paraplegia than in able-bodied persons. History, physical examination, and diagnostic tests are used to establish a working diagnosis and rule out diagnoses such as fracture, acromioclavicular separation, and traumatic rotator cuff tear. Still, it is important to maintain a high index of suspicion for neurologic causes, such as syringomyelia and cervical radiculopathy, and referred pain from the cervical spine. Treatment is prescribed as appropriate for the working diagnosis.

If the diagnosis is new-onset impingement, rotator cuff tendinitis, or rotator cuff tear, treatment should follow the general principles outlined below under "Chronic Shoulder Pain."

Although the directed treatment of acute shoulder pain is essentially the same as with the general population, the effects of shoulder pain—secondary disability and handicap—are not. Compared with the general population, several unique features are noted: (1) relative rest is often not possible, (2) "bad habits" and "damaging patterns of use" are frequently related to environment and accessibility issues, (3) pain might interfere with basic ADLs and mobility, (4) secondary problems, particularly skin breakdown, are frequent complications of shoulder pain, and (5) psychosocial problems and depression are common with the onset of secondary disabilities caused by shoulder pain.

Chronic shoulder pain in individuals with paraplegia: Impingement and rotator cuff arthropathy. The initial evaluation of chronic shoulder pain should include ruling out systemic disease, such as rheumatoid arthritis, or neurologic causes, such as syrinx and radiculopathy, and establishing a working diagnosis. It is often difficult to distinguish musculoskeletal diagnoses such as subacromial bursitis, impingement syndrome, acromioclavicular degenerative joint diseases, biceps tendinitis, rotator cuff tendinitis, and small rotator cuff tears. This is because one or several of these entities occur concomitantly in individuals with SCI and chronic shoulder pain. It is also important to establish the functional impairments, such as restricted range of motion, weakness, and instability, as well as a pathologic diagnosis because treatment is often directed at the functional impairment rather than the pathophysiologic process.

We recommend a conservative program of treatment for impingement and rotator cuff tears. For both shoulders, the goals of our program are to strengthen intact muscles, achieve muscular balance, optimize function, and avoid further injury. Overall goals also include pain management and the maintenance of functional skills while optimizing body mechanics. Many of these interventions aim at minimizing impingement and poor biomechanics when reaching overhead and using good position of the pectoral girdle when weightbearing and pushing the wheelchair. We have achieved these goals in many individuals with paraplegia and documented rotator cuff tears. As discussed above, there is little research to support one approach over another. Therefore, the following program was developed using biomechanics, the anatomy and physiology of joints, trial and error, and common sense.

The program includes the following four general principles:

1. Eliminate damaging patterns. A thorough functional evaluation is done to identify all aspects of daily living and work that involve biomechanically deleterious activities. Any position of overhead reaching (particularly weighted), abduction over 90°, and hyperabduction are modified. Wheelchair push mechanics and the manner of stowing the wheelchair into the car are optimized. Any habits that use damaging patterns are replaced with biomechanically sound techniques.

2. Optimize posture. This intervention is based on the theory that sitting posture is intimately related to shoulder function, particularly during reaching activities. The goal of optimizing posture is to eliminate kyphosis, a forward head, and rounded shoulders and achieve normal alignment of the shoulder, head, and spine. Wheelchair set-up is a critical intervention to accomplish this goal and often entails a positive angle of the seat plane with respect to the floor and lowering the backrest. Stretching shortened anterior shoulder muscles and strengthening available postural muscles are also frequently recommended.

3. Achieve a balanced shoulder. Many individuals who always use a wheelchair develop anterior hypertrophy of the shoulder musculature. Therefore, the goal of achieving a balanced shoulder usually involves stretching the anterior shoulder muscles and strengthening the lengthened, and weaker, posterior muscles. This includes strengthening external rotators and posterior scapular muscles.

4. Educate patients. A mainstay of the program involves patient education. Basic biomechanical principles are reviewed with an emphasis on avoiding reaching and impingement by modifying the environment, using biomechanically sound transfers, and the need for the stretching/strengthening component of the program. Health maintenance with a particular focus on weight loss and the cessation of smoking are also stressed.

Conclusion of Case

The patient was found to have posture that is quite common in individuals with paraplegia, including round shoulders with hypertrophied, short anterior muscles and lengthened, weak posterior muscles, and a head-forward position. The functional history revealed several detrimental activities, such as biomechnically poor transfers and reaching overhead throughout the day.

Prescription

- Goals: Control pain, balanced shoulder, full restoration of function.

- Control pain: ibuprofen, relative rest (2 days).

- Teach new activities and issue equipment to eliminate damaging patterns and bad habits (e.g., because the patient was transferring to the bottom of the bathtub, a tub bench was issued with transfer training to the tub bench).

- Optimize posture.

- Stretching program to lengthen anterior musculature.

- Strengthening program that targets posterior musculature.

- Shoulder protection and prevention program for the uninvolved shoulder.

Follow-up. The patient has been followed for 5 years and has had no further shoulder problems.

Conclusions

Given the high estimated prevalence of shoulder pain in individuals with paraplegia, there is a remarkably lack of research into the specific musculoskeletal pathologies, their natural history, and treatment of these shoulder problems. Research is essential because shoulder function is so directly related to functional independence for individuals with an SCI. Individuals with an SCI are now living into their eighth and ninth decades. Using the upper extremities for weightbearing for 50 years or more has created fascinating biomechanical challenges to limbs that are designed primarily for prehension and mobility. The anatomic changes that occur, the clinical relevance of those changes, and the appropriate interventions in the aging SCI population are largely unknown. Finally, conservative rehabilitation principles such as we have outlined should be used to optimize function of the involved shoulder and prevent injury to the uninvolved shoulder.

CHRONIC ELBOW PAIN: LATERAL EPICONDYLITIS

Case Study

Case history. A 44-year-old right-handed woman is referred for treatment of left elbow pain. She reports that the pain is located in the lateral elbow region and is worse when gripping and lifting objects. The pain has been present for about 3 months even though she has only recently sought medical evaluation. She reports some pain relief with two tablets of over-the-counter ibuprofen three times a day. She has no symptoms elsewhere in the left or the right upper extremity. She has not received any treatment to date. Her job involves the use of small power tools on an assembly line.

Physical examination. Point tenderness is noted just distal to the left, lateral epicondyle. Reported pain is increased with grasp and resisted wrist extension. Passive wrist flexion is found to be 70° on the right and 80° on the left. No weakness is noted in the right upper extremity.

Working diagnosis. Lateral epicondylitis, also known as tennis elbow.

Diagnostic evaluation. None.

Introduction and Epidemiology

Lateral epicondylitis is one of the most common musculoskeletal disorders seen by physicians. It bears a number of names, each of which implies a known cause or pathophysiology. Despite the high prevalence, its pathophysiology remains controversial, and the most common treatments have little literature to support their use.

Although the disorder has been associated with tennis, it also has a high prevalence in certain occupations and is common in the general population. The prevalance in tennis players has been estimated to be 14%, with 40% of all tennis players reporting a history of lateral epicondylitis.[53] Fewer than half of tennis players seek medical attention. A 14% prevalance also has been reported in gas- and waterworks employees.[116]

Etiology and Pathophysiology

The pathoanatomy of lateral epicondylitis remains controversial. Most theories invoke functional overload of the connective tissue structures originating from the lateral epicondyle as the inciting event. Intrinsic risk factors for the development of overuse injuries include increased age, prior injury, decreased flexibility, and decreased strength. Specific patterns of muscle activation have been noted in patients with lateral epicondylitis. Some investigators have proposed that inflammation plays an important role in the early development of the disorder.

Tendinosis.   The pathologic process in chronic cases of lateral epicondylitis is best described as tendinosis or tendinopathy, because there is no evidence of an acute inflammatory response in reported cases. Abnormalities are nearly universal in the tendinous origin of the extensor carpi radialis brevis, with many cases also involving the extensor digitorum. The histopathologic changes, involving disorganized collagen fibers, immature fibroblasts, and immature vascular elements, are described as an angiofibroblastic tendinosis.[97] In addition to these histologic changes, abnormalities can be visualized with MRI. The characteristic findings include increased signal and thickening at the common extensor origin on the lateral epicondyle.[59]

The underlying pathophysiology has been hypothesized to be due to ischemia of the involved structures or due to a direct mechanical effect from tensile stresses. These changes are thought to represent an incomplete healing response and failed adaptation to increased demands on the connective tissue structures.

Although an inflammatory response has not been demonstrated, the cases examined have primarily included persons with chronic symptoms who are undergoing surgical treatment. It remains possible that a significant inflammatory component exists early in the disorder, and thus there is a rationale for treatments directed at reducing inflammation.

Clinical Features and Differential Diagnosis

Lateral epicondylitis has a number of characteristic symptoms and signs. There is generally a subacute onset of symptoms, but a single period of excessive activity occasionally may result in an acute onset. Pain is noted in the lateral elbow region and is increased with forceful gripping. Local tenderness on palpation over the lateral epicondyle is characteristic for the disorder. In addition, resisted wrist or finger extension produces an increase in pain.

Literature Review: Treatments Directed toward Known Abnormalities

The literature on the treatment of lateral epicondylitis presents little to no evidence to support the use of most conventional treatments.[76] Many studies have similar methodologic flaws. A primary limitation of many studies is a lack of adequate control groups. Although the natural history of the disorder is unknown, few studies include an untreated control group, which is a significant problem for a disorder in which patients have symptoms lasting a few days to a few years. Because the chronicity of the disorder and the population from which the subjects are recruited vary so much between studies, it is impossible to compare treatment results between studies.

The characteristics of the treatments make it difficult in many cases to include an adequate placebo treatment, because patients will often be aware that they have received placebo treatment. Many patients will not consent to a study in which they may receive no treatment. Consequently, most studies have compared treatments. With a lack of an untreated control group, it is impossible to determine whether the treatments are equally beneficial or equally ineffective.

Treatment options for lateral epicondylitis can be considered as being directed at one or more of the proposed contributing factors or known pathophysiologic processes. They broadly can be considered as being prescribed to treat inflammation, abnormalities of connective tissue (tendinopathy), abnormalities of range of motion, or abnormalities of muscle activation or biomechanics.

Treatment directed toward inflammation. As noted above, there is no evidence for an inflammatory cell response in the area of tendinopathy. However, because these cases have almost exclusively involved chronic lateral epicondylitis undergoing surgery, inflammation may play a role earlier. Specific treatments directed toward the inflammatory component of the disorder include ice, NSAIDs, ultrasound, and local corticosteroid injection. No specific NSAID has been shown superior to another or, for that matter, to placebo. Ultrasound is covered in detail in the following section addressing treatment for tendinosis. Studies of corticosteroid injection have the same methodologic flaws described above and have failed to demonstrate long-term improvement over other treatment modalities.

Treatment directed at tendinopathy (ultrasound). Based on its ability to increase blood flow and tissue extensibility, ultrasound is frequently used to treat lateral epicondylitis. It is theorized that the biologic effects of ultrasound can promote remodeling of the areas of abnormal tendon, through either a direct effect on fibroblasts and the production of collagen fibers or an indirect effect through improved blood flow. In addition, increased extensibility of connective tissue structures has been demonstrated following ultrasound treatment; therefore, limitations in passive range of motion may be eliminated through stretching in conjunction with ultrasound.

A number of studies have examined whether ultrasound is effective in promoting resolution of the condition, and the results are contradictory. One study that demonstrated the beneficial effects of ultrasound included a group of 76 patients who had symptoms of lateral epicondylitis for at least 1 month.[9] Patients were randomly assigned to receive ultrasound or placebo ultrasound. A total of 63% of the ultrasound-treated group had a satisfactory outcome, defined as full functional recovery with no more than minor ache or tenderness, but only 29% of placebo-treated patients showed satisfactory outcome. Significantly greater improvement in grip strength was also measured in the ultrasound-treated group.

Most studies on treatment with ultrasound, however, have not demonstrated beneficial effects. Lundeberg et al.[82] studied 99 patients with lateral epicondylitis as the working diagnosis; satisfactory outcome occurred in 36% of patients treated with ultrasound, 30% of patients treated with placebo ultrasound, and 24% of patients treated with rest. The difference between ultrasound and placebo ultrasound was not statistically significant, but the difference between ultrasound and rest was significant. The authors concluded that the placebo effect in part explains the response to ultrasound. Based on the sample size, it is impossible to rule out a small beneficial effect from ultrasound separate from the placebo effect.

These two studies demonstrate dissimilar response rates to ultrasound treatment despite similar inclusion criteria, similar treatment, and similar outcome measures. Due to the limited information provided on the patient recruitment process, it is unclear whether the patients were truly similar with respect to chronicity and severity of symptoms. In addition, lack of blinding of the persons rating the patients' responses may have been a significant factor.

If ultrasound is to be used as treatment, it should be a portion of a comprehensive prescription and not the sole treatment. It is typically used at a frequency of 1.0 MHz, an intensity of 1–2 W/cm^2, and an application time of 10 minutes, and it is repeated twice per week for 4–6 weeks. If stretching is part of the therapy prescription, it should be performed immediately after ultrasound treatment.

Treatment directed at decreased wrist range of motion (stretching). Although stretching exercises for muscles acting at the wrist have been emphasized in the treatment of lateral epicondylitis, no well-controlled studies have been performed on the effects of conventional stretching or on pre- and posttreatment measurement of wrist range of motion. In fact, restricted wrist range of motion in conjunction with lateral epicondylitis has only recently been reported. Compared to the unaffected side, a decrease of 4–8° of wrist flexion is seen for both active and passive motion.[129] (Solveborn 1996). Less consistently, decreased wrist extension and forearm pronation and supination were noted for both active and passive motion. These decreases in range are likely a result of the primary pathologic process and are unlikely to be a primary contributor to the disorder.

Based on these range restrictions, an argument can be made to include a stretching program in the prescription with a goal of improving range of motion to match the unaffected side. A range of motion program includes active range of motion with passive stretch at the end range for wrist flexion and extension, forearm pronation and supination, and elbow flexion and extension. The exercises are performed three times daily with sets of 20 repetitions for each movement.[139] If ultrasound is being performed, the period immediately following a treatment should be used for stretching.

Treatment directed at abnormal biomechanics of wrist and elbow movement: counterforce braces and modification of technique. A number of factors have been identified that predispose individuals to the development of overuse injuries. Although factors such as age and history of previous injury cannot be modified, factors such as strength deficits and patterns of muscle activation have clearly been shown to differ in patients with overuse injuries and are amenable to treatment. In many cases it is impossible to determine whether these abnormalities are a primary factor contributing to the disorder or whether they are a secondary effect. Weakness and patterns of muscle activation are treated with strengthening, alteration of technique, or use of braces to modify muscular action.

In light of DeSmet's finding that individuals with lateral epicondylitis have decreased grip strength versus the unaffected side,[29] strengthening of wrist extensors has been proposed as treatment. The grip strength deficit is most pronounced when the elbow is held in extension. There are two problems with DeSmet's study. First, the strength deficit might have been a preexisting condition—a predisposing factor for the development of the disorder—rather than the primary pathologic process. It also does not show whether the weakness is on the basis of pain inhibition resulting in submaximal contraction or whether true muscular weakness has developed. Still, strengthening exercises might be efficacious by way of achieving a balanced joint, and they also may be helpful in stimulating a healing response within the area of tendon abnormality. Since the extensor carpi radialis brevis and extensor digitorum are most frequently involved, these muscles are invariably included in strengthening programs. Forearm pronators and supinators, elbow flexors and extensors, wrist flexors, and extrinsic finger muscles also should be included in the strengthening program, because all of these muscles cross the elbow. Strengthening of more proximal muscles should also be considered, because they form part of the kinetic chain for upper extremity movement, and deficits in strength of more proximal muscles may contribute to poor mechanics and result in compensatory movement in distal parts of the limb.

Most studies of patterns of muscle activation and biomechanics in lateral epicondylitis have examined variations in technique for tennis players, specifically for the single-handed backhand stroke. Variations in technique between expert and novice players have been examined, because there is a greater prevalence of lateral epicondylitis in novice players. At ball contact, novice players hold their wrists in a slight degree of wrist flexion, and this flexion increases after contact, indicating eccentric contraction of wrist extensors.[10] In contrast, expert players strike the ball with the wrist extended, and the wrist extensors contract concentrically with ball impact. Numerous studies in humans and animals have documented significantly greater muscle damage resulting from eccentric versus isometric or concentric contraction; therefore, this difference in technique constitutes a potential factor in the development of lateral epicondylitis in novice players. In a study comparing recreational tennis players with and without lateral epicondylitis, significantly higher electromyographic (EMG) activity in the wrist extensors has been demonstrated.[72] Consequently, changes in stroke technique and measures to limit the force of muscular contraction have been advocated.

The use of a strap around the proximal forearm is considered by many to be effective treatment for lateral epicondylitis. The straps have been called *counterforce braces, forearm support bands,* and *tennis elbow bands.* They are made of relatively inelastic materials and can be adjusted by the patient to achieve the desired tension and compression. Burton[19] found that more than 80% of patients with lateral epicondylitis showed increased pain-free grip strength with use of a strap.

The most widely accepted explanation for pain relief is that the strap prevents normal expansion of the extensor muscles on active contraction. Decreased muscle expansion would result in less tension generation by the muscle and thus limit the degree of tissue overload. Other theories propose either a redistribution of tensile forces away from the lateral epicondyle or a reflex effect from sensory stimulation of the skin.

There is conflicting evidence on the ability of counterforce braces to limit muscular contraction. In a study of persons without symptoms of lateral epicondylitis, the duration of EMG activity in wrist extensor muscles was decreased during tennis backhand strokes by application of a brace.[52] In addition, wrist and elbow angular acceleration during the backhand swing was decreased with brace use. However, maximal isokinetic wrist extensor torque is on average increased by 11% with strap use in patients with lateral epicondylitis.[135] This effect was noted at an isokinetic angular velocity of 120° per second but not at 30° per second.

Although the evidence does not clearly demonstrate a reduction in wrist extensor torque or grip strength with brace use, the treatment has become accepted and patients commonly report symptomatic improvement with use. Thus, it is likely that the benefits are derived from an effect other than restriction of muscular expansion. Controversy remains over the optimal wearing schedule. The brace is usually worn during symptomatic activities in cases of moderate severity and is worn continuously during waking hours in more severe cases.

In addition to counterforce braces, a number of technique changes have been recommended for tennis players with lateral epicondylitis. The wrist should be in a position of extension on backhand strokes at the time of ball contact. Attaining this wrist position will require the player to achieve proper positioning of the entire body before ball impact. A change to a two-handed technique for backhand shots will decrease the stress on structures involved in lateral epicondylitis. In addition to modification of muscular activity, technique and equipment changes may decrease vibration, which is thought to be an additional factor contributing to lateral epicondylitis. Vibration is minimized with a central ball impact rather than peripheral impact, and less grip strength is required to prevent the racquet from rotating when the impact is on the long axis of the racquet. Changing racquet materials also may reduce the vibration transmitted following ball impact.

Other treatments. Manipulation and friction massage has been advocated as an effective treatment[27] and was compared with corticosteroid injection in a recent study.[144] Short-term pain relief was significantly better in the group treated with corticosteroid injection, but the injected group demonstrated a higher recurrence rate at 1 year of follow-up. Because the study used unblinded patient assessment and no placebo injection was used in the group treated with manipulation, the results are difficult to generalize.

Conclusion of Case

At the end of your initial visit, you write the following prescription:

Prescription

- Goals: Control pain and inflammation, begin to restore mobility.

- Continue with NSAIDs.

- Counterforce brace.

- Ice massage to painful areas four or five times daily for 3 days, then as needed.

- Referral to therapist for education/home exercise program as follows: (1) stretching program to wrist extensors and (2) strengthening program to forearm (pronators, supinators), wrist (flexors, extensors), finger extensors, and grip.

It was recommended that the patient continue to take the NSAID because it had been providing some pain relief, presumably through its analgesic properties rather than antiinflammatory properties. Corticosteroid injection was not considered.

The patient was referred to a physical therapist for instruction in a stretching program, with emphasis on stretching of wrist extensors. A home program for upper extremity strengthening was prescribed that included strengthening of wrist extensors and flexors, finger extensors, grip, and forearm rotation. She was also given a counterforce brace and advised to wear it while at work and during other activities that exacerbated her pain. She noted gradual improvement in her symptoms over 2 months.

CHRONIC WRIST PAIN IN INDIVIDUALS WITH PARAPLEGIA: OVERUSE INJURIES OF THE WRIST

Case Study

Case history.   Mr. Z is a 46-year-old right-handed man who works as a medical clerk and has had a history of T5 paraplegia for 25 years. He complains of worsening left wrist pain over the past 6 months. He is unable to identify a specific event or date of onset; rather, he feels that the onset was insidious. He recalls having similar symptoms on several occasions in the past but states that the pain has been gradually worsening with each episode. Pain is worse when pushing his manual wheelchair and more marked during transfers to and from his wheelchair. Pain is localized to a region on the dorsum of the wrist, on the ulnar aspect of the extensor pollicis longus tendon. The patient is concerned that he can no longer function at his job, because wrist pain interferes with his ability to transfer into his automobile. In addition, he is an avid outdoorsman and has not been able to propel over rough surfaces as required on camping and fishing trips.

Physical examination.   No significant swelling, erythema, or asymmetry. There is moderately severe tenderness to palpation at the junction of the distal radius and proximal carpal bones. No tenderness is present at the base of the snuffbox or on palpation of any of the extensor tendons. Finkelstein's maneuver, Tinel's sign, and Phalen's maneuver are negative. Wrist dorsiflexion was moderately limited by pain to approximately 45°. Wrist flexion was within normal limits with slight pain at end range. Passive radial deviation (abduction) was also limited by pain 10° (normal is 20°). Ulnar deviation was within normal limits at 35°. The rest of the examination of both upper extremities and neurologic examination was normal.

Working diagnosis.   Osteoarthritis of the wrist.

Diagnostic evaluation.   Initial radiographs and bone scan did not reveal a stress fracture. A small hypertrophic ridge at the dorsal scaphoid rim is seen on the lateral view, performed in slight flexion.[31]

Introduction and Epidemiology

Repetitive motion disorders of the wrist can be frustrating for the patient and clinician due to the chronicity of the symptoms and the fact that it is difficult to establish a specific diagnosis.[115] Thus, designing a treatment program is more difficult.

This frustration is compounded further in an individual who is in a manual wheelchair and uses the upper extremities for all mobility. Rest, often prescribed for repetitive motion disorders, is difficult or impossible for manual wheelchair users. Thus, these persons are often faced with the choice of inactivity or remaining active but dealing with pain.

This section presents a therapeutic approach for long-term management of articular wrist pain. It is not intended to be a comprehensive overview of the relative effectiveness of various modalities for soft tissue problems at the wrist. Special emphasis is placed on the impact and complexity of wheelchair use and weightbearing on treatment approaches.

The high prevalence of carpal tunnel syndrome in SCI, reported as 49–73%, is well described,[44,117,123] as is the increased incidence of shoulder impingement and rotator cuff abnormalities.[35,44,123,148] The wrist joint has received less attention as the site of overuse or repetitive trauma.

Reporting on the incidence of all causes of wrist and shoulder pain, Subbarao et al. found that 64% of respondents had wrist pain and that upper extremity changes often led to the requirement for wheelchair modification.[137] However, they did not investigate the incidence of wrist pain specifically related to joint pathology, and it is not reported in other literature. They suggested that future research should focus on new methods of wheelchair propulsion and transfer techniques that lessen stress and cumulative trauma on the wrist and shoulders.

Etiology and Pathophysiology

Appreciation of Wolff's law is important in the pathogenesis and treatment of overuse injuries of the wrist. As discussed above, bone and the nonosseous connective tissues normally respond to mechanical loads in an adaptive manner. Longitudinal growth in bones, increased bone mass, increased density and diameter of collagen fibers in tendon and ligament, and increased amount and type of proteoglycans in dense connective tissues have all been demonstrated as a normal response to applied mechanical forces. Conversely, immobilization has been found to negatively affect bone, tendon, ligament, and cartilage both structurally and biomechanically.[20,86,113] The application of these principles to repetitive motion disorders is an active area of investigation.

Wrist injury may result from a single high-force trauma or from repetitive stresses involving smaller forces.[115] By definition, repetitive motion injuries pertain to the latter and occur at the wrist following repetitive microtrauma, which eventually overwhelms the normal adaptive capabilities of the loadbearing tissues.[108]

Pathogenesis of wrist joint overuse injury in manual wheelchair users. During axial loading of the wrist joint, about 80% of the load is borne through the radius and lateral carpal bones—primarily the scaphoid—with the remainder through the ulna/triangular fibrocartilage/medial carpal complex. If the triangular fibrocartilage is excised, the percentage borne through the radius increases to 94%.[61]

It has been proposed that wrist pain in some manual wheelchair users may be analogous to syndromes that occur in competitive gymnasts. One such injury, termed *gymnast's wrist* or *dorsal radiocarpal impingement syndrome,* involves the dorsal aspect of the radiocarpal joint.[104] A similar injury is scaphoid impaction syndrome.[31,61]

In gymnasts, a number of other sites of pathology have been identified. Mandelbaum et al.[86] described the articular wrist pain syndrome occurring in male and female collegiate gymnasts, most frequently associated with the pommel horse in male gymnasts and the beam and vault in female gymnasts. Increased forces of compression, rotation, and distraction in the distal aspects of the upper extremity were cited as potential causes of this syndrome. In Mandelbaum's study, subjects with and without wrist pain (pain during compression and impaction) were evaluated by MRI, cine MRI, and arthroscopy. In subjects with pain, ligamentous tears, tears in the triangular fibrocartilate complex, and secondary chondromalacia in the ulnalunate, ulnatriquetrum complex and radioscaphoid articulations were seen. Subjects with pain also had significantly increased positive ulnar variance (e.g., the head of ulna is distal to the radius) relative to controls.

A literature review by Dobyns and Gabel[31] described several acute and chronic soft tissue and osseous injuries in gymnasts, including scaphoid and ulnar impaction syndromes, carpal chondromalacia, and carpal instability. Distal radius physeal stress reactions from compressive forces were also noted. In all injuries, the primary load was compressive, and the most frequent position for application of that load was dorsiflexion.

Similar to gymnasts, the wrist in manual wheelchair users is also subjected to high mechanical stresses. A common posture during transfers, for example, is with the wrist at the end range of extension, often combined with compressive loading. The wrist is also in a similar position during wheelchair propulsion and crutch use, but the wrist is not in as extreme a position of extension.[142] Wrist pathologies also have been identified in individuals who use manual wheelchairs. Static carpal instability has been demonstrated in symptomatic individuals with long-standing paraplegia who have not had an antecedent acute injury. The prevalence appears to be associated with the duration of upper extremity weightbearing, demonstrating a relationship between carpal instability and repetitive loading of the distal upper extremity.[123] A study by Blankstein demonstrated radiographic wrist pathology in 55% of individuals with chronic SCI of 5 years or longer.[11] The most common locations were at the trapeziometacarpal and radioscaphoid joints. Range of motion in flexion-extension was significantly reduced compared to controls.

Clinical Features and Presentation

A history of acute trauma should be sought. If none is found, specific positions and activities causing pain should be carefully noted. The patient's lifestyle and any change in activity level are important concerns, as is the impact of the patient's pain with ADLs and vocational and avocational pursuits. It is also important to try to characterize the mechanical loads and technique during weightbearing activities. How often does a person do transfers? What distances are pushed each day? What are the vocational activities and demands? What is the posture of the upper extremity during transfers and wheelchair pushing? Does the person perform injurious activities and habits (e.g., biomechanically poor transfers from the bottom of the tub or into a vehicle) that can be modified or eliminated?

Although changes are often not visible, inspection for anatomic irregularities or tissue swelling is performed. Palpation for sites of tenderness is particularly important and also should be performed during joint motion and mobility assessment to detect articular irregularities and crepitus. Common sites of pathology that might be tender include the radioscaphoid joint and the scaphoid palpated at the floor of the carpal tunnel. Range of motion in all planes of movement should be assessed because restrictive range is an important finding. Tests for instability should be performed when indicated and soft tissue restrictions among wrist articulations noted. Strength and range of motion of the entire upper extremity should be assessed, because compensation for more proximal deficits might be the source of the wrist problem. Neurologic examination of the involved and contralateral extremity should be performed to rule out central or peripheral nerve pathology. Finally, the patient should be assessed during functional activities to evaluate technique, dynamic rhythm, and smoothness of movement.

Because of its tenuous blood supply and the high incidence of nonunion, it is imperative to rule out a fracture of the scaphoid. Plain radiographs should not be relied upon if a stress fracture is suspected. Bone scan may be indicated if there is clinical suspicion or if symptoms persist beyond 2 weeks of initiation of appropriate rehabilitation interventions.[113] Arthrography remains the gold standard for evaluation of the radioscaphoid and lunate joint but may have less value in chronic lesions. MRI is a rapidly improving, noninvasive, and sensitive means for detecting both ligamentous and cartilaginous injuries.[24]

Differential Diagnosis and Classification

The differential diagnosis of chronic wrist pain includes tendon problems, including deQuervain's disease or tenosynovitis of other dorsal compartments,[104] and ligamentous and capsular pathologies, stress fractures, the arthritides, compartment syndromes, ganglions at the level of the wrist, nerve entrapments about the wrist, nonspecific pain syndromes, and referred pain.

A common example of repetitive motion injury of a tendon is deQuervain's disease.[61] The literature is replete with epidemiologic studies on tenosynovitis and peritendinitis of the wrist-forearm region in people whose occupation requires manually strenuous tasks with high repetitiveness and the use of high forces.[83,127] Stress fractures are more common in the lower extremity but also might occur in the upper extremity.[108] Although sometimes classified separately from other overuse injuries, articular injuries resulting from weightbearing are also common, as previously discussed in gymnasts and wheelchair users.[61] Others have included bony injuries from repetitive trauma, such as the impaction syndromes and physeal injuries.[108]

Literature Review: Rehabilitation of Wrist Joint Overuse Injuries

The best treatment for wrist injuries in individuals who use a wheelchair is prevention. As noted above, according to Wolff's law, tissues respond in a positive and adaptive way to increased mechanical forces. The amount of stress tolerated before adaptive mechanisms are overwhelmed by tissue injury is related to several factors. These relate to work performed (e.g., frequency, magnitude, and types of forces involved), the environment (e.g., how high are objects in the house and at work, are overheight transfers into a vehicle required), and individual factors such as the age, health, physical characteristics, and fitness of the person. Because sudden increases in activity are often associated with injury, the safest approach is to gradually increase activity to allow tissues to accommodate to increases in stress.[47,111] This can be said equally of manual wheelchair users and athletes.

Treatment directed at decreasing mechanical forces. Articular wrist pain in manual wheelchair users may be akin to that in athletes in that the use of "relative rest" as a treatment modality may significantly hinder the patient's goals and life. In elite athletes, reduction in training time can impair competitiveness. In manual wheelchair users, inability to use the upper extremities normally can mean loss of ability to carry out ADLs.

The use of a sliding board, while not reducing the total force required to perform transfers, may allow a single large force transfer to be broken down into several events with smaller force. Training of an individual for careful technique and hand placement are imperative in this setting.

Treatment directed at inflammation. NSAIDs, on a scheduled basis for up to 2 weeks and then as needed, are helpful to control pain and decrease articular inflammation. Long-term use is not advisable, especially in patients with SCI, due to the increased risk of renal injury.[77] The need for prolonged NSAID use should suggest incorrect diagnosis or treatment, such as failure to correct biomechanical problems such as flexibility or strength imbalance.

Icing of the wrist is an essential component of treatment. Icing provides analgesia as well as reduction in inflammation. Icing generally should be performed several times daily for 10–20 minutes per session in the acute period. A side effect of icing can be joint stiffness until temperature returns to baseline.

If edema is present, compression is added to the prescription and is more effective than icing alone.[113] Overuse injuries typically do not present with significant edema. With marked edema, suspicion should be raised for an occult stress fracture or soft tissue strain.

Various heating modalities can be effective in elevating superficial tissue temperatures. Heat aids mobilization, provides analgesia, and increases local circulation. Paraffin is especially attractive because skin temperatures can be elevated to 125–130°F without skin burns.[112] In addition, patients with chronic pain can perform this modality at home with the use of paraffin, mineral oil, a double boiler, and a thermometer.

Ultrasound has the advantage of heating deeper structures. With all modalities, clinicians should be aware of contraindications, and care should be taken to avoid use on anesthetic areas to decrease the risk of burns.

Treatment directed at hypermobility. For periods of inactivity, especially at night, splinting should be prescribed to allow joint rest and prevent wrist hyperextension or flexion during sleep. A static wrist-hand orthosis or dorsiflexion splint is appropriate for this purpose.[68] The splints are usually fabricated in approximately 15–20° of dorsiflexion. However, if dorsal wrist impingement is occurring, the position of comfort may be more toward neutral. A static volar wrist orthosis may not limit dorsiflexion adequately if a sturdy dorsal strap is not present.

Wrist taping can be useful to limit wrist hyperextension and prevent dorsal radiocarpal or dorsal carpal impingement but still allow adequate functional range of motion for daily activities. Taping probably also provides joint proprioceptive feedback, but it is generally not believed to significantly affect wrist stability. Alternatively, an elastic wrist cuff ("gym cuff") or a specialized adhesive bandage may be used for the same purpose.[104] Wrist cock-up splints can be used for immobilization but are not functional for wheelchair propulsion.

Treatment directed at increasing range of motion. Heating and stretching soft tissues allows the collagen of ligaments to stress-relax and creep, improving its viscoelastic properties.[113] Reports vary on the effect of stretching on muscle. Some have reported that it can increase muscle length,[47] and others suggest that the absolute length of muscles does not change but the length-tension curve is shifted such that the exponential portion of the curve is achieved at higher tensions. The reasons for stretching muscles and soft tissues on the wrist joint are probably twofold: (1) to maintain maximal joint range of motion to prevent ensuing contracture, and (2) that improving the viscoelastic properties of the tissues lessens stress on the joint during activity.

Both sides of the joint should be stretched to maintain balance. Active assisted range of motion allows more vigorous stretching than active range of motion alone. Stretching is optimally performed on warm tissues, and stretch should be prolonged for 15–30 seconds.

Treatment directed at muscle imbalance. Patients should be evaluated for muscle imbalance across the wrist. Strengthening of wrist (and probably finger) flexors makes sense to improve the joint's ability to limit hyperextension via eccentric contraction of wrist flexors. The goal is improved dynamic support during activities in which wrist hyperextension may occur. To maintain balance of forces across the joint, wrist extensor strength should be maintained.

Fingertip push-ups are another activity that has been suggested for wrist rehabilitation and may serve to improve dynamic wrist control. These exercises are possible for manual wheelchair users if excessive lower extremity contractures are not present. Additional benefits might include improved dynamic shoulder strength and stretching of the anterior aspect of the hip.

Arm ergometry can improve upper extremity endurance and enhance overall fitness while avoiding high-impact forces encountered during wheelchair propulsion.

Handcycles are an expensive but entertaining alternative form of exercise that can provide similar benefits.

Other treatments. The effects of wrist mobilization are not well known. The goal of mobilization is to restore normal joint play by stretching tissues that cross joints and thereby improve the normal joint gliding movements that occur during use.

Assessment for and correction of errors in technique should begin early to alleviate factors that may be the cause of the primary pathologic process, interfere with recovery, and hinder the rehabilitation process. Activity modification aimed at correcting errors in technique may be the most critical component of the rehabilitation process in terms of ensuring long-term improvement in functional status. Eliminating injurious activities and correcting improper technique will sometimes eliminate all symptoms, but it is usually not so simple. Referral should be to skilled occupational and physical therapists who are familiar with proper wheelchair propulsion and set-up, posture, and transfer techniques and who have the training and ability to evaluate the patient during functional activities to detect errors.

Prescription Writing
Prescription—Initial Visit (Initial Phase)

- Goals: Control pain/inflammation, begin to restore mobility.

- Relative rest (no vigorous or uphill wheelchair propulsion) for 3–5 days.

- Sliding board or assistance for transfers.

- Ibuprofen: three times daily with food or antacid for 10 days.

- Ice massage to painful areas four to five times daily for 3 days, then as needed.

- Resting wrist-hand orthosis at night, elastic wrist bandage or taping during the day.

Prescription—Second Visit (Subacute Stage)

- Goals: Restore mobility, begin strength training, correct errors in technique.

- Passive range of motion: wrist and finger flexion/extension, pronation/supination.

- Begin wrist flexion isometric exercises, then follow with isotonic exercises.

- Begin functional activities assessment with emphasis on wrist, elbow, and trunk position during transfers and wheelchair propulsion.

- May engage in moderate wheeling.

- Dynamic stabilization with slow push-ups.

- Arm ergometry, 30 minutes daily.

- Wean use of night splints.

- Continue daytime elastic brace for more vigorous or prolonged activity.

Conclusion of Case

Serial functional activities assessments confirm that Mr. Z tends to allow excessive dorsiflexion during transfers. His propulsion technique was noted to be rather uncontrolled, resulting in rapid and excessive dorsiflexion combined with radial deviation.

The physical therapist found that Mr. Z's wheelchair sitting posture was contributing to his wrist pain. He tended to sit in a slouched, round-shouldered, head-forward position, with his scapulae abducted, a forward-facing glenoid, and relative internal rotation of the upper extremities. This results in compensatory movements in the distal extremity that consist of excessive dorsiflexion and radial deviation at the wrist during the "cocking phase" of wheelchair locomotion. The therapist changed the patient's seating and gave him a home program that included strengthening of scapular retractors and other posterior shoulder musculature while stretching the anterior shoulder musculature.

The final phase of the patient's rehabilitation involves maintenance of gains in strength, range of motion, endurance, and improved technique for functional tasks. The involvement of an ergonomics specialist should be considered in problematic cases. The patient should leave therapy thoroughly educated in the biomechanical and ergonomic principles of pain-associated activities.

Wrist pain in the weightbearing upper extremity of the manual wheelchair user presents a difficult diagnostic and therapeutic challenge. Accurate diagnosis aids in prescription of appropriate therapeutic interventions. A comprehensive approach to rehabilitation takes into account the patient's age, overall medical status, prior activity level, lifestyle, and vocational and avocational goals.

The incidence and exact nature of articular wrist pain syndromes in persons who use manual wheelchairs has not been fully appreciated. Further studies would be helpful to better characterize exact sites of pathology, provide radiographic correlates, and reveal pathoanatomic findings. Studies evaluating forces involved in manual wheelchair propulsion have been carried out.[117] Wheelchair propulsion and transfers are felt to be associated factors in the development of wrist pain.[137] These and other types of studies will be helpful in determining what characteristics of these activities lead to overuse injuries in this population.

CHRONIC KNEE PAIN IN A PROFESSIONAL BASKETBALL PLAYER

Case Study

Case history. A 30-year-old right-handed professional basketball player complains of bilateral anterior knee pain that started 3 weeks ago. When he is not playing he feels a diffuse soreness just below his kneecaps. The pain is most severe when he squats or lands from a jump. The center on the basketball team was injured, and the patient was switched to the center position from forward last month. The patient thinks he has been jumping more often and higher than ever in the past. The patient also reports that he is adjusting to home life with his new wife and has been away from the "training table" and may have gained some weight. The team was sold last year and now is run by a new coaching and trainer staff. They practice at a new gym that has a linoleum surface over concrete.

Physical examination. A tired-appearing muscular man sitting with knees extended as the clinician takes the history. There is no gross evidence of atrophy or lower extremity asymmetry. On close inspection of the left vastus medialis obliquus, there may be less muscle mass than on the right. There are two prominent firm contender protrusions at the tibial tuberosities, left larger than right. There is no tenderness or redness there. There is no effusion that can be palpated in the suprapatellar or quadriceps bursa bilaterally. There is no evidence of static or dynamic patellar misalignment. Patellar movement reveals no crepitus or apprehension. Measurement of the leg lengths from the anterior superior iliac spine to the crest of the medial malleolus revealed that the right limb was 3.5 cm shorter than the left. The Q angle was 12 on the right and 14 on the left (normal < 10). On palpation of the patellar tendon there is tenderness and some bumpy irregularity at its origin from the inferior patellar pole. There is no abnormality in femorotibial alignment. There is no knee instability in anterior or posterior stress or with lateral and medial bending. Review of gait showed no abnormality. A deep kneebend increased pain at the inferior patellar poles bilaterally.

Working diagnosis. Patellar tendinitis.

Diagnostic evaluation. Plain radiographs of the knees are normal.

Introduction, Epidemiology, and Pathophysiology

Patellar tendinitis, or "jumper's knee," is the second most common injury in basketball and accounts for the most time loss in the game.[75] A high incidence of jumper's knee is also noted in sports such as the high jump, long jump, and volleyball.[37] The maximal amount of mechanical strain is put on the tendon during the deceleration phase of the landing with knees flexed. During this time the quadriceps femoris muscle is overcoming the force of gravity by eccentrically contracting.[143] The hardness of the training surface and the amount of strain placed on the patellar tendon are risk factors for the condition. Knee misalignment also can contribute to risk for patellar tendinitis.[8,38] Functional imbalance of the lower extremity musculature can contribute to overstrain of the knee extensor system. Weak iliopsoas, gluteus maximus, and rectus abdominis muscles along with tight hamstrings have been demonstrated to contribute to extensor mechanism overuse in cinematographic analyses of basketball jumps.[130] There is some evidence that the amount and number of strain cycles across the patellar tendon during a given period can contribute to the risk of developing the clinical syndrome. Volleyball players that train four or more times per week are more likely to develop symptoms that suggest overstrain of the patellar tendon.[37,38] There is some suggestion of the ability to adapt to the repetitive strain if the proper dose of tension is applied through the patellar tendon. There is a higher risk for occurrence upon abrupt return to activity following breaks in the training process.[38]

Jumper's knee was first described by Blazina et al. as tendinitis of the patellar tendon or quadriceps tendon at the inferior or superior pole of the patella.[12] The definition has since been expanded to include pathologic changes of the bone tendon junction between the patellar tendon and the tibial tuberosity. The cause is repeated sudden high tensile force across the tendon that is transmitted to sites of origin or insertion. This occurs with forceful eccentric contraction of the quadriceps as the patient lands from a jump. Repetitive microtrauma results in tendinopathies of the quadriceps and patellar tendons. The most common location is proximal patellar tendinitis, or Sinding-Larsen-Johansson disease (65%), frequently occurring at the origin from the inferior patellar pole in the 20- to 40-year-old age group. Quadriceps tendinitis is located at the proximal patellar pole at the insertion of the quadriceps tendon and accounts for 25% of cases, usually in patients older than 40. The third presentation is Osgood-Schlatter disease, which occurs in children or adolescents due to patellar tendon microtrauma-induced inflammation at the aphophysis where it inserts with the tibial tuberosity. This condition typically presents in males in only one knee, with high predilection for the left knee. This sidedness has been attributed to left-foot dominance, which is common in right-handed individuals.[2]

The many anatomic, physiologic, and kinesiologic factors that might contribute to patellar tendinitis include bony factors, such as excessive torsional deformity of the femur or tibia, lateral position of the patella, and pes planus, and soft tissue abnormalities, such as an increased Q angle, atrophy of vastus medialis oblique muscle, and tight lateral retinaculum.

Clinical Features and Presentation

The situation of a basketball player experienced in the forward position rapidly switching to compete with tall centers from other teams would be expected to contribute to an increase in compensatory jumping. Other hints come from changes in his social roles, the immediate environment (shoes), and the intermediate environment (basketball court floor). The increased body weight from recent diet change adds to eccentric loading of the patellar tendon in landing from jumps.

Differential Diagnosis

A systematic review of the history, physical examination, and diagnostic tests leads to a working and differential diagnosis. A childhood history of knee pain could fit with his anthropomorphic features and stresses at the proximal patellar tendon (Sinding-Larsen-Johansson disease) or tibial insertion (Osgood-Schlatter disease). Other possible causes of anterior knee pain include Hoffa's disease, bursitis, plica inflammation, tumor, and osteomyelitis.

Literature Review

Patients often present to medical care when symptoms are most severe, at acute exacerbations of conditions maintained by overuse. Relief of the pain from injury or inflammation at the site of pathology is addressed first. The knee can be cooled by applying a bag of crushed ice to the knee under an elastic wrap to allow some movement during treatment. Nonsteroidal and antiinflammatory agents should be advanced to reach antiinflammatory doses as tolerated. Depending on the severity, immobilization can be done with full knee extension and nonweightbearing with crutch ambulation.[90] The time of immobilization should be limited to a few days because the tensile strength and elastic modulus of the unloaded patellar tendons in animal models occur as soon as 1 week after injury.[100]

In the subacute phase of treatment, inflammation and pain are reduced. Emphasis shifts to minimization of secondary impairments, avoidance of disuse atrophy, and prevention of reconditioning. Low-resistance high-repetition knee extension exercise provides a stimulus to promote collagen remodeling and strengthening of bony attachments. Cyriax[27] has promoted friction massage with firm digital pressure over the tendon with movement back and forth in a direction perpendicular to the direction of desired collagen deposition. Flexibility is achieved with open chain active range of motion and gentle sustained stretch in end range of the hamstrings, gastrocsoleus, quadriceps, and tibialis posterior.

As the physiologic processes producing patellar tendon strain are undermined and compensation for secondary impairments has begun, task-specific activity is emphasized to refine performance and develop techniques that minimize risk for training reinjury. Limited jumping is resumed up short steps to emphasize the leap and reduce the eccentric forces of landing. Plyometric techniques are used to focus the patient's attention on eccentric hip extension and gastrocsoleus contraction in landing from high jumps. Strengthening can resume at tensions less than the threshold for tendon damage. In eccentric contraction, in which the muscle is stretched during contraction, the individual sarcomere cross bridges develop greater resistance and therefore greater force than in concentric contraction performed at comparable velocity.[146] Kinetic energy is dissipated at the landing through joints above and below the knee to reduce instantaneous forces across the patellar tendon. The balance of eccentric muscle contraction in landing can be further trained using a Pogo stick, which has been shown to strengthen the quadriceps more effectively than isometric methods.[25] A prescribed number of bounces can provide a gradual dosed resumption of dynamic stress along the patellar tendon. Titration of instantaneous forces and repetitions can potentially promote adaptation of the tissues. Forces below the threshold for injury stimulate collagen formation and deposition along force lines. Continued strength training with the goal of stronger ballistic concentric contractions in jumps is expected to achieve more competitive sports performance.[109]

Rehabilitation Program and Prescription Writing

The components of the rehabilitation program must be orchestrated to meet the critical patient needs at each phase of intervention. Immediately after the injury or at the time of severe exacerbation, it is important to prescribe a program that interrupts the injury process and reduces inflammation.

Prescription—Initial Visit (Initial Phase)

- Diagnosis: patellar tendinitis, left worse than right.

- Goals: Control pain/inflammation.

- Train patient in four-point gait.

- Apply crushed ice to both knees for 30 minutes five times a day.

- Give antiinflammatory medication in antiinflammatory doses.

- Immobilize with patellar Air cast or McConnell infrapatellar taping.

- Avoid stairs, hills, and forceful eccentric quadriceps contraction.

Prescription—Second Visit (Subacute Stage)

- Regain and retain flexibility.

- Active unrestricted range of motion.

- Passive range of motion.

- Stretch hamstrings, quadriceps, gastrocsoleus, toe flexors, and hip flexors.

- Unloaded exercise (open kinetic chain):
  Open chain table exercises.
  Quadriceps sets, straight leg raises without ankle leading.

- Strengthen compensatory muscle groups.

- Strengthen gastrocsoleus with repeated standing plantar flexion then to loaded one-leg standing wall slides, balance board, leg presses.

Conclusion of Case

The last stage of the rehabilitation program will involve a strengthening program that develops maximal eccentric and concentric strength of the erector spinae muscles, hip extensors, and gastrocsoleus. Plyometric exercises are then applied to prepare for competitive games. If problems continue, recommendations regarding team roles that are consistent with anthropomorphics and abilities will be pursued.

REFERENCES

1. Abramson DI, Burnett C, Bell Y, et al: Changes in blood flow, oxygen uptake, and tissue temperatures produced by therapeutic physical agents. I. Effect of ultrasound. Am J Phys Med 39:51–62, 1960.
2. Antich T, Lumbardo S. Clinical presentation of Osgood-Schlatter disease in the adolescent population. J Orthop Sports Ther 7:1–10, 1985.
3. Aronen JG: Shoulder rehabilitation. Clin Sports Med 4:477–493, 1985.
4. Aronen JG, Regan K: Decreasing the incidence of recurrence of first-time anterior shoulder dislocations with rehabilitation. Am J Sports Med 12:283–291, 1984.
5. Barber DB, Gall NG: Osteonecrosis: An overuse injury of the shoulder in paraplegia: Case report. Paraplegia 29:423–426, 1991.
6. Basmajian JV: Muscles Alive: Their Functions Revealed by Electromyography. Baltimore, Williams & Wilkins, 1967, pp 196–200.
7. Bayley JC, Cochran TP, Sledge CB: The weight-bearing shoulder: The impingement syndrome in paraplegics. J Bone Joint Surg 69A:676–678, 1987.

8. Beckman M, Craig R, Lehman RC: Rehabilitation of patellofemoral dysfunction in the athlete. Clin Sports Med 8:841–861, 1989.
9. Binder A, Hodge G, Greenwood AM, et al: Is therapeutic ultrasound effective in treating soft tissue lesions? BMJ 290:512–514, 1985.
10. Blackwell JR, Cole KJ: Wrist kinematics differ in expert and novice tennis players performing the backhand stroke: Implications for tennis elbow. J Biomech 27:509–516, 1994.
11. Blankstein A, Shmueli R, Weingarten I, et al: Hand problems due to prolonged use of crutches and wheelchairs. Orthop Rev 14:29–34, 1985.
12. Blazina M, Kerlan R, Jobe FW, et al: Jumper's knee. Orthop Clin North Am 4:655–678, 1973.
13. Bodne D, Quinn SF, Murray WT, et al: Magnetic resonance images of chronic patellar tendinitis. Skeletal Radiol 17:24–28, 1988.
14. Boker DJ, Hawkins RJ, Huckell GH, et al: Results of nonoperative management of full-thickness tears of the rotator cuff. Clin Orthop 294:101–110, 1993.
15. Brown LP, Niehues SL, Hurrah A, et al: Upper extremity range of motion and isokinetic strength of the internal and external shoulder rotators in major league baseball players. Am J Sports Med 16:577–585, 1988.
16. Brunet, ME, Haaddad RJ, Porsche EB: Rotator cuff impingement in sports. Phys Sports Med 10:86–94, 1982.
17. Burkhardt SS: Arthroscopic treatment of massive rotator cuff tears: Clinical results and biomechanical rationale. Clin Orthop 267:45–56, 1991.
18. Burnham RS, May L, Nelson E, et al: Shoulder pain in wheelchair athletes: The role of muscle imbalance. Am J Sports Med 21:238–242, 1993.
19. Burton AK: Grip strength and forearm straps in tennis elbow. Br J Sports Med 19:37–38, 1985.
20. Buschbacher RM: Deconditioning, conditioning, and the benefits of exercise. In Braddom RJ (ed): Physical Medicine and Rehabilitation. Philadelphia, WB Saunders, 1996, pp 687–710.
21. Chan AK, Sigelmann RA, Guy AW: Calculations of therapeutic heat generated by ultrasound in fat-muscle-bone layers. Biomed Eng 21:280–284, 1973.
22. Chard MD, Cawston TE, Riley GP, et al: Rotator cuff deneration and lateral epicondylitis: A comparative histological study. Ann Rheum Dis 53:30–34, 1994.
23. Clain MR, Baxter DE: Achilles' tendinitis. Foot Ankle Int 13:482–487, 1990.
24. Cole AJ, Sacco DC, Ho CP, Holland BA: Imaging studies for the physiatrist. In Braddom RL (ed): Physical Medicine and Rehabilitation. Philadelphia, WB Saunders, 1996, pp 206–238.
25. Colon V, Mangine R, et al: The Pogo stick in rehabilitating patients with patellofemoral chondrosis. J Rehabil (1), 1988.
26. Cook EE, Gray VL, Savinar-Nogue, et al: Shoulder antagonistic strength ratios: A comparison between college-level baseball pitchers and nonpitchers. J Orthop Sports Phys Ther 8:451–461, 1987.
27. Cyriax J: Textbook of Orthopaedic Medicine, Vol. 2, 11th ed. London, Bailliere Tindall, 1984.
28. DeCaro JJ, Feuerstein M, Hurwitz TA: Cumulative trauma disorders among educational interpreters: Contributing factors and intervention. Am Ann Deaf 137:288–292, 1992.
29. DeSmet L, Fabry G: Grip strength in patients with tennis elbow: Influence of elbow position. Acta Orthop Belg 62:26–29, 1996.
30. DiGiovine NM, Jobe FW, Pink M, et al: An electromyographic analysis of the upper extremity in pitching. J Shoulder Elbow Surg 1:15–25, 1992.
31. Dobyns JH, Gabel GT: Gymnast's wrist. Hand Clin 6:493–505, 1990.
32. Downing DS, Weinstein A: Ultrasound therapy of subacromial bursitis: A double-blind trial. Phys Ther 66:194–199, 1986.
33. Eisele S: A precise approach to anterior knee pain: More accurate diagnoses and specific treatment programs. Phys Sports Med 19:127–139, 1991.
34. Ellenbecker TS, Davies GJ, Rowinski MJ: Concentric versus eccentric isokinetic strengthening of the rotator cuff: Objective data versus functional test. Am J Sports Med 16:64–69, 1988.
35. Escobedo EM, Hunter JC, Hollister MC, et al: MR imaging of rotator cuff tears in individuals with paraplegia. Am J Roentgenol 168:912–923, 1997.

36. Fernandez-Palazzi F, Rivas S, Mujica P: Achilles' tendinitis in ballet dancers. Clin Orthop 257:257–261, 1990.
37. Ferretti A: Epidemiology of jumper's knee. Sports Med 3:289–295, 1986.
38. Ferretti A, Puddu G, Mariani PP, Neri M: The natural history of jumper's knee: Patellar or quadriceps tendinitis. Int Orthop 8:239–242, 1985.
39. Frisbie JH, Aguilera EJ: Chronic pain after spinal cord injury: An expedient diagnostic approach. Paraplegia 28:460–465, 1990.
40. Fukuda H, Hamada K, Yamanaka K: Pathology and pathogenesis of bursal side rotator cuff tears viewed from en-block histologic sections. Clin Orthop 254:75–80, 1990.
41. Fulkerson JP: Disorders of the Patellofemoral Joint. Baltimore, Williams & Wilkins, 1997.
42. Gacon G, Deidier C, Rhenter JL, Minaire P: Ectopic bone formation in neurological lesions. Rev Chir Orthop Reparatrice Appar Mot 64:375–390, 1978.
43. Gelberman RH, Woo SI, Lothringer K, et al: Effects of early intermittent passive mobilization tendons. J Hand Surg 7:170–175, 1982.
44. Gellman H, Sie I, Waters RL: Late complications of the weight-bearing upper extremity in the paraplegic patient. Clin Orthop 233:132–135, 1988.
45. Gersten JW: Effect of ultrasound on tendon extensibility. Am J Phys Med 34:362–369, 1955.
46. Glaesener JJ, Maske A, Peterson W, Steinberg K: Traumatic paraplegia with injury of the upper extremity—effects on the success of rehabilitation. Rehabilitation 31:224–230, 1992.
47. Glennon TP: Rehabilitation of repetitive motion disorders of the wrist. In Gordon SL, Blair SJ, Fine LJ (eds): Repetitive Motion Disorders of the Upper Extremity. Rosemont, IL, American Academy of Orthopaedic Surgeons, 1995, pp 449–453.
48. Glousman R, Jobe FW, Tibone JE, et al: Dynamic electromyographic analysis of the throwing shoulder with glenohumeral instability. J Bone Joint Surg 70A:220–226, 1988.
49. Goldstein B, Young J, Escobedo E: Rotator cuff repairs in individuals with paraplegia: Are failed repairs common? Am J Phys Med Rehabil 76:316–322, 1997.
50. Goodfellow J, Hungerford DS, Zindel M: Patello-femoral joint mechanics and pathology: Functional anatomy of the patello-femoral joint. J Bone Joint Surg 58B:287, 1976.
51. Gordon EE, Kowalski K, Fritts M: Protein changes in quadriceps muscle of rat with repetitive exercises. Arch Phys Med Rehabil 48:296–303, 1967.
52. Groppel JL, Nirschl RP: A mechanical and electromyographical analysis of the effects of various joint counterforce braces on the tennis player. Am J Sports Med 14:195–200, 1986.
53. Gruchow HW, Pelletier D: An epidemiologic study of tennis elbow. Am J Sports Med 7:234–238, 1979.
54. Harding DC, Brandt KD, Hillbery BM: Minimization of finger joint forces and tendon tensions in pianists. Med Probl Perform Artists 4:103–108, 1989.
55. Harris BA, Leffert RD: The role of physical therapy in rehabilitation of the shoulder. In Rowe CR (ed): The Shoulder. New York, Churchill Livingstone, 1988.
56. Hawkins RJ, Bokor DJ, Angelo RL, Huckle G: Full thickness tears of nonoperative management. Presented at the meeting of the American Shoulder and Elbow Surgeons, Las Vegas, NV, February 1989.
57. Hellebrandt FA, Houtz SJ, Patridge MJ, et al: The Chandler table: Analysis of its rationale in the mobilization of the shoulder joint. Phys Ther Rev 35:545–556, 1955.
58. Herberts P, Kadefors R: A study of painful shoulder in welders. Acta Orthop Scand 47:381–387, 1976.
59. Herzog RJ: Magnetic resonance imaging of the elbow. Magn Reson Q 9:188–210, 1993.
60. Hitchcock TF, Light TR, Bunch WH, et al: The effect of immediate controlled mobilization on the strength of flexor tendon repairs. Trans ORS 11:216, 1986.
61. Howse C: Wrist injuries in sport. Sports Med 17:163–175, 1994.
62. Hudak PL, Cole DC, Haines AT: Understanding prognosis to improve rehabilitation: The example of lateral elbow pain. Arch Phys Med Rehabil 77:586–593, 1996.
63. Hughes CJ, Weimar WH, Sheth PN, Brubaker CE: Biomechanics of wheelchair propulsion as a function of seat position and user-to-chair interface. Arch Phys Med Rehabil 73:263–269, 1992.
64. Hughes M, Neer CS II: Glenohumeral joint replacement and postoperative rehabilitation. Phys Ther 55:850–858, 1975.

65. Hughston JC: Patellar subluxation: A recent history. Clin Sports Med 8:153–162, 1989.
66. Ilfeld FW, Field SM: Treatment of tennis elbow: Use of a special brace. JAMA 195:67–70, 1966.
67. Inaba MK, Piorkowski M: Ultrasound in treatment of painful shoulders in patients with hemiplegia. Phys Ther 52:737–741, 1972.
68. Irani KD: Upper limb orthoses. In Braddom RL (ed): Physical Medicine and Rehabilitation. Philadelphia, WB Saunders, 1996, pp 321–332.
69. Jobe FW, Tibone JE, Perry J, et al: An EMG analysis of the shoulder in throwing and pitching: A preliminary report. Am J Sports Med 11:3–5, 1983.
70. Kannus P, Jozsa L: Histopathological changes preceding spontaneous rupture of a tendon. J Bone Joint Surg 73A:1507–1525, 1991.
71. Kazar B, Relovszky E: Prognosis of primary dislocation of the shoulder. Acta Orthrop Scand 40:216–224, 1969.
72. Kelley JD, Lombardo SJ, Pink M, et al: Electromyographic and cinematographic analysis of elbow function in tennis players with lateral epicondylitis. Am J Sports Med 22:359–363, 1994.
73. Kiefhaber TR, Stern PJ: Upper extremity tendinitis and overuse syndromes in the athletic. Clin Sports Med 11:39–55, 1992.
74. Kottke FJ, Pauley DL, Ptrak RA: The rationale for prolonged stretching for correction of shortening of connective tissue. Arch Phys Med Rehabil 47:345–352, 1966.
75. Kunkel S: Basketball injuries and rehabilitation. In Buschbacher R, Braddom RL (eds): Sports Medicine and Rehabilitation: A Sports-Specific Approach. Philadelphia, Hanley & Belfus, 1994, pp 95–109.
76. Labelle H, Guibert R, Joncas J, et al: Lack of scientific evidence for the treatment of lateral epicondylitis of the elbow. J Bone Joint Surg 74B:646–651, 1992.
77. Laskowski ER: Concepts in sports medicine. In Braddom RL (ed): Physical Medicine and Rehabilitation. Philadelphia, WB Saunders, 1996, pp 915–937.
78. Lee M, Haq AM, Wright V, Longton EB: Periarthritis of the shoulder: A controlled trial of physiotherapy. Physiotherapy 59:312–315, 1973.
79. Lehmann JF, DeLateur BJ, Warren CG, et al: Heating of joint structures by ultrasound. Arch Phys Med Rehabil 49:28–30, 1968.
80. Lehmann JF, McMillan JA, Brunner GD, et al: Comparative study of the efficiency of short-wave, microwave, and ultrasonic diathermy in heating the hip joint. Arch Phys Med Rehabil 40:510–512, 1959.
81. LeVeau BF, Rogers C: Selective training of the vastus medialis muscle using EMG biofeedback. Phys Ther 60:1410–1415, 1980.
82. Lundeberg T, Abrahamsson P, Haker E: A comparative study of continuous ultrasound, placebo ultrasound, and rest in epicondylalgia. Scand J Rehabil Med 20:99–101, 1988.
83. Luopajarvi T, Kuorinka I, Virolainen M, Holmberg M: Prevalence of tenosynovitis and other injuries of the upper extremities in repetitive work. Scand J Work Environ Health 5(Suppl 3):48–55, 1979.
84. Macnab I, McCulloch J: Neck Ache and Shoulder Pain. Baltimore, Williams & Wilkins, 1994, pp 465–488.
85. Maitland GD: Treatment of the glenohumeral joint by passive movement. Physiotherapy 69:3–7, 1983.
86. Mandelbaum BR, Bartolozzi AR, Davis CA, et al: Wrist pain syndrome in the gymnast: Pathogenetic, diagnostic, and therapeutic considerations. Am J Sports Med 17:305–317, 1989.
87. Matsen FA, Lippitt SB, Sidles JA, Harryman DT: Practical Evaluation and Management of the Shoulder. Philadelphia, WB Saunders, 1994.
88. Miyashita K, Shiomi S, Itoh N, et al: Epidemiological study of vibration syndrome in response to total hand-tool operating time. Br J Ind Med 40:92–98, 1983.
89. Moss R, Dawson ML: A biomechanical analysis of patellofemoral stress syndrome. J Athlet Train 27:64–69, 1992.
90. Nelson KA: The use of knee braces during rehabilitation. Clin Sports Med 9:799–811, 1990.
91. Neer CS II: Impingement lesions. Clin Orthop 173:70–77, 1983.
92. Neer CS II, McCann PD, MacFarlane EA, et al: Earlier passive motion following shoulder arthroplasty and rotator cuff repair: A prospective study. Orthop Trans 11:231, 1987.
93. Nicholas JJ: Joint and soft tissue injection techniques. In Braddon RL (ed): Physical Medicine and Rehabilitation. Philadelphia, WB Saunders, 1996, pp 503–513.
94. Nichols PJR, Norman PA, Ennis J: Wheelchair user's shoulder. Scan J Rehab Med 11:29–32, 1979.

95. Nicholson GG: The effects of passive joint mobilization on pain and hypomobility associated with adhesive capsulitis of the shoulder. J Orthop Sports Phys Ther 6:238–246, 1985.

96. Nirschl RP: Shoulder tendinitis. Presented at the American Academy of Orthopedic Surgeons Symposium on Upper Extremity Injuries in Athletes. Washington, DC. St. Louis, CV Mosby, 1986.

97. Nirschl RP: Elbow tendinosis/tennis elbow. Clin Sports Med 11:851–870, 1992.

98. Nirschl RP: Tennis elbow tendinosis: Pathoanatomy, nonsurgical and surgical management. In Gordon SL, Blair SJ, Fine LJ (eds): Repetitive Motion Disorders of the Upper Extremity. Rosemont, IL, American Academy of Orthopaedic Surgeons, 1995.

99. Occupational Injuries and Illnesses in the United States, 1992. Washington, DC, US Department of Labor, Bureau of Labor Statistics, 1994, gov doc no L2.2:OC1/153.

100 Ohno K, Yasuda K, Yamamoto N, et al: Effects of complete stress-shielding on the mechanical properties and histology of in situ frozen patellar tendons. J Orthop Res 11:592–602, 1993.

101. Ohry A, Brooks ME, Steinbach TV, Rozin R: Shoulder complications as a cause of delay in rehabilitation of spinal cord injured patients: Case reports and review of the literature. Paraplegia 16:310–316, 1978.

102. Pappas AM, Zawacki RM, McCarthy CF: Rehabilitation of the pitching shoulder. Am J Sports Med 13:223–235, 1985.

103. Pattern RM: Overuse syndromes and injuries involving the elbow: MR imaging findings. AJR 164:1205–1211, 1995.

104. Pecina MM, Bojanic I: Overuse Injuries of the Musculoskeletal System. Boca Raton, FL, CRC Press, 1993.

105. Pentland WE, Twomey LT: The weight-bearing upper extremity in women with long-term paraplegia. Paralegia 29:521–530, 1991.

106. Pentland WE, Twomey LT: Upper limb function in persons with long-term paraplegia and implications for independence. Part I. Paraplegia 32:211–218, 1994.

107. Pezzullo D, Whitney SL: Patellar tendinitis: Jumper's knee. J Sports Rehabil 1:56–68, 1992.

108. Pitner MA: Pathophysiology of overuse injuries in the hand and wrist. Hand Clin 6:355–364, 1990.

109. Podolsky A, Kaufman K, Cahalan TD, et al: The relationship of strength and jump height in figure skaters. Am J Sports Med 18:400–405, 1990.

110. Powers CM, Newsam CJ, Gronley JK, et al: Isometric shoulder torque in subjects with spinal cord injury. Arch Phys Med Rehabil 75:761–765, 1994.

111. Press JM, Weisner SL: Prevention: Conditioning and orthotics. Hand Clin 6:383–392, 1990.

112. Prokop LL: Upper extremity rehabilitation: Conditioning and orthotics for the athlete and performing artist. Hand Clin 6:517–524, 1990.

113. Reid DC: Sports Injury Assessment and Rehabilitation. New York, Churchill Livingstone, 1992, pp 1053–1129.

114. Richardson AB: Overuse syndromes in baseball, tennis, gymnastics, and swimming. Clin Sports Med 2:379–389, 1983.

115. Riley SA: Wrist pain in adult athletes. Postgrad Med 98:147–154, 1995.

116. Ritz BR: Humeral epicondylitis among gas- and waterworks employees. Scand J Work Environ Health 21:478–486, 1995.

117. Robertson RN, Boninger ML, Cooper RA, Shimada SD: Pushrim forces and joint kinetics during wheelchair propulsion. Arch Phys Med Rehabil 77:856–864, 1996.

118. Robinson MD, Hussey RW, Ha CY: Surgical decompression of impingement in the weightbearing shoulder [published erratum appears in Arch Phys Med Rehabil 74:467, 1993]. Arch Phys Med Rehabil 74:324–327, 1993.

119. Rockwood CA: The management of patients with massive defects in the rotator cuff. Presented at the annual meeting of the Mid-American Orthopedic Association. Orlando, FL, 1986.

120. Rodgers, MM, Gayle GW, Rigoni SF, et al: Biomechanics of wheelchair propulsion during fatigue. Arch Phys Med Rehabil 75:85–93, 1994.

121. Roels J, Martens M, Mulier JC, Burssens A: Patellar tendinitis (jumper's knee). Am J Sports Med 6:362–368, 1978.

122. Rothstein JM, Lamb RL, Mayhew TP: Clinical uses of isokinetic measurements: Critical issues. Phys Ther 67:1840–1844, 1987.

123. Schroer W, Lacey S, Frost FS, Keith MW: Carpal instability in the weight-bearing upper extremity. J Bone Joint Surg 78A:1838–1843, 1996.

124. Shamberg S, Stiens SA, Shamberg A: Personal enablement through environmental modifications. In O'Young BJ, Young MA, Steins SA (eds): Physical Medicine and Rehabilitation Secrets. Philadelphia, Hanley & Belfus, 1997, pp 86–93.

125. Sie IH, Waters RL, Adkins, RH, Gellman H: Upper extremity pain in the postrehabilitation spinal cord injured patient. Arch Phys Med Rehabil 73:44–48, 1992.

126. Silfverskiold J, Waters RL: Shoulder pain and functional disability in spinal cord injury patients. Clin Orthop 272:141–145, 1991.

127. Silverstein B: Epidemiologic and psychologic laboratory studies. In Gordon SL, Blair SJ, Fine LJ (eds): Repetitive Motion Disorders of the Upper Extremity. Rosemont, IL, American Academy of Orthopedic Surgeons, 1995, pp 3–76.

128. Snyder-Mackler L, Epler M: Effect of standard and Aircast tennis elbow bands on integrated electromyography of forearm extensor musculature proximal to the bands. Am J Sports 1989 17:278–281,

129. Solveborn SA, Olerud C. Radial epicondylalgia (tennis elbow): Measurement of range of motion of the wrist and the elbow. J Orthop Sports Phys Ther 23:251–257, 1996.

130. Sommer H: Patellar chondropathy and apicitis and muscle imbalances of the lower extremities in competitive sports. Sports Med 5:386–394, 1988.

131. Spiker J: Comprehensive management of patellofemoral pain. J Sports Rehabil 1:258–263, 1992.

132. Stiens S, Golstein B: Rehabilitation of the shoulder after repetitive motion injury. In Gordon SL, Blair SJ, Fine LJ (eds): Repetitive Motion Disorders of the Upper Extremity. Rosemont, IL, American Academy of Orthopedic Surgeons, 1995.

133. Stiens SA, Haselkorn J, Peters DJ, Goldstein B: Rehabilitation intervention for patients with upper extremity dysfunction: Challenges of outcome evaluation. Am J Ind Med 29:590–601, 1996.

134. Stiens SA, O'Young BJ, Young MA: The person, disablement, and the process of rehabilitation. In O'Young BJ, Young MA, Stiens SA (eds): Physical Medicine and Rehabilitation Secrets. Philadelphia, Hanley & Belfus, 1997, pp 1–4.

135. Stonecipher DR, Catlin PA: The effect of a forearm strap on wrist extensor strength. J Orthop Sports Phys Ther 6:184–189, 1984.

136. Stratford PW, Levy DR, Gauldie S, et al: The evaluation of phonophoresis and friction massage as treatments for extensor carpi radialis tendinitis: A randomized controlled trial. Physiother Can 41:93–99, 1989.

137. Subbarao JV, Chintam R, Rao MS, Nemchausky B: Nontraumatic dislocation of shoulder with rupture of axillary vessel branch in a paraplegic patient: A case report. J Am Paraplegia Soc 13:15–17, 1990.

138. Subbarao JV, Klopstein J, Turpin R: Prevalence and impact of wrist and shoulder pain in patients with spinal cord injury. J Spinal Cord Med 18:9–13, 1995.

139. Thomas DR, Plancher KD, Hawkins RJ: Prevention and rehabilitation of overuse injuries of the elbow. Clin Sports Med 14:459–477, 1995.

140. Townsend H, Jobe FW, Pink M, et al: Electromyographic analysis of the glenohumeral muscles during a baseball rehabilitation program. Am J Sports Med 19:264–272, 1991.

141. Verhaar JAN, Walenkamp GHIM, van Mameren H, et al: Local corticosteroid injection versus Cyriax-type physiotherapy for tennis elbow. J Bone Joint Surg 77B:128–132, 1995.

142. Waters RL, Sie IH, Adkins RH: The musculoskeletal system. In Whiteneck GG, et al (eds): Aging with Spinal Cord Injury. New York, Demos Publications, 1993, pp 53–72.

143. Weinstabl R, Scharf W, Firbas W: The extensor apparatus of the knee joint and its peripheral vastic: Anatomic investigation and clinical relevance. Surg Radiol Anat 11:17–22, 1989.

144. Weiser HI: Painful primary frozen shoulder under local anesthesia. Arch Phys Med Rehabil 58:406–408, 1977.

145. Westfall D: Anterior knee pain syndrome: Role of the vastus medialus oblique. J Sports Rehabil 1:317–325, 1992.

146. White D: Muscle mechanics. In Alexander RM, Goldspink G (eds): Mechanics and Energetics of Animal Locomotion. London, Chapman and Hall Ltd 23–56.
147. Wilson CL, Duff GL: Pathological study of degeneration and rupture of the supraspinatus tendon. Arch Surg 47:121–135, 1943.
148. Wing PC, Tredwell SJ: The weightbearing shoulder. Paraplegia 21:107–113, 1983.
149. Wingate L: Efficacy of physical therapy for patients who have undergone mastectomies: A prospective study. Phys Ther 65:896–900, 1985.
150. Woo SL, Gomez MA, Sites TJ, et al: The biomechanical and morphological changes of the medial collateral ligament of the rabbit after immobilization and remobilization. J Bone Joint Surg 69A:1200–1211, 1987.
151. Woo SL, Matthews JV, Akeson WH, et al: Connective tissue response to immobility. Correlative study of biomechanical and biochemical measurements of normal and immobilized rabbit knees. Arthritis Rheum 18:257–264, 1975.
152. Wooten ME, Kadaba MP, McCann PD, et al: Electromyographic and kinematic analysis of shoulder rehabilitation exercises. Trans ORS 14:569, 1989.
153. World Health Organization: International Classification of Impairments, Disabilities, and Handicaps. Geneva, World Health Organization, 1980.
154. Wylie EJ, Chakera TM: Degenerative joint abnormalities in patients with paraplegia of duration greater than 20 years. Paraplegia 26:101–106, 1988.

VIVIANE UGALDE, MD

TISSA KAPPAGODA, MBBS, PhD

DAVID R. GATER, MD, PhD

19

Exercise Prescription for Postmenopausal Women

Exercise is eschewed by many people. Many women have been socialized to believe that exercising is considered nonfeminine and undesirable. Thus, it is not surprising that postmenopausal women are unfamiliar and unaccustomed to exercise. However, lack of exercise is not unique to women; more than 54% of adults in 1991 reported having little or no regular leisure physical activity.[52] Factors that predict continuation of exercise are myriad but often include the perception that one is doing something healthy, that physical activity helps to avoid musculoskeletal injury, and that tangible improvements in physical capacity and well being are occurring. Guidance in proper exercise techniques and education regarding risks and benefits of exercise are needed to maintain lifelong exercise habits.

Menopause is characterized by a loss of reproductive function and accompanying endocrine changes, including the absence of cyclic estrogen secretion. Decreases in circulating estrogen lead to changes such as thinning of the vaginal wall and the lower urinary tract. Along with changes in pelvic muscle and ligament strength and elasticity, these factors can lead to stress incontinence. Changes in cardiac risk profiles also occur in the estrogen-replete individual with increases in lipidemia and blood pressure. There is a steady loss of bone mass after the age of 35, with more rapid losses occurring in the immediate postmenopausal period.[71]

This chapter discusses the physiology unique to postmenopausal women in the context of cardiovascular responses and musculoskeletal adaptations. Pertinent literature is examined in the context of level of significance for a translation into clinical recommendations. Level 1 significance is based on large randomized, controlled trials (RCT) with low risk of error. Level 2 studies are RCTs with moderate to high risk of error. Levels 3 and 4 are nonrandomized trials with concurrent or historical controls. Level 5 is a case series with no control.[60] Armed with the knowledge of appropriate exercise prescription, health professionals may then educate and motivate women toward healthier lifestyles.

CARDIOVASCULAR RESPONSES TO EXERCISE

The cardiovascular system adapts to a bout of physical exercise by increasing the cardiac output and directing a significant portion of it to exercising muscles. An increase of four- to fivefold occurs as a result of increases in heart rate and stroke volume. However, at any given level of activity, the cardiac output is the product of the heart rate and the stroke volume. The relationship between these two parameters is not linear. The stroke volume increases during the initial stages of activity until the heart rate reaches 110–120 bpm. As the severity of exercise increases and the heart rate exceeds this value, the stroke volume remains relatively steady until the subject is exhausted.[2]

The increase in stoke volume observed during the early stages of exercise is due to a combination of the Starling mechanism and an enhanced level of activity in the sympathetic nerves to the heart.[68] When the degree of exertion increases the heart rate beyond 110–120 bpm, stroke volume is maintained by an increased ability of the ventricles to relax. This enhanced compliance is central to maintenance of the cardiac output. The increase in heart rate occurs first as a result of withdrawal of the restraining influence of the vagi and later as a result of increased activity of the sympathetic nerves.

Concurrent with these changes in the heart are adaptations in the peripheral circulation. Sympathetic nerve activity is enhanced, tending to increase vascular tone and diminish blood flow to nonexercising organs, except for the brain. However, blood flow to exercising muscles increases approximately 20- to 40-fold, resulting in a reduction in overall peripheral vascular tone.[59] The current consensus is that the increase in sympathetic nerve activity is in part due to activation of reflexes originating from exercising muscles.[29] These physiologic adaptations to acute exercise break down when the demands for thermal regulation take precedence over maintenance of the cardiac output.

The changes in the cardiovascular system are accompanied by other adaptive mechanisms involving the respiratory system. The ventilatory rate, tidal volume, and minute ventilation increase, and the airway resistance is reduced. The resulting increase in alveolar ventilation facilitates an increase in oxygen consumption and elimination of carbon dioxide. However, respiratory adaptations do not impose a limit on exercise capacity in normal subjects.

CONCEPT OF PHYSICAL FITNESS

The overall capacity for exercise is widely accepted as a measure of cardiorespiratory fitness. Under laboratory conditions, exercise capacity is expressed in terms of the maximum oxygen consumption. The rationale for this proposition is the relationship between the maximum stroke volume (SV_{max}) and the maximum oxygen consumption ($VO_{2\ max}$).

$$\text{Cardiac output } (Q)_{max} = \text{Heart rate } (HR)_{max} \times SV_{max} \tag{1}$$

In accordance with the Fick principle,

$$Q_{max} = VO_{2\ max} / \text{A-V difference}_{max} \tag{2}$$

By combining equations 1 and 2,

$$VO_{2\ max} / \text{A-V difference}_{max} = HR_{max} \times SV_{max} \tag{3}$$

Thus,

$$VO_{2\,max} = HR_{max} \times SV_{max} \times \text{A-V difference}_{max} \qquad (4)$$

A-V difference is the difference in the oxygen content of arterial and mixed venous blood. The HR_{max} and the maximum A-V difference are relatively independent of the level of cardiorespiratory fitness.

Therefore,

$$VO_{2\,max} = SV_{max} \times \text{Constant} \qquad (5)$$

General fitness implies more than cardiorespiratory fitness. Muscle strength and endurance are important components, as are flexibility, body composition, neuromuscular coordination, and balance.

EFFECT OF EXERCISE TRAINING

Habitual exercise results in significant changes in the cardiovascular response to exercise. Taken collectively, these changes are termed the training response. Briefly, the most significant effect is an improvement in overall exercise capacity, which is indicated by an increase in maximum oxygen consumption, which in normal sedentary subjects is approximately 15–20%. From the equations given above, it is evident that an increase in maximum oxygen consumption could be achieved only through a significant increase in maximum stroke volume. In the peripheral circulation, a reduction in vascular resistance is observed.

At submaximal levels of exertion, there is a reduction in heart rate. Since there are no significant concurrent changes in oxygen consumption or cardiac output, it follows that exercise training also results in an increase in stroke volume at submaximal levels of activity.[24]

EFFECT OF AGING

With increasing age, cardiovascular adaptations to exercise alter. The maximum heart rate and oxygen consumption are reduced. The maximum cardiac output declines with age at the rate of approximately 1% per year. Part of this decline could be attributed to underlying subclinical disease processes. In addition, other central (i.e., cardiac) and peripheral factors (i.e., declining muscle mass) could play important roles. For instance, it has been suggested on the basis of both human and animals studies that the sensitivity of adrenergic receptors diminishes with age, thereby resulting in a decline in maximum heart rate. Longitudinal studies indicate that with increasing age, cardiac muscle mass is increased and ventricular compliance decreased.[38] It is likely that a combination of these factors contributes to a reduction in maximum stroke volume in older subjects. In one of the few longitudinal studies of $VO_{2\,max}$ in women, no decline in $VO_{2\,max}$ was found when expressed in terms of lean body mass (LBM). Body weight remained constant, but percent body fat increased with a concomitant decrease of LBM. Thus, the reduction of absolute $VO_{2\,max}$ was due to the relative loss of muscle mass. Despite the decreases in aerobic power, the active women were able to increase their walk time to exhaustion, indicating that positive practical functional gains were made over 6 years.[53] Blood pressure and total vascular resistance increase, requiring more cardiac work for the same amount of cardiac output compared to younger persons. During training, adaptation and recovery from exercise proceeds at a lower rate with aging.[63]

EFFECT OF GENDER

Most differences in exercise response between women and men can be attributed to differences in body size (Table 1). Morphologic changes that occur after puberty lead to a greater peak LBM in men of up to 1.4 times that of women, larger heart and left ventricle size in men, and increased body fat percentage in women. Early studies of physiologic differences were criticized for comparing sedentary females with more active males. However, even with corrections for body fat percentage and LBM some physiologic differences remain. The principle difference in the response to exercise that could be attributed to gender is a reduction in overall exercise capacity, which is reflected in a 8.6% reduction in maximum oxygen consumption and lower maximum stroke volume in women. Recalling the equation $VO_{2\,max} = SV \times HR \times A\text{-}V$ difference, one can determine the sources for variation in $VO_{2\,max}$. The difference in stroke volume is likely due to larger heart and left ventricle size in men and a 12% greater blood volume due to greater body size, leading to increased end-diastolic volume.[48] Women also have lower hemoglobin content and lower arterial oxygen content, contributing to a lower arteriovenous oxygen difference. All of these factors likely contribute to the difference in $VO_{2\,max}$. There may be other sex-linked differences in oxygen transport and utiliza-

TABLE 1. Differences in Exercise Response Between Men and Women

Female Physiologic Differences from Males*	% Difference
$VO_{2\,max}$	8.6% less
Blood volume	12% less
Lean body mass	15% less
Relative % body fat (age 15–59)	4–8% more
Relative % body fat (age 60–69)	1–3% more
Muscle biopsy fiber area	15% less
Stroke volume	Decreased
A-V difference†	Decreased
Peak heart rate	None
Minute ventilation	None
Heat acclimatization	None
Cardiovascular training responses	None
Soft tissue injury rate	Controversial

*When matched for activity level, lean body mass, and percentage of body fat
†The difference in the oxygen contents of arterial and mixed venous blood

tion that can explain the remaining difference in $VO_{2\,max}$.[48] There is no gender difference for peak heart rate, which varies primarily due to age. However, the heart rate for an absolute level of submaximal exercise is higher in women. An explanation is that for the same cardiac output, women have higher heart rates due to the lower stroke volume relative to men. There are no differences in ventilatory rate or acclimatization to heat stress.[48,72]

The blood pressure response to exercise is enhanced with aging, but this effect can be attenuated by training to a greater degree in men. Estrogen replacement in older women appears to have a favorable effect on the blood pressure response to exercise.[43] However, in a multicenter RCT of 875 postmenopausal women, systolic blood pressure was unaffected by estrogen replacement. The women experienced significant and favorable response to lipid profiles and lowered fibrinogen levels.[50] Another comparison of active and sedentary postmenopausal women found that abdominal adiposity measured as waist circumference was the primary predictor of systolic blood pressure (SBP) and that estrogen replacement was predictive of diastolic blood pressure.[69]

In general, the responses to exercise training are similar in men and women regardless of age. In many urban societies, cultural barriers prevent older women from undertaking exercise training programs. Such attitudes probably explain the paucity of controlled studies that have attempted to define the effect of exercise training in elderly women. Nevertheless, even in the limited studies that have been reported, the usual training responses could be demonstrated in elderly females in their sixth, seventh, and eighth decades of life.[19,53] However, exercise prescriptions should take cognizance of the higher heart rates for a given submaximal workload and the relative lack of mobility experienced by many elderly women. Regardless of these differences, postmenopausal women benefit from exercise in reduced mortality compared to sedentary controls.[37] Exercise also can positively affect the cardiac risk profile by increasing high-density lipoproteins (HDL),[31] reducing systolic blood pressure (SBP), improving insulin sensitivity, and changing body composition. Exercise is especially important in light of the fact that cardiovascular diseases are the leading cause of death in women.

SPECIFIC EXERCISE PROGRAMS

In a rare level 1 trial comparing varying intensities of treadmill walking in men and women ages 50–65, improvements were demonstrated in $VO_{2\,max}$, body composition, and HDL levels. Of note, the home-based high-intensity exercisers maintained the best compliance compared to the class-based or the home-based low intensity groups. Greater HDL improvements were seen with more frequent, moderate-intensity exercise (5 days per week) than with the group that exercised at higher intensity 3 days per week.[31] Numerous level 3 studies demonstrate significant improvements in $VO_{2\,max}$ with various regimens in postmenopausal women. High-intensity dynamic exercise of 30-minute sessions, three or four times per week, have led to increases of 9–17% in $VO_{2\,max}$, but rates in controls declined.[14,23,46,65] Postmenopausal women respond favorably to dynamic exercise, improving their cardiac risk profile. For a more thorough review of the literature pertaining to therapeutic exercise and health status, the reader is referred to Haskell.[26]

EXERCISE RECOMMENDATIONS

For general health and cardiovascular risk reduction, an accumulation of 30 minutes or more daily (at least 10 minutes duration) of moderate-intensity activity is recommended for sedentary individuals. For those already at that activity level, additional health and fitness benefits can be achieved by participating in more vigorous activity. Higher intensity, longer duration activity can be performed three times per week. It appears that weight loss and an increase of HDL cholesterol is related to absolute intensity (i.e., number of calories per minute), and an increase in aerobic or cardiovascular capacity is related to relative intensity (i.e., percent $VO_{2 max}$ or HR_{max}).[26] One should particularly consider in older sedentary adults the need to slowly increase activity over a longer period to reach the recommended levels compared to young sedentary adults.

MUSCULOSKELETAL ADAPTATIONS

OSTEOPOROSIS

Osteoporosis affects 25 million Americans, 30-50% of all postmenopausal women, and 50% of persons older than 75. Complications of osteoporosis that present the greatest morbidity and mortality are 1.3 million fractures per year.[8,57] The risk of hip fracture is fivefold if the bone mineral density (BMD) falls below 2.5 standard deviations from the mean of young normal subjects.[13] It also has been demonstrated that an increase in BMD of 3–5% reduces the fracture rate by 20%.[66] Osteoporosis is loss of bone mass per unit volume with retention of a normal mineral-to-matrix ratio. Trabecular bone, which makes up 20% of skeletal mass, is located in the vertebral bodies, the femoral neck, and the distal radius. In osteoporosis, trabecular bone is lost first, followed by cortical bone, which makes up the remaining 80% of the skeleton.

Exercise has been proposed both as a treatment and as a prophylactic measure for osteoporosis. Cross-sectional studies consistently demonstrate greater total body and regional BMD in active versus sedentary women.[15,21,32,73] Longitudinal prospective trials have focused on the measurement of BMD of the spine, hip, and wrist as an outcome measure. More recent work also has looked at other factors contributing to fracture risk, such as balance, strength, neuromuscular reflexes, and circumstances of the fall. Many of these factors can be improved with exercise.

To determine the level of significance of trials, the following factors were considered:[60] (1) the study design was randomized and controlled; (2) the variables of years postmenopausal, age, height, weight, calcium and estrogen intake, and current and prior activity levels were controlled; (3) the exercise protocol was structured and monitored for compliance, intensity, and progression; (4) site-specific loading of the bone corresponded with BMD measurements; (5) the protocol lasted at least 9 months; and (6) acceptable techniques were used for BMD reproducible measurements. To stimulate an osteogenic response in the bone, it is known that the intensity of the load, the area of application of the load, and the relative newness of the activity for the person are important factors.[66]

Exercise interventions have used a variety of types. Resistive exercises require muscle contraction against a resistance, which can include free weights, resistance machines (Nautilus, Universal, Keiser), elastic bands, and water. Intensity of resistance machines and free weights is often expressed in terms of a percentage of one repetition maximum (1RM). 1RM is the maximum weight a person can lift one time. Dynamic exercise is continuous and relies on oxygen for energy production. Examples include walking, aerobic dancing, jogging, running, pool running, and jumping. Intensity of dynamic exercise is often expressed in percentage of $VO_{2 \, max}$. Unique to exercise for BMD, the force of activity and its action on the bone are considered in nonimpact versus impact exercises. The intensity of force is estimated with force plates or implanted force transducers, and it is expressed in terms of multiples of body weight.

The remainder of this section reviews exercise regimes and resultant effects on the wrist, spine, and hip. The type, intensity, frequency, and duration are evaluated to allow incorporation into recommendations for exercise prescription. Emphasis is placed on trials of postmenopausal women, because premenopausal women have greater response to exercise if not amenorrheic.[16]

Few exercise trials of level 1 significance demonstrate an increase in BMD in the radius, particularly within ranges that would effectively reduce fracture risk, i.e., increases of 3–5% BMD (Table 2). Level 1 trials of exercise alone have failed to demonstrate any significant change at the wrist. The combination of resistance exercise with Nautilus equipment and estrogen has demonstrated increases of 3–4%, while estrogen alone was associated with maintenance of BMD.[57,55] Thus, exercise and estrogen causes a synergistic effect.[47] In women who are estrogen-replete, high-intensity resistance exercise with Universal weights did not demonstrate any significant change from controls.[56] As expected, an exercise trial of walking alone did not find BMD changes at the wrist.[42] Criticism of studies using exercise alone includes the nonspecificity of the exercise to the targeted area one is measuring for an osteogenic response. Obviously, walking and lifting weights is not enough of an osteogenic stimulus for the forearm. One study that attempted to address this issue used a set of specific upper extremity exercises designed to load the radius with tensile, bending, compressive, and torsional loads.[3] These exercises included hanging from a bar for a tensile load, weightbearing activities in a quadruped position for a bending load, wall push-ups for compressive loads, and twisting motions of pronation and supination for torsional loads. Although the groups were nonrandomized, they did demonstrate an increase of 3.8% in BMD after 5 months. Further research is needed to clarify the role these specific loading exercises may play in future exercise prescriptions for postmenopausal women.

Level 3 and 4 studies have provided conflicting results at the wrist. The use of combinations of interventions also makes interpretation more difficult. At least two studies that include pre- and postmenopausal women have demonstrated either maintenance or a slowing of the rate of decline in BMD.[54,65] These studies included dynamic exercise mixed with elastic bands for resistance or a combination of elastic bands, light weights, and push-ups. On the contrary, two other studies using mat, quadruped exercises or a progressive resistance dumbbell program for 8–10 months combined with an aerobics dance or walk/run regimen demonstrated no effect on BMD at the

TABLE 2. Trials Demonstrating the Effects of Exercise on the Radius and Wrist

Type of Exercise	Author	% Change in Bone Mineral Density	Exercise Protocol	Duration (Months)	No.	Mean Age
LEVEL I - EXERCISE ALONE						
Resistance	Pruitt et al.[56]	No change	Universal Gym weights	9	27	53–56
Dynamic	Martin et al.[42]	No change	Walking	12	76	57–60
Impact	None					
LEVEL I - EXERCISE + ESTROGEN						
Resistive	Notelovitz et al.[47]	4.1% increase	Nautilus weights	12	20	43–46
Dynamic	Prince et al.[55]	2.7% increase	Low-impact aerobics	24	162	55–56
Impact	None					
LEVEL III - EXERCISE ALONE						
Dynamic + Light	Presinger et al.[54]	Maintenance (no attenuation)	Walk, jog, gym balls, Therabands	36	146	59–62
Resistance	Smith et al.[65]*	Maintenance	Aerobics, light weights	48	142	50
	Krolner[36] et al.[†]	No change	Walk, run, quadruped mat exercise	8	31	61
	Peterson et al.[51]*	No change	aerobics vs. free weights	12	59	49–55
	Rikli et al.[58†]	No change	Aerobics, dumbbells	10	31	72
Impact	Ayalon et al.[3]	3.8% increase	5 loading exercises to the forearm	5	40	62–63

*Pre- and postmenopausal subjects
†Experimental and controls groups with some members on estrogen

wrist.[36,58] Currently, existing studies have not demonstrated significant increases in BMD of the radius with exercise alone. Brisk walking and nonspecific, high-intensity resistance exercise has been proven to not be beneficial in increasing or maintaining wrist BMD.[42,56] In combination with estrogen, high-intensity resistance exercise does provide appropriate increases in BMD to provide fracture risk reduction in the distal forearm.[47] Further study of specific loading exercises must be performed to definitively demonstrate increases in BMD by exercise alone.

While hip fractures are associated with the highest mortality from osteoporosis, it has been difficult to demonstrate a response to exercise (Table 3). A level 1 study by Nelson et al. is the only exercise intervention to demonstrate a small increase (0.9%) in BMD in the femur in sedentary, estrogen-replete, postmenopausal women. A program using progressive weight training with Keiser pneumatic resistance of three sets of eight repetitions at 80% 1RM was performed 2 days per week for 1 year.[45] Opposing these findings is an RCT of similar design by Pruitt et al. using Universal weight training with one set of 10–12 repetitions maximum, 3 days a week for 9 months. This study failed to demonstrate any significant difference in BMD compared to controls.[56] Perhaps the difference was due to differences in total workload, as illustrated by the strength gains of 76% in Nelson's study compared to 36% in Pruitt's study. A study of weight resistance training at 70% 1RM for 1 year also failed to demonstrate a significant change in BMD of the femur.[64] This study, however, recruited women who were already active, thereby making it less likely to demonstrate a change in BMD. Resistance exercise appears promising but thus far requires very high intensity for a minimal increase in BMD. An encouraging fact from Nelson's study was a low injury rate with good compliance.

If traditional resistance exercises do not stimulate increases in BMD, high-impact exercise should. Bassey and Ramsdale designed an RCT with heel drops to allow 2.5–3 times the body weight at a specific rate to allow for the greatest osteogenic effect.[5] An implanted force transducer in the hip of two exercisers demonstrated 1.5–1.75 times the body weight with a heel drop compared to 3–3.5 with a jump. Unfortunately, the exercisers did not demonstrate any changes in BMD compared to controls after 1 year. The implanted transducer was helpful in demonstrating that forces estimated from a force plate are not completely accurate in vivo.

There are two level 3 studies using dynamic, high-impact exercise that produced conflicting results. Kohrt et al. have demonstrated an increase in BMD in the femur of 1.6% with exercise alone and 2.6% when combined with estrogen replacement. The women walked, jogged, and climbed stairs at 65–85% of maximal heart rate for 45 minutes a day at least 3 days a week for 9 months.[33] However, Nelson demonstrated that walking with leaded waist belts at 75–85% of maximal heart rate for 50 minutes 4 days a week for 1 year did not provide an adequate osteogenic or preserving stimulus to the femur.[46] The difference in osteogenic response may lie in the relative "newness" of the activity to sedentary women and in the rate the force was applied on the femur. In Kohrt's study, the women were encouraged to jog at least every third lap and also to climb stairs. While adding waist weights would increase ground reaction forces, the rate of application of the force would be slower relative to the force incurred while

TABLE 3.   Trials Demonstrating the Effects of Exercise on the Femur and Hip

Type of Exercise	Author	% Change in Bone Mineral Density	Exercise Protocol	Duration (Months)	No.	Mean Age
LEVEL I - EXERCISE ONLY						
Resistance	Nelson et al.[45]	0.9% increase	80% 1RM Keiser pneumatic	12	39	57–61
	Pruitt et al.[56]	No change	Universal Gym weights, 15 rep max	9	27	53–56
Impact	Bassey et al.[5]	No change	50 heel drops/day	12	44	54–55
LEVEL II & III - EXERCISE ONLY						
Resistance	Smidt et al.[64]*	No change	70% 1RM	12	49	55–57
Dynamic/Impact	Nelson et al.[46]		Walk with leaded waist belts			
LEVEL III - EXERCISE + ESTROGEN						
Dynamic/Impact	Kohrt et al.[33]	1.6–2.6%	Walk, jog, stair-climb	9	32	65–67

*Mixture of active and sedentary subjects

jogging. These positive changes seen in femoral BMD are relatively new. Even premenopausal women, who typically demonstrate more response to exercise than postmenopausal women, have not shown increases at the hip.[67] Recent studies in pre-menopausal women have provided encouraging results, illustrating that when adequate force is applied in an appropriate fashion, increases in BMD will occur.[28,41] In summary, BMD in the hip can be increased with high-intensity resistance training of greater than 80% 1RM. Heel drops do not provide an adequate osteogenic response. There is an indication that high-impact dynamic exercise, especially when combined with estrogen, can lead to clinically significant increases in the hip, but further study is needed for clarification.

Vertebral bodies contain up to 66% trabecular bone and are more likely to demonstrate measurable responses to exercise training. There are several level 1 and 2 studies demonstrating increases in BMD (Table 4). The greatest gains in BMD (8.4%) again are found with combinations of resistance exercise and estrogen.[47] With exercise alone, increases of 1–1.6% in BMD can be seen with high-intensity weight training protocols, i.e., 80% 1RM.[45,56] High-impact exercise with 50 heel drops compared to low-impact activity did not demonstrate any significant change in BMD.[5] Walking at 70–85% of maximal heart rate did not cause any change from baseline or compared to controls.[42] This confirmed a prior level 4 study that walking alone is not adequate to stimulate protective increases in BMD in the spine.[10]

Level 3 studies of the spine indicate clinically significant increases, mild increases, maintenance, or no change from controls in BMD, depending on the type and intensity of the exercise (see Table 4). High-impact exercise appears to increase BMD by 5.2–6.1% with a combination of walking, jogging, and climbing stairs at 70–90% of $VO_{2\ max}$.[14] Other nonrandomized studies demonstrate modest increases of 1–2.2% with dynamic exercise, such as walking at the anaerobic threshold or with water calisthenics.[27,70] A small sample of exercisers using low- and high-impact aerobics demonstrated maintenance of BMD while the controls continued to lose bone mineral.[23] A walking program with leaded waist belts also demonstrated maintenance of BMD.[46] Resistance training using 30% of 1RM and 70% 1RM failed to demonstrate significant differences from controls. The 30% 1RM is likely of insufficient intensity to cause an osteogenic response.[61,64] Smidt's study with weight resistance training at 70% intensity may still be of inadequate force.[64] The study design also recruited active women and allowed women taking estrogen to be placed in both groups, which may have affected the outcome.

Level 1 studies with premenopausal women also reveal similar results in the spine. Weight resistance training of levels of 70–75% 1RM stimulated BMD increases.[41,67] Nonrandomized studies using weight resistance of 70–60% 1RM failed to demonstrate any change from controls.[20] Running[67] and jumping/stair-stepping[28] also demonstrated increases. Thus, it appears that intensities of greater than 70% 1RM with resistance training causes a positive effect on lumbar vertebral body BMD. There are indications in the literature that dynamic exercise, such as aerobics, step aerobics, stair climbing, and walking at the anaerobic threshold may provide modest increases in BMD in postmenopausal women. Running, climbing stairs, and jumping with forces

TABLE 4. Trials Demonstrating the Effects of Exercise on the Spine and Vertebral Bodies

Type of Exercise	Author	% Change in Bone Mineral Density	Exercise Protocol	Duration (Months)	No.	Mean Age
LEVEL I - EXERCISE ONLY						
Resistance	Nelson et al.[45]	1% increase	80% 1RM Keiser pneumatic	12	39	57–61
	Pruitt et al.[56]	1.6% increase	Universal Gym weights, 15 rep max	9	27	53–56
Dynamic	Martin et al.[42]	No change	Walking	12	76	57–60
Impact	Bassey et al.[5]	No change	50 heel drops/day	12	44	54–55
LEVEL I - EXERCISE + ESTROGEN						
Resistance	Notelovitz et al.[47]	8.5% increase	Nautilus, 8 rep max	12	20	43–46*
LEVEL II - EXERCISE ONLY						
Resistance	Sinaki et al.[61]	No change	30 1RM,	24	65	56
	Smidt et al.[64]**	No change	70% 1RM,	12	49	55–57
Dynamic Impact	Grove et al.[23]†	Maintained	High- vs low-impact aerobics	12	15	54–56

LEVEL III–IV · EXERCISE ONLY

Resistance	Tsukahara et al.[70]	1.6–2.2% increase	Water calisthenics	12	97	60–64
Dynamic	Hatori et al.[27]	1.1% increase	Walking at anaerobic threshold	7	33	56–58
	Cavanaugh et al.[10‡]	No change	Walking	12	17	55–57
	Krolner et al.[36]	3.5% increase	Walk, run, quadruped mat exercises	8	31	61
Dynamic/Impact	Dalsky et al.[14§]	5.2–6.1% increase	Walk, jog, stair-climb	9	35	62
	Nelson et al.[46]		Walk with leaded waist belts	12	36	60

LEVEL III · EXERCISE + ESTROGEN

Dynamic/Impact	Kohrt et al.[33]	2-6% increase	Walk, jog, stair-climb	9	32	65-67

*Surgical Menopause
**Poor control for variables of estrogen replacement and activity level
†Poor control for variable of estrogen replacement
‡Compared active subjects to sedentary controls
§Poor control for variable of estrogen replacement

two to six times the body weight clearly demonstrate increases in spinal BMD in pre-menopausal women.

High-intensity resistive exercise appears to mildly increase BMD in hip and spine in postmenopausal women. There are indications that high-impact dynamic exercise may also cause similar changes in BMD, but level 1 studies need to be performed. At this point, exercise cannot be recommended in place of estrogen therapy for attenuation of bone mass loss in menopausal women.[1] In combination with estrogen, BMD increases become clinically significant in the range that could reduce fracture risk by 20%. Some may consider taking estrogen alone given the maintenance of BMD seen in longitudinal studies[47,55] and the epidemiologic data that describes a reduction in fracture risk of 50% with estrogen replacement.[13] However, taking estrogen alone does not confer the other benefits gained from exercise—namely, reduction of cardiovascular disease risk and improvements in strength and coordination, which have been associated with reduction of the risk of falls and further reduction in the risk of hip fractures.

Factors besides BMD that have been associated with the risk of hip fracture include physical inactivity, muscle weakness, and a history of falls.[13] The way a person falls, laterally landing directly on the trochanter versus falling backward, is an independent risk factor for hip fractures.[22] Muscle weakness, poor balance, and low muscle mass

---

TABLE 5. Risk Factors for Osteoporosis[29]

Menopause before age 45
Family history of fractures in elderly women
Corticosteroid use
Chronically low calcium intake
Thin/small bones
Caucasian or Asian descent
Sedentary lifestyle
Cigarette smoking
Excessive alcohol consumption
Advanced age

TABLE 6. Risk Stratification with Bone Mass Measurement*

Group I	Group II	Group III
BMD≤1 SD below peak normal mean	BMD > 1 SD and ≤ 2.5 SD below peak normal and/or 1 osteoporotic fracture	BMD > 2.5 SD below peak normal mean and/or 2 or more osteoporotic fractures

BMD = Bone mineral density; SD = Standard deviation
*Women with fewer than three risk factors do not need BMD measurement and are placed in Group I. Adapted from Bonner FJ: Exercise presented at the 58th annual meeting of the American Academy of Physical Medicine and Rehabilitation, Chicago, October 10–13, 1996.

TABLE 7. Physical Medicine Program for Patients with Osteoporosis

Education	Group 1	Group 2	Group 3
	Risk Factors and Environmental Hazards	Same	Same
Appropriate pharmacologic management	?	Estrogen or alendronate	Estrogen or alendronate
Nutritional counseling	Calcium 1500 mg/day	Same	Same
Stretching	Pectoral, shoulder girdle, soft tissue restrictions	Same	Same
Back extensor strengthening	Prone exercises, progress to machine	Same	Supervised with slow progression
Abdominal strengthening	Supine, bilateral leg flexion-extension	Supine, single leg flexion-extension	Isometric contraction of abdomen, pelvic tilt
Upper extremity strengthening	Push-ups, military press, Therabands (moderate resistance)	Wall push-ups, medium Therabands, hand putty	Progress to light Theraband, wand resistance, putty
Lower extremity strengthening	Leg presses	Isometrics	Isometrics
Dynamic activities	Jog/run/aerobics/ Nordic track	Acute - pool therapy, walk, Nordic track, aerobics	Pool therapy, walk
Balance and transfer techniques	Double and single leg support balance for 30 seconds	Same as Group 1, transfer and gait training as needed, consider hip protectors	Balance for 15 seconds, same as Group 2
Proper lifting techniques	Avoid spinal flexion, lift with legs	Same	Same, avoid loads over 10 pounds
Posture correction	Stretching and strengthening as above	Same, may benefit from posture training system (PTS) brace	Same, may need thoracolumbosacralorthosis for acute compression fractures
Pain control		Heat, ice, TENS, braces, rest, medications, psychologic support	Same, may also benefit from facet and/or intercostal nerve blocks

Adapted from Bonner FJ: Exercise prescription for osteoporosis. Presented at the 58th annual meeting of the American Academy of Physical Medicine and Rehabilitation, Chicago, October 10–13, 1996.

are all risk factors for falls in the elderly.[45] Several of the aforementioned trials improved strength[5,45,56,58,61,64] and dynamic balance.[5,45] Use of functional tasks for training produced significant improvements in balance, strength, flexibility, and functional mobility.[62] In postmenopausal women, gains in factors other than BMD have been shown to reduce the risk of falls and hip fractures as well as to directly translate into improvements in activities of daily living. In addition, muscle strengthening of the back extensors may provide improvement in posture, reducing factors that contribute to the development of kyphosis.[61] Outside the realm of this discussion, but worthy of mention, are devices that pad the trochanteric area of the hip to dissipate forces from a side-landing fall.[40] A combination of these interventions should ultimately reduce the morbidity and mortality associated with falls in postmenopausal women.

As a result of this research, physiatrists at Allegheny Graduate Hospital in Pennsylvania have devised a comprehensive rehabilitation program for women (Tables 5–7) that has three major pathways based on risk stratification. If a woman has less than three risk factors, she proceeds to group 1 for a prevention program. If she demonstrates greater than three risk factors, she is assessed with BMD measurements, allowing for fracture risk stratification into groups 1–3. The beauty of this program is the incorporation of balance training and review of functional transfer techniques, lifting and biomechanics, posture correction, counseling on environmental hazards, pain control, and nutritional counseling. Although more specific recommendations regarding exercise prescription require further definition, similar programs that address this multifaceted problem will become the focus of clinical care of persons with osteoporosis.

Although all of the studies reported some musculoskeletal injuries that led to attrition in the sample size, factors such as losing interest and moving away were more frequent reasons for attrition. Even with 80% 1RM, or in persons with actual osteoporosis,[11,36] acceptance was high for the activities and no new fractures were demonstrated. Compliance rates were high for the 12- to 18-month programs. Those of 2–4 years duration had problems with maintaining compliance.

In summary, for positive increases in BMD that reach clinically significant reductions in fracture risk, exercise must be of sufficient intensity (80% 1RM, eight repetitions, three sets, twice per week) and appropriate loading, include a variety of activities to provide better osteogenic response, and be of sufficient duration with a lifelong commitment to maintain the benefits. Exercise in combination with estrogen yields the greatest increases in BMD. Maintenance of BMD may be accomplished with exercise alone by high-impact activities but is less likely with walking. More research is needed to determine more specific recommendations for exercise prescription. Current research is focusing on skeletal-specific force application and rate of application. The implication is that briefer, more frequent bouts of skeletal loading may be the prescription of choice.[4]

OSTEOARTHRITIS

Osteoarthritis (OA) commonly affects the elderly population, with radiographic findings occurring in 75% of persons older than 70.[39] Data from the Framingham cohort reveal that OA of the knee is associated with age, female sex, obesity, prior injury, occupational knee bending, and physical labor.[17] Equally important, the Framingham data found that habitual physical activity did not increase one's risk of developing knee OA.[25] Supporting this concept is a longitudinal controlled study of runners that demonstrated no increased prevalence of symptomatic knee OA, but women did develop asymptomatic osteophytes and sclerosis. The runners visited physicians less often and had less disability than controls.[39] Published reports are inadequate for several reasons, such as methodologic problems of defining early OA, a lack of longitudinal results, RCTs with exercise of prolonged duration, inadequate quantitation of actual activity levels and relying instead on recall or self-reports of activity, and probable bias introduced by the self-selecting nature of the exercise or sport. The current consensus is that persons with clinically normal joints have no increased risks of OA with exercise while persons with deformities, congenital abnormalities, or prior injuries that alter joint biomechanics in a subtle manner are at risk for accelerating OA. The intensity of the exercise and degree of impact also may be key factors.[39]

Can persons with OA exercise in any fashion? Remaining mobile and as active as possible is an important part of any arthritis program. It is well recognized that inactivity will exacerbate the symptoms of stiffness and lead to muscle disuse, which lessens the ability of the muscle to unload the joint, thereby furthering the degenerative process. In an RCT of 102 patients with knee OA, those randomized to the 8-week walking program had significant increases in walking distance and functional status, had decreased pain by 27%, and required less medication.[34] In a case series of patients with OA of the knee, a 3-month program of strengthening and stretching lead to 9–39% increases in strength and endurance as well as improvements in functional activities, such as rising from a chair, climbing stairs, and walking speed.[18] It appears that habitual activity does not increase one's risk for developing OA. Regarding knee OA, walking and strengthening exercises can improve function and pain levels.

INJURY

Postmenopausal women experience soft tissue injuries that can be as inhibiting as OA. They experience a higher prevalence of plantar fasciitis, metatarsalgia, and meniscal injury than younger women.[44] Common athletic injuries in women include breast soreness due to vertical and circular motion of the breasts during exercise, patellofemoral dysfunction, bunions, and shin splints. Lumbar, tibia, pelvic, and metatarsal stress fractures are seen often in runners.[71] Many of the exercise trials mentioned previously used a variety of methods to reduce musculoskeletal injury, including emphasizing warm-up periods, stretching, and using slow progression over several months to build up to higher intensity exercise.

EXERCISE PRESCRIPTION

When considering an exercise prescription one must be familiar with the physiology, health status, and fitness profile of the individual, including risk stratification. Generalizations may be used as a guide but should be modified to the individual. Training can improve the health and fitness level of an individual. Important concepts of training include overload and specificity. In addition to health status and fitness profile, components of exercise prescription include objectives, resources, contraindications, mode or type of exercise, intensity, duration, frequency, progression, and length of intervention.

HEALTH STATUS AND FITNESS PROFILE

The need for exercise testing in this population is controversial. There is no level 1 evidence to support screening exercise testing in healthy, asymptomatic individuals. There is level 2 evidence that exercise testing is appropriate in asymptomatic men older than 40 under certain conditions, but it is not recommended in women.[63] If a woman has had prior cardiac events or other cardiac risk factors, she should be referred for an evaluation by a physician. Complaints of typical anginal chest pain in women are helpful diagnostically, especially in older women, and should be investigated prior to beginning an exercise program. Atypical chest pain is more difficult, but a negative exercise stress test is helpful. A positive test with atypical chest pain requires further testing given the high rate of false positives in this population.[9] A predictor of high risk of sudden death, coronary artery disease, and left ventricular dysfunction is a maximum heart rate of less than 120 beats per minute achieved during testing. In persons older than 64, the degree of SBP increase was the best predictor of mortality.[9] For more recent information, the reader is referred to the latest consensus statement by the American College of Cardiology/American Heart Association regarding guidelines for exercise testing and prescription.

There is no firm consensus on the use of BMD measurements for fracture risk stratification. Currently, a reasonable approach would use BMD testing for persons with three or more risk factors.[7]

OBJECTIVES

In addition to some of the goals listed below, the objectives also should include goals the individual sets forth.

1. To retard bone loss or to recover from prior losses of BMD.

2. To maintain or improve strength, balance, and coordination to reduce fall risk and improve activities of daily living (maintain independent function).

3. To improve cardiovascular responses and increasing HDL cholesterol levels, thereby reducing coronary artery disease risk.

4. To increase LBM and reduce body fat percentage, allowing improvements in cardiovascular responses and reducing the likelihood of OA of the knee.

Literature regarding mode, intensity, duration, frequency, progression, and length of the exercise intervention have been discussed in previous sections. There are many unknowns regarding these components of exercise prescription for both cardiovascular health and especially for BMD. Future research will be needed to further define the specific "dose" of exercise that is needed to maintain health.

EXAMPLE EXERCISE PRESCRIPTION

Health Status

A sedentary 60-year-old caucasian woman presents with an interest in becoming more active after hearing a report on women's health on the radio. She has mild hypertension and hyperlipidemia that are controlled with diet and medication. She has no other cardiac risk factors. She has some residual pain and restrictions in motion of her right shoulder from a gardening injury 10 years ago. Her family history is positive for hip fracture in her mother and maternal aunt. Medications include an antihypertensive, estrogen, and 1500 mg of calcium daily. Activity and hobbies include reading, light gardening, and knitting. The functional history is notable for an independent status in activities of daily living and community mobility. She notes that it is difficult to keep up with her grandchildren, and she experiences shortness of breath after walking six blocks. Her medical history is otherwise remarkable. Her physical examination reveals an apparently healthy woman with a resting blood pressure of 140/87, resting pulse of 80, and a normal cardiopulmonary examination. Musculoskeletal examination reveals head forward posture with decreased shoulder retraction. She also demonstrates reduced range of motion of right shoulder abduction to 110. Her examination is otherwise unremarkable.

Risk Stratification

She has three cardiac risk factors: hypertension, hyperlipidemia, and sedentary lifestyle. Two of the factors have been identified early and are well controlled with medication. She has no history of angina. She does not need an exercise stress test for risk stratification. However, because of her lifelong sedentary status, an exercise treadmill test could be used to determine a maximal heart rate to better determine a more appropriate exercise intensity. She demonstrates poor exercise capacity with a $VO_{2\,max}$ of 20 ml/kg/min. She tolerates the test well but stops after 5 minutes. No abnormalities are noted on electrocardiogram, and she achieves 94% of her maximal predicted heart rate of 150. Her history reveals three risk factors for osteoporosis, including postmenopausal status, family history, and sedentary lifestyle. Dual-energy x-ray absorptiometry demonstrates BMD 1.25 standard deviation below the mean at the radius and the second through fourth lumbar vertebral bodies. Her femoral neck and intertrochanteric areas measured 1.6 standard deviations below the mean. Radiographs of her right shoulder reveal no evidence of OA or osteophytes of her acromion that would predispose her to continued impingement problems in her shoulder.

Goals and Resources

The goals of an exercise program would be to modify the risk factor common to both cardiac and skeletal morbidity—sedentary lifestyle. She also would like to lose

15 pounds. She enjoys going to the mall and has heard of a group of women who meet three times a week to walk. Her other interests include gardening and bicycling.

Mode

To achieve improvements in cardiovascular endurance, mall walking is appropriate. This activity may also attenuate her BMD loss[27] and may cause some increase in BMD due to the hormone replacement treatment,[33] especially if she later adds jogging and stair-climbing to her program. Initially, she may alternate days of walking with bicycling to provide cross-training and reduce the risk of musculoskeletal injury. Resistance exercise also should be included to assist with BMD and overall strength with three sets of eight repetitions. Specific resistance exercises are hip extension, knee extension, lateral pull-down, back extension, and abdominal flexion.[45] One might question the appropriateness of abdominal flexion, as it may increase the risk of vertebral compression fractures. However, while exercises can be associated with large forces across the vertebral bodies, in Nelson's group of postmenopausal women whose BMD was near the fracture threshold of 1.0 g/cm^2, there were no reported injuries or fractures to the spine or femur actually increasing BMD by 1%.[45] Upper extremity BMD may be increased with upper extremity resistance training of the biceps, triceps, pectorals, and grip.[47] Overhead weight training such as the military press, pull-over, or lateral pull-down should be avoided initially until her shoulder range and strength improves. Strengthening of internal and external shoulder rotators should be performed to help rehabilitate her shoulder. If she was not taking estrogen, one might consider push-ups (wall, then progress to floor), quadruped exercises, torsional grip exercises, and hanging from a chin-up bar once her range of motion was restored.[3] Flexibility training, especially of the pectoral muscles and anterior shoulder girdle muscles, is important for maintaining upright posture, as is generalized stretching to prevent injury. Balance training also will be recommended.

Intensity

The patient is taught how to take her own pulse. Her target heart rate (THR) is initially calculated by the Karvonen method of heart rate reserve = 60% × (maximum heart rate achieved on exercise testing − resting heart rate) + resting heart rate. THR = 0.60(150 − 80) + 80 = 122. This is equal to 53% of her $VO_{2\,max}$.[63] She can then be transitioned up to 75–85% of her maximal predicted heart rate (0.75 × 160, 0.85 × 160) over 2 months. Stairs are added after 3 months. Her 1RM is determined, and initially she is set up to work at 50% 1RM for 1 week, 60% 1RM for 1 week, and 80% 1RM thereafter for resistance training.

Duration and Frequency

Cardiovascular benefits can be gained by at least 10 minutes of continuous moderate activity three times a day for 5–7 days per week.[26] Initially, a sedentary person may be able to tolerate only 4–5 minutes of dynamic exercise. By adding 2 minutes onto the 5 minutes with each additional session, over 2–3 weeks she should be up to 30–35 minutes of continuous exercise. However, to reap skeletal benefits, exact duration and frequency is unclear. In the previously described studies that demonstrated positive effects on BMD, dynamic exercise was performed at a greater intensity, 20–45 minutes continuously, 3–7 days per week. Time also must be allowed for warm-up and cool-down, each lasting 5–10 minutes. The older and less fit person should spend more time on warm-up and cool-down. Resistance exercise is recommended to be performed 2–3 times per week.

Progression

With dynamic exercise, progression is built into the prescription. As a training effect occurs, the heart rate will decrease over time as the stroke volume improves. Thus, if the person performs activity to maintain THR, she eventually will need to walk, jog, or climb stairs faster. Another means of progression for dynamic exercise is to begin at 60% of heart rate reserve, adding gradual increases every 2 weeks for 2 months until the endpoints of 70–85% of maximal heart rate (0.7 × 160, 0.85 × 160) are reached. The total amount of exercise performed is equal to the duration × frequency × intensity, and it should increase by only 10% per week.[63] For resistance exercise, reevaluation of 1RM every 4 weeks is reasonable. Another method is to use a resistance that allows 10–15 repetitions. Once a particular resistance level is easily performed at 10–15 repetitions, the resistance is increased. No clear endpoint was discussed in resistance training programs for BMD.

Length of Intervention

Cardiovascular and skeletal adaptations to exercise are reversible with detraining.[14,63] Therefore, maintenance of dynamic impact exercise should be performed at least 3 times a week.[14] Moderate intensity activity for cardiovascular health should be maintained 5–7 days a week. Regardless, continued physical activity for health benefit should continue for the lifetime of the individual. However, as the person ages and health status changes, the exercise prescription will need to be modified. Interestingly, new information regarding bone adaptations also may lead to more emphasis being placed on changing modes of exercise. This would expose the skeleton to differently applied forces, resulting in an osteogenic stimulus. For example, a woman who has run for many years might switch to step aerobics.[4] Further study is needed to allow more specific recommendations.

CONCLUSION

Exercise is a worthwhile endeavor that should be encouraged for all postmenopausal women. Dynamic exercise at moderate intensity, such as walking daily, should reduce the risk of cardiovascular diseases. Additionally, resistance training has been shown to improve bone mineral density. A combination of these activities improves strength and balance, further reducing the risk of hip fracture and enabling maintenance of an independent lifestyle with aging.

REFERENCES

1. American College of Sports Medicine: Position stand on osteoporosis and exercise. Med Sci Sports Exerc 27:i–vii, 1995.
2. Astrand PO, Rodahl K: Textbook of Work Physiology—Physiological Basis of Exercise, 3rd ed. New York, McGraw-Hill, 1986.
3. Ayalon J, Simkin A, Leichter I, Raifmann S: Dynamic bone loading exercise for postmenopausal women: Effect on the density of the distal radius. Arch Phys Med Rehabil 68:280–283, 1987.
4. Bailey D: Osteoporosis Symposium. Presented at the 44th annual meeting of the American College of Sports Medicine, Denver, May 28–31, 1997.
5. Bassey EJ, Ramsdale SJ: Weight-bearing exercise and ground reaction forces: A 12-Month RCT of effects on BMD in healthy postmenopausal women. Bone 4:469–476, 1995.
6. Berlin JA, Colditz GA: A meta-analysis of physical activity in the prevention of coronary heart disease. Am J Epidemiol 132:612–628, 1992.
7. Bonner FJ: Exercise prescription for osteoporosis. Presented at the 58th annual meeting of the American Academy of Physical Medicine and Rehabilitation, Chicago, October 10–13, 1996.
8. Browner WS, Seeley DG, Vogt TM, Cummings SR: Non-trauma mortality in elderly women with low bone mineral density. Lancet 338:355–358, 1991.
9. Bryant BA, Limacher MC: Exercise testing in selected patient groups: Women, the elderly, and the asymptomatic. Prim Care 21:517–534, 1994.
10. Cavanaugh DJ, Cann CE: Brisk walking does not stop bone loss in postmenopausal women. Bone 9:201–204, 1988.
11. Chow R, Harrison J, Dornan J, et al: Prevention and rehabilitation of osteoporosis: Exercise and osteoporosis. Int J Rehabil Res 12:49–56, 1989.
12. Cononie CC, Graves JE, Pollack ML, et al: Effect of exercise training on blood pressure in 70- to 79-year-old men and women. Med Sci Sports Exerc 23:505–511, 1991.
13. Cummings SR: Treatable and untreatable risk factors for hip fracture. Bone 18:165S–167S, 1996.
14. Dalsky GP, Stocke KS, Ehsani AA, et al: Weight-bearing exercise training and lumbar bone mineral content in postmenopausal women. Ann Intern Med 108:824–828, 1988.
15. Dook JE, James SC, Henderson NK, Price RI: Exercise and BMD in mature female athletes. Med Sci Sports Exerc 29:291–296, 1997.
16. Drinkwater BL, Bruemmer B, Chestnut CH: Menstrual history as a determinant of current bone density in young athletes. JAMA 263:545–548, 1990.
17. Felson D: The epidemiology of knee osteoarthritis: Results from the Framingham Osteoarthritis Study. Semin Arthritis Rheum 20(suppl 1):42–50, 1990.
18. Fisher NM, Gresham GE, Abrams M, et al: Quantitative effects of physical therapy on muscular functional performance in subjects with osteoarthritis of the knees. Arch Phys Med Rehabil 74:840–847, 1993.
19. Foster VL, Humeg J, Byrnes WC, et al: Endurance training for elderly women: Moderate versus low intensity. J Gerontol 44:M184–M188, 1990.
20. Gleeson PB, Protas EJ, Leblanc AD, et al: Effects of weight lifting on BMD in premenopausal women. J Bone Min Res 5:153–158, 1990.
21. Greendale GA, Barrett-Conner E, Edelstein S, et al: Lifetime leisure exercise and osteoporosis: The Rancho Bernardo Study. Am J Epidemiol 141:951–959, 1995.
22. Greenspan SL, Myers ER, Maitland LA, et al: Fall severity and BMD as risk factors for hip fracture in ambulatory elderly. JAMA 271:128–133, 1994.
23. Grove KA, Londeree BR: Bone density in postmenopausal women: High impact vs low impact exercise. Med Sci Sports Exerc 24:1190–1194, 1992.
24. Haennel RG, Teo KK, Guinney AH, Kappagoda CT: Effects of hydraulic circuit training on cardiovascular function. Med Sci Sports Exerc 21:605–612, 1991.
25. Hannan MT, Felson DT, Anderson JJ, Naimark A: Habitual physical activity is not associated with knee osteoarthritis: The Framingham Study. J Rheumatol 20:704–749, 1993.
26. Haskell WL: Health consequences of physical activity: Understanding and challenges regarding dose-response. Med Sci Sports Exerc 26:649–660, 1994.

27. Hatori M, Hasegawa A, Adachi H, et al: The effects of walking at the anaerobic threshold level on vertebral bone loss in postmenopausal women. Calcif Tissue Int 52:411–414, 1993.
28. Heinonen A, Kannus P, Sievanen H, et al: Randomized controlled trial of effect of high-impact exercise on selected risk factor for osteoporotic fractures. Lancet 348:1343–1347, 1996.
29. Kaplan MS: Osteoporosis: Pathophysiology and Management in the 90's [course]. Presented at the 54th annual meeting of the American Academy of Physical Medicine and Rehabilitation, San Francisco, November 13–17, 1992.
30. Kaufman MP, Longhurst JC, Rybicki RJ, et al: Effects of static muscular contraction on impulse activity of groups III and IV afferents in cats. J Appl Physiol 55:105–112, 1983.
31. King AC, Haskell WL, Young DR, et al: Long-term effects of varying intensities and formats of physical activity on participation rates, fitness, and lipoproteins in men and women aged 50 to 65 years. Circulation 91:2596–2604, 1995.
32. Kirk S, Sharp CF, Elbaum N, et al: Effect of long distance running on bone mass in women. J Bone Min Res 4:515–522, 1989.
33. Kohrt WM, Snead DB, Slatopolsky E, Birge SJ: Additive effects of weight-bearing exercise and estrogen on BMD in older women. J Bone Min Res 10:1303–1311, 1995.
34. Kovar PA, Allegrante JP, Mackenzie CR, et al: Supervised fitness walking in patients with OA of the knee. Ann Intern Med 116:529–534, 1992.
35. Krall EA, Dawson-Hughes B: Walking is related to bone density and rates of bone loss. Am J Med 96:20–26, 1994.
36. Krolner B, Toft B, Nielsen SP, Tondevold E: Physical exercise as prophylaxis against involutional vertebral bone loss: A controlled trial. Clin Sci 65:541–546, 1983.
37. Kushi LH, Ree RM, Folsom AR, et al: Physical activity and mortality in postmenopausal women. JAMA 277:1287–1292, 1997.
38. Lakatta EG: Changes in cardiovascular function with aging. Eur Heart J 11(suppl C):22–29, 1990.
39. Lane NE, Buckwalter JA: Exercise: A cause of osteoarthritis? Rheum Dis Clin North Am 19:617–633, 1993.
40. Lauritzen JB, Petersen MM, Lund B: Effect of external hip protectors on hip fractures. Lancet 341:11–13, 1993.
41. Lohman T, Going S, Pamenter R, et al: Effects of resistance training on regional and total BMD in premenopausal women: A randomized prospective study. J Bone Min Res 10:1015–1024, 1995.
42. Martin D, Notelovitz M: Effects of aerobic training on BMD of postmenopausal women. J Bone Min Res 8:931–936, 1993.
43. Martin WH, Ogawa T, Kohrt WM, et al: Effects of aging, gender, and physical training on peripheral vascular function. Circulation 84:654–664, 1991.
44. Matheson GO, Macintyre JG, Taunton JE, et al: Musculoskeletal injuries associated with physical activity in older adults. Med Sci Sports Exerc 21:379–385, 1989.
45. Nelson ME, Fiatarone MA, Morganti CM, et al: Effects of high-intensity strength training on multiple risk factors for osteoporotic fractures. JAMA 272:1909–1914, 1994.
46. Nelson ME, Fisher EC, Dilmanian FA, et al: A 1-Y walking program and increased dietary calcium in postmenopausal women: Effects on bone. Am J Clin Nutr 53:1304–1311, 1991.
47. Notelovitz M, Martin D, Tesar R, et al: Estrogen therapy and variable-resistance weight training increase bone mineral in surgically menopausal women. J Bone Min Res 6:583–590, 1991.
48. O'Toole ML: Gender differences in the cardiovascular response to exercise. In Douglas PS (ed): Heart Disease in Women. Philadelphia, FA Davis, 1989, pp 17–33.
49. Owens JF, Matthews KA, Wing RR, Kuller LH: Can physical activity mitigate the effects of aging in middle-aged women? Circulation 85:1265–1270, 1992.
50. PEPI Trial: Effects of estrogen/progestin regimens on heart disease risk factors in postmenopausal women. JAMA 273:199–208, 1995.
51. Peterson SE, Peterson MD, Raymond G, et al: Muscular strength and bone density with weight training in middle-aged women. Med Sci Sports Exerc 23:499–504, 1991.
52. Physical activity and cardiovascular health. NIH Consensus Statement Dec 18–20; 13(3):1–33, 1995.

53. Plowman SA, Drinkwater BL, Horvath SM: Age and aerobic power in women: A longitudinal study. J Gerontol 34:512–520, 1979.

54. Presinger E, Alacamlioglu Y, Pils K, et al: Therapeutic exercise in the prevention of bone loss: A controlled trial with women after menopause. Am J Phys Rehabil 74:120–123, 1995.

55. Prince R, Smith M, Dick I, et al: Prevention of postmenopausal osteoporosis-A comparative study of exercise, calcium supplementation and hormone-replacement therapy. N Eng J Med 325:1189–1195, 1991.

56. Pruitt LA, Jackson RD, Bartels RL, Lehnhard HJ: Weight training effects on BMD in early postmenopausal women. J Bone Min Res 7:179–185, 1992.

57. Riggs BL, Melton LJ: Involutional osteoporosis. N Engl J Med 314:1676–1686, 1986.

58. Rikli RE, McManis BG: Effects of exercise on bone mineral content in postmenopausal women. Res Q Exerc Sport 3:243–249, 1990.

59. Rowell LB: Human Cardiovascular Control. New York, Oxford University Press, 1992.

60. Sackett DL: Rules of evidence and clinical recommendations on the use of antithrombotic agents. Chest 95:2S–4S, 1989.

61. Sinaki M, Wahner HW, Offord KP, Hodgson SF: Efficacy of non-loading exercises in prevention of vertebral bone loss in postmenopausal women: A controlled trial. Mayo Clin Proc 64:762–769, 1989.

62. Skelton DA, McLaughlin AW: Training functional ability in old age. Physiotherapy 82:159–167, 1996.

63. Skinner JS: Exercise Testing and Exercise Prescription for Special Cases, 2nd ed. Philadelphia, Lea & Febiger, 1993.

64. Smidt G, Lin S, O'Dwyer K, Blanpied R: The effect of high-intensity trunk exercise on bone mineral density of postmenopausal women. Spine 17:280–285, 1992.

65. Smith EL, Gilligan C, Mcadam M, et al: Deterring bone loss by exercise intervention in premenopausal and postmenopausal women. Calcif Tissue Int 44:312–321, 1989.

66. Snow C: Osteoporosis Symposium. Presented at the 44th annual meeting of the American College of Sports Medicine, Denver, May 28–31, 1997.

67. Snow-Harter C, Bouxsein ML, Lewis BT, et al: Effects of resistance and endurance exercise on bone mineral status of young women: A randomized exercise intervention trial. J Bone Min Res 7:761–769, 1992.

68. Starling EH: Linacre Lecture on the Law of the Heart. London, Longmans, Green & Co. Ltd., 1918.

69. Stevenson ET, Davy KP, Jones PP, et al: Blood pressure risks factors in healthy postmenopausal women: Physical activity and hormone replacement. J Appl Physiol 82:652–660, 1997.

70. Tsukahra N, Toda A, Goto J, Ezawa I: Cross sectional and longitudinal studies on the effect of water exercise in controlling bone loss in Japanese postmenopausal women. J Nutr Sci Vitaminol 40:37–47, 1994.

71. Wells CL: Women, Sport and Performance—A Physiological Perspective, 2nd ed. Champaign, IL, Human Kinetics Books, 1991.

72. Wilmore JH: Importance of differences between men and women for exercise testing and exercise prescription. In Skinner JS: Exercise Testing and Exercise Prescription for Special Cases, 2nd ed. Philadelphia, Lea & Febiger, 1993, pp 41–56.

73. Zylstra S, Hopkins A, Erk M, et al: Effect of physical activity on lumbar spine and femoral neck bone densities. Int J Sports Med 10:181–186, 1989.

TANJA L. KUJAC, MD

ARJUN SHANKAR

KAMALA SHANKAR, MD

20

Computer Injury, Posture, and Exercise Prescription

The number of physical complaints related to computers and visual display terminals (VDTs) has been increasing. Most of these complaints and related injuries involve the neck, lower back, wrists, forearms, and hands. There also appears to be a higher prevalence of computer-related injuries in women. Upper extremity disorders are often grouped together for claim purposes as cumulative trauma disorders of the upper extremities. A number of articles have appeared in the popular press regarding the rise in workplace injuries related to the use of computers. However, there have not been many large-scale studies to determine the extent of these injuries; nor have there been many studies analyzing patients' premorbid physical complaints prior to excessive computer use. Although computer-related disorders appear to be on the rise, they represent a small fraction of all work-related claims. It is important to distinguish computer-related pain from actual disability, as the latter is much less common.[7] Also, nonspecific computer-related musculoskeletal complaints are far more common than complaints with precise diagnoses.

The history of the current keyboard layout, the QWERTY, is rather enlightening. The QWERTY was designed by Christopher Sholes in 1867.[9] Because early typewriters had a tendency to jam with fast typing, it made sense to place some of the commonly used keys in awkward positions to slow the typist. Thus, the most commonly used letters (e, t, o, a, h, n) were dispersed on all three lines. Amusingly, the letter "r" was moved to a more awkward position on the top row as an early sales pitch. Thus, all the letters of the word *typewriter* appeared on the top row and could be typed more quickly for demonstration.[9]

The QWERTY design requires as much work on the weakest—fifth—digits as it does of the strongest—second—digits. Also, although most people are right-handed, an estimated 60% of typing workload is typed by the left hand. Although the QWERTY design is awkward and injury-provoking, change to a new keyboard layout is unlikely in the near future.[9]

Computer injuries occur in the hands, wrists, forearms, shoulders, and, most commonly, in the neck. This chapter summarizes injuries related to computer use, treatments, therapeutic exercises, and ergonomically correct posture to prevent and eliminate symptoms.

HAND INJURIES

DeQuervain's disease is related to excessive keyboard use. DeQuervain's disease is a stenosing tenosynovitis also known as first compartment tendinitis, with inflammation of the abductor pollicis longus and extensor pollicis brevis tendons. Although this disorder is most commonly associated with repetitive pinching motions, strain on these tendons has occurred in typists, because the thumb is abducted and extended to avoid hitting the space bar.[32] One source called this the "alienated thumb phenomenon"[29] (Fig. 1). Other secondary hand strains also have been noted; the alienated thumb adds tension to the hand, making hand flexion more difficult because the flexors are contracting against contracting extensors.[29] Volar carpometacarpal joint capsule strain at the base of the thumb also occurs, because the thumb is maintained in the plane of the palm with the hand pronated and ulnar deviated. DeQuervain's disease is also prevalent in the thumb that is used to hit the space bar, indicating that this tendinitis can result from excessive space bar tapping or strain from avoiding the space bar. Ulnar deviation that is common with keyboard use also can cause tension in the first dorsal compartment, leading to irritation of these tendons. There have been reports of focal dystonias, also known as occupational cramps, leading to deQuervain's disease.[29] Cramping causes patients to hold their thumb in uncontrolled task-specific abduction and extension, leading to tendon irritation.[29] This focal deQuervain's disease is also more prevalent among typists who tend to press the keys with excessive force. Because

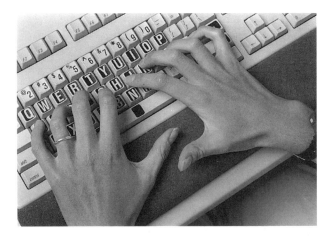

FIGURE 1. The alienated thumb phenomenon.

computer keys are not cushioned, there is a definite endpoint, and excessive force can be translated to first compartment tendons. Wrist injury also may ensue.

One maneuver to help delineate deQuervain's tendinitis is the Finkelstein test. The patient places the flexed thumb in the flexed fingers and then deviates the wrist to the ulnar side. Pain implies that a tenosynovitis exists in the first compartment. Patients also may have palpable tenderness at the lateral border of the anatomic snuffbox.

Treatment includes rest and activity alteration, such as several hours a day of no keyboard use. Nonsteroidal antiinflammatory drugs (NSAIDs) in the acute phase can help eliminate inflammation. Splinting may be necessary in severe cases. Steroid injections have provided some relief when injected into the tendon sheath. For severe refractory cases, surgical release of the tendon sheaths may be necessary.[4] The need for better cushioning of the endpoint in computer keyboards has been recommended as a means of prevention.[29]

Focal dystonia is a focal degradation of fine hand movements that can be very disabling to computer users.[6] This condition results from dual contraction of agonists and antagonists, as seen electromyographically.[8] With the use of instruments, the fingers may pull uncontrollably into flexion or extension. Work tasks may become impossible because subjects begin having trouble starting, sequencing, and controlling the force necessary for the task or for similar tasks with other instruments, such as toothbrushes.[6] One theory to explain focal dystonia is that forceful end range movements carried out under conditions of high demand result in cortical learning. This rapid stimulation may be interpreted simultaneously by the brain so that stimulus to one digit is interpreted as stimulation to multiple digits. Rapid stimulation also may cause serious sensory and motor cortical confusion.[26] This theory may explain the impairments seen for stereognosis as well as loss of motor control in patients with focal dystonia.[6]

Focal dystonia is not easily treated. Initially, NSAIDs, heat, and phonophoresis may be helpful.[16] Some relief, albeit temporary, can be obtained with botulinum toxin injections.[5] Physical therapy, spinal cord stimulation, and surgery all provide only temporary relief. Physical therapists also should perform a tactile sensory examination. If tactile interpretive problems are identified, patients should receive sensory discrimination activities that may help restore accuracy and speed processing.[6]

Another observed hand keyboard injury is weakness of the flexor digiti minimi.[29] With excessive keyboard use, subjects tend to hyperextend and abduct the fifth digit to gain better access to outlying keys (Fig. 2). Also, the fifth fingers are more heavily used for *shift* and *enter* keys than the more dextrous second and third fingers.[7] Patients have been noted to have weak flexor digiti minimi believed to result from overextension and flexor disuse.

There have not been extensive studies on this overextension injury or its treatment. Relaxation techniques of the long extensors have been suggested as has retraining subjects on more equal use of flexors with extensors of the fifth digit.[29] One review noted that ulnar deviation could be corrected by changing the shape of the keyboard.[7] Conventional keyboards cause the forearms to be internally rotated and the wrists to be in ulnar deviation. There are proposals to divide keyboards in half to reduce strain, an arrangement that has been used with success in jet fighter aircraft.[7] Even though the QWERTY layout is ergonomically undesirable and causes more strain on the fifth digits, changing the keyboard layout is unlikely given the millions of keyboards in use.

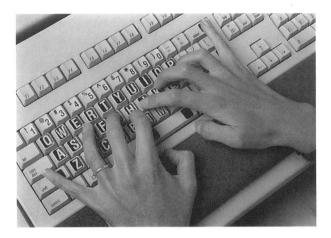

FIGURE 2.   Chronic abduction and extension of fifth digits.

Other noted hand strains related to chronic keyboard use involve adaptations to hyperextendable finger joints (Fig. 3). Pascarelli and Kella observed subjects adapting for hypermobility by hyperextending their hands with increased use of the extensor digitorium to provide stiffening and therefore stability of the fingers.[29] This causes increased strain on the extensors. Hypermobility of finger joints also has been noted to affect the wrist. Long fingernails are thought to contribute to finger hyperextension. Because the wrist is forced to compensate by flexing and extending for hypermobile finger joints, adaptations can be made for hypermobility. Keeping fingers slightly more flexed to keep joints from hyperextending can compensate these hypermobile joints.[29]

Pascarelli and Kella also observed mouse users. Although there were not enough

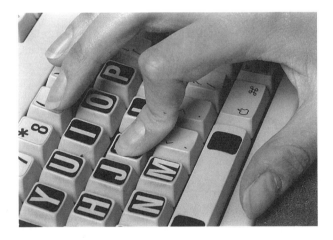

FIGURE 3.   Hyperextendable joints.

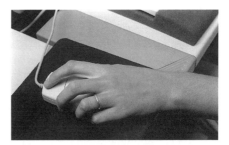

FIGURE 4. Thumb and index finger strain resulting from excessive mouse use.

TABLE 1. Hand Exercises

Hyperextend fingers with opposite hand
Hold fingers maximally abducted and straight for 10 seconds until stretch tension is felt; repeat
Flex fingers at the knuckles and hold for 10 second; repeat

---

patients to draw firm conclusions, it was believed that prolonged tight gripping of the mouse with excessive use of the index finger may lead to fatigue (Fig. 4). First dorsal interosseous strain with excessive metacarpal joint extension and radial deviation has been noted.[29] More studies are needed to confirm these findings. Chair adjustment so the forearm is parallel to the floor can prevent extreme hand extension associated with this strain.[34] Although mouse-related injuries are currently a small fraction of all computer injuries and not thoroughly studied, there seems to be an especially rapid increase in mouse-related claims.[15]

The literature has discussed arm and hand strains related to ulnar deviations of the hands, and to the nonuse of lower arm supports during keyboard use. The importance of taking rest breaks and not substituting the use of lower arm supports for these breaks has been emphasized.[2] Another study has noted a dose-response relationship between working at the video display station and increased hand and wrist symptoms, again implying the importance of rest breaks.[3] Table 1 lists useful exercises to perform during rest breaks.

WRIST INJURIES

More reported wrist injuries pertain to the development of carpal tunnel syndrome (CTS). There also have been mentions of occupational overuse of fingers thought to place patients at risk for developing CTS. Overuse of the keyboard is thought to lead to forearm fatigue, causing typists to hyperextend their wrists to rest their hands while typing which can lead to wrist irritation and ensuing CTS.[20] CTS, a cumulative trauma disorder, is reportedly increasing among computer users, especially those who now type faster with improved technology.[7, 20] Ergonomic risk factors include increased repetition, vibration, and increased force. Excessive dorsiflexion of the wrists along with repeated forearm muscle cause results in friction and shearing of the flexor tendons in the carpal tunnel (Fig. 5). The basic wrist position of keyboard users is wrist dorsiflexion, with the wrists resting on the desktop and the fingers arched for proximal key use. This is called the leaner position.[29] The shearing force also may occur at the extensor tendons as they pass under the extensor retinaculum. The shearing force is created as pressure in the carpal tunnel increases. Pressure in the carpal tunnel increases as the force exerted by the tendons increases with vertical hand/wrist angle, i.e., wrist extension. Also, forces are further increased by coactivated muscles. Pressure in the tunnel is minimal when the hand is in a wrist-neutral position, i.e., with the hand slightly flexed in ulnar deviation. Forces on the median nerve and tendons increase as the hand moves vertically from dorsal extension through palmar flexion. It is thought that these vertical extension/flexion movements of chronic keyboard use cause more irritation to the tendons and the median nerve than ulnar and radial deviations of the hands.[20] Irritation at the carpal tunnel also may result from constant ulnar deviation of the hands. Ulnar deviation occurs as the shoulders are locked and protracted and the elbows are held close to the body. Substantial increases in intracarpal pressure occur when the hand is ulnar deviated greater than 20% or radially deviated greater than 20%.[20] Striking the keys with excessive force translates the force proximally, leading to irritation of tendons and the median nerve as they pass through the carpal tunnel.[29]

A number of manual tests exist that aid in the diagnosis of CTS. Phalen's test is carried out by having patients maximally flex their wrists over the edge of a table with the elbows flexed. This position will cause compression between the proximal edge of the transverse carpal ligament and the flexor tendons. Patients with CTS usually get numbness and tingling in the median nerve distribution within 12 minutes in this position. Tinel's test can be done by lightly tapping over the median nerve and assessing for numbness and tingling in the nerve distribution.[27] Other helpful tests are the reverse

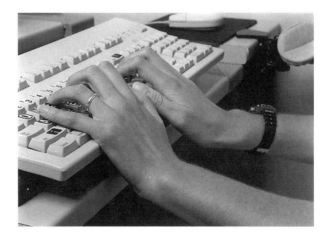

FIGURE 5. Hyperextension of the wrists resulting from poor posture and wrist support.

Phalen's test and the tethered median nerve stress test. A useful screening method for early detection of CTS is the ratio of the wrist to finger sensory nerve conduction velocity to the wrist to palm sensory conduction velocity.[25] Confirmation of nerve injury can be made by electromyography (EMG).

Treatment of CTS includes hand splinting in 0–30° of extension, diuretics, NSAIDs, and corticosteroid injections. There are some reports that pyridoxine (vitamin B_6) may be helpful.[27] Surgery is indicated for chronic, refractory cases.

A number of ergonomic modifications exist that may be useful in reducing the incidence of keyboard-related CTS. One approach to reducing wrist hyperextension is the use of negative-slope keyboard support systems (NSKS). With the NSKS, the keyboard is slightly tilted inferior from the user. One field test performed in Australia noted that there were major reductions in the incidence of CTS with use of the NSKS.[31] Some positive results have occurred with the use of an NSKS, but this keyboard is not frequently recommended in ergonomically correct keyboard demonstrations. By having the keyboard in a negative slope, subjects could obtain a more wrist-neutral posture.[20] One study has shown a decline in performance and no significant improvement in comfort with the use of split keyboards.[11] Another intervention is the use of wrist rests. Interestingly, although these rests are commonly recommended to avoid hyperextension of the hand, studies have shown that they can be more detrimental than helpful.[28] Subjects tend to have increased shoulder and neck muscle activity with the use of wrist rests as they raise their arms to avoid uncomfortable pressure on their arms.[18] Also, carpal tunnel pressure can be increased more than 120%.[21] There also have been reports of increased compression on the ulnar nerve as it passes through Guyon's canal. Full motion forearm supports have been developed that allow horizontal movements while providing arm support. There has not been enough research studying improvements in hand/wrist posture.

Ulnar nerve entrapment also has been associated with repetitive hand injury.[12] Occupational overuse can lead to compression of the ulnar nerve in Guyon's canal, which is bordered medially by the pisiform bone and laterally by the hook of the hamate. Patients present with a positive Tinel's sign, pain, paresthesias, decreased sensation, weakness, and, rarely, atrophy in the ulnar nerve distribution. One would also expect to have some positive EMG findings.[27] Treatments consist of decreased activity, ergonomic changes, NSAIDs, splinting, possibly physical therapy, corticosteroid injections, and possibly surgery.

Less common injuries associated with repetitive injury include anterior and posterior interosseus nerve syndromes. Table 2 lists some useful preventive exercises.

TABLE 2. Wrist Exercises

Flex hand with opposite hand to maximum stretch and hold for 30 seconds; repeat twice.
Repeat above exercise with hand extension.
Lock fingers and press palms together moving hands in circular motions.

FOREARM AND ELBOW INJURIES

An injury associated with jobs requiring repetitive hand use is flexor carpi ulnaris tendinitis.[6] One study noted an increase in problems with dynamic position sense in patients with this and other types of distal upper extremity tendinitis. To test for this disorder, one assesses for pain elicited by having the patient flex the hand in a neutral position and resist extension and radial deviation. Other signs of a tendinitis are inflammation and swelling.

Although specific ergonomic changes have not been identified for this disorder, the usual treatments for an acute tendinitis can be employed, including rest and NSAIDs.

Lateral epicondylitis, also known as tennis elbow, has been associated with computer injuries and other repetitive manual activities. Irritation occurs at the extensor insertions with ongoing repetitive use of the wrist extensors, primarily the extensor carpi radialis brevis.[4] Repetitive flexion-extension of the wrist and pronation-supination of the forearm are thought to be the most common contributing activities. Tenderness is present over the lateral epicondyle. Pain can be maximally produced by having the patient make a fist with pronation of the forearm while radially deviating the wrist.

Treatment involves decreasing repetitive stress, especially repetitive flexion-extension and forearm pronation-supination. NSAIDs, hot packs, ultrasound, ice, and corticosteroid injections may be helpful. Forearm bands have recently become popular. Their purpose is to alleviate tension at extensor insertion sites at the lateral epicondyle and prevent full muscular forearm expansion.[4]

Radial sensory deficits also have been associated with computer use. With poor posture, i.e., the wrists overextended with the forearms pronated, the extensor carpi radialis longus moves closer to the brachialis tendon, causing compression of the radial sensory nerve as it runs between the two tendons.[19] Thus, the patient may be experiencing decreased sensation in the radial sensory distribution of the hand. Proper wrist alignment can help eliminate these symptoms.

Pronator teres syndrome has been associated with computer overuse. The forearms tend to overpronate when the index fingers perform much of the typing, causing proximal entrapment of the median nerve between the two heads of this shortened pronator muscle. Patients may complain of weakness in the median nerve distribution of the hand.[19]

Patients also may get an extensor digitorum communis tendinitis as a result of the tendons being irritated by constant movement under the dorsal retinaculum. There are increased shear forces under this retinaculum when the wrists are overextended, as is commonly the case.[19]

SHOULDER AND NECK INJURIES

The normal position for typing is with the shoulders flexed, abducted, and slightly elevated by contraction of the trapezius and other shoulder muscles. The neck is usually in a few degrees of flexion. Placement of the screen too close or too far from the subject may result in unnecessary neck flexion or extension. Neck pain and stiffness can result with increased flexion of the head (inclination), and constant neck muscle contraction can lead to headaches.[22] Significant increases in neck flexion beyond 20–30° have been noted with work shifts of 2 hours due to increased fatigue. One study reported that painful/stiff neck or shoulders in subjects increased from 48% at 1–2 hours of work to 65% at 6–8 hours of work.[13] A decrease in head/neck flexion angle with more flexible work schedules has been found.[22] The flexion angle was lowest (mean 30.2°) for flexible work schedules and highest (mean 36.5°) for schedules of 50 minutes of work with a 10-minute break per hour. There also was an increased number of extension/flexion episodes with the latter schedule, which can lead to cervical radiculopathy.[22] Rapid cervical spine strain of the extensors results from this excessive forward head position.[1] A number of articles note that it is not necessarily the rest breaks that help eliminate shoulder and neck complaints but, rather, exercise breaks, and frequent changes in position exhibited lower levels of postural discomfort. This is also supported by findings of ongoing neck and shoulder complaints in patients working at ergonomically correct stations who did not change positions frequently.[22] Some shoulder complaints could be eliminated by minimizing flexion/abduction of the upper arm in the shoulder joints. It is recommended that elbows be flexed 90° while at the keyboard to prevent upper arm elevation. Interestingly, studies have shown differences in postural shoulder strain with different levels of mental strain. One study concluded that, due to the higher computational demands of more complex tasks, there was increased shoulder muscle tension with tasks that required increased mental effort.[35] Full motion forearm supports can help maintain this position; by supporting the forearms, referred strain to the shoulders is minimized.[20]

Fatigue is not the only reason for poor head position. The stress on the cervical spine results mainly from head position, and this is influenced by both visual requirements and posture of the trunk. In the upright trunk position, rapid fatigue of the cervical extensors occurs with neck flexion exceeding 30°. Also, VDT being situated too low promotes increased head flexion. The proper position of the screen is at arm's length, with the top of the monitor aligning with the top of the subject's head. Hourly breaks are recommended, during which the subject can perform neck exercises (Figs. 6–24).

The neck can be rotated from side to side and then flexed and rotated again from side to side.[10] Circular arm motions can be performed to promote full range of the shoulders. Note the various exercises in Figures 6–24 for the neck and shoulders.

Cervical radiculopathy has been associated with repetitive head motions that are common at VDTs. Patients will complain of pain, paresthesias, decreased sensation, and possibly weakness and atrophy in cervical nerve root distributions.[12] Treatments include work breaks, NSAIDs, muscle relaxants, physical therapy, epidural injections, and possibly surgery. Physical therapy includes cervical traction as well as passive exercises that advance to active stretching and flexibility. Patients then engage in strengthening and stabilization.[4]

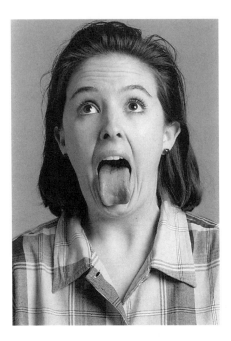

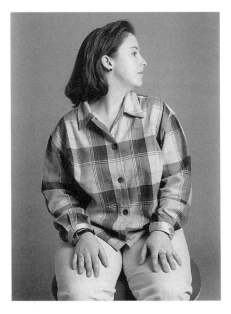

FIGURE 6. Raise eyebrows, open mouth wide, and extend tongue to stretch facial muscles.

FIGURE 7. Turn chin to the left to stretch the right neck and hold 15 seconds. Repeat and change sides.

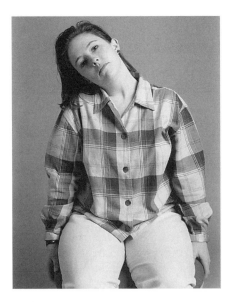

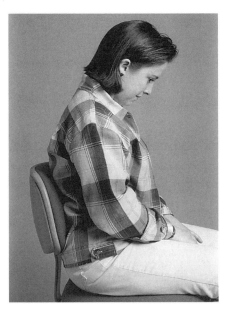

FIGURE 8. Tilt head to the right side to stretch muscles on the side of the neck. Hold for 15 seconds. Repeat and change sides.

FIGURE 9. Tilt head forward to stretch muscles of the back of the neck. Hold 15 seconds. Repeat. Pain with this exercise indicates overstretching.

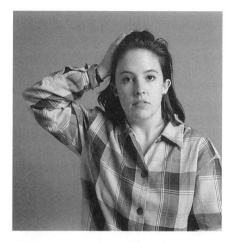

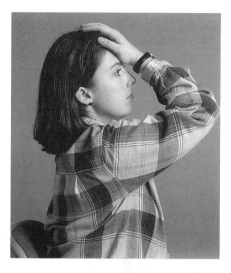

FIGURE 10. Bend head to the side into resisted force applied by the palm of the hand. Hold 20–30 seconds. Engage the neck in full range of motion and repeat.

FIGURE 11. Flex head against resisted force applied by hand. Hold 20–30 seconds. Engage the neck in full range of motion and repeat.

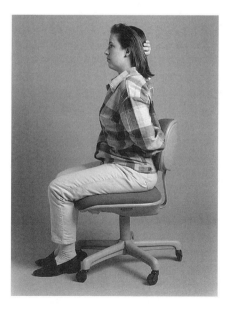

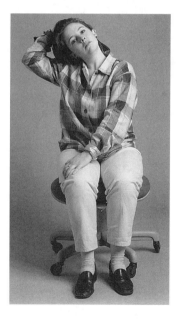

FIGURE 12. To stretch the neck and one shoulder, extend head back against force of applied palm while extending opposite arm behind back. Hold 15 seconds, change sides, and repeat.

FIGURE 13. Grasp back of head and pull head into flexion to one side and rotation to the opposite side. Hold 15 seconds, repeat, and change sides.

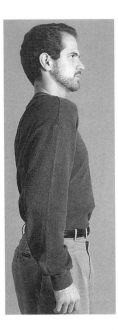

FIGURE 14. Rotate shoulders 360° for 15 seconds. Reverse direction and repeat.

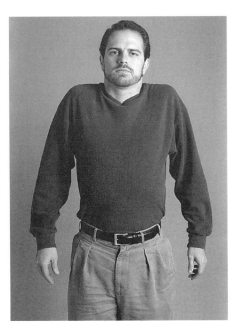

FIGURE 15. To help relieve tension in the shoulders and neck, shrug shoulders toward ears. Hold for 5 seconds and repeat.

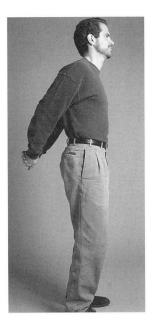

FIGURE 16. To stretch the shoulders and arms, interlace fingers behind the back and extend arms up. Hold 15 seconds and repeat.

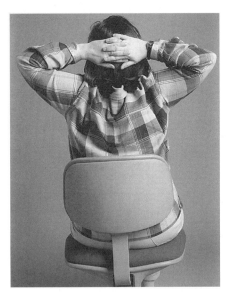

FIGURE 17. Interlace fingers behind the head and extend elbows back until stretching is felt in both shoulders. Hold 15 seconds and repeat.

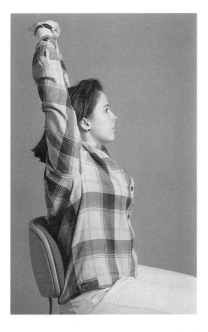

FIGURE 18. Interlace fingers with palms facing the ceiling and extend arms above the head until stretch is felt in both shoulders. Hold 15 seconds and repeat.

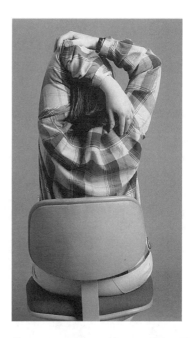

FIGURE 19. Grasp elbow with opposite hand behind the head and pull elbow to contralateral side until a stretch is felt in shoulder and upper arm. Hold 15 seconds and repeat.

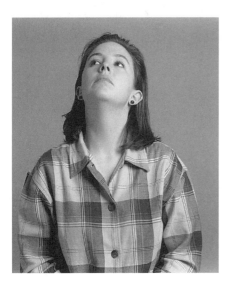

FIGURE 20. Extend head back until a stretch is felt. Hold 15 seconds and repeat.

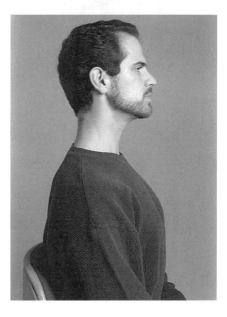

FIGURE 21. Lengthen neck by raising head vertically. Hold for 15 seconds and repeat.

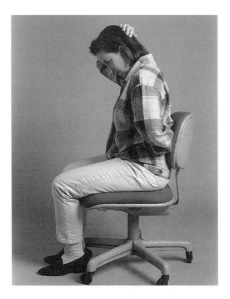

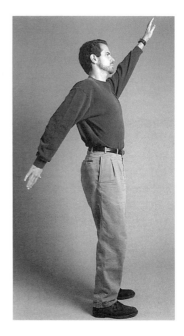

FIGURE 22. Pull head into flexion with one hand while extending the other arm behind the back to stretch the neck and one shoulder. Hold 15 seconds and repeat.

FIGURE 23. Extend one arm maximally while flexing the other arm maximally to stretch the shoulders. Hold 15 seconds, repeat, and change sides.

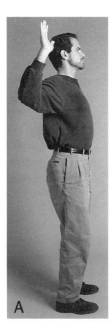

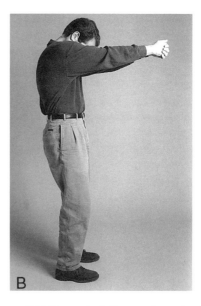

FIGURE 24. *A*, Flex elbows 90 ° and abduct and extend arms. Hold 15 seconds. *B*, Flex arms forward and clasp hands while flexing the head and hold 15 seconds. Repeat. This exercise stretches the neck, shoulders, and arms.

BACK INJURIES

Although there is ambiguity in the literature about sitting erect versus sitting reclined, it is generally agreed that the erect position is more ergonomically correct. Enough lower back support should be supplied to the patient so that the ears, shoulders, and hips align vertically (Fig. 25). Although this erect position is considered ergonomically correct, EMG studies of the back have shown that erector spinae muscle activity was greater in the erect spine, suggesting more back stress than in a slightly reclined patient. The normal erect seated position causes the lumbar to straighten from its normal lordotic curve. Also, the reclined spine is considered to reduce strain on vertebral discs and back muscles as opposed to the forward slouched position, which increases tension on ligaments, discs, and facet joints of the vertebrae.[2,34] Trunk flexion in the seated position increases posterior force on vertebral discs, which can promote disc prolapse.[7] Why increased pressure on discs causes pain is still debated. Thus, an ergonomically correct chair would include a lower, slightly reclined backrest that would allow for lower back lordosis with some reclining. This sloping backrest allows for transfer of weight from the upper back to the backrest. The recline should be minimal to avoid promoting neck flexion. Static contractions of the erector spinae muscles cause erector spinae fatigue sooner than dynamic work. This static work may be induced by attempting to sit erect without a backrest. Excessive static contractions may impair blood flow and cause an accumulation of waste products that together produce inflammation that accompanies pain, and pain can exacerbate muscle tension, creating a continuous cycle.[7] The importance of proper pelvic rotation using the psoas muscle instead of the commonly used back extensors also has been emphasized. Use of the back extensors for pelvic rotation leads to rapid muscle fatigue.[10] Exercise programs should include point immobilization, moderate aerobics to increase circulation, and muscle strengthening of the trapezius and the erector spinae muscles.[7] Stretching exercises are shown in Figures 26 and 27. Patients should be taught how to massage their

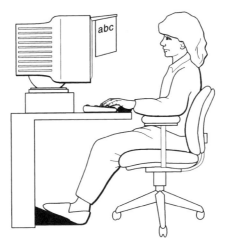

FIGURE 25. Correct ergonomic posture.

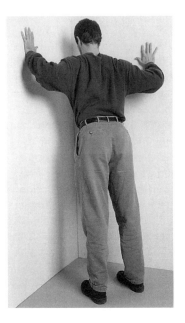

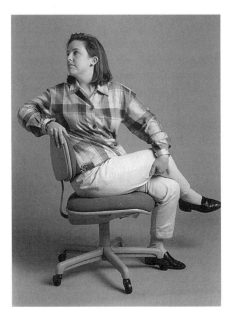

FIGURE 26. To stretch the upper back, place arms on the walls of a corner and lean into the wall keeping the back straight. Hold 15 seconds and repeat.

FIGURE 27. To stretch the back and thigh, sit in a chair and twist the torso to one side with legs crossed while pulling the leg to the opposite side. Hold 15 seconds and repeat.

neck, shoulders, and lower back and be instructed to perform this therapy several times a day. Exercise sessions should be 30–60 minutes in duration three to four times a week. Short rests averaging 5–10 minutes an hour are also recommended. Workers should alternate with tasks that are more active and require less sitting. Studies have shown that even though an electric typewriter requires the use of more force than an electric keyboard, the trapezius load in keyboard users is greater. This observation suggests that musculoskeletal disorders may be caused not only by the visual characteristics of the terminals but also on the overall nature of the work of keyboard operators, i.e., added psychological stresses.[2]

LOWER EXTREMITY INJURIES

Prolonged sitting at any job can promote decreased circulation and increased edema of the lower extremities, which may cause pain to the legs. It has been suggested that seating pads with minimal vibration or, also, constantly changing configurations may help alleviate symptoms. There are a number of ergonomically correct postures for the lower extremities. The feet should be flat so that weight is correctly distributed, and high heels should be avoided. There should be plenty of leg room to promote frequent mov-

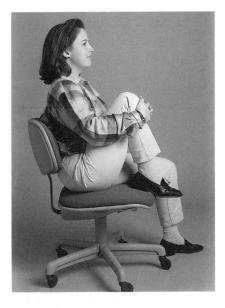

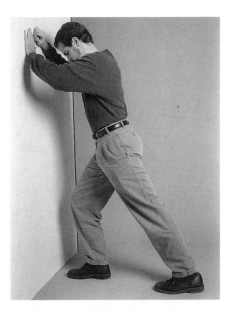

FIGURE 28. To stretch one thigh, sit in a chair and flex one hip, pulling knees toward chest. Hold 15 seconds, repeat, and change sides.

FIGURE 29. To stretch the calf, lean into a wall with one leg extended with heels on the ground. Hold 15 seconds, repeat, and change sides.

ing.[10] Subjects can do squats and bends every 1–2 hours to stretch the legs and increase circulation in the lower extremities.[10] Subjects should use a foot rest for lower leg support if the feet do not touch the ground when the rest of the body is in an ergonomically correct position (see Fig. 25). Exercises for the lower extremities are shown in Figures 28 and 29.

EYE STRAIN

Studies have shown that the preferred viewing distance from the screen is 60–90 cm and that the average distance of resting point accommodation is 80 cm. When a monitor is too close to the viewer, the ciliary muscles have to work two and a half times harder to focus an image on a screen. Exercises to reduce eye strain include blinking, rolling the eyes in gentle circles, and refocusing on other objects far away. People who wear bifocals should wear a separate pair of glasses to prevent neck hyperextension as a result of viewing the screen through the lower part of the glasses.[10] Another useful tip is to position the screen to provide minimal glare and to position lights directly on documents rather than on the screen. Mesh glare guards are not recommended because they are difficult to keep clean and make characters blurry and more difficult to read.[23]

PSYCHOSOCIAL STRESS

Importantly, psychosocial factors appear to contribute to musculoskeletal disorders among computer users. Higher incidences of musculoskeletal complaints have been noted in subjects who have more intellectually demanding work.[20]

Psychosocial factors also may play an important role in computer-related musculoskeletal symptoms. One study correlated lower levels of coworker support with more severe complaints of hand and arm weaknesses.[29] Differences also have been observed in frequency of musculoskeletal complaints among computer operators in different ethnic groups.

YOUNG COMPUTER USERS

Emphasis should be placed on teaching children proper computer posture, because poor habits start early and people are beginning to use computers at earlier ages. In a survey of 127 middle school students conducted in 1996, 57% worked at a computer at least 3 hours a week, 80% said that the way they sit could be affecting their posture, and 36% said they made an attempt to maintain good posture (unpublished data). The question arises concerning how many children know what proper computer posture is. Children spend many hours sitting in the classroom and playing at the computer. Education on proper sitting should be started in primary and middle school years to prevent poor posture.

DISABLED COMPUTER USERS

There are number of computer-adaptive devices for handicapped individuals. With the voice recognition system, for example, a person can speak into a system that is programmed to recognize one's voice and record the information as written text. Verbal commands such as *delete* and *print* also may be recognized.[4] Perhaps when some of

---

TABLE 3. Proper Computer Ergonomics

Align top of monitor with top of head
Position screen at arm's length
Position lights and screen to prevent glare
Use document holder to prevent the need to look down
Shoulders should be relaxed and aligned vertically with ears and hips
Chair should provide lumbar support
Elbows should be flexed 90°
Wrists should be straight to 5° of extension, with use of wrist supports if necessary
Hips should be flexed 80–90°, preferably with knees slightly below the hips
Feet should be supported on the floor or on a support to accommodate proximal posture
Take 5–10 minutes rest breaks every hour to perform stretching exercises

---

TABLE 4. Basic Principles of Preventing Computer-Related Injury

---

Education on proper ergonomic principles
Learning relaxation techniques, including frequent breaks and stretching exercises
Environmental manipulation, including reducing distracting noises and creating a relaxing work
  atmosphere

---

these devices for disabled individuals become more accessible, persons with computer-related injuries such as CTS will be able to use them.

CONCLUSION

With the exponential increase in the use of computers in jobs and schools, proper ergonomics (Table 3) and stretching exercises are imperative to prevent computer-related injuries (Table 4). Once a computer-related injury is identified, treatment should be sought immediately to prevent permanent disability.

REFERENCES

1. Andersson GBJ: Biomechanical aspects of sitting: An application to VDT terminals. Behav Info Technol 6:257–269, 1987.
2. Bergqvist U, Wolgast E, Nilsson B, Voss M: Musculoskeletal disorders among visual display terminal workers: Individual, ergonomic, and work organizational factors. Ergonomics 38:763–776, 1995.
3. Bernard B, Sauter S, Fine L, et al: Job task and psychosocial risk factors for work-related musculoskeletal disorders among newspaper employees. Scand J Work Environ Health 20:417–426, 1994.
4. Braddom RL (ed): Physical Medicine and Rehabilitation. Philadelphia, WB Saunders, 1996.
5. Brin MF: Interventional neurology: Treatment of neurological conditions with local injection of botulinium toxin. Arch Neurobiol 54:173–189, 1991.
6. Byl N, Wilson F, Merzenich M, et al: Sensory dysfunction associated with repetitive strain injuries of tendinitis and focal hand dystonia: A comparative study. J Orthop Sports Phys Ther 23:234–244, 1996.
7. Carter JB, Banister EW: Musculoskeletal problems in VDT work: A review. Ergonomics 37:1623–1648, 1994.
8. Cohen L, Hallett M: Hand cramps: Clinical features and EMG patterns in focal dystonia. Neurology 38:1005–1012, 1988.
9. Diamond J: The curse of the qwerty. Discover 34–42, April 1997.
10. Doheny M, Linden P, Sedlak C: Reducing orthopaedic hazards of the computer work environment. Orthop Nurs 14:7–15, 1995.
11. Douglas SD, Happ AJ: Evaluating performance discomfort, and subjective preference between computer keyboard designs. Human-computer interaction—applications and case studies. Proceedings of the 5th International Conference on Human-Computer Interaction. 2:1064–1069, 1993.
12. Downs DG: Non-specific work-related upper extremity disorders. Am Fam Physician 55:1296–1302, 1997.
13. Evans J: Office conditions influence VDU operator's health. Health and Safety at Work 34–36, December 1985.
14. Fernstrom EA, Ericson MO: Upper-arm elevation during office work. Ergonomics 39:1221–1230, 1996.

15. Fogleman, Brogmus G: Computer mouse use and cumulative trauma disorders of the upper extremities. Ergonomics 38:2465–2475, 1995.
16. Fry H: Overuse syndromes in musicians 100 years ago: A historical review. Med J Aust 146:620–625, 1986.
17. Gerard MJ, Armstrong TJ, Foulke JA, Martin BJ: Effects of key stiffness on force and the development of fatigue while typing. Am Ind Hyg Assoc J 57:849–854, 1996.
18. Hagberg M, Wegman D: Prevalence rates and odds ratios of shoulder–neck diseases in different occupational groups. Br J Ind Med 44:602–610, 1987.
19. Reference deleted.
20. Hedge A, Powers J: Wrist postures while keyboarding: Effects of a negative slope keyboard system and full motion forearm supports. Ergonomics 38:508–517, 1995.
21. Horie S, Hargens A, Rempel D: Effect of keyboard wrist rest in preventing carpal tunnel syndrome. Proceedings of the American Public Health Association. Annual Meeting 319, 1993.
22. Karwowski W: The effects of computer interface design on human postural dynamics. Ergonomics 37:703–724, 1994.
23. Larson N, MacLeod D, Kennedy E: An ergonomics guide for computer users. Can J Infect Control 10:9–14, 1995.
24. Mellion MB (ed): Sports Medicine Secrets. Philadelphia, Hanley & Belfus, 1994.
25. Murata K, Araki, Okajima F, Saito Y: Subclinical impairment in the median nerve across the carpal tunnel among female VDT operators. Int Arch Occup Environ Health 68:75–79, 1996.
26. Newmark J, Hockberg F: Isolated painless manual incoordination in musicians. J Neurol Neorosurg Psychiatry 50:291–295, 1987.
27. O'Young B, Young M, Stiens S (eds): PM&R Secrets. Philadelphia, Hanley & Belfus, 1997.
28. Parsons CA: Use of wrist rest by data input VDU operators. Contemp Ergon 319–321, 1991.
29. Pascarelli E, Kella J: Soft-tissue injuries related to use of the computer keyboard. J Occup Med 35:522–532, 1993.
30. Scalet E: Strain and injury. In Scalet EA, Stewart TFM, McGee K (eds): VDT Health and Safety: Issues and Solutions. Lawrence, KS, Ergosyst Associates, 1987.
31. Stack B: Keyboard RSI: The Practical Solution. Hobart, Meuden Press, 1987.
32. Tintinalli JE, Ruiz E, Krome R: Emergency Medicine. New York, McGraw Hill, 1996.
33. Twitchell TE: Sensory factors in movement. J Neurophysiol 17:250–254, 1954.
34. Villanueva MB, Sotoyama M, Jonai H, Saito S: Adjustments of posture and viewing parameters of the eye to changes in the screen height of the visual display terminal. Ergonomics 39:933–945, 1996.
35. Wersted M, Bjorklund R: Shoulder muscle tensions induced by two VDU-based tasks of different complexity. Ergonomics 34:137–150, 1991.

ROBERT P. PANGRAZI, PhD

CHARLES B. CORBIN, PhD

21

Exercise and Youth

Much has been written about the fitness and physical activity of children. However, guidelines and recommendations for children and youth are often based on less than scientific information. Exercise prescription models designed for adults are commonly directly applied to youth. This chapter presents a brief history of fitness and physical activity as it applies to children and youth, which sets the stage for the discussion of prescription of physical activity guidelines designed specifically for children and youth.

A few definitions are needed so the discussion is based on a common understanding of terms. *Physical activity* is an umbrella term that covers all types of activity. It is defined in this chapter as "any bodily movement produced by skeletal muscles that results in energy expenditure."[45]

Exercise describes "planned, structured, and repetitive bodily movement done to improve or maintain one or more components of physical fitness"[45] and is a subset of physical activity. Exercise is usually goal-related and designed to enhance components of physical fitness such as strength, endurance, flexibility, and aerobic capacity.

Physical fitness for youth is usually defined as an outcome(s) measured with a fitness test, most commonly the Fitnessgram[19] or the President's Challenge.[50] Therefore, a physically fit youth is defined as one who meets criteria measured by one of these two tests.

Children describes youth between the ages of 5 and 12; *youth* are age 6–18 years; and *teens* or *adolescents* are age 13–18 years.

Product refers to an expected outcome, specifically, a fitness outcome. As described in the physical fitness definition above, it is measured by a fitness test and the sole objective is to measure physical performance in a single frame of time.

Authors' Note: This chapter draws from previously published papers by the authors. Several sections of the chapter include passages from references 24–27 and 43. The authors express their appreciation to the *President's Council on Physical Fitness and Sports Physical Activity and Fitness Research Digest*, the *Journal of Physical Education, Recreation, and Dance*, and the Council on Physical Education for Children of the American Alliance for Health, Physical Education, Recreation, and Dance for granting permission to use portions of these previously published materials. The authors also wish to thank Dr. Greg Welk, who contributed to the preparation of some of the cited papers.

Process is defined as ongoing and continuous participation in physical activity. The process of activity can be measured, but the focus of attention is given to regular (daily) participation in some type of physical activity. Often, emphasis is placed on lifestyle activities that will carry over into adulthood.

Based on these definitions, it is clear that the authors view physical activity and physical fitness as different concepts. Although they are often used interchangeably, they need to be viewed separately. There are a number of misconceptions about fitness and activity that prevent adults from assessing the needs of youth correctly. Below we address some key issues that affect prescription of activity for youth and offer a better understanding of their fitness status.

A HISTORY

In 1879 a German physician named Behnke warned of the danger of vigorous physical activity among children.[33] He cautioned adults to restrict activity among children because of the "natural disharmony" between the development of the size of the heart muscle and the size of the large vessels. He suggested that the blood vessels develop at a relatively slower rate than the heart muscle, making the vessels unable to accommodate the faster growing heart. He concluded that the exercising child would be in "grave danger" as a result of high blood pressure and accompanying circulatory problems.

Physical and health educators perpetuated this myth, as did supposed experts in child growth and development.[32,62,64] A widely used textbook in elementary school physical education warned ". . . the heart increases greatly in size during this growth period (11–14 years), with veins and arteries developing much more slowly. The heart, therefore, should not be overtaxed with heavy and too continuous activity."[62] As late as 1967, Hurlock's text on adolescent development indicated that until late adolescence when the size of the blood vessels catches up with the size of the heart, ". . . too strenuous exercise may cause an enlargement of the heart and result in valvular disease."[32] Apparently these experts had cited other experts, each of whom had relied on Behnke's 1879 research.

The myth of children being unable to perform vigorous exercise persisted in the literature well into the 1960s even though data debunking the ideas of Behnke had been published in 1937. Karpovich reexamined Behnke's data and showed that a simple mathematical error had been made.[33] Although the circumference of the artery of children is proportionally small compared to the size of the heart, the blood-carrying capacity of the artery is proportional to increases in heart size. Behnke assumed that the blood-carrying capacity of the artery could be measured using the circumference of the artery when, in fact, it is the cross-sectional area of the interior of the artery that is critical. Karpovich was not the only one to debunk the "child heart" myth. Boas conducted studies with exercising children that led him to conclude that during vigorous exercise the muscles will "flag" so that the child will "collapse before the heart is called for its last ounce of effort."[14]

Even though research discredited the notion that children were incapable of vigorous exercise, many educators were skeptical about prescribing strenuous activity for children well into the 1960s. Texts for elementary school physical educators began to include sections documenting the cardiovascular capabilities of children[21] and repudiating earlier incorrect statements. Still, not all physical educators were convinced of the capabilities of children, as evidenced by the fact that the 600 yard run/walk, which was introduced in 1958, continued as the measure of cardiovascular fitness for children in the 1965 and 1975 national youth fitness battery.[3] Many physical educators apparently still felt that children were not physically able to run long distances or to perform endurance activities.

During the 1960s and early 1970s, human subjects committees were appointed to ensure that safe practices were followed in research projects. These committees were somewhat reluctant to approve studies that involved exercising children. An example was an initial rejection by a human subjects committee for a study of the heart rates of children using telemetry during runs of various distances.[22] The committee felt that children should be stopped from running if heart rates exceeded 170 beats per minute (bpm) and if distances exceeded 600 yards. It was necessary to educate the committee members, which included physicians. More than a few committee members were concerned about heart murmurs and the rheumatic fever that was responsible for many of the murmurs. However, by the time the study was reviewed, rheumatic fever had been virtually eliminated with the use of antibiotics. The study was ultimately approved even though heart rates often exceeded 200 bpm and distances were as long as 800 yards.

In 1980 longer runs became part of national physical fitness test batteries for children.[2] Only after much research, such as that proposed and first rejected by a human subjects committee, did experts feel that it was appropriate for children to perform vigorous physical activity.

As this overview shows, the topics of fitness and activity for youth often lead to discussions filled with strong opinions and few facts. Adults can quickly become emotional about the current plight and decline of America's youth. In addition, most of the discussions about children are based on an adult perspective. Many adults believe that youth have the same needs as adults and that they should reach these adult standards. This chapter reviews the current body of knowledge related to youth and activity gives a clearer picture of their actual activity patterns based on existing research.

THE FITNESS OF AMERICAN YOUTH

Since the early 1950s, when the results of studies using the Kraus-Weber test were reported, it has been assumed by many that American children and youth are low in physical fitness. The results of this famous study led to a *Sports Illustrated* article entitled "The Report That Shocked the President."[17] Over the past 40 years, the popular media have reinforced the notion that American children are unfit. However, recent research suggests that our children and youth are much fitter than previously reported.

A complete report of the status of child and youth fitness was recently published.[23] When compared to the most recent criterion referenced standards, most children and youth did quite well on fitness tests. On all health-related fitness tests, most children and youth were considered fit. When data from the last four national surveys of youth fitness conducted by the American Alliance of Health, Physical Fitness, Recreation, and Dance (AAHPERD) and the President's Council on Physical Fitness and Sports were compared, it was found that youth of today are just as fit, if not more fit than youth of the 1950s, 1960s, and 1970s.

Interestingly, many people continue to believe that most youth are unfit even though no longitudinal data support this belief. The reason for a lack of longitudinal data is that definitions of physical fitness changed over the years. The first AAHPERD Youth Fitness Test (AAHPER at the time) included many skill-related fitness test items. Recently health-related fitness (HRF) has been emphasized in national fitness test batteries because improvement in these components contributes to good health and feelings of well being. Not only have the test items changed, but standards for rating have changed. Today it is clear that an exceptionally high performance on fitness test does not necessarily reflect good health, especially when the performance is based on skill-related fitness tests such as the 50-yard dash and long jump. Evidence suggests that more moderate amounts of health-related physical fitness activity is enough to contribute to good health.[13,61]

There is one exception to the fitness status of today's teenagers. Because none of the four national surveys measured body fatness, it is impossible to compare the body composition of children participating in previous youth fitness tests. However, recent studies have shown that American children and youth today are slightly fatter than they were 20 years ago,[29,54] but at least 80% of American children still meet health-related fitness standards for body fatness.[36]

HEREDITY, TRAINABILITY, AND MATURATION: LIMITING FACTORS

Research has shown that a significant amount of fitness test performance is explained by heredity.[15,16] It is clear that heredity and maturation strongly impact fitness scores.[16,42] In fact, these factors may have more to do with youth fitness scores than activity level. Lifestyle factors, such as nutrition, and environmental factors, such as heat, humidity, and pollution, also can influence test performance. The important point is that fitness improvement and performance is substantially limited by factors that cannot be controlled or mediated.

Some youngsters have a definite advantage on tests because of the types of muscle fibers they inherit. Others inherit a predisposition to perform well on tests. For instance, some untrained children score better and some trained children do not score as well as others simply because of their genetic predisposition.

Heredity, however, represents more than an inherited ability that predisposes youngsters to high performance. "Trainability" is another major factor that is inherited.[16] Trainability allows some people to receive more benefit from training (regular physical activity) than others. Figure 1 illustrates the point. Child A does the same activity as child B throughout a semester. Child A shows dramatic improvement immediately, but child B does not. Child A simply responds more favorably to training than child B. Child A inherited a system that is responsive to exercise. Child A not only gets

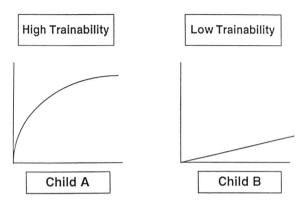

FIGURE 1. Variation in trainability. When both children participate in the same activities, child A will respond more favorably to training.

fit and scores well on the test but gets feedback that tells him or her that "the activity works—it makes me fit." Child B scores poorly, receives no feedback, and concludes that "activity doesn't improve my fitness, so why try?" However, child B *will* improve in fitness—it will just take longer and the amount of improvement may be less. The patterns shown here are only two examples; there are many degrees of trainability.

Should it be assumed that there is little use in helping students to become more active? Certainly not. Regardless of the role of heredity in the fitness performance and trainability of youth, all can benefit from regular physical activity. Some children will need more encouragement and positive feedback because their improvement will be in smaller increments and of a lesser magnitude.

Age and maturation also affect fitness test performance. Although it is apparent to most professionals that some youngsters mature faster than others, what is often forgotten is the importance of maturation in relationship to performance. If two youngsters are the same age and gender, but one is physiologically older (advanced maturation), the more mature youngster probably will perform better on tests. Fitness norms show that children also do better on fitness tests as they age. In such cases, fitness test scores for an active child might be lower than those of a more mature and less active youngster. Maturation can override the effects of activity among young children. As youth reach their high school years, maturation becomes less of a mediating factor on physical performance.

Age also plays a role in fitness performance.[42] Older children are often more mature than younger children. The biggest differences occur when immature children are in the same group as postpubescent children. Older students will perform better than younger children in the same grade.

FITNESS AND ACTIVITY

Many adults believe that fitness in youngsters is primarily a reflection of the amount of activity children perform on a regular basis. Physical activity does has some positive effect on the fitness of children, but assuming that youngsters who score high on fitness tests are active and those who do not score well are inactive is a mistake. Physical activity is an important variable in fitness development for adults, but other factors are of equal or greater importance for children and youth.

What accounts for the low relationship between physical activity and fitness among youth?[46,47,53] In addition to differences in structure, trainability, maturation, and age, another factor is that children are more homogeneously active than adults. Rowland has shown the high activity levels of children compared to adults.[56] Even the least active child is rarely totally sedentary and the most active child does not run marathons. Accordingly, the most active child will not move ahead of less active children on fitness tests based on activity alone. Further, if all children are encouraged to be active and take up the challenge, they will show improvement, but position in the group will not likely change much. Once it is understood that activity and fitness are not highly correlated, it is important to understand the implications of this weak association.

Assuming that a child is inactive based on scores on a fitness test creates unforeseen problems. Youth want to perform well in front of their peers. Most youngsters who are encouraged to do regular exercise to improve their fitness scores take this challenge seriously. When fitness tests are given, they expect to do well on the tests if they have been exercising regularly and, conversely, others expect them to do well. If, however, they receive scores that are lower than expected or lower than other children, they may become disappointed. They are especially discouraged if an adult concludes that their relatively low fitness status is a reflection of inactivity. Similarly, assuming youngsters who make high scores on fitness tests are more active than others also may lead to incorrect conclusions. Youngsters who are genetically gifted may be inactive but perform well on fitness tests. If not taught otherwise, these gifted youngsters learn that it is possible to be fit and healthy without being active.

Fitness tests are best used when they educate youngsters about the status of their physical fitness. Since fitness tests have limitations, care should be used in recommending fitness testing for remedial problems. Before fitness tests are prescribed, a clear understanding of the purpose for testing should be defined. The three major uses of fitness testing are (1) to learn the process of evaluating one's personal fitness level, (2) to discover one's personal best physical performance, and (3) to evaluate the goals of the institution.

The most useful approach for use with most youth is the process of *personal fitness evaluation*. This approach is student-centered, concerned with the process of fitness testing, and places less emphasis on performance scores. With this technique, students are asked to find a friend with whom they feel comfortable. They work with the friend to help each other develop a fitness profile. The Fitnessgram test[19] is best used for personal fitness evaluation because it utilizes criterion-referenced health standards. Each student strives to reach personal health standards rather than an arbitrary standard that is unrelated to health. The goals is to teach students the process of fitness testing so they can evaluate their health status during adulthood without a supervisor. The results are the property of the student and are not posted or shared with other students. The self-testing program is an educational endeavor; it allows for more frequent evaluation because it can be done quickly and informally.

The *personal best* approach may appeal to gifted performers and to students who want to measure their maximum performance. The objective is to achieve a maximum score in each of the test items that are normative-based. This type of program has been in place for years for most fitness tests, with a number of awards[50] offered to high-level performers. This is a formal testing program as compared to the self-testing approach discussed above. It mandates that test items be performed correctly, following test protocol exactly. Since this program requires maximal performance, it may not be motivating to less capable students and requires a considerable amount of time to complete. Some students are threatened and fear embarrassment of failing to perform well in front of peers. Students can feel less threatened if they can choose to participate in a personal best testing session or decide to avoid such testing. Testing opportunities can be offered after or before school and on a weekend when school is not in session.

The third approach, *institutional evaluation*, entails evaluating the fitness levels of students to see if the school is reaching its desired objectives. Institutional objectives are closely tied to the physical education curriculum. If the curriculum being taught to students is adequate and the goals are reasonable, students should be able to reach institutional goals. A common approach is to establish a percentage of the student body that must meet or exceed criterion-referenced health standards for a fitness test. If the percentage is below established institutional objective standards, the curriculum should be modified to increase the percentage of students meeting the health standards.

Because institutional evaluation affects teachers and curriculum offerings, it should be done in a formal and standardized manner. A common approach is to train a team of parents to administer tests throughout the system. This ensures accuracy and consistency across all schools in the district. Each test item is reviewed separately, because it is possible that objectives are being reached for some but not all items. To avoid testing all students every year, many institutions only evaluate students during their fifth-, eighth-, and tenth-grade years. This minimizes the amount of formal testing youngsters have to endure during their school career.

When the three different approaches for testing are reviewed, the personal fitness evaluation is most likely the most meaningful to students. It focuses on the process of evaluation rather than a product expressing a one-time performance. It can be done in the least amount of time, is educational, and can be done frequently. In addition, little instructional time is lost, and youth learn to evaluate their personal fitness, a skill that will serve them for a lifetime.

PHYSICAL ACTIVITY OR FITNESS?

An important question to consider is whether the focus of activity prescription should be placed on physical fitness performance or participation in regular activity. The issue is one of product versus process. Asking the question of "how many, how fast, or how far" places emphasis on the product of fitness. Product orientation has been used for years, as evidenced by the nationwide focus on fitness testing and performance. In contrast, prescribing moderate daily activity that all youngsters can accomplish places the focus on the process of participation in regular physical activity. A process focus involves activity and participation rather than fitness scores and award systems. Young exercisers who focus on the product of fitness often burn out or become discouraged after a short time. For example, when running against the clock, improvement continues to the point at which it is impossible to go any faster. This lack of improvement becomes discouraging to a product-oriented student. In like fashion, emphasizing product outcomes with youth causes them to become discouraged if they fail to reach goals their peers have reached.

All youth have the right to a lifetime of physical activity and health. When youth fail to learn how to live an active lifestyle, they may not become active and healthy adults. A study conducted by the U.S. Department of Health and Human Services[52] showed that about half of American children were not acquiring enough knowledge and skill to develop a healthy cardiovascular system. The same studies showed that only about a third of America's youth participate in organized physical education programs. A statement issued by the American Academy of Pediatrics reported that children ages 2–12 spend about 25 hours a week watching television.[1] Even in school programs, children may spend only 1 hour a week in an organized physical education lesson. Emphasis must be placed on developing habits that carry over to out-of-school activities. The school cannot develop patterns of activity alone; active lifestyles need to be encouraged at home and by medical professionals.

PRESCRIPTION MODELS

THE EXERCISE PRESCRIPTION MODEL

The health fitness movement for adults began to gain momentum in the 1960s. Paul Dudley White, physician for President Eisenhower during the 1950s, emphasized the health value of physical activity,[49] and his national visibility brought attention to the health benefits of activity. The classic 1953 study of Morris et al.[38] on London transportation workers provided good evidence for the health value of physical activity.[38] By the early 1960s, Taylor and colleagues had added to the body of literature supporting the value of physical activity for health.[60] Rehabilitation programs for cardiac patients using physical activity were gaining credibility due to the work of pioneers such as Hellerstein and Wolffe. The exercise prescription model (EPM) was developed and served as the basis for most cardiovascular exercise for the next two decades.

During the late 1950s and 1960s, considerable work was conducted regarding the EPM in an attempt to define the intensity and frequency of short-duration exercise required to promote gains in cardiovascular fitness as measured by $VO_{2\ max}$. Karvonen's classic research identified the threshold of training and provided a basis for the EPM.[34] By 1966, widely used exercise physiology texts cited Karvonen's formula for fitness development. DeVries, for example, cited the work of Karvonen and noted that exercise must be performed at 60% of heart rate reserve.[28] This guideline is similar to rules of thumb advocated for performance improvement by swimming and track coaches of the era. Whatever the original reasons for research concerning the EPM and the related concepts of threshold of training and target zone heart rates, the major emphasis in exercise prescription was on performance improvement ($VO_{2\ max}$) as opposed to health enhancement.

By the 1970s, the EPM and its focus on high-intensity and short-duration activity (using percentage of maximum heart rate or oxygen consumption as the criterion for intensity) was firmly established for adults. In 1972, the American Heart Association published an exercise testing and training handbook.[6] By 1978, the quickly emerging American College of Sports Medicine (ACSM) published its first position statement outlining the frequency, intensity, duration, and mode of exercise prescription necessary to produce cardiovascular fitness gains for adults.[4] The statement was updated in 1990,[5] and, most recently, the American Heart Association released recommendations for physical activity programs for all Americans.[7]

The EPM and the exercise guidelines based on this model have been useful and effective. For young adults of Western cultures, exercise programs based on the EPM are useful because cardiovascular fitness can be achieved without a major time commitment. Improved fitness can be accomplished by performing continuous exercise on as few as three days per week. This allows busy people to fit moderate- to high-intensity exercise into their otherwise sedentary lifestyles. In addition, the EPM is particularly effective for athletes and those interested in optimal physical performance.

Ironically, EPM—the model for prescribing adult physical activity that gained the greatest attention—was quite different than the type of activity that seemed effective for public health promotion. Although the epidemiologic literature suggested that exercise of longer duration and relatively low intensity reduced the risk of heart disease,[38,60] the type of exercise prescription gaining notoriety was shorter in duration and of higher intensity.

Because improvement in cardiovascular fitness (rather than the reduction of health risk) was central to the EPM, measures of cardiovascular fitness were of particular importance. The 12-minute run developed by Cooper to test the cardiovascular fitness of military personnel was popularized for the general public in the book *Aerobics*.[20] Shorter runs were developed for children and, in 1980, the health-related physical fitness test that included a mile run was adopted by AAHPERD.[2] By 1985, all of the major national fitness tests included a distance run of at least a mile. The ability of children to perform vigorous physical activity was acknowledged. In the absence of specific research to guide recommendations, the EPM was used to design exercise programs for children. Professionals had come full circle. Instead of fearing for the health of children who participated in vigorous exercise, guidelines for physical activity were similar to those designed for adults.

A LIFESTYLE PHYSICAL ACTIVITY MODEL: THE NEW STRATEGY

In July 1992 the Centers for Disease Prevention and Control (CDC) and ACSM, in cooperation with the President's Council on Physical Fitness and Sports, issued a statement acknowledging the importance of lifestyle physical activity as a means of reducing disease risk.[18] The recommendation is to accumulate throughout the day a minimum of 30 minutes of moderate-intensity physical activity over most days of the week. Examples of such activities are climbing stairs, gardening, raking leaves, dancing, and walking. Activity also can come from planned exercise or recreation such as jogging, playing tennis, swimming, cycling, and walking 2 miles daily.[18]

Blair and colleagues have called this "new strategy" the lifestyle exercise model.[12] Haskell, in a 1994 lecture to ACSM, also advocated the adoption of a lifestyle exercise model he called the physical activity health paradigm.[30] This chapter refers to this model as the lifetime physical activity model (LPAM). Strong scientific evidence exists to support the LPAM.[30] The work of Paffenbarger and colleagues showed that the expenditure of 2000 kcal per week resulted in a significant reduction in morbidity and mortality among Harvard alumni.[39–41] Those who expended 2000–3500 kcal per week attained the optimal value from exercise. The studies of Harvard men showed that lifestyle activities such as climbing stairs, walking, doing physically active household activities, and participating in active sports helped reduce disease risk not only for heart disease but for cancer and other types of hypokinetic conditions. Leon and colleagues, studying a different group of adults, found that a 1500-kcal per week expenditure through moderate-intensity physical activity produced similar health benefits to those found for the Harvard alums.[35] Based on a literature review, Haskell suggested 150 kcal per day (1050 kcal per week) as the minimum threshold for lifestyle exercise.[30] These studies have demonstrated that health benefits accrue from lower-intensity, longer-duration exercise.

Based on research at the Cooper Institute for Aerobics Research, Blair has proposed that adults expend 3 kilocalories per kilogram of body weight per day (kcal/kg/day) in physical activity to achieve the benefits of regular physical activity.[11] This standard is similar to the one used by previous researchers to classify people as "very active"[37] and amounts to about 200 kcal per day for a 150-pound person. The kcal/kg/day standard allows individuals to calculate the caloric expenditure (based on their body weight) required to obtain health benefits. The physical activity necessary to expend 1000–2000 calories per week or 3 kcal/kg/day is the basis on which the CDC/ACSM guidelines for lifestyle physical activity were developed.

The LPAM differs from the EPM in several ways. First, the LPAM focuses on the amount of physical activity necessary to produce health benefits as associated with reduced morbidity and mortality rather than fitness and performance benefits. While the LPAM promotes fitness as it relates to good health, it does not focus on fitness performance, as does the EPM. Moderate- to high-intensity exercise of shorter duration as outlined by the EPM was designed to promote changes on fitness tests such as $VO_{2\,max}$. Second, the LPAM recognizes the value of a wide range of physical activities that expend calories throughout the day rather than requiring a single session of continuous moderate to vigorous physical activity. Finally, the LPAM acknowledges that some activity is better than none at all and that, up to a point, progressively increasing amounts of physical activity provide added health benefits.

The shift of the LPAM from the EPM does not mean, however, that the EPM is no longer a useful model. For young adults with limited amounts of time, moderate to vigorous physical activity is still an effective approach to achieving health benefits. For those who are interested in enhancing fitness for relatively high-level performance, such as in sports or for active careers such as in law enforcement or the military, the EPM is also an effective model. However, the type of exercise prescribed in the EPM is not necessarily the best approach for the general population that wants to receive substantial health benefits.[61]

CHILDREN AND THE EXERCISE PRESCRIPTION MODEL

Just as most physical activity recommendations for adults have been based on the EPM for the past 20–30 years, recommendations for children have been based principally on guidelines evolving from the EPM. Rowland concluded that children need to follow the same exercise prescription as adults to achieve cardiovascular fitness.[55] Using Karvonen's heart rate reserve method for calculating target heart rates, Sady estimated a heart rate of 159 as the threshold for aerobic exercise for most children.[57] These results and the findings of other studies have served as the basis for recommendations suggesting that children need to perform 20–30 minutes of continuous moderate to vigorous physical activity (MVPA) at least three times a week. Typically heart rate standards are used as the indicator of MVPA. Recommendations vary but, in general, heart rates advocated are 140 bpm and higher.

Using heart rate standards as indicators has caused several researchers to conclude that many, if not most, children are inactive. Some examples illustrate the point. Using heart rates above 140 bpm for 20 minutes of continuous exercise as the criterion of MVPA, Armstrong and Bray found 77% of the boys and 88% of the girls they studied to be inactive by this measure.[9] In another study of younger children, Armstrong, Balding, Gentle, and Kirby found 61% of boys and 66% of girls to be inactive.[8] Using observation techniques to assess 20 minutes of MVPA as the standard, Sleap and Warburton found 86% of children to be inactive, and Baranowski, Hooks, Tsong, Cieslik, and Nader found 89.6% of children to be inactive.[10,59] In another study involving 177 trials of day-long monitoring of children averaging 703 minutes a day, Welk found 17% of children to have heart rates above 140 bpm for 20 consecutive minutes. If the EPM were used to evaluate activity, it would be easy to conclude that most children are inactive.[63]

Using data from the same studies but applying standards that are more consistent with the LPAM, a different conclusion is reached. When minutes of physical activity during the day are determined for these same studies, the data of Armstrong et al. show that, on the average, boys were active 45 minutes and girls 31 minutes of each day (above 140 bpm but not consecutive minutes).[8] In a second study, Armstrong and Bray found younger boys were active 68 minutes and girls 59 minutes each day.[9] Similarly, children studied by Baranowski et al. performed 60–70 minutes of activity per day even though 89% would be classified as inactive by the EPM standard.[10] A total of 86% of the children Sleap and Warburton studied were inactive in terms of EPM exercise, but, on average, they participated in 88 minutes of activity.[59] Data from Welk's study using activity and heart rate monitors at the same time showed that 99% of boys and 98% of girls exceeded an energy expenditure of 4 kcal/kg/day, a standard that is slightly higher than the 3 kcal/kg/day advocated by proponents of the LPAM.[63]

It is apparent that the same children who fail to meet activity standards based on the EPM generally meet standards established for the LPAM. Rather than judge children as inactive based on MVPA data, it seems more reasonable to suggest that EPM is an inappropriate model for judging activity levels of most children. Children are sporadic exercisers who alternate between vigorous activity and rest. They are high-volume exercisers who generally do not engage in continuous high-intensity exercise. Table 1 lists concepts and implications concerning physical activity and children.

APPROPRIATE ACTIVITY MODELS FOR CHILDREN

The following statements provide the basis for the selection of the specific physical activity recommendations made in this chapter. As discussed above, the models used to determine appropriate physical activity (exercise) for adults are not necessarily the most appropriate ones for planning activity for children. A 1994 consensus statement concerning physical activity for adolescents recommended a minimum of 30 minutes of moderate physical activity most days of the week and involvement in more vigorous activity at least three days per week for 20 minutes.[58] The consensus statement uses one recommendation based primarily on the LPAM (30 minutes of moderate physical activity most days of the week) and one recommendation based on the EPM (20 minutes of moderate to vigorous physical activity three days a week). The first of the two recommendations is well suited to children (age 5–12) and provides a basis for the recommendations made here. The second recommendation is appropriate for adolescents

TABLE 1. Physical Activity and Children: Basic Concepts

Concept	Implication
Young animals, including humans, are inherently active.	Children will be active if given encouragement and opportunity.
Children are concrete rather than abstract thinkers.	Children are often unwilling to persist in activity if they see no concrete reason to do so.
The relationship between activity and fitness is small among children.	Children may receive little feedback for their efforts in some activities.
Childhood activity is often intermittent and sporadic in nature.	Children will not likely do prolonged exercise without rest periods.
Total volume is a good indicator of childhood activity.	Given the opportunity, many children will perform relatively large volumes of intermittent physical activity.
Physical activity patterns vary with children of different developmental and ability levels.	Young children are not attracted to high-intensity exercise but highly skilled older children may see its value for enhancing performance in sports.

Adapted from Corbin CB, Pangrazi RP: Toward an understanding of appropriate physicial activity levels of youth. President's Council on Physical Fitness and Sports Physical Activity and Fitness Research Digest 1(8):1—8, 1994.

(age 13–18) but is not recommended for universal application to younger youth (see following section).

As discussed above, the LPAM and its recommendations for the volume of activity as determined by calories expended over time is best suited for use with children. The recommendation for 30–60 minutes of activity (total volume) for children and youth is similar to the caloric expenditure recommendations for adults above and slightly higher than the minimum recommendation made for adolescents by a panel of experts. This slightly higher recommendation as well as the inclusion of an additional recommendation of more than 60 minutes of activity on most days of the week is based on the following points:

1. Adult recommendations are based primarily on the energy expenditure necessary to reduce risk of chronic disease. The adult recommendation (and the one for adolescents) is a minimum—not an optimal—amount. Expenditure of 1000–2000 calories and up to 3500 calories per week gives extra benefits. The recommendation of 1 hour or more is within these limits.

2. Children are inherently active. Most young children perform more than minimum amounts of activity. They become less active as they grow older. Promoting relatively high activity levels (by volume) in childhood provides a buffer when activity levels begin to decrease.

3. Childhood is the time of learning skills. Children and youth learn skills through involvement in physical activity. It is important for children and youth to experience activities in all areas of the physical activity pyramid and for all parts of health-related physical fitness, not just aerobic or cardiovascular fitness. Time must be devoted to teaching physical skills so children reach a level of competency that allows them to use such skills during adulthood.

4. Calories expended in childhood and youth can help control body fatness, which can be a problem for children and youth. Children who are active when they are young are more likely to be active adults.[47,51] With higher caloric intake being a characteristic of modern society, a higher caloric output is perhaps the best remedy.

GUIDELINES FOR APPROPRIATE PHYSICAL ACTIVITY FOR CHILDREN

Based on the unique needs and interests of children, the following guidelines are presented for children ages 6–12.[24]

Guideline 1: Elementary school children should accumulate at least 30–60 minutes of age-appropriate physical activity on all or most days of the week. Previous sections of this report provide the basis for making this recommendation. It is appropriate for all preadolescent children.

Guideline 2: An accumulation of more than 60 minutes and up to several hours per day of appropriate activities is encouraged for school-age children. For reasons outlined elsewhere in this chapter, children will typically need to spend more than 30–60 minutes in activity each day. Activities of a physical nature should constitute a relatively large part of the child's day, including some periods that are more vigorous. In a typical day it should not be unusual for the time accumulated in physical activity to exceed 60 minutes and to total several hours. This guideline urges greater overall time involvement for children, with total volume of activity emphasized.

Guideline 3: Some of the child's activity each day should be for periods of 10–15 minutes or more and include moderate to vigorous activity. This activity typically will be intermittent in nature and involve alternating moderate to vigorous activity with brief periods of rest and recovery. Continuous moderate to vigorous physical activity lasting more than 5 minutes are rare among children younger than 13. Because typical activities of children involve sporadic bursts of energy, a greater time involvement rather than a greater intensity of continuous involvement is recommended. Three to six or more activity sessions spaced throughout the day may be necessary to accumulate adequate activity time for elementary school children. For older children (10–12), some of these periods should include 10–15 minutes of moderate to vigorous activity alternated with brief rest or recovery periods. If continuous activity is prescribed for children, the reasons should be made clear because children are concrete, not abstract, thinkers.

Guideline 4: Extended periods of inactivity are discouraged for children. More information for this guideline is contained in the section that follows.

Guideline 5: A variety of physical activities selected from the Physical Activity Pyramid (Fig. 2) are recommended. The Physical Activity Pyramid is a method of classifying physical activities.

In the following sections, each of the different categories of physical activity from the Physical Activity Pyramid is discussed, and applications for young children (age 5–9) and older children (age 10–12) are outlined. In general, the Physical Activity Pyramid encourages participation in activities at the lowest levels of the pyramid. Age, current fitness level, developmental level, and other factors such as hereditary predispo-

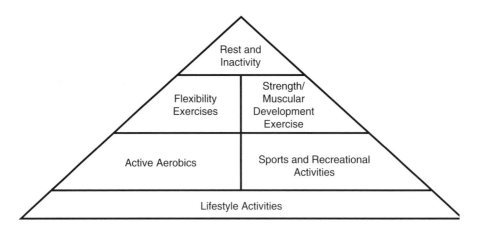

FIGURE 2. The Physical Activity Pyramid. (Adapted from Corbin CB, Lindsey R: Fitness for Life, 4th ed. Glenview, IL, Scott Foresman/Addison-Wesley, 1997.)

sition will determine the optimal amounts of activity from different levels of the pyramid for different individuals or groups of individuals.

PHYSICAL ACTIVITY PYRAMID LEVEL 1: LIFESTYLE ACTIVITIES

Activities that require large muscle activity as part of typical daily routine are considered to be lifestyle physical activities. Examples are walking to or from school, climbing the stairs, raking the leaves, and doing chores around the house that require more than a little calorie expenditure. Riding a bicycle as transportation is an example, as are physical activities such as digging, lifting, and other activities performed as part of daily work. For children, active play involving large muscles is considered to be lifestyle activity. Lifestyle activities are at the base of the pyramid because an accumulation of daily minutes of involvement in these activities has been shown to have positive health benefits. These activities are widely accessible and relatively easy to perform for people of all ages.

Recommendations for Young Children

The greatest portion of accumulated minutes of physical activity for children age 5–9 will typically come from lifestyle activities. Lifestyle activities for this age include active play and games involving the large muscles of the body. Climbing, tumbling, and other activities that require lifting the body or relocating the body in space are desirable when they can be performed safely. Activities are typically performed intermittently rather than continuously. They normally involve few rules and little formal organization. Lifestyle activities such as walking to school and being involved in household chores are appropriate.

Recommendations for Older Children

As with young children, a large portion of accumulated minutes of physical activity for children age 10–12 typically will come from lifestyle activities, which include active play and games involving the large muscles of the body. Activities are typically intermittent in nature, and older children are more likely to be involved in continuous activities than younger children. Walking to school and being involved in household chores are appropriate.

PHYSICAL ACTIVITY PYRAMID LEVEL 2: ACTIVE AEROBICS

Activities that can be done for relatively long periods without stopping are generally considered to be aerobic in nature. For optimal health benefits, some of these activities should be done at least at a moderate level. Examples of moderate activity are brisk walking, jogging or running, biking, swimming, and hiking.

Recommendations for Young Children

Participation in some aerobic activities is appropriate when it is not expected that children will participate in them continuously for a long duration. Most appropriate are intermittent aerobic activities such as recreational swimming, family walking, or aerobic activities that are included in the lifestyle activity category. Participation in continuous aerobic activities for 15 minutes or more is not recommended for this age group.

Recommendations for Older Children

Participation in aerobic activities of longer duration than for young children is appropriate for this age group; however, participation in continuous aerobic activities of long duration should not be emphasized. Because many children will not voluntarily choose to participate in continuous activity, it is important to clearly outline reasons for performing such activities. Intermittent involvement in aerobic activities is appropriate (several shorter bouts followed by rest) and is preferred by many children of this age. Note: Physical activity guidelines for adolescents recommend three days per week of 20 minutes of continuous moderate to vigorous physical activity. While some children in the 10–12 age group may *choose* to meet this guideline, it is not a basic recommendation at this age level.

PHYSICAL ACTIVITY PYRAMID LEVEL 2: ACTIVE SPORTS AND RECREATIONAL ACTIVITIES

Sports such as tennis, soccer, racquetball, and basketball and recreational activities such as canoeing and waterskiing are included in this category. Some activities such as bowling and golf are also included because, even though they require relatively low energy expenditure, they have health benefits when included as part of a total physical activity program. Recreational activities such as board games are not generally considered to be part of this category.

Recommendations for Young Children

Active sports are most appropriate for the older children, but the younger may choose to participate. Sports should be modified to meet their developmental level. In general this type of activity should be only a small part of the child's daily activity. Although age-appropriate recreational activities such as fishing or boating with the family are appropriate for young children, they are not typically high in energy expenditure. It is important for children of this age to spend time learning basic skills that are prerequisites for performing sports and other activities, such as catching, throwing, jumping, running, and striking objects.

Recommendations for Older Children

Because this is the age at which the largest number of children and youth are involved in sports, a greater amount of time will be dedicated to this type of activity. Modifications are necessary to make the activities most suitable for this age. An emphasis on conditioning for sports is premature for most children in this age group because of the low relationship between fitness and physical activity.[48] More of the time spent in this type of activity should be dedicated to learning skills and playing games rather than conditioning. Age-appropriate recreational activities that have a lifetime emphasis or that can be done with family and friends are encouraged.

PHYSICAL ACTIVITY PYRAMID LEVEL 3: EXERCISES FOR FLEXIBILITY

Exercises and physical activities designed and performed specifically to increase the length of muscles and connective tissues and to improve range of joint motion are included in this category. Some activities at lower levels in the pyramid may contribute to the development of flexibility, but specific exercises are often necessary to develop this part of fitness, even for the most active people.

Recommendations for Young Children

In general, the amount of time spent on flexibility exercises for young children need not be great. Children are more flexible than adults, and flexibility exercises therefore will be relatively easy for most children. Some formal stretching exercises can be used to illustrate the importance of this fitness component and to help maintain flexibility levels. Active play activities such as tumbling and climbing are encouraged for development of flexibility.

Recommendations for Older Children

Older children need not spend much time with this type of exercise, but it is reasonable for them to spend more time on flexibility exercises than younger children. Older children, especially boys, begin to lose flexibility. Some regular stretching is appropriate in the form of flexibility exercises or activities that promote flexibility, such as tumbling and stunts.

PHYSICAL ACTIVITY PYRAMID LEVEL 3: EXERCISES FOR STRENGTH AND MUSCULAR ENDURANCE

Exercises and physical activities designed and performed specifically to increase strength (the amount of weight one can lift) and muscular endurance (the ability to persist in muscular effort) are included in this category. Some activities at lower levels in the pyramid may contribute to the development of these parts of muscle fitness, but extra exercises are often necessary to build strength and muscular endurance, even for the most active people.

Recommendations for Young Children

Participation in some basic exercises as part of a physical education class or a regular family fitness program is appropriate. However, so long as children are accumulating adequate daily amounts of the activities from lower levels in the pyramid it is not necessary for them to spend large amounts of time performing organized calisthenics on a regular basis. Formal resistance training is not recommended. Calisthenics, as part of modified youth sports programs, should be kept to a minimum for children of this age. Overload of the muscles and bones can adequately be accomplished in activities such as those in lower levels of the pyramid.

Recommendations for Older Children

Exercises for strength and muscle endurance will be emphasized more for older children than for younger children. Older children can develop strength and muscular endurance using formal weight training. However, other activities are generally better suited to the needs of most children. Activities that require children to move and lift their own body weight, including participation in active play, games, and sports that require muscle overload, are desirable for older children. Formal conditioning exercises using body weight are appropriate, especially when alternative exercises are offered to allow all children to be successful. Formal exercises and conditioning programs as part of youth sports programs or other activity programs should not typically constitute a major part of activity periods, although children who are highly motivated may benefit from greater exposure to these activities.

PHYSICAL ACTIVITY PYRAMID LEVEL 4: REST AND INACTIVITY

Total sedentary living as well as activities involving little large muscle activity such as computer games is included in this category. Reading, watching television, and participating in other relatively inactive recreational activities have their own benefits. Abstinence from these activities is unnecessary if there is adequate involvement in other activities in the pyramid.

Recommendations for Young and Older Children

Both young and older children need some private time to be involved in play of types other than in activities using the large muscles. However, long periods of sedentary living—not typically a characteristic of children—should be discouraged. For older children, the time between activity periods can be shorter than for younger children.

GUIDELINES FOR PHYSICAL ACTIVITY FOR ADOLESCENTS

As noted earlier, a consensus statement has been issued concerning appropriate physical activity for adolescents.[58] The specific guidelines follow:

Guideline 1: All adolescents should be physically active daily, or nearly every day, as part of play, games, sports, work, transportation, recreation, physical education, or planned exercise, in the context of family, school and community activities.[58]

The consensus statement states: "Adolescents should do a variety of physical activities as part of their daily lifestyles. These activities should be enjoyable, involve a variety of muscle groups, and include some weight bearing activities. The intensity or duration of the activity is probably less important than the fact that energy is expended and a habit of daily activity is established. Adolescents are encouraged to incorporate physical activity into their lifestyles by doing such things as walking up stairs, walking or riding a bicycle for errands, having conversations while walking with friends, parking at the far end of parking lots, and doing household chores."[58]

Guideline 2: Adolescents should engage in three or or more sessions per week of activities that last 20 minutes or more at a time and that require moderate to vigorous levels of exertion.[58]

"Moderate to vigorous activities are those that require at least as much effort as brisk or fast walking. A diversity of activities that use large muscle groups are recommended as part of sports, recreation, chores, transportation, work, school physical education, or planned exercise. Examples include brisk walking, jogging, stair climbing, basketball, racquet sports, soccer, dance, swimming laps, skating, strength (resistance) training, lawn mowing, strenuous housework, cross-country skiing, and cycling."[58]

Guideline 1 for adolescents is similar to guideline 1 for children and focuses primarily on level 1 of the Physical Activity Pyramid. Guideline 2 encourages more vigorous activity. Adolescents then, are encouraged to do more sustained physical activity than children. They are encouraged to select from level 2 (active aerobics and active sports and recreational activities) and level 3 of the pyramid (muscle fitness and flexibility exercises) because these activities are more appropriate for adolescents than children. The guideline for avoiding extended periods of physical activity is as appropriate for adolescents as for children.

GUIDELINES FOR PROMOTING PHYSICAL ACTIVITY

A number of approaches can be used to increase the possibility of students being interested in activity. How fitness activities are presented contributes to the attitudes students develop about being active for a lifetime. The following suggestions are for educators and others involved in the well being of youth.

PROVIDE TIME FOR ACTIVITY IN THE SCHOOL SETTING

Since youth spend many of their waking hours in schools, it is reasonable to expect that schools and physical education can play a significant role in meeting the recommendations in this chapter. Regular physical education programs (preferably daily) should provide a significant amount of the time in activity necessary to meet the guidelines in this chapter. In addition to physical education, opportunities should be provided for children to participate in regular physical activity throughout the school day, i.e., recess and short activity periods.

INDIVIDUALIZE ACTIVITIES

Lifetime activity is a personal choice. Students who are unable to exercise or play certain sports well may not develop positive attitudes toward activity. Experiences should be presented so that youngsters can determine the workload that best suits their needs. Too often, adults set one dosage for all students, such as the mile run or 25 push-ups, only to see most students fail. Instead of specifying speed and number of repetitions, one can use time to set workload and ask students to do the best they can within the time limit. People dislike and fear experiences they perceive to be forced upon them for an external source. Voluntary long-term exercise is a more probable result when individuals are internally driven to do their best. Experiences that allow students to control the intensity of their workouts offer better opportunity for the development of positive attitudes toward activity.

EXPOSE YOUNGSTERS TO A VARIETY OF PHYSICAL ACTIVITIES

Presenting a variety of opportunities avoids the monotony of performing the same activities week after week and increases the likelihood that students will experience activities they find enjoyable. Activities also should be presented with a purpose. Activities must go beyond cursory instruction; there must be an opportunity for repetition and quality learning. Youngsters are willing to accept activities they dislike if they know they will have a chance to experience the ones they enjoy in the near future.

FOCUS FEEDBACK ON PROCESS RATHER THAN PRODUCT

For too many years, feedback about activity has focused on the product of how many, how fast, and how difficult. Students who were genetically limited but gave their best efforts often received little feedback. Instead of reinforcing only youth who score the highest, one should direct feedback to students who are doing their best. Some youth will never be able to run as fast or perform as many repetitions of exercises as more gifted students; however, if they do their best the activity is of great benefit to them. The process of activity is being involved, doing one's best, and participating regularly. Provided in a positive manner, feedback can stimulate children to extend their participation to outside the confines of physical education class.

TEACH PHYSICAL SKILLS

During physical activity, students should be able to learn new physical skills. Skills are tools that many adults use to maintain health and fitness. Many individuals maintain fitness through skill-based activities such as tennis, badminton, swimming, golf, basketball, aerobics, and bicycling. Students will have a much greater propensity to continue activities into adulthood if they feel competent. In fact, perceptions of competence are an important determinant of future physical activity. School programs must graduate students with requisite entry skills in a variety of activities.

BE AN ACTIVE ROLE MODEL

Appearance, attitude, and actions speak loudly about adults and their values regarding fitness. Adults who display physical vitality, take pride in being active, participate in activities with students, and are fit positively influence youngsters to maintain an active lifestyle. Living a lifestyle is part of teaching it. Take time to tell students why you chose to be active and how you structure activity into your daily routine.

CARE ABOUT THE ATTITUDES OF STUDENTS

Pull students toward a lifetime of activity rather than pushing them into a short-term fitness experience. Too often, adults want to force fitness on children to "make them fit." Short-term fitness training does not equate to lifetime fitness. If youngsters are trained without concern for their feelings, the result is often that children learn to dislike activity. Once developed, a negative attitude is difficult to change. This does not mean that youngsters should be allowed to avoid activity, but it implies that the physical activity experience should be a positive one designed to teach students about their personal abilities. Activity works best when it is a challenge rather than a threat. Whether an activity is a challenge or a threat depends on the perceptions of the learner, not the instructor. Help students design activity goals that are within the realm of challenge.

ENCOURAGE POSITIVE APPROACHES TO LIFETIME ACTIVITY

Help youth learn about the values of different activities and how to develop personal workouts they can *accomplish*. When students successfully accomplish activities, they develop a system of self-talk that looks at their exercise behavior in a positive light and minimizes self-criticism. Particular attention should be given to students who have special needs, such as those who are obese, inactive, or possess physical or mental disabilities.

PROMOTE ACTIVITY IN MANY ENVIRONMENTS

The school environment restricts the activity level of youngsters, who spend most of their time sitting in a classroom. Students need to know about the many possibilities for activity outside of school, such as community recreation centers, YWCAs, and Boys and Girls Clubs. Educators can show leadership by coordinating and promoting activity experiences at their schools. There is time for activity before, during, and after the formal school day. Lunch-hour intramural programs can be designed to help less able students become participants. Teaching active playground games encourages students to be active during their free time. Activity at home can be encouraged through an activity-monitoring program.

CONSIDER LIFETIME ACTIVITIES THAT ENDURE

Certain activities are more likely to become lifestyle activities than others. There is some evidence that if the following activity conditions are met, exercise becomes positively addicting and a necessary part of one's life. These steps imply that many individual activities, including walking, jogging, hiking, and biking, are activities that students will use for fitness during adulthood.

- The activity is usually best if it is noncompetitive; the student chooses and wants to do it.

- It must not require a great deal of mental effort.

- The activity can be done alone, without a partner or teammates.

- Students must believe in the value of the exercise for improving health and general welfare.

- Participants must believe that the activity will become easier and more meaningful if they persist. To become addicting, the activity must be done for at least 6 months.

- The activity should be accomplished in such a manner that the participant is not self-critical.

REFERENCES

1. American Academy of Pediatrics: Sports Medicine: Health Care for Young Athletes. Elk Grove Village, IL, AAP, 1991.
2. American Alliance of Health, Physical Education, Recreation, and Dance: Health Related Physical Fitness Test Manual. Reston, VA, American Alliance of Health, Physical Education, Recreation, and Dance, 1980.
3. American Association of Health, Physical Education, and Recreation: Youth Fitness Testing Manual. Washington, DC, American Association of Health, Physical Education, and Recreation, 1958.
4. American College of Sports Medicine: The recommended quantity and quality of exercise for developing and maintaining cardiorespiratory and muscular fitness of healthy adults. Med Sci Sports Exerc 10:vix, 1978.
5. American College of Sports Medicine: The recommended quantity and quality of exercise for developing and maintaining fitness of health adults. Med Sci Sports Exerc 22:265–274, 1990.
6. American Heart Association: Exercise Testing and Training of Apparently Healthy Individuals: A Handbook for Physicians. Dallas, American Heart Association, 1972.
7. American Heart Association: Medical/scientific statement on exercise: Benefits and recommendations for physical activity programs for all Americans. Circulation 86:2726–2730, 1992.
8. Armstrong N, Balding J, Gentle P, Kirby B: Patterns of physical activity among 1116 year old British children. BMJ 301:203–205, 1990.
9. Armstrong N, Bray S: Physical activity patterns defined by continuous heart rate monitoring. Arch Dis Child 66:245–247, 1991.
10. Baranowski T, Hooks P, Tsong Y, et al: Aerobic physical activity among third to sixth grade children. Dev Behav Pediatr 8:203–206, 1987.
11. Blair SN: C.H. McCloy Research Lecture: Physical activity, physical fitness, and health. Res Q Exerc Sport 64:365–376, 1993.
12. Blair SN, Kohl HW, Gordon NF: Physical activity and health: A lifestyle approach. Med Exerc Nutr Health 1:54–57, 1992.
13. Blair SN, Kohl HW, Paffenbarger RS, et al: Physical fitness and all-cause mortality. JAMA 262:2395–2401, 1989.
14. Boas EP: The heart rate of boys during and after exhausting exercise. J Clin Invest 10:145–151, 1931.
15. Bouchard C: Discussion: Heredity, fitness and health. In Bouchard C, Shepard RJ, Stephens T, et al. (eds): Exercise, Fitness and Health. Champaign, IL, Human Kinetics, 1990, pp 147–153.

16. Bouchard C, Dionne FT, Simoneau J, Boulay M: Genetics of aerobic and anaerobic performances. Exerc Sport Sci Rev 20:27–58, 1992.
17. Boyle RH: The report that shocked the President. Sports Illustrated, August 15, 1995, pp 30–33.
18. Centers for Disease Control and American College of Sports Medicine: Summary statement: Workshop on physical activity and public health. Sports Med Bull 28(4):7, 1994.
19. Cooper Institute for Aerobics Research: The Prudential Fitnessgram Test Administration Manual. Dallas, Cooper Institute for Aerobics Research, 1992.
20. Cooper KH: Aerobics. New York, M. Evans, 1968.
21. Corbin CB: Becoming Physically Educated in the Elementary School. Philadelphia, Lea & Febiger, 1969.
22. Corbin CB: Relationships between PWC and running performance of young boys. Res Q 43:235–238, 1972.
23. Corbin CB, Pangrazi RP: Are American children and youth fit? Res Q Exerc Sport 63:96–106, 1992.
24. Corbin CB, Pangrazi RP: Guidelines for Appropriate Physical Activity for Elementary School Children: A Position Statement of the Council for Physical Education for Children. Reston, VA, American Alliance for Health, Physical Education, Recreation, and Dance, 1998.
25. Corbin CB, Pangrazi RP: How much physical activity is enough? J Phys Educ Rec Dance 67(4):33–37, 1996.
26. Corbin CB, Pangrazi RP: Toward an understanding of appropriate physical activity levels of youth. President's Council on Physical Fitness and Sports Physical Activity and Fitness Research Digest 1(8):1–8, 1994.
27. Corbin CB, Pangrazi RP: What you need to know about the Surgeon General's Report on Physical Activity and Health. President's Council on Physical Fitness and Sports Physical Activity and Fitness Research Digest 2(6):1–8, 1996.
28. DeVries HA: Physiology of Exercise for Physical Education and Athletics. Dubuque, IA, WC Brown, 1966.
29. Gortmaker SL, Dietz WH, Sobol AN, Wehler CA: Increasing pediatric obesity in the U.S. Am J Dis Child 14:535–540, 1987.
30. Haskell WL: Health consequences of physical activity: Understanding and challenges regarding dose response. Med Sci Sports Exerc 26:649–660, 1994.
31. Haskell WL: Physical activity and health: Need to define the required stimulus. Am J Cardiol 5:4D–9D, 1985.
32. Hurlock EB: Adolescent Development. New York, McGraw-Hill, 1967.
33. Karpovich PV: Textbook fallacies regarding the development of the child's heart. Res Q 8:33–39, 1937.
34. Karvonen MJ: The effects of vigorous exercise on the heart. In Rosenbaum FF, Belknap EL (eds): Work and the Heart. New York, PB Hoebner, 1959.
35. Leon AS, Connett J, Jacobs DR, Rauramaa R: Leisure-time physical activity levels and risk of coronary heart disease and death. JAMA 258:2388–2395, 1987.
36. Looney MA, Plowman SA: Passing rates of American children and youth on the Fitnessgram criterion-referenced physical fitness standards. Med Sci Sports Exerc 61:215–223, 1990.
37. Montoye HJ: How active are modern populations? Academy Papers 21:34–45, 1987.
38. Morris JN, Heady J, Raffle P, et al: Coronary heart disease and physical activity of work. Lancet ii:1053–1057, 1111–1120, 1953.
39. Paffenbarger RS, Hyde RT, Wing AL, Hsueh RT: Physical activity, all-cause mortality, and longevity of college alumni. N Engl J Med 314:605–613, 1986.
40. Paffenbarger RS, Hyde RT, Wing AL, Steenmetz CH: A natural history of athleticism and cardiovascular health. JAMA 252:491–495, 1984.
41. Paffenbarger RS, Wing AL, Hyde RT: Physical activity as an index of heart attack risk in college alumni. Am J Epidemiol 108:161–175, 1978.
42. Pangrazi RP, Corbin CB: Age as a factor relating to physical fitness test performance. Res Q Exerc Sport 61:415–418, 1990.
43. Pangrazi RP, Corbin CB, Welk GJ: Physical activity for children and youth. J Phys Educ Rec Dance 67(4):38–43, 1996.

44. Pate RR, Baranowski T, Dowda M, Trost S: Tracking of physical activity in young children. Med Sci Sports Exerc 28:92–96, 1996.
45. Pate R, Pratt M, Blair S, et al: Physical activity and public health. JAMA 273:402–407, 1995.
46. Pate RR, Dowda M, Ross JG: Associations between physical activity and physical fitness in American children. Am J D Child 144:1123–1129, 1990.
47. Pate RR, Ross JG: Factors associated with health-related fitness. J Phys Educ Rec Dance 58(9):93–96, 1987.
48. Payne VG, Morrow JR Jr.: Exercise and $VO_{2\ max}$ in children: A meta-analysis. Res Q Exerc Sport 64:305–313, 1993.
49. Pomroy WC, White PD: Coronary heart disease in former football players. JAMA 167:711–714, 1958.
50. President's Council on Physical Fitness and Sports: The President's Challenge: Physical Fitness Program Packet. Washington, DC, President's Council on Physical Fitness and Sports, 1996.
51. Raitakari OT, Porkka KVK, Taimela S, et al: Effects of persistent physical activity and inactivity on coronary risk factors in children and young adults. Am J Epidemiol 140:195–205, 1994.
52. Ross JG, Gilbert GG: The national children and youth fitness study: A summary of findings. J Phys Educ Rec Dance 56(1):45–50, 1985.
53. Ross JG, Pate RR, Caspersen CJ, et al: Home and community in children's exercise habits. J Phys Educ Rec Dance 58(9):85–92, 1987.
54. Ross JG, Pate RR, Lohman TG, Christenson GM: Changes in body composition of children. J Phys Educ Rec Dance 58(9):74–77, 1987.
55. Rowland TW: Aerobic response to endurance training in prepubescent children: A critical analysis. Med Sci Sports Exerc 17:493–497, 1985.
56. Rowland TW: Exercise and Children's Health. Champaign, IL, Human Kinetics, 1990.
57. Sady SP: Cardiorespiratory exercise training in children. Clin Sports Med 5:493–514, 1986.
58. Sallis JF, Patrick K, Long BL: An overview of international consensus conference on physical activity guidelines for adolescents. Pediatr Exerc Sci 6:299–301, 1994.
59. Sleap M, Warburton P: Physical activity levels of 5–11 year old children in England as determined by continuous observation. Res Q Exerc Sport 63:238–245, 1992.
60. Taylor HL, Klepetar E, Keys A, et al: Death rates among physically active and sedentary employees of the railway industry. Am J Public Health 52:1697–1707, 1962.
61. U.S. Department of Health and Human Services: Physical Activity and Health: A Report of the Surgeon General. Atlanta, Centers for Disease Control and Prevention, National Center for Chronic Disease Prevention and Health Promotion, 1996.
62. Van Hagen WV, Dexter G, Williams JF: Physical Education in the Elementary School. Sacramento, California State Department of Education, 1951.
63. Welk GJ: A comparison of methods for the assessment of physical activity in children [doctoral dissertation]: Tempe, AZ, Arizona State University, 1994.
64. Young E: Hygiene in the Schools. Philadelphia, WB Saunders, 1923.

NIRMALA N. NAYAK, MD
KEN RANDALL, MPT
KAMALA SHANKAR, MD

22

Exercise in the Elderly

For many years exercise has been recognized as a significant component of a healthy lifestyle. Until recently most studies on exercise have focused on younger adults. However, convincing data now exist that regular exercisers have lower morbidity and mortality rates, even when exercise is initiated later in life. Paffenbarger found that increasing one's activity level can reduce mortality rates, even when exercise is started after age 60 and as late as 75.[40] The Framingham Heart Study showed that moderately active older women had significantly lower mortality rates after 10 years than their less active peers.[48]

Exercise prescription for the elderly is challenging in that many factors are often involved, including medical limitations and psychological considerations. Normal aging changes in the neuromuscular, musculoskeletal, cardiovascular, and pulmonary systems will affect functional capacity. Table 1 lists some of the physiologic changes associated with aging.[45] Additionally, decreased sensory and cognitive awareness, postural changes, motivation, and perceived levels of fatigue all affect the potential for rehabilitation and should be assessed prior to initiating exercise programs.[3]

Brummel-Smith proposed three classifications in which age-related changes could be grouped: biologic, psychological, and social.[10]

Biologic changes include changes in muscle strength and in cardiac and pulmonary function that necessitate mild-intensity activity levels.

Psychological changes affect learning and motivation. For patients requiring a slower learning rate, repetition of directions and activities is recommended. It is important to consider the individual's lifelong activity level and sensitivity toward the learning of new tasks. These factors, including self-motivation and dedication to recovery, determine the success of an exercise program.

Social considerations include ageist attitudes of health care professionals and others that may preclude an appropriate exercise program.

Table 2 lists the primary benefits of exercise.[29]

Exercises for improving cardiac and pulmonary function are especially important in the elderly because most conditions causing morbidity and mortality are related to these two organ systems. The Centers for Disease Control and Prevention and the

TABLE 1. Physiologic Changes Associated with Aging

Organ System	Physiologic Changes
Skeletal System	Disc degeneration, osteoarthritis, kyphosis, and osteoporosis resulting in postural changes, including decreased height and joint range of motion.
Muscular System	Decreased size of muscle cells, decreased number of muscle fibers, increase in interstitial fat and collagen resulting in decreased strength and endurance.
Nervous System	Central nervous system cortical atrophy and nerve cell loss results in prolonged reaction time and impaired memory and cognition. Decreased myelination in the peripheral nervous system results in decreased conduction velocities.
Cardiovascular System	Vessel wall stiffness and myocardial hypertrophy results in decreased cardiac output and coronary bloodflow with an increase in blood pressure.
Endocrine System	Decreases in growth hormone secretion, estrogen, and androgen result in decreased weight, infertility in women, and loss of tumescence in men.
Respiratory system	Decreases in elasticity, parenchyma, and the number of alveoli result in decreased lung capacities.

TABLE 2. Benefits of Exercise in the Elderly

Maintain activities of daily living
Increase strength, flexibility, and endurance
Maintain community involvement and socialization
Maintain self-esteem
Improve quality of life

American College of Sports Medicine have suggested that 24% of elderly persons are completely sedentary and another 54% are suboptimally active.[2,12]

CARDIOVASCULAR AGING AND EXERCISE

Several modifications in cardiac structure occur with aging and result in physiologic, anatomic, and microscopic changes. Important among these are clinically measurable changes such as decreased contractility of the myocardium. The age-related increase in deposition of connective tissue and myocyte hypertrophy likely produces an increase in the ventricular wall thickness, which in turn contributes to the increase in wall stiffness.[37] This increased stiffness of the myocardium impairs ventricular diastolic relaxation and increases end diastolic pressure. This suggests that exercise-induced increases in heart rate would be less tolerated in older people.

In addition, a number of alterations in the vasculature have been observed in the elderly. The aorta dilates, elongates, and loses elasticity. These changes produce an increase in systolic pressure, to a lesser extent in diastolic pressure, and an increase in pulse pressure. The increase in left ventricular thickness is concomitant with the rise in systolic blood pressure.

Age-related decline in heart rate (HR) is well established.[6] The cause of this is multifactorial, but most significant is the decrement in the adrenergic reaction. Reductions in maximal oxygen uptake ($VO_{2\,max}$), cardiac output, stroke volume, and stroke index have been observed with increasing age,[7,9,18,25,43] especially in persons with heart disease. The healthy aging human heart maintains cardiac output through the Starling effect by increasing stroke volume. The cardiac output at rest and with exercise is mediated by a rise in stroke volume with a decrease in heart rate that is a compensatory and efficient response. During exercise, however, both stroke volume and heart rate rise to support the increasing cardiac output.[9,25,44] The increase in stroke volume is a function of an increase in end diastolic volume. However, because end diastolic volume does not increase with maximal exercise to the same extent in older versus younger subjects, the increase in ejection fraction with exercise is smaller in elderly individuals.

Aerobic exercise capacity, usually measured by $VO_{2\,max}$, declines about 10% per decade.[5,28] However, older athletes who maintain competitive levels of training have only half the expected rate of decline.[28]

Activity programs for the elderly with cardiac disease must be tailored to the person's age, fitness level, and overall health status. Improvement in functional capacity can be achieved with regular exercise, which also can lead to increased strength and muscle mass, loss of fat, and maintenance of an optimal body composition. The goal of the exercise program should be to limit the deterioration in functional capacity so that an independent active lifestyle can be maintained.

GUIDELINES FOR EXERCISE PRESCRIPTION

Guidelines for prescribing exercise for the elderly patients with cardiac disease are outlined below.

Warm-up and cool-down periods may be longer in older individuals. At rest, only 15–20% of the total blood volume is delivered to the muscles, but during vigorous exercise up to 75% of the blood flow may be diverted. Adequate warm-up allows a gradual redistribution of blood flow to the muscles, which in turn increases elasticity of the connective tissue and other muscle components.[15] These changes should theoretically reduce soft tissue injuries. Optimally 15–20 minutes should be devoted and should involve primarily large muscle groups such as the calf, hamstring, quadriceps, lower back, and proximal shoulder girdle muscles.

The same muscles are involved in the cool-down period, which lasts 10–15 minutes. A gradual slowing of activity for washout and metabolism of byproducts such as lactate, avoids venous pooling in the legs, and reduces the likelihood of syncope.

Typical warm-up and cool-down exercises include bent-knee sit-ups, bent-knee single leg lifts, shoulder shrugs, presses, and circles. Standing toe touches with knees locked, straight-leg sit-ups, double leg lifts, deep knee bends, and full head rolls should be avoided.

Intensity of exercises can be monitored on the basis of an individual or a combination of parameters, which commonly include HR, rate of perceived exertion (RPE), and energy expenditure expressed as a MET (1.5 Kcal/min = 1 MET). Intensity of exercise is always prescribed within a range regardless of what method is used.

Using HR as a guideline, exercises can be monitored to progress to goals of 40–70% of maximal HR (220 minus age). A second method is to use HR reserve or HR range, which is the percentage difference between maximum HR and resting HR. HR range correlates well with functional capacity, i.e., 60–80% of HR corresponds to 60–80% of functional capacity.

A high level of correlation has been noted between ratings on the Borg scale of perceived exertion and physiologic parameters such as VO_2 and heart rate.[23] RPE is a 15-point scale ranging from 6 to 20, in which 12–13 corresponds to 60% of HR range and 16 corresponds to 80% of HR range. For optimal results, exercises should be targeted for an RPE of 12–16 (somewhat hard to hard). When starting an exercise program, RPE is best used in conjunction with HR. After developing a knowledge of the HR–RPE relationship, HR can be monitored less frequently and RPE can be used as the primary monitoring method.

Using energy consumption as a monitor for conditioning exercises is best done by alternating periods of high- and low-intensity exercises. The exercises or activities should result in the desired range of energy expenditure. Exercise intensity in mets is directly related to speed of movement or measurable resistance. Environmental factors such as temperature, surface grade, and type of clothing could modify the energy expenditure. However, maintaining the desirable exercise intensity in a steady state activity such as walking and cycling in a changing environment can be done by monitoring HR or RPE.

Frequency of exercise depends in part on the duration and intensity of exercise. It can vary from daily to three to five times a week. Based on functional capacity, the following guidelines may be used:[3]

< 3 METs: 5 minutes of exercise several times daily

3–5 METs: at least twice daily as tolerated

> 5 METs: 3 times a week on alternate days

Weightbearing and nonweightbearing exercises can be alternated.

Rate of progression of exercise usually starts from conditioning to improvement and then to maintenance phase.

Conditioning exercises start with low-level aerobic activities for 3 minutes, after which the pulse is checked and the exercises adjusted to higher or lower intensity. The goal is to reach 10–15 minutes of aerobic exercise. When the HR decreases for a given exercise intensity, the activities are progressed to a higher level. Depending on the rate of adaptation of the participants, this phase generally lasts 4–10 weeks. The goals of exercise are to (a) acclimatize all the organ systems to the chosen activities, (b) develop a regular exercise habit, (c) learn to monitor the exercise intensity accurately, and (d) perfect the appropriate skill.

The improvement phase incorporates a gradual increase in duration and intensity, with goals of achieving 40–85% of $VO_{2\,max}$ range. The duration of any given activity is increased to 20–30 minutes of the exercise. This phase can last 4–6 months.

The maintenance phase of the exercise has been reached when a satisfactory level of cardiorespiratory fitness has been achieved and the participant is no longer interested in increased conditioning. The same routine can continue as in the previous phase, or variable, more enjoyable activities may be substituted.

Physical activity in the elderly must address a number of distinctive features applicable to this age group.

- The warm-up and cool-down periods should be longer. The warm-up allows readiness of the musculoskeletal and cardiorespiratory system for exercise.[54] Cool-down activities allow for gradual lowering of the heat load of exercise and of the exercise-induced peripheral vasodilatation.

- Longer rest periods are required between exercise sessions to allow enough time for the heart rate to return to resting levels, which in the elderly takes longer than in younger individuals.

- Risk for musculoskeletal complications with exercise increases significantly in the elderly. Safe and effective physical conditioning without adverse effects to the musculoskeletal system is brisk walking, the pace and distance of which can be gradually increased. Enclosed shopping malls provide ideal walking sites.

- The environment in which exercise is done is important to avoid hypothermia and hyperthermia as well as dehydration. Skin blood flow decreases with aging, resulting in impairment of sweating and temperature regulation during physical activity.[54]

MEDICATION USE AND EXERCISE

Since the elderly are the major users of prescription drugs, awareness of drugs' effects on exercise capacity is of utmost importance. Commonly prescribed medications such as antihypertensive agents, antidepressants, major tranquilizers, and diuretics may be associated with orthostatic hypotension, which can result in falls. Diuretics can also exacerbate dehydration, causing electrolyte imbalance and producing myalgias and muscle cramping. β-blockers can impair glucose uptake by the exercising muscle, which decreases the availability of substrate for aerobic metabolism. This results in an increase in lactic acid production, causing muscle soreness. Hyperthermia and dehydration during exercise may be exacerbated by psychotropic drugs, which are known to affect thermoregulation.

CHRONIC LUNG DISEASE AND EXERCISE

Chronic obstructive pulmonary disease (COPD), which is common in the elderly, causes a significant decrease in exercise endurance. An excess of mucus production and loss of elasticity are common in smokers. Exercise has been shown to improve overall conditioning and prevent further deterioration. One study suggests improvement in diaphragmatic breathing with exercise.[52] There is controversy regarding improvement in aerobic capacity with training in patients with COPD. However, more recent studies in patients with moderate COPD have shown significant reductions in lactate production with concurrent decrease in ventilation with exercise.[12] These physiologic effects occur without any appreciable improvement in pulmonary function or arterial blood gases in patients with COPD.[1,12,17,39]

Patient selection for exercise is important to achieve optimal results. Screening of potential candidates should include a baseline physical examination, pulmonary function testing, arterial blood gases (if appropriate), a chest radiograph, a resting and exercise electrocardiogram, and an exercise tolerance test with measurements of oxygen saturation and cardiorespiratory responses.

Patients who are clinically stable and report breathlessness despite optimal use of bronchodilators are good candidates for exercise training.

Training is individualized based on the test results. Aerobic training is achieved using large muscles such as during walking, stair-climbing, treadmill use, and leg and arm ergometry. Training intensity is monitored using the Borg scale and is regulated primarily on the basis of symptom tolerance. HR target training in this group of patients is less reliable than in the general population.[8]

The goals of the exercise program are to improve exercise capacity and reduce breathlessness.

GUIDELINES FOR EXERCISE IN PATIENTS WITH PULMONARY DISEASE

- Cycling, walking, and swimming are desirable. Upper body exercises such as running or arm cranking are not recommended because of the high ventilation required at a given power output.[19]

- For patients with forced vital capacity (FVC) and forced expiratory volume (FEV_1) between 60 and 80% of predicted value, exercise intensity should be maintained at a level requiring a ventilatory rate less than 75% of patient maximal exercise ventilation.

- For patients more severely limited with FVC and FEV_1 below 60% of predicted value, exercise intensity should be regulated using a dyspnea scale, as follows:

1. mild, noticeable to patient but not observer
2. mild, some difficulty, noticeable to observer
3. moderate difficulty, but patient can continue
4. severe difficulty, patient cannot continue

- Some severely limited patients require supplemental oxygen during exercise, which has been demonstrated to improved exercise performance. Oxygen should be administered at high flow rates at FIO_2 (fractional concentration of oxygen in inspired gas) of 24–28%.

- Modifications in the duration and frequency of exercise may be necessary, e.g., if 20–30 minutes of continuous exercise cannot be tolerated, two 10-minute sessions can be scheduled.

The final phase of the exercise program is the maintenance phase. Following improvement in exercise capacity, patients are encouraged to continue training on a stationary bicycle or treadmill at home. Support groups are recommended to help patients derive psychosocial benefits, which include improved self-esteem, greater independence, and the freedom to participate in a greater range of activities of daily living.[38]

MUSCULOSKELETAL AGING AND EXERCISE

Alterations in body composition occur in aging that result in a decrease in lean body mass and an increase in percentage of body fat. Total body water decreases, urinary creatinine levels decline, and the resting metabolic rate is lower in older individuals.[19,20]

Significant losses in maximal force production (muscle strength) occur with aging.[4,13,15] Muscle strength appears to be well maintained up to the fifth decade of life, after which the decline amounts to 15% per decade, in the sixth and seventh decades.[15,27,31]

The decline in muscle strength with aging can be attributed to loss of muscle mass, some alteration of the muscles' capacity to generate force, or to a combination of these mechanisms. More studies support the notion that loss of muscle mass is the major factor in age-related decline in muscle strength and is more important than deterioration in the contractile capacity of the muscle.[24,34] There is no preferential loss of type 1 or type 2 muscle fibers with age;[34] both types are equally affected. However, there appears to be reduction in type 2 fiber area (both type 2a and 2b) with age, which accounts for the significant decrease in muscle size and strength.[33]

Loss of bone mass occurs with aging and is more evident in women than in men. It is estimated that women older than 35 lose bone mass at a rate of 1% per year and that men lose bone mass starting at about age 55, approximately 10–15% by age 70.[20] Bone loss can be exacerbated in the elderly by other factors, such as diabetes mellitus, lack of hormones in menopausal women, renal impairment, and immobility.

The greatest effect on alleviating the rate of osteoporotic fractures may be not as a direct result of exercise on bone strengthening but rather on exercise's potential to improve muscle strength and possibly balance and or gait,[14] thereby reducing the incidence of falls.

EXERCISE PRESCRIPTION FOR PATIENTS WITH OSTEOPOROSIS AND OSTEOPENIA

■ Regular weightbearing is essential for maintenance of bone mass although the amount of such activity necessary has not been determined. The National Osteoporosis Foundation recommends a prevention program of 45–60 minutes of weightbearing exercise four times a week.

■ Bone mineral density of the spine is correlated with the strength of spine extensors and, therefore, maintaining muscular strength of the spine muscles is important.[51] Because exercises that place flexion forces on the vertebrae tend to cause an increase in the number of vertebral fractures, flexion exercises for the spine should be avoided.

■ Patients with osteoporosis should engage in 1 hour of weightbearing exercises four times a week, including walking and climbing stairs.

■ Although aquatic exercises and swimming improve cardiovascular fitness, they do not improve bone mass. They may be beneficial for symptomatic relief of back pain associated with spine fractures.

■ An exercise program alone is less successful than the combination of exercise and estrogen regimen in minimizing bone loss in postmenopausal women. Therefore, exercise should not be considered a substitute for hormone replacement at menopause.

COMMON PROBLEMS IN AGING

There are many medical diagnoses that require specific exercise programs. These programs vary widely in how and why they are employed. We focus on two of the most prevalent and encompassing conditions: falls and deconditioning.

FALLS

Falls and decreased mobility are major concerns for the elderly. Statistics on falls and resulting injuries to the elderly are alarming. The incidence of falls in the community-dwelling elderly is 25% at age 70 and 35% after age 75.[11] While death is a less frequent consequence of falling, complications caused by falls are the leading cause of death from injury in men and women older than 65.[46] Interestingly, a cluster of falls has been observed in some older individuals during the months preceding death.[26]

Given the risk and associated emotional and monetary costs, falls are of significant concern for the elderly, their families, and the health care system. The importance of falls lies in their impact on an older person's function, health, and independence.

Falls can be the result of underlying physical and cognitive dysfunctions, medications, and environmental hazards.[13] Fall prevention begins with patient and family education on safety and modification of the environment to reduce hazards. Appropriate assistive devices such as canes and walkers also are beneficial in preventing falls. Walkers that are equipped with a seat for rest breaks work well for patients with limited endurance.

Exercise is key in fall prevention. Functionally, the limitations of decreased joint mobility and muscle strength, reduced range of motion, impaired coordination, and gait deviations can predispose the elderly to falls. Research has indicated that lower extremity weakness, particularly at the ankle and knee, is significantly associated with recurrent falls in the elderly.[55] It is only logical to conclude that strengthening exercises are helpful in reducing falls. Specific strengthening and balance exercises can help prevent falls by improving overall strength and coordination, balance response, reaction time, and awareness of safe ambulation practices.[32] In a recent study, Province looked at elderly subjects in community dwellings and nursing homes who were given intervention with exercises to improve balance. Compared to controls, subjects assigned to an exercise intervention were less likely to fall in the follow-up period.[42]

Some elderly patients can tolerate progressive resistive exercise programs for strengthening. Others perform better with more functional approaches to strengthening, including reaching, scooting, sit to stand, and ambulation. Progression can include stairs, single-limb stance, and marching in place. Specifically, balance exercises address three areas of posture control: response to perturbation, weight shifting, and anticipatory adjustments to limb movements.[30] In the clinic, exercises for improving the motor component of balance should focus on challenging the patient's balance in the following three areas:

1. **Response to perturbation.** While in a standing or Rhomberg (feet together) position, the patient is nudged from the sternum, side, or back. This challenges the patient's ability to respond appropriately and return the center of gravity over the base of support. The patient can practice various strategies, including bending at the hip, ankle, or knee.

2. **Weight shifting.** From a standing position, the patient can progressively shift weight from side to side until able to stand on a single limb. This trains the patient to move voluntarily versus reactively, as in the previous area.

3. **Anticipatory adjustments to limb movements.** From a standing position, the patient can reach for an object and place it on a table or at his side, or the patient can swing one leg. In doing so, the patient is forced to adjust his posture in anticipation of the limb movement to maintain the center of gravity over the base of support.

To address the sensory component of balance, the sensory input to the patient can be modified by blocking vision or providing a nonlevel or moving surface on which the patient is standing. Tilt boards, BAPS (biomechanical ankle platform system) boards and KATS (kinesthetic ability trainers) are quite effective (Fig. 1). Foam pads

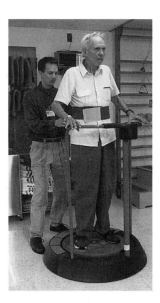

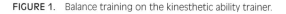

FIGURE 1. Balance training on the kinesthetic ability trainer.

can be used to disrupt information to the soles of the feet or the ankles, thus forcing the patient to rely more on visual cues to maintain balance.[49] Our patients improve most rapidly when their balance is truly challenged. Obviously, patients vary with the amount of surface perturbation and sensory modification they can handle. However, once the patient's limits are determined, a safe environment can be created to allow the patient to become unsteady and immediately correct appropriately. Safety belts and handrails are ideal for balance training and activities (Fig. 2).

The overall goal of each of these balance activities and exercises is to improve the motor and sensory components of balance. This improvement will translate into improved function and independence for the patient.

DECONDITIONING

When hospitalized for acute or chronic medical illness, the frail elderly are at high risk for becoming deconditioned. Additionally, a sedentary lifestyle can lead to deconditioning. Deconditioning is simply the physiologic changes produced from inactivity or low activity that result in decreased function.

Siebens states that deconditioning is the multiple changes in organ system physiology that are induced by inactivity and reversed by activity.[50] Regardless of the primary diagnosis, deconditioning is prevalent among the elderly. Therefore, we should combat deconditioning with exercise for both prevention and treatment. However, studies have shown that while exercise improves physical conditioning in older persons, it takes longer to achieve those results. It is therefore important to adhere to safety precautions. Activities and exercises that involve the large lower extremity muscle groups have been found to be the most beneficial for physical conditioning.[22] To prevent de-

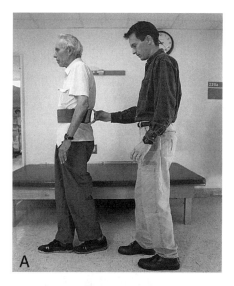

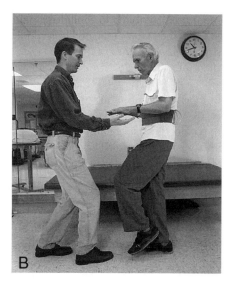

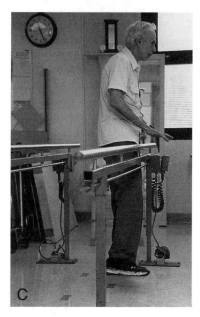

FIGURE 2. Balance training in the Rhomberg stance position (A), with a single-limb stance (B), and by side-stepping in parallel bars (C).

conditioning, Vorhies recommends that exercises be performed 3–5 days per week, with multiple rest breaks during each session.[53]

Perhaps the biggest challenge in prescribing exercise to elderly patients is finding a program in which they will participate and will continue to participate. An interesting study performed in 1986 revealed that older persons lack the confidence of their younger counterparts.[41] When given an unsolvable problem, the younger subjects felt that they were not trying hard enough, but the older subjects claimed that they were unable to solve the problem. On subsequent tests, the younger subjects tried harder and the older subjects gave up. It is therefore important to set and establish obtainable goals for geriatric exercise programs. For a severely deconditioned patient, a goal such as being able to walk 20 feet with a walker is good in that it is obtainable, easily recognized, and can serve as a motivating force for the patient. In a separate study, Mento et al. found that the best performance in difficult tasks occurred when a specific goal was set by the elderly subject himself.[36] This highlights the importance of having the patient help to choose the exercises for an exercise program.

There are several outstanding ways to exercise the elderly deconditioned patient. Initially, having the patient perform activities of daily living is a smart and functional way to begin exercise. Dressing, transferring, and bathing can be extremely taxing on the severely deconditioned patient but are highly beneficial. Progression to an exercise program that incorporates endurance, strength, and flexibility is ideal. Endurance exercises include walking, biking, swimming, and extremity ergometer aids (Fig. 3). Strengthening can be accomplished with rubber tubing, ankle/wrist weights, pulley systems, Kinetron systems, and closed chain lower extremity exercises such as squats or stair stepping (Figs. 4 and 5). Finally, flexibility should be addressed before and after each session through a stretching program.

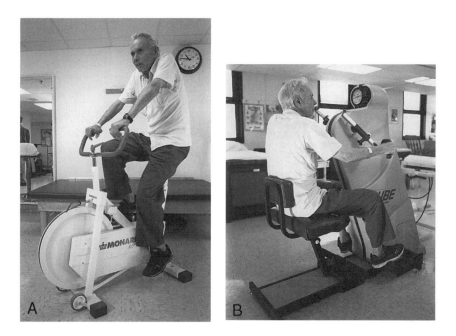

FIGURE 3. Endurance exercise on the stationary bicycle (A) and on the upper extremity ergometer (B).

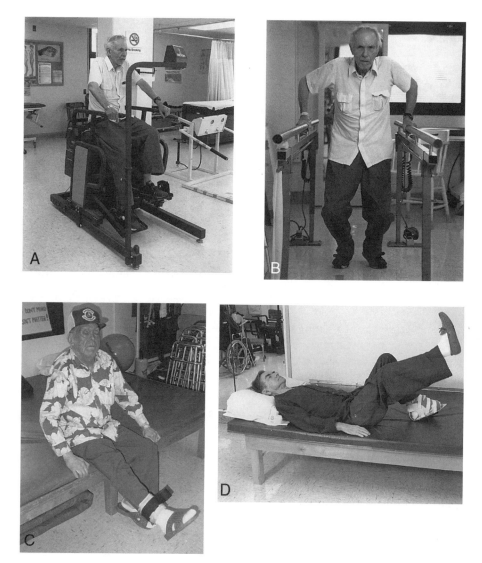

FIGURE 4. Lower extremity strengthening on the Kinetron machine (A), with partial squats in the parallel bars (B), with ankle weights (C), and with mat exercises (D).

AQUATIC THERAPY

Another excellent therapeutic exercise is aquatic therapy. Aquatic, or pool, therapy refers to an exercise swimming pool program supervised by a physical therapist or medical professional. Pool therapy for the more independent elderly participant can be performed in group sessions. For the more dependent elderly, individual pool therapy

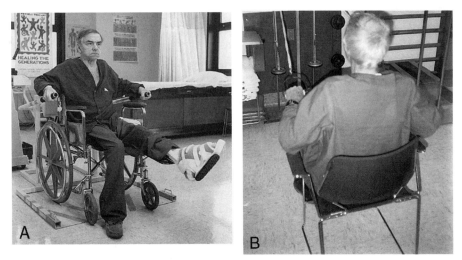

FIGURE 5. Upper extremity strengthening on the rickshaw machine (*A*) and with a wall pulley system (*B*).

can offer an outstanding setting for recovery from injury or simply reconditioning. In all cases it is important that patients be evaluated beforehand to screen for safety and assess goals. Goals may include improving or maintaining endurance, balance, strength, and joint range of motion.

The primary benefits of pool exercise include gravity elimination and the positive effect of water buoyancy, which may result in decreased pain and joint compression.[35] These factors also can contribute to increased muscle relaxation and allow for a greater level of aerobic exercise than could be tolerated on land. This is especially valuable for the deconditioned patient or patients with severe arthritis, cardiopulmonary compromise, or orthopedic problems. In studying patients with rheumatoid arthritis, Danneskoid-Samsoe and colleagues found that, following an 8-week pool exercise program, patients exhibited significant increases in isokinetic and isometric lower extremity strength.[16] Additionally, significant improvements in aerobic capacity occurred following the 8-week program.

In our clinic elderly patients have reacted positively to the warm water environment the pool offers. In general the patients appear to move and breathe more easily. We use a hands-on patient education style that focuses on helping patients learn how to improve their own mobility. With this program we are able to provide a comfortable exercise setting that is designed to decrease pain while improving posture, mobility, and endurance.

PATIENT COMPLIANCE

Regardless of the setting, elderly patients may be less compliant with their exercise program, often because they are unwilling to comply or because they have pain or fatigue. However, with a positive attitude and ingenuity on the part of the therapist, many of these obstacles can be overcome. In our practice, where we prescribe and instruct ex-

TABLE 3. Techniques to Improve Patient Compliance

Show Respect
  Address the patient formally, using Mr., Mrs., or Ms.
  Listen to discover interests and dislikes.
Communicate and Discuss
  Work together to create an exercise program that is beneficial, enjoyable, and relatively pain-free.
Mirror
  Perform the exercise with the patient when able. This will create an outstanding visual cue as well as
    improve motivation.
Rest
  Allow frequent rest breaks.
  At regular intervals, ask the patient to relay their perceived exertion level.
Home Programs
  When issuing home exercise programs, limit the number of exercises to 6 or fewer.
  Involve family members to improve compliance.
  Issue large illustrated photocopies of exercises.
Encourage
  Encourage the patient to continue with exercise and develop a routine at home that incorporates an
    aerobic activity, if possible.
Resource Information
  Provide information on community resources available for exercise and support groups.

ercise for the elderly in inpatient and outpatient settings, the techniques described in Table 3 are usually successful.

As mentioned above, recent studies continue to provide convincing data that exercise can improve health and function of the elderly. Encouraging results also have been found in a study by Sforzo on exercise detraining. Despite interruptions in formal exercise, patients were able to retain newly gained muscular strength for at least 5 weeks. This suggests that elderly patients should realize the ease with which they can restart their exercise programs even though they have missed several days or weeks.[47] Designing an exercise program that will be enjoyable, beneficial and safe is the true challenge in prescribing exercise for the elderly. Regardless of the disability, beneficial exercise programs can be created for the geriatric patient.

ACKNOWLEDGMENTS   We gratefully acknowledge the assistance of Virginia Carrillo for typing this manuscript and Paula Schwartz, DO, for assistance with screening the reference material.

REFERENCES

1. Alpert JS, Bass H, Szucs MM, et al: Effects of physical training on hemodynamics and pulmonary functional rest and during exercise in patients with chronic obstructive pulmonary disease. Chest 66: 647–651, 1975.

2. American College of Sports Medicine: ACSM's Guidelines for Exercise Testing and Prescription. Baltimore, Williams & Wilkins, 1995.
3. American College of Sports Medicine: Guidelines for Exercise Testing and Prescription, 4th ed. Philadelphia, Lea & Febiger, 1991.
4. Aniansson A, Hedberg M, Henning GB, Grimby G: Muscle morphology, enzymatic activity and muscle strength in elderly men: A follow-up study. Muscle Nerve 9:585–591, 1986.
5. Astrand I: Aerobic work capacity in men and women with special reference to age. Acta Physiol Scand 49(suppl 169):1–90, 1960.
6. Astrand P, Rodahl K: Textbook of Work Physiology, 3rd ed. New York, McGraw Hill, 1986.
7. Becklake M, Frank H, Dagenais G, et al: Age changes in myocardial function and exercise response. J Appl Physiol 20:938–947, 1965.
8. Belman MJ: Exercise in chronic obstructive pulmonary disease. Clin Chest Med 7:585–587, 1986.
9. Brandfonbrenner M, Landowne M, Shock N: Changes in cardiac output with age. Circulation 12:557–566, 1955.
10. Brummel-Smith K: Rehabilitation of the geriatric patient. In Hazzard W, Andreas R, Bierman E (eds): Principles of Geriatric Medicine and Gerontology, 2nd ed. New York, McGraw-Hill, 1990.
11. Campbell AJ, Reinken J, Allan BC, et al: Falls in old age: A study of frequency and clinical factors. Age Ageing 10:264–270, 1981.
12. Casaburi R, Patessio P, Ioli F, et al: Reductions in exercise lactic acidosis and ventilation as a result of exercise training in patients with chronic obstructive lung disease. Am Rev Respir Dis 143:9–18, 1991.
13. Christiansen J, Juhl E (eds): The prevention of falls later in life. Danish Med Bull 34(suppl):1–24, 1987.
14. Cunningham DA, Morrison D, Rice CI, Cooke C: Aging and isokinetic plantar flexion. Eur J Appl Physiol 56:24–29, 1987.
15. Danneskoid-Samsoe B, Kofod V, Munter J, et al: Muscle strength and functional capacity in 78–81 year old men and women. Eur J Appl Physiol 52:310–314, 1984.
16. Danneskoid-Samsoe B, Lynberg K, Risum T, Telleng M: The effect of water exercise therapy given to patients with rheumatoid arthritis. Scand J Rehabil Med 19:31–35, 1987.
17. Degre S, Sergysels R, Messin R, et al: Hemodynamic responses to physical training in patients with chronic lung disease. Am Rev Respir Dis 110:395–402, 1974.
18. Dehn M, Bruce R: Longitudinal variations in maximal oxygen intake with age and inactivity. J Appl Physiol 33:805–807, 1972.
19. Evans WJ: Exercise and muscle metabolism in the elderly. In Hutchinson M, Munro HN (eds): Nutrition and Aging. New York, Academic Press, 1986, pp 179–191.
20. Fleg JL, Latatta EG: Role of muscle loss in the age associated reduction in $VO_{2\ max}$. J Appl Physiol 65:1147–1151, 1988.
21. Fletcher GF, Balady G, Froelicher VF, et al: Exercise standards. A statement of healthcare professionals from the American Heart Association. Circulation 91:580–615, 1995.
22. Fletcher G, Froelicher V, Hartley L, et al: Exercise standards. A statement for health professionals from the American Heart Association. Circulation 82:2286–2322, 1990.
23. Franklin BA, Buchal M, Hollingsworth V, et al: Exercise prescription. In Strauss RH (ed): Sports Medicine, 2nd ed. Philadelphia, WB Saunders, 1991.
24. Frontera WR, Hughes VA, Lutz KJ, Evans WJ: A cross sectional muscle strength and mass in 45 to 78 year old men and women. J Appl Physiol 71:644–650, 1991.
25. Gerstenblith G, Lakatta E, Weisfeldt M: Age changes in myocardial function and exercise response. Prog Cardiovasc Dis 19:1–21, 1976.
26. Gryfe CI, Amies A, Ashley MJ: A longitudinal study of falls in an elderly population. I. Incidence and morbidity. Age Ageing 6:201–210, 1977.
27. Harries UJ, Bassey EJ: Torque velocity relationships for the knee extensors in women in their 3rd and 7th decades. Eur J Appl Physiol 60:187–190, 1990.
28. Heath GW, Hagberg JM, Ehsani AA, et al: A physiologic comparison of younger and older endurance athletes. J Appl Physiol 51:634–640, 1981.
29. Heath G: Exercise programming for the older adult. In Blair S, Painter P, Pate R (eds): Resource Manual for Guidelines for Exercise Testing and Prescription. Philadelphia, Lea & Febiger, 1988.

30. Horak FB: Clinical measurement of postural control in adults. Phys Ther 67:1881–1885, 1987.
31. Larrson L: Morphological and functional characteristics of the aging skeletal muscle in man. Acta Physiol Scand Suppl 457:1–36, 1978.
32. Lewis CB, Bottomly JM: Geriatric Physical Therapy. Norwalk, CT, Appleton & Lange, 1994.
33. Lexell J, Downham DY: What is the effect of aging on Type 2 muscle fibers? J Neurol Sci 107:250–251, 1992.
34. Lexell J, Taylor C, Sjostrom M: What is the cause of aging atrophy? Total number, size and proportion of different fiber types studies in whole vastus lateralis muscle from 15 to 83 year old men. J Neurol Sci 84:275–294, 1988.
35. McNeal RL: Aquatic therapy for patients with rheumatic disease. Rheum Dis Clin North Am 16:915–929, 1990.
36. Mento A, Steele RP, Karren RJ: A metaanalytic study of the effects of goal setting on task performance: 1966–1984. Organ Behav Hum Decis Process 39:52, 1987.
37. Nichols WW, O'Rourke MF, Avolio AP, et al: Effects of age on ventricular vascular coupling. Am J Cardiol 55:1179–1184, 1985.
38. O'Donnell DE, Webb KA, McGuire MA: Older patients with COPD: Benefits of exercise training. Geriatrics 48:59–62, 1993.
39. Paez PN, Phillipson EA, Masangkay M, Sproule BJ: The physiologic basis of training patients with emphysema. Am Rev Respir Dis 95:944–953, 1967.
40. Paffenbarger RS Jr, Hyde RT, Wing AL, et al: The association of changes in physical-activity level and other lifestyle characteristics with mortality among men. N Engl J Med 328:538–545, 1993.
41. Prohaska T, Pontiam IA, Teitleman J: Age differences in attributions to causality: Implications for an intellectual assessment. Exp Aging Res 10:111–117, 1984.
42. Province MA, Hadley EC, Hornbrook MC, et al: The effects of exercise on falls in elderly patients: A pre-planned meta-analysis of the FICSIT trials. JAMA 273:1341–1347, 1995.
43. Raven P, Mitchell J: The effect of aging on the cardiovascular response to dynamic and static exercise. In Weisfeldt M (ed): The Aging Heart. New York, Raven Press, 1980, pp 269–296.
44. Rodenheffer RJ, Gerstenblith G, Becker LC, et al: Exercise cardiac output is maintained with advancing age in healthy human subjects. Cardiac dilatation and increased stroke volume compensated for a diminished heart rate. Circulation 69:203–213, 1984.
45. Rossman I: The anatomy of aging. In Rossman I (ed): Clinical Geriatrics, 2nd ed. Philadelphia, JB Lippincott, 1979, pp 3–22.
46. Sattin RW: Falls among older persons: A public health perspective. Annu Rev Public Health 13:489–508, 1992.
47. Sforzo GA, McManis BG, Black D, et al: Resilience to exercise detraining in healthy older adults. J Am Geriatr Soc 43:209–215, 1995.
48. Sherman SE, D'Agostino RB, Cobb JL, Kannel WB: Does exercise reduce mortality rates in the elderly? Experience from the Framingham Heart Study. Am Heart J 128:965–972, 1994.
49. Shumway-Cook A, Horak FB: Assessing the influence of sensory interaction on balance. Phys Ther 66:1548–1550, 1986.
50. Siebens H: Deconditioning. In Kemp B, Brummel-Smith K (eds): Geriatric Rehabilitation. Boston, Little, Brown & Co., 1990.
51. Sinaki M, McPhee MC, Hodgson SF: Relationship between bone mineral density of spine and strength of back extensors in healthy postmenopausal women. Mayo Clin Proc 61:116–122, 1986.
52. Stamford B: Exercise and chronic airway obstruction. Phys Sport Med 19:189–190, 1991.
53. Vorhies D, Riley BE: Deconditioning. Clin Geriatr Med 9:745–763, 1993.
54. Wenger NK: Physical inactivity and coronary heart disease in elderly patients. Clin Geriatr Med 12:79–88, 1996.
55. Whipple RH, Wolfson LI, Amerman P: The relationship of knee and ankle weakness to falls in nursing home residents: An isokinetic study. J Am Geriatr Soc 35:13–20, 1987.

INDEX

Page numbers in **boldface type** indicate complete chapters.